Vascular Dementia

Current Clinical Neurology

Daniel Tarsy, MD, Series Editor

Parkinson's Disease and Nonmotor Dysfunction, edited by ***Ronald F. Pfeiffer and Ivan Bodis-Wollner,*** *2005*

Movement Disorders Emergencies: *Diagnosis and Treatment*, edited by ***Steven J. Frucht and Stanley Fahn,*** *2005*

Inflammatory Disorders of the Nervous System: *Pathogenesis, Immunology, and Clinical Management*, edited by ***Alireza Minagar and J. Steven Alexander,*** *2005*

Neurological and Psychiatric Disorders: *From Bench to Bedside*, edited by ***Frank I. Tarazi and John A. Schetz,*** *2005*

Multiple Sclerosis: *Etiology, Diagnosis, and New Treatment Strategies*, edited by ***Michael J. Olek,*** *2005*

Seizures in Critical Care: *A Guide to Diagnosis and Therapeutics*, edited by ***Panayiotis N. Varelas,*** *2005*

Vascular Dementia: *Cerebrovascular Mechanisms and Clinical Management*, edited by ***Robert H. Paul, Ronald Cohen, Brian R. Ott, and Stephen Salloway,*** *2005*

Handbook of Neurocritical Care, edited by ***Anish Bhardwaj, Marek A. Mirski, and John A. Ulatowski,*** *2004*

Atypical Parkinsonian Disorders, edited by ***Irene Litvan,*** *2004*

Handbook of Stroke Prevention in Clinical Practice, edited by ***Karen L. Furie and Peter J. Kelly,*** *2004*

Clinical Handbook of Insomnia, edited by ***Hrayr P. Attarian,*** *2004*

Critical Care Neurology and Neurosurgery, edited by ***Jose I. Suarez,*** *2004*

Alzheimer's Disease: *A Physician's Guide to Practical Management*, edited by ***Ralph W. Richter and Brigitte Zoeller Richter,*** *2004*

Field of Vision: *A Manual and Atlas of Perimetry*, edited by ***Jason J. S. Barton and Michael Benatar,*** *2003*

Surgical Treatment of Parkinson's Disease and Other Movement Disorders, edited by ***Daniel Tarsy, Jerrold L. Vitek, and Andres M. Lozano,*** *2003*

Myasthenia Gravis and Related Disorders, edited by ***Henry J. Kaminski,*** *2003*

Seizures: *Medical Causes and Management*, edited by ***Norman Delanty,*** *2002*

Clinical Evaluation and Management of Spasticity, edited by ***David A. Gelber and Douglas R. Jeffery,*** *2002*

Early Diagnosis of Alzheimer's Disease, edited by ***Leonard F. M. Scinto and Kirk R. Daffner,*** *2000*

Sexual and Reproductive Neurorehabilitation, edited by ***Mindy Aisen,*** *1997*

Vascular Dementia

Cerebrovascular Mechanisms and Clinical Management

Edited by

Robert H. Paul, PhD

Department of Psychiatry and Human Behavior, Brown Medical School, Providence, RI

Ronald Cohen, PhD

Department of Psychiatry and Human Behavior, Brown Medical School, Providence, RI

Brian R. Ott, MD

Department of Neurology, Memorial Hospital of Rhode Island, Pawtucket, Rhode Island; Department of Clinical Neurosciences, Brown Medical School, Providence, RI

Stephen Salloway, MD

Department of Neurology, Butler Hospital; Department of Clinical Neurosciences, Brown Medical School, Providence, RI

HUMANA PRESS TOTOWA, NEW JERSEY

999 Riverview Drive, Suite 208
Totowa, New Jersey 07512

humanapress.com

This publication is printed on acid-free paper. ∞
ANSI Z39.48-1984 (American Standards Institute) Permanence of Paper for Printed Library Materials.

Cover illustration: Derived from Fig. 4 in Mousa S. A., Fareed, J., Iqbal, O., and Kaiser, B. (2003) In *Methods in Molecular Medicine, vol. 93: Anticoagulants, Antiplatelets, and Thrombolytics* (Mousa, S. A., ed.), Humana Press, Totowa, NJ, p. 146.

Production Editor: Wendy S. Kopf
Cover Design: Patricia F. Cleary

For additional copies, pricing for bulk purchases, and/or information about other Humana titles, contact Humana at the above address or at any of the following numbers: Tel.: 973-256-1699; Fax: 973-256-8314; E-mail: humana@humanapr.com, or visit our Website: http://humanapress.com

Printed in the United States of America. 10 9 8 7 6 5 4 3 2 1
e-ISBN: 1-59259-824-2
Library of Congress Cataloging-in-Publication Data

Vascular dementia : cerebrovascular mechanisms and clinical management / edited by Robert H. Paul ... [et al.].
p. ; cm. -- (Current clinical neurology)
Includes bibliographical references and index.
ISBN 1-58829-366-1 (alk. paper)
1. Vascular dementia.
[DNLM: 1. Dementia, Vascular--physiopathology. 2. Dementia, Vascular--therapy. WM 220 V3318 2004] I. Paul, Robert H. II. Series.
RC388.5.V3659 2004
616.8'1--dc22

2004008302

Series Editor's Introduction

The understanding and treatment of dementia remains one of the greatest challenges facing the contemporary clinical neuroscientist. This is obviously not surprising given the complex infrastructure that forms the basis for what we consider the higher brain functions of memory, language, thought, abstract reasoning, motivation, and emotion. Progressive dementia is, by and large, a disorder of the aging brain. Running parallel to the aging of brain tissue is aging of the cerebrovascular system, which is necessary to meet the brain's demand for a large volume of blood flow. Therein lies the problem that has historically been put very simply: is dementia a result of a primary degenerative disease of the brain or a result of a progressive impairment in it's blood supply? The 19th-century view was that dementia resulted from vascular insufficiency. Later, with more sophisticated neuropathology, the concept arose that dementia was caused by a primary neurodegenerative process which attacked cortical neurons. However, well into the latter part of the 20th century, the popular concept that cerebral arteriosclerosis—commonly known as "hardening of the arteries"—was the basis for dementia continued to hold sway. Eventually, however, Alzheimer's disease became the principal culprit and even found its way into the popular lexicon. Appearing to confirm the neurodegenerative view, there quickly followed the discovery of additional neuropathologic and clinical entities such as Lewy body dementia, frontotemporal dementia, progressive supranuclear palsy, and corticobasal degeneration to name just a few.

As indicated by the editors of this volume, the pendulum appears to have swung too far from vascular dementia. Even while knowledge of the primary degenerative disorders was evolving, more respectable concepts of arteriosclerotic dementia, such as multi-infarct dementia and subcortical dementia, began to emerge. Binswanger's disease even made a respectable comeback. Until recently however, Alzheimer's disease and vascular dementia continued to be considered distinctive with a polarization of opinion as to which of these was more important etiologically. As it turns out, the truth may lie somewhere in the middle. The editors of this volume are of this mindset and have collected a group of distinguished experts who provide the clinical and laboratory evidence that vascular dementia is a genuine entity and that a mutually exclusive separation between primary degenerative and vascular dementias is difficult to support. Going further, if one accepts the concept of vascular dementia, the existence of a "mixed dementia" must also be considered. In the end, the question remains as to whether vascular and degenerative dementias simply coexist or whether there is an important pathophysiologic interaction between the two processes. *Vascular Dementia: Cerebrovascular Management and Clinical Management* lays out the guidelines for understanding this debate and points the way to future research which should clarify the question, lead to better understanding of the cause of these disorders, and produce effective methods for their prevention and treatment.

Daniel Tarsy, MD
Department of Neurology
Beth Israel Deaconess Medical Center
Harvard Medical School
Boston, MA

Preface

The intent of Vascular Dementia: Cerebrovascular Mechanisms and Clinical Management is to address the many recent advances in cardiovascular and cerebrovascular medicine and the impact of these on the lives of older adults by examining the state-of-the-art research on vascular dementia (VaD). A distinguishing feature of this work is its interdisciplinary nature. We have assembled work from contributors in multiple related fields, including both human and animal studies, in order to advance our collective understanding of VaD. A second distinguishing feature is that we have devoted one-third of our text to the examination of the interactions between VaD and Alzheimer's disease (AD). We believe that this combined approach will enhance patient care, as well as promote future research.

One may ask whether yet another summary of work in the field of VaD is necessary, given the number of review papers and recent texts devoted to the topic. However, it is important to note that research conducted over the recent "Decade of the Brain" has brought to light both consensus and controversy regarding the identity of VaD, and as a result the field is in constant flux. No better example of this could be scripted than the topics of discussion at a recent international conference on VaD. Attended by many prolific contributors to the field, the debates were charged and the range of discussion was provocative. In one open forum debate, the very existence of VaD as a construct was under question. Data from autopsy studies were presented which argued that pure VaD was such a rare phenomenon that the construct barely warranted clinical and research attention. By contrast, in a separate debate, the discussion focused on whether all cases of sporadic AD were manifestations of VaD. This bipolar conceptualization of VaD is the primary impetus behind our book.

In addition, though AD has been the central focus of research for several decades, the pendulum has begun to move towards a greater interest in cerebrovascular disease. This likely reflects the ever-growing population of older adults with cerebrovascular disease, as well as studies conducted in recent years describing important interactions between vascular disease and the expression of cognitive deficits in AD. There is now a growing consensus that clear, clinical, and pathological distinctions between these two conditions sometimes cannot be made in individual patients. We are certainly not the first group to describe this pending paradigm shift, as others (i.e., Roman, Hachinski, et al.) have offered this observation in public forum. However, it is from our own observations and empirical studies that we came to appreciate this conceptualization of dementia research, and eventually concluded that the time was right to synthesize the literature in an effort to move science forward.

Vascular Dementia: Cerebrovascular Mechanisms and Clinical Management is divided into six sections. Part I is focused on introducing VaD as a construct. Part II describes the basic mechanisms associated with aging that may have an important role in the development of VaD. Part III identifies the impact of VaD on cognitive status, psychiatric health, and the ability of patients to complete important activities of daily living. Part IV describes the application of neuroimaging methods to investigate VaD, with particular attention directed toward both functional and structural imaging methods. Part V is devoted to the topic of interactions between VaD and AD. Finally, Part VI reviews pharmacological management of VaD. This section also addresses the impact of VaD on perceived quality of life of patients and caregiver burden, two rarely addressed issues in the scientific community.

We developed the book to be of interest to both clinicians and basic scientists. The topics covered are broad in nature and capture work from both the bench and the exam room. Chapters are also provided that address issues likely new to those who practice or conduct research within a circumscribed specialty area. The contributors have skillfully identified the important discoveries of the previous years, explored where this field of research is currently headed, and emphasized the critical topics that require a more intensive research focus. Overall, we hope the book will serve as a valuable reference for the current state of knowledge regarding VaD as well as a guide for future studies.

Robert H. Paul, PhD
Ronald Cohen, PhD
Brian R. Ott, MD
Stephen Salloway, MD

Contents

Contributors

MARK S. ALOIA, PhD • *Department of Psychiatry and Human Behavior, Brown Medical School, Providence, RI*
CLIVE BALLARD • *Wolfson Research Centre, University of Newcastle upon Tyne, Newcastle, UK*
PATRICIA A. BOYLE, PhD • *Department of Neurology, Boston University School of Medicine, Boston, MA*
ADAM M. BRICKMAN, MPhil • *Department of Psychiatry and Human Behavior, Brown Medical School, Providence, RI*
JEFFREY BROWNDYKE, PhD • *Department of Psychiatry and Human Behavior, Brown Medical School, Providence, RI*
DEBORAH CAHN-WEINER, PhD • *Department of Psychiatry and Human Behavior, Brown Medical School, Providence, RI*
RONALD COHEN, PhD • *Department of Psychiatry and Human Behavior, Brown Medical School, Providence, RI*
ANELYSSA D'ABREU, MD • *Department of Clinical Neurosciences, Brown Medical School, Providence, RI*
JENNIFER DUNCAN DAVIS, PhD • *Department of Psychiatry and Human Behavior, Brown Medical School, Providence, RI*
SOPHIE DESBIENS, BS • *Department of Biomedical Engineering, Boston University, Boston, MA*
JOHN E. DONAHUE, MD • *Division of Neuropathology, Department of Pathology, Brown Medical School, Providence, RI*
TIMO ERKINJUNTTI, MD • *Memory Research Unit, Department of Neurology, Helsinki University Central Hospital, Helsinki, Finland*
MARGARET M. ESIRI, MD • *Department of Clinical Neurology, University of Oxford; Department of Neuropathology, Oxford Radcliffe NHS Trust, Oxford, UK*
MARC FISHER, MD • *Department of Neurology, University of Massachusetts Medical School, Worcester, MA*
KELLY D. GARRETT, PhD • *Utah State University, Logan, UT*
SERGE GAUTHIER, MD • *MCSA Alzheimer's Disease Research Unity, McGill Center for Studies on Aging, McGill University, Montreal, Canada*
PAULA GRAMMAS, PhD • *Department of Pathology and the Oklahoma Center for Neuroscience, University of Oklahoma Health Sciences Center, Oklahoma City, OK*
JOHN GUNSTAD, PhD • *Department of Psychiatry and Human Behavior, Brown Medical School, Providence, RI*
VLADIMIR HACHINSKI, MD, FRCP(C), DSC • *Department of Clinical Neurological Sciences, University of Western Ontario, London Health Sciences Centre, London, Ontario, Canada*
EBRAHIM HAROON, MD • *Department of Psychiatry and Biobehavioral Sciences, UCLA School of Medicine, Los Angeles, CA*
ANGELA LEE JEFFERSON, PhD • *Department of Psychiatry and Human Behavior, Brown Medical School, Providence, RI*
KURT A. JELLINGER, MD • *Institute of Clinical Neurobiology and University of Vienna, Vienna, Austria*
ELIZABETH M. JONAK, PhD • *Yerkes National Primate Center, Emory University, Atlanta, GA*
RAJ KALARIA • *Wolfson Research Center, University of Newcastle upon Tyne, Newcastle, UK*
JASON E. KANZ, PhD • *Department of Psychiatry, University of Iowa Carver College of Medicine, Iowa City, IA*

ROSE ANNE KENNY • *Wolfson Research Center, University of Newcastle upon Tyne, Newcastle, UK*
GEORGE A. KUCHEL, MD • *University of Connecticut Center on Aging, University of Connecticut Health Center, Farmington, CT*
ANAND KUMAR, MD • *Department of Psychiatry and Biobehavioral Sciences, UCLA School of Medicine, Los Angeles, CA*
KELLY L. LANGE, MD • *Department of Psychology, San Diego State University and Department of Psychiatry, School of Medicine, University of California at San Diego, San Diego, CA*
HELEN LAVRETSKY, MD • *Department of Psychiatry and Biobehavioral Sciences, UCLA School of Medicine, Los Angeles, CA*
DAVID J. LIBON, PhD • *Department of Psychiatry, Center for Aging, School of Osteopathic Medicine, University of Medicine and Dentistry of New Jersey, Stratford, NJ*
LEWIS A. LIPSITZ, MD • *Division on Aging, Harvard Medical School, Hebrew Rehabilitation Center for Aged, Beth Israel Deaconess Medical Center, Boston, MA*
JOSÉ G. MERINO, MD, MPhil • *Department of Neurology, University of Florida, Shands Jacksonville, Jacksonville, FL*
WILLIAM P. MILBERG, PhD • *Department of Psychiatry, Harvard Medical School and West Roxbury Department of Veteran Affairs Medical Center, Boston, MA*
DAVID J. MOSER, PhD • *Department of Psychiatry, University of Iowa Carver College of Medicine, Iowa City, IA*
MARK B. MOSS, PhD • *Department of Anatomy and Neurobiology and Department of Neurology, Boston University School of Medicine, Boston, MA and Yerkes National Primate Center, Emory University, Atlanta, GA*
DAN MUNGAS, PhD • *Department of Neurology, University of California at Davis, Sacramento, CA*
ZSUZSANNA NAGY, MD • *Department of Pharmacology, University of Birmingham, Birmingham, UK*
BRIAN R. OTT, MD • *Department of Clinical Neurosciences, Brown Medical School, Providence, RI*
ROBERT H. PAUL, PhD • *Department of Psychiatry and Human Behavior, Brown Medical School, Providence, RI*
DANA L. PENNEY, PhD • *Department of Neurology, Lahey Clinic, Burlington, MA*
REBECCA E. READY, PhD • *Department of Psychiatry and Human Behavior, Brown Medical School, Providence, RI*
KENNETH ROCKWOOD, PhD • *Geriatric Medicine Research Unit, Queen Elizabeth II Health Science Center, Dalhousie University, Halifax, Nova Scotia, Canada*
GUSTAVO C. ROMÁN, MD • *Geriatric Research Education and Clinical Center, Department of Neurology, University of Texas Health Science Center at San Antonio and the Audie L. Murphy Memorial Veterans Administration Hospital, San Antonio, TX*
STEPHEN SALLOWAY, MD, MS • *Departments of Clinical Neurosciences and Psychiatry and Human Behavior, Brown Medical School; Department of Neurology, Butler Hospital, Providence, RI*
STEPHEN SCHEINTHAL, DO • *Department of Psychiatry, Center for Aging, School of Osteopathic Medicine, University of Medicine and Dentistry of New Jersey, Stratford, NJ*
MAGDY SELIM, MD, PhD • *Department of Neurology, Harvard Medical School, Beth Israel Deaconess Medical Center, Boston, MA*
JORGE M. SERRADOR, PhD • *Division on Aging, Harvard Medical School, Beth Isreal Deaconess Medical Center, Boston, MA*
MARY BETH SPITZNAGEL, MS • *Department of Psychiatry and Human Behavior, Brown Medical School, Providence, RI*
SALLY STEPHENS • *Wolfson Research Center, University of Newcastle Upon Tyne, Newcastle, UK*
EDWARD G. STOPA, MD • *Division of Neuropathology, Department of Pathology, Brown Medical School, Providence, RI*

LAWRENCE SWEET, PhD • *Department of Psychiatry and Human Behavior, Brown Medical School, Providence, RI*
ROD SWENSON, PhD • *Department of Neuroscience, University of North Dakota School of Medicine, Grand Fords, ND*
DAVID F. TATE, PhD • *Department of Psychiatry and Human Behavior, Brown Medical School, Providence, RI*
GEOFFREY TREMONT, PhD • *Department of Psychiatry and Human Behavior, Brown Medical School, Providence, RI*
SHARON X. C. YANG, MD • *University of Connecticut Center on Aging, University of Connecticut Health Center, Farmington, CT*
BRIAN D. ZIPSER, MD • *Division of Neuropathology, Department of Pathology, Brown Medical School, Providence, RI*

I Introduction

1

The Aging Population and the Relevance of Vascular Dementia

Kelly L. Lange and Robert H. Paul

1. INTRODUCTION

Changes occur in nearly every body system with advanced age. Many adults successfully negotiate these transitions; nevertheless, physiologic changes and disease processes emerge with longer lifespan. Numerous age-related changes in physical and psychological conditions can be addressed with advances in medical procedures and pharmacological treatment; however, there are inevitable consequences of prolonging life and the immediate effects on individuals extend to their families, the healthcare system, and society at large. In short, increased longevity introduces several financial and medical challenges and has ramifications for quality of life in a large proportion of the world population.

The significance of health among the elderly remains a paramount concern because of their changing demographics. In 2000, 35 million people in the United States were at least 65 yr old, accounting for one of every eight Americans, with similar figures represented in most developed countries. Projections about the growth of this group indicate an expected doubling of the older population by 2030 to 70 million individuals, with individuals over the age of 65 accounting for one of every four Americans. As recently as the past decade (between 1990 and 2000) the number of adults aged 65 or older increased by 12% *(1)*. The increased prevalence of the older generation raises important questions about their physical and mental health.

Many older individuals express significant concern about potential loss of cognitive function and the development of dementia with advanced age. By no means is this a focus restricted to modern society. Impaired thinking ability associated with advanced age was recognized by the Egyptians in 2000 BC, and some records suggest that dementia was so ubiquitous among the elderly that it was considered a "normal" aspect of the aging process by Plato and other scholars of the day. This assertion was debated then with no less vigor than it is currently (*see* ref. *2*). History aside, there is no question regarding the overwhelming prevalence of the condition today. Currently, more than 4 million individuals in the United States are diagnosed with dementia, and the expected prevalence is predicted to top 16 million by 2050 if the primary contributors to dementia are not controlled. The current individual and societal costs of dementia are no less striking, and the magnitude of these effects will continue to parallel the changing demographics throughout the coming years.

Determining the etiology of dementia in the elderly has been a moving target. In the not-too-distant past, cerebrovascular disease (CVD) was identified as the primary etiology of dementia. Early French neurologists described discrete vascular lesions in the brain that were presumed to underlie declines in mental functions. Binswanger promulgated this model in 1894, reporting that arteriosclerosis and associated reductions in brain perfusion were responsible for mental decline in older adult-

From: *Current Clinical Neurology*
Vascular Dementia: Cerebrovascular Mechanisms and Clinical Management
Edited by: R. H. Paul, R. Cohen, B. R. Ott, and S. Salloway © Humana Press Inc., Totowa, NJ

hood *(3)*. Research during the next 100 yr focused nearly exclusively on CVD as the culprit underlying dementia in the elderly. Terms were introduced to describe the nature of vascular lesions in the centrum semiovale (e.g., leukoariosis) and grey matter, as well as terms to describe the construct of dementia associated with vascular disease (e.g., multiinfarct dementia).

The scientific focus on CVD during the 1800s occurred near the same time that plaques and tangles were first described in the medical literature. Interestingly, these newer neuropathological abnormalities were believed to be relatively uncommon. Alzheimer himself declared that the plaques and tangles described in his report were likely a rare finding *(2)*, and this position was maintained until the late 1970s. In the wake of scientific conferences and meetings that convened soon thereafter, Alzheimer's disease (AD) took center stage as the driving force behind dementia research and clinical practice for the next 20 yr. This focus on AD has begun to expand, and there is renewed interest in additional contributors to dementia, including CVD, and related interest in cardiovascular disease as a contributor to CVD. One impetus underlying this reenergized focus on cardiac and CVD is associated with the advancing age of the baby boomer population in the United States, as well as the general world population. The prevalence and incidence of this older population, coupled with advances in medicine and associated increases in life expectancy among individuals who suffer severe cardiac disease and stroke, have resulted in significant numbers of older individuals living with chronic, incurable, vascular-related morbidity. In effect, the prevalence of stroke increased by nearly 20% during the 1990s, and stroke is now one of the most common neurologic diseases and a leading cause of disability in Western countries *(4)*. The prevalence of vascular dementia (VaD) remains somewhat difficult to determine, but most studies rank VaD as the third most common type of severe cognitive impairment in the elderly, after AD and Lewy body dementia (*see* Chapter 17).

The personal effect of stroke and VaD is noteworthy. Data obtained from the Framingham Heart Study cohort indicate that 20% of an individual's life expectancy after age 50 is comorbid with cardiovascular disease, and individuals who experience a stroke lose as many as 12 yr from their life expectancy *(5)*. Among individuals with dementia associated with vascular disease, life expectancy is significantly shortened compared to the general population. Individuals who are diagnosed with VaD have an estimated median survival of 3.1 yr after the onset of dementia, a rate that is comparable to that of individuals diagnosed with probable AD *(6)*.

Quality of life (QOL) among individuals with VaD has not been extensively studied (*see* Chapter 24 for review), and most of our current understanding of QOL in the elderly has been heavily borrowed from other dementia literature. However, there are several key aspects of VaD that may differentially affect QOL, including preserved insight and significant motor and sensory dysfunction. Consequently, it is possible that individuals with VaD experience significant reductions in life satisfaction compared to other patient populations.

The benefits of further developing our understanding of the natural history of VaD are obvious at both the individual and the societal levels. Unlike other forms of degenerative dementia, VaD is believed to be preventable for many individuals via control over cardiac and vascular risk factors (e.g., hypertension). Obviously, this does not apply to some individuals (e.g., patients with cerebral autosomal dominant arteriopathy with subcortical infarcts and leukoencephalopathy [CADASIL]), and the application of this position for the remainder of the population remains dependent on a more comprehensive understanding of the factors that either promote or provide protection from the development of VaD. The following chapters shed light on these factors by synthesizing the current state of knowledge regarding VaD. However, it is important to recognize that the field of dementia research is dynamic and fluid, and it should be anticipated that new scientific and clinical data will emerge with time that will add significantly to our current conceptualizations of VaD and related syndromes. Ideally, this book will promotes these scientific advances.

REFERENCES

1. Federal Interagency Forum on Aging-Related Statistics. Available at Website: http://agingstats.gov/tables%202001/Tables-population.html#Indicator%20. Accessed April 28, 2004.
2. Boller F, Forbes MM. History of dementia and dementia in history: an overview. J Neurol Sci 1998;158:125–133.
3. Binswanger O. Die abgrenzung der allgemeinen progressiven paralyse. Berl Klin Wochenschr 1894;49:1103–1105; 50:1137–1139; 52:1180–1186.
4. Carolei A, Sacco S, De Santis F, Marini C. Epidemiology of stroke. Clin Exp Hypertens 2002;24:479–83.
5. Peteers A, Mamun AA, Willekens F, Bonneux L. A cardiovascular life history. A life course analysis of the original Framingham Heart Study cohort. Eur Heart J 2002;23:458–466.
6. Wolfson C, Wolfson DB, Asgharian M, et al. A reevaluation of the duration of survival after the onset of dementia. N Engl J Med 2001;344:1111–1116.

2

Clinical Forms of Vascular Dementia

Gustavo C. Román

1. INTRODUCTION

The presence of vascular dementia (VaD) is largely unrecognized and untreated in the elderly *(1,2)*. The typical history is that of an elderly parent or grandparent who fails to regain the previous level of function and independence after a stroke. More often, in the absence of the heralding stroke symptoms, the family notices that the patient has become depressed and apathetic, exhibits personality changes, experiences social inhibition, and has slowing mental capacity and sluggish motor activities with the inability to solve simple daily problems. Walking becomes deliberate, insecure, with a shuffling character and short steps; patients become unsteady on their feet and may take frequent falls. Often, the patient also suffers from urinary urgency, stress incontinence, and nocturia. Patients are no longer able to perform simple activities of daily living (ADLs), such as using the bathroom, showering, getting dressed, cooking, shopping, participating in rehabilitation activities and exercise routines, or performing more complex tasks, such as using the telephone or balancing a checkbook. Frequently, these changes occur after a surgical procedure, such as abdominal surgery, knee or hip replacement, or coronary artery bypass graft (CABG).

The primary care physician is often surprised to find normal or minimally impaired results in the Mini-Mental State Examination *(3)* (MMSE) or the Cambridge cognitive capacity scale (CAMCOG) *(4)*, which is the cognitive portion of the Cambridge Mental Disorders of the Elderly Examination (CAMDEX). The physician may conclude that the patient is depressed, or "deconditioned," after hospitalization, and these symptoms are dismissed as part of a slow convalescence. Nonetheless, the overall net result is dementia, i.e., the loss of cognitive function and the dependency on others for ADLs. The MMSE and the CAMCOG test memory and other posterior cortical functions that are specifically designed to detect Alzheimer's disease (AD), which is a cortical dementia. Therefore, most screening tests for dementia are completely insensitive to alterations of executive function, a cognitive domain localized in prefrontal-subcortical circuits selectively impaired in subcortical forms of VaD *(5)*. This chapter reviews these and other clinical differences between AD and VaD.

2. DEFINITIONS

Vascular dementia: Vascular dementia (VaD) is the loss of cognitive functions to a degree that interferes with ADLs, resulting from ischemic or hemorrhagic cerebrovascular disease (CVD) or from cardiovascular or circulatory disturbances that injure brain regions that are important for memory, cognition, and behavior *(1)*. VaD is the second most common form of dementia after AD, accounting for approximately 20% of dementia cases worldwide *(6)*. Globally, VaD is more common in men, especially before age 75—in contrast with AD that predominates in women—and is

From: *Current Clinical Neurology*
Vascular Dementia: Cerebrovascular Mechanisms and Clinical Management
Edited by: R. H. Paul, R. Cohen, B. R. Ott, and S. Salloway © Humana Press Inc., Totowa, NJ

more prevalent in populations that are affected by cerebral small-vessel disease, such as Asians, Blacks, and Hispanics. In keeping with the predictions of increasing burden of stroke and heart disease in the near future *(7)*, VaD will probably become the most common cause of senile dementia, both by itself and as a contributor to other degenerative dementias *(8)*.

Vascular cognitive impairment: Vascular cognitive impairment (VCI) is a recently coined term to signify any degree of cognitive loss caused by CVD, including vascular dementia *(9,10)*. However, by analogy with mild cognitive impairment (MCI) resulting from AD *(11)*, the term *VCI* is better reserved for patients with risk factors for CVD and some degree of cognitive loss short of dementia. Intrinsic to the VCI concept is the hope that appropriate prevention and treatment of CVD can prevent VaD development. Although this is an appealing undertaking, there have been difficulties in providing a strict definition of VCI and operational diagnostic criteria. The concept of VCI suffers from the same problems once criticized in VaD; i.e., the notion is too wide and too vague for a precise operative definition. Furthermore, as demonstrated in the Canadian Study on Health and Aging *(12,13)*, some patients with a diagnosis of VCI no dementia (VCI-ND) improved with time, indicating that progression from VCI to VaD may not always be a unidirectional pathway. There is growing evidence that preventive measures to decrease the vascular burden on the brain may also decrease VaD, as well as AD *(14)*. This may be achieved by controlling hypertension and cardiac disease, lowering lipids with the use of statins, by decreasing homocysteine, with smoking cessation, and with a Mediterranean diet, among other factors. Moreover, it is hoped that by preventing CVD, the onset of symptomatic AD can be delayed, thereby decreasing the overall burden of dementia.

Mixed dementia: The boundaries between VaD and AD recently have become indistinct. The belief that CVD may lead to cognitive decline and dementia in the elderly has been around since 1672, when Thomas Willis first described cases of postapoplectic dementia. Less well recognized is that *silent* strokes and incomplete white matter ischemia—documented by modern brain imaging—are also strongly associated with cognitive loss, behavioral changes, and VaD. During most of the past two centuries, it was widely held that atherosclerotic dementia was the sole cause of senile dementia. It was only in the 1980s that AD was declared the most common form of dementia in the elderly. However, most elderly patients with dementia who are autopsied will have amyloid plaques and neurofibrillary tangles, the typical brain lesions of AD, localized in the hippocampal regions (Braak Stages I–III), coexisting with cerebrovascular lesions, such as large and small strokes, hemorrhages, arteriolosclerosis, lacunes, microinfarcts, and ischemic leukoencephalopathy. CVD is required to "amplify" the clinical expression of AD pathology beyond the stage of amnestic MCI (Braak Stage III). This explains why almost 20% of cases pathologically defined by Consortium to Establish a Registry for Alzheimer Disease (CERAD) criteria as AD do not have clinical dementia. Conversely, more than half of the octogenarians without dementia meet CERAD criteria for pathologically confirmed AD *(15)*. On the other hand, Hénon and colleagues *(16,17)*, have also shown that in patients with bona fide postapoplectic VaD, preexisting amnestic deficits occurred in 16% of cases, suggesting that the underlying AD had not progressed beyond Stage III, which is clearly insufficient to produce clinical dementia. Evidence from the Nun Study *(18)* also concluded that lacunes increase more than 20 times the risk of clinical expression of dementia at early Braak stages that are insufficient to produce dementia. Moreover, in pathologically confirmed cases of "mixed" dementia (AD+CVD, AD+VaD), there is a significant *inverse* relationship between the severity of CVD and Braak stage *(19–22)*. In all these patients, VaD is the defining cause of the dementia. In addition, population-based studies have shown that silent lacunes are extremely common in the elderly. Longstreth et al. *(23)* showed the presence of one or more silent lacunes in approximately one-fourth of the 3,660 participants in the Cardiovascular Health Study (CHS) aged 65 and older that underwent cerebral magnetic resonance imaging (MRI). Recently, in the Rotterdam cohort, Vermeer et al. *(24)* demonstrated that the presence of lacunes, particularly in the thalamus, more than doubled the risk of dementia (hazard ratio = 2.26, 95% CI, 1.09–4.70). Small-vessel disease may be the most common mechanism to convert from MCI into AD in persons over the age of 70 yr *(8)*.

Table 1
Risk Factors for Vascular Dementia

• Advanced age	• Long-term, untreated arterial hypertension
• Isolated systolic hypertension in the elderly	• Diabetes mellitus
• Cigarette smoking	• Hyperlipidemia
• Hyperhomocysteinemia	• Hyperfibrinogenemia
• Congestive heart failure	• Atrial fibrillation
• Other cardiac arrhythmias	• Complicated stroke
• Recurrent stroke	• Orthostatic hypotension
• Obstructive sleep apnea	• Major surgery in the elderly
• Coronary artery bypass graft surgery	

The weight of the evidence validates the hypothesis that CVD is the most important cause of dementia in the elderly, both by itself and as a catalyst for the conversion of low-grade AD to dementia. As customarily done in neuroepidemiological studies *(25)*, patients with AD+CVD should be included among the VaDs and not in the AD category. Moreover, to this group of patients we must add the thousands of cases with cognitive loss and VaD resulting from cerebral hypoperfusion complicating cardiac and circulatory diseases. The evidence presented notwithstanding, it should be emphasized that AD is not primarily a vascular disease as postulated by de la Torre *(26)*.

3. CLINICAL FORMS OF DEMENTIA

3.1. *When to Suspect VaD*

Typically, patients with VaD are not found in memory disorder clinics, because memory loss is a less prominent manifestation of this syndrome. This must be considered when extrapolating figures of dementia prevalence from hospital- or office-based data. This also explains the alleged rarity of VaD in neuropathologically examined specimens from brain banks of AD clinics *(27)*. Primary care settings (family physicians and geriatricians) are the main referral source of patients with VaD. These cases occur among patients affected by coronary artery disease (CAD), stroke, diabetes mellitus, transient ischemic attacks (TIAs), arterial hypertension, cigarette smoking, increased homocysteine, and hyperfibrinogenemia. VaD affects elderly persons with systolic hypertension, congestive heart failure (CHF), atrial fibrillation and other cardiac arrhythmias, orthostatic hypotension, or obstructive sleep apnea (*see* Table 1).

Poststroke VaD also occurs among patients recovering from recurrent strokes in rehabilitation services and stroke clinics. Likewise, VaD secondary to cerebral hypoperfusion is seen in cardiac rehabilitation patients after myocardial infarction (MI) *(28)* or among patients convalescing from major surgery, particular hip fracture repair *(29)*. Approximately 26% of patients discharged from the hospital after treatment for CHF have significant cognitive decline *(30)*. Patients with severe cognitive dysfunction usually have worse left ventricular dysfunction and systolic blood pressure levels below 130 mmHg. Cognitive decline resulting from cerebral embolism and hypoperfusion is also frequently found in patients' post-CABG surgery *(31–33)*. Patients with VaD and severe behavioral manifestations (apathy, agitation, and uninhibited behavior) are usually seen by geriatric psychiatrists, who have coined the terms *vascular depression* and *depression-executive dysfunction syndrome of late life* for this clinical syndrome *(34,35)*.

3.2. *Cortical and Subcortical Dementias*

Clinicians divide the dementia syndrome into two main types, *cortical* and *subcortical,* according to the clinical features and the pattern of neuropsychological impairment. The prototypical cortical

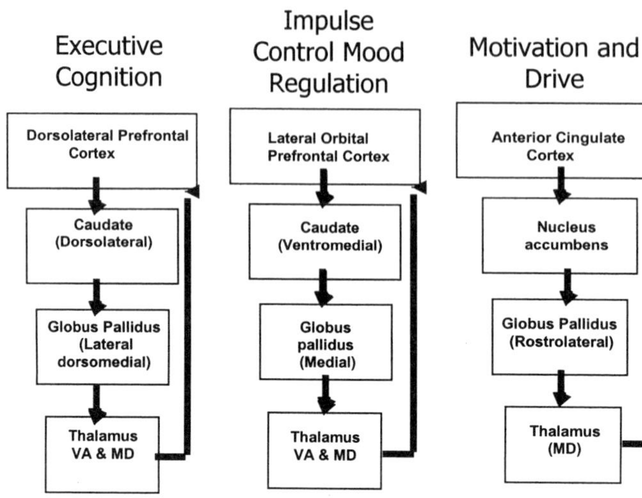

Fig. 1. Frontal-subcortical-thalamic circuits: the prefrontal cortex is connected to the striatum and thalamus in parallel but separate circuits that help regulate behavior; there is topographic mapping of caudate and thalamus. A typical feature of these prefrontal cortico-subcortical circuits is that an injury anywhere in a circuit can produce a major deficit and small subcortical lesions can mimic large cortical lesions.

dementia is AD that manifests preponderantly with early and severe memory disturbances, aphasia, agnosia, and apraxia resulting from lesions involving posterior cortical association regions. In sharp contrast, VaD manifestations, a typical subcortical dementia, include slowing of cognition and motor function owing to executive control *(5)*, along with prominent alterations of gait *(36)*, speech, affect, and mood. The manifestations mentioned result from the interruption by ischemic lesions of frontal cortico-subcortical circuits (*see* Fig. 1) for executive control of memory, language, mood, constructional skills, motivation, and socially responsive behaviors *(37–42)*.

Unfortunately, there is a dearth of bedside executive function tests *(42)*. Commonly used tests include Luria's kinetic melody *(43)*, the Clock Drawing Test and Executive Function (CLOX) *(44)*, and the trail test part B *(45)*, as well as verbal fluency tasks and similarities tests in the Modified Mini-Mental State (3MS) *(46)* and the Cognitive Abilities Screening Instrument (CASI) *(47)*. Clinical experience indicates that frontal system involvement is common in VaD and is a constant component of subcortical VaD.

4. CLINICAL FORMS OF VAD

VaD is a complex neuropathological entity resulting from several causal vascular lesions with numerous clinical manifestations (*see* Table 2). However, according to Román *(48)*, the clinical syndromes of VaD may be divided simply into two main groups, *acute* and *subacute*, according to the temporal profile of clinical presentation.

4.1. *Acute-Onset (Poststroke) VaD*

Acute-onset VaD (also called poststroke, postictal, or postapoplectic VaD) includes patients with new-onset dementia after a clinically eloquent acute cerebrovascular event. The causal stroke is either a single strategic stroke resulting from occlusion (or rupture) of a large-size vessel or a symptomatic subcortical lacunar stroke caused by occlusive small-vessel disease. The older term *multistroke dementia* (MID) is sometimes used when VaD develops after recurrent large-vessel strokes. Table 3

Table 2
Clinical and Pathological Forms of Vascular Dementia

Large-vessel dementia	
Mechanisms	• Artery-to-artery embolism • Thrombosis/occlusion of extracranial or intracranial cerebral arteries • Cardiogenic embolism
Multi-infarct dementia	• Multiple large complete infarcts, cortico-subcortical in location, usually with perifocal incomplete infarction involving the white matter
Strategic infarct dementia	• Single brain infarct in functionally critical areas of the brain (angular gyrus, thalamus, basal forebrain, posterior cerebral artery, and anterior cerebral artery territories)
Small-vessel dementia	
Mechanisms	• Endothelial dysfunction appears to be the final common pathway of hypertension, diabetes, smoking, aging, and other risk factors for small-vessel brain disease
Subcortical ischemic VaD	• Binswanger's disease • CADASIL • Lacunar dementia or lacunar state *(état lacunaire)* • Multiple lacunes with extensive perifocal incomplete infarction
Cortical-subcortical	• Hypertensive and arteriolosclerotic angiopathy • Cerebral amyloid angiopathies • Other hereditary forms • Collagen-vascular disease with dementia • Moyamoya • Cerebral sinus/venous thrombosis
Ischemic-hypoperfusive dementia	
Border-zone infarction	• Restricted injury resulting fromdue to selective vulnerability
Ischemic leukoencephalopathy	• Incomplete white-matter infarction
Hemorrhagic dementia	
	• Traumatic subdural hematoma • Subarachnoid hemorrhage • Cerebral hemorrhage • Hematological factors

Abbr: VaD, vascular dementia; CADASIL, cerebral autosomal dominant arteriopathy with subcortical infarcts and leukoencephalopathy.

summarizes the main risk factors for poststroke MID. It has been estimated that approximately 20% of patients older than 65 yr who suffer an ischemic stroke develop poststroke VaD *(49–51)*.

Clinically, large-vessel forms of poststroke VaD may resemble the cortical dementias in the accumulation of stroke-related cortical cognitive deficits, such as agnosia, apraxia, alexia, aphasia, often without motor deficit *(52,53)*. The latter cases result from relatively unusual (strategic) ischemic strokes that involve single branches of the middle cerebral artery (MCA), the anterior (ACA), or the posterior cerebral artery (PCA) and their branches *(52,53)*. For example, strokes of the left posterior parietal branch of the MCA with ischemia of association areas in the posterior portions of the superior and inferior parietal lobules, including the supramarginal gyrus, usually produce cortical sensory loss with astereognosia, agraphesthesia, and proprioceptive loss, Wernicke's aphasia, and Gerstmann's syndrome with right-left disorientation, finger agnosia, acalculia, and agraphia *(53)*.

Table 3
Main Risk Factors for Poststroke Vascular Dementia

1. Age	Older age
2. Education	Lower educational level
3. Personal factors	Lower income, current smokers
4. Genetic factors	Family history of dementia
5. Stroke type	Recurrent strokes
6. Stroke location	Left-sided lesions, "strategic strokes" (i.e., posterior association areas, such as gyrus angularis; posterior cerebral artery territories, including paramedian thalamic artery territory, inferomedial temporal lobes, and hippocampus; watershed or border-zone infarcts mainly involving superior frontal and parietal regions; bilateral anterior cerebral artery territories, anterior choroidal artery strokes, and basal forebrain lesions; and frontal white matter lesions). Inferior capsular genu stroke producing diaschisis of frontal lobes and cerebellum.
7. Stroke volume	Lesions larger than 50–100 mL of tissue destruction, large perilesional incomplete ischemic areas involving white matter, larger periventricular white matter ischemic lesions.
8. Stroke complications	Hypoxic and ischemic complications of acute stroke (i.e., seizures, cardiac arrhythmias, aspiration pneumonia, and hypotension).
9. Stroke manifestations	Dysphagia, gait limitations, and urinary impairment.

However, amnesia is not present and, despite, the multiple deficits, with time many of these patients recover their independence in ADLs and no longer fulfill the National Institute of Neurological Disorders and Stroke-Association Internationale pour la Recherche et l'Enseignement en Neurosciences (NINDS-AIREN) criteria for dementia *(54)*. This contrasts the memory loss and the usual deterioration of AD with time. When stroke patients recover and return to functional capacity or are left with isolated poststroke cognitive deficits, they are usually classified under the heading VCI.

Nonetheless, there are VaD cases with amnesia as a prominent feature resulting from interruption by ischemic injury of portions of the circuit comprising the hippocampus, fornix, mamillary body, mammillothalamic tract, anterior thalamus *(55,56)*. Memory loss may also occur with mediobasal forebrain damage *(57)*. Sometimes the amnestic manifestations of the lesions mentioned may be confused clinically with AD. A brief summary of the main features of acute-onset VaD associated with large-vessel stroke follows.

4.1.1. Posterior Cerebral Artery

Brandt and colleagues *(58)*, found that approximately 25% of patients with infarctions in the PCA territory present with amnesia as a result of damage to the hippocampus, isthmus, entorhinal and perirhinal cortex, and parahippocampal gyrus. Lesions that are more limited may occur with territorial infarctions of the anterior or posterior choroidal arteries. Unilateral lesions cause material-specific memory loss (verbal amnesia with left-sided lesions and loss of visuospatial memory and memory for locations with lesions on the right side), whereas bilateral damage gives rise to global amnesia *(53,57)*. In some patients with mesial temporal lobe lesions (hippocampus and its projections), episodic anterograde amnesia—similar to that of AD—may be observed *(58)*. These patients are unable to encode and consolidate new verbal material, facts; events, short stories, names, and concepts their but working memory and procedural memory are intact; confabulations are uncommon *(53,57,59)*.

Visual signs in more than 80% of patients usually accompany the memory deficits in PCA strokes. These include homonymous hemianopsia, color agnosia, and visual agnosia. Left-sided lesions may have transcortical sensory aphasia, pure alexia, or alexia without agraphia. Spatial disorientation may be prominent with right-sided lesions. Anton's syndrome of cortical blindness with anosognosia occurs with bilateral occipital lesions. Bilateral parietooccipital infarctions above the calcarine fissure may result in Balint's syndrome with simultagnosia, optic ataxia, and ocular apraxia; prosopagnosia occurs with bilateral occipital ischemia below the calcarine fissure.

4.1.2. Basal Forebrain Infarction

Lesions of the mesial temporal lobe and thalamus causing memory and other cognitive deficits may interrupt cholinergic projections to these regions *(60)*. However, in humans, a single study of 12 patients with MID failed to find changes in the nucleus basalis of Meynert (nbM) *(61)*. Direct ischemic injury of the cholinergic nuclei in the basal forebrain has been documented in patients with subarachnoid hemorrhage from ruptured aneurysms of the anterior communicating artery (AComA), usually after surgical repair *(62,63)*. The damage results from aneurysmal bleeding and from sacrifice of perforating branches of the AComA or proximal ACA at the time of surgery. After surgical repair of an aneurysm of the AComA, Phillips et al. *(64)* found severe anterograde amnesia for verbal or visuospatial material, along with severe apathy, lack of initiative and spontaneity, and executive dysfunction. Postmortem neuropathological lesions were found in midline basal areas, rostral to the anterior commissure and lamina terminalis, destroying the medial septal nuclei (Ch1), the vertical portion (Ch2) of the nucleus of the diagonal band of Broca (ndbB), the nucleus accumbens, and adjacent areas. Damage to the cholinergic neurons in the septal nucleus and ndbB determine the persistence of the amnesia *(63,64)*.

From the clinical viewpoint, most patients with AD have severe anterograde episodic amnesia with extremely poor recall of verbal material. Although a similar type of amnesia may result from localized strokes, in general, most subjects with VaD perform better on story recall and word list learning (California and the Rey verbal learning tests); also, in contrast with AD patients, they are usually able to respond to cues and have superior free recall and relatively minor deficits of verbal long-term memory *(65)*. Patients with VaD retain speech and calculation longer than those with AD.

4.1.3. Thalamic VaD

This peculiar form of VaD, described originally by Castaigne et al. *(66,67)*, occurs after paramedian thalamic ischemic strokes. Lesions involve the anterior (polar) thalamus *(68,69)* in territories irrigated by the polar thalamic artery, which is a branch of the posterior communicating artery, or the medial and central thalamus involving the dorsomedial nucleus (DMn) and the mamillothalamic tract *(70)*. The latter two structures are irrigated by the paramedian thalamic artery which is a branch of the basilar-PCA. For Van der Werf et al. *(70)*, the critical lesion in the production of thalamic amnesia is the damage of the mamillothalamic tract, which projects into the anterior nuclei of the thalamus and then to the cingulate cortex.

All patients have a depressed level of consciousness that gradually improves within days to weeks, revealing impairments in attention, motivation, initiative, executive functions, and memory, as well as dramatic verbal and motor slowness and apathy *(71)*. Gaze abnormalities are common and include vertical gaze paresis, medial rectus paresis, and absent convergence. Dysarthria and mild hemiparesis may be present when the lesions extend to the subthalamic and midbrain tegmentum in the superior paramedian mesencephalic artery territory, which may arise adjacent to or from a common trunk with the paramedian thalamic artery.

Left thalamic lesions are accompanied by memory deficits more often than right-sided lesions; verbal and, occasionally, visual memory loss are present with left-sided lesions and visual amnesia with right-sided lesions. Global amnesia occurs with bilateral lesions or in those with simultaneous damage to the mamillothalamic tract and the inferior thalamic peduncle. These patients have severe anterograde episodic amnesia plus retrograde amnesia; i.e., both the encoding of new memories and retrieval of new and old memories are affected, but motor learning and implicit memory are intact *(53)*. The severe attentional and motivational deficits play a role in the amnesia *(68,71)*.

4.1.4. *Inferior Genu Stroke*

A clinical syndrome, which is closely related to thalamic VaD, was described by Tatemichi and colleagues *(72,73)* in patients with a lacunar infarction in the inferior genu of the internal capsule. This characteristic—albeit relatively uncommon—syndrome is manifested by a sudden change in cognitive function, often associated with fluctuating attention, confusion, abulia, striking psychomotor retardation, inattention, executive dysfunction, and other features of frontal lobe dysfunction but with mild focal findings, such as hemiparesis or dysarthria. Memory loss was present in all cases: left-sided infarcts had severe verbal memory loss and right-sided infarcts caused visuospatial memory loss *(74,75)*.

Lacunar strokes of the inferior genu of the internal capsule result from involvement of anterior perforators arising from the internal carotid artery (ICA) or from the ACA. These arteries are commonly affected by hypertension and other forms of small-vessel disease and could be an unrecognized cause of cognitive deficits. For instance, Ghika et al. *(76)* found neuropsychological deficits in up to 34% of patients with lacunes in the territory of deep perforators of the ICA system identified by brain computed tomography (CT).

Furthermore, a lacunar stroke involving the inferior genu of the internal capsule causes ipsilateral blood flow reduction to the inferior and medial frontal cortex *(72,73,77)* and to the ipsilateral temporal lobe and contralateral cerebellar hemisphere *(77)*, by a mechanism of diaschisis. These lesions in the genu of the inferior capsule may sever corticothalamic and thalamocortical fibers in the thalamic peduncles, which detach from the internal capsule to enter the thalamus at its rostral and caudal poles and along its dorsal surface. The *anterior thalamic peduncle* connects the DMn with the cingulate gyrus, prefrontal, and orbitofrontal cortex. The *inferior thalamic peduncle* connects the thalamus with orbitofrontal, insular, and temporal cortex, as well as with the amygdala, via the ansa peduncularis and the amygdalofugal pathway. The last two named also contain cholinergic fibers from the nbM (Ch4) and may have an effect in reducing blood flow. Thus, lacunar infarctions in the region of the inferior genu cause both frontal behavioral effects and memory loss associated with functional deactivation of the ipsilateral frontal and temporal cortex.

Finally, there are also rare amnesic syndromes with subcortical lesions interrupting frontal networks, separate from the traditional Papez circuit or the Delay-Brion memory system *(56)*.

4.1.5. *Caudate Strokes*

The loss of memory observed with caudate strokes is characterized by recall difficulties even with cues but with normal recognition *(53)*. These features, along with the typical abulia *(78,79)*, probably result from interruption of frontal connections. Frontal and temporal hypoperfusion in these cases may conceivably result from interruption of cholinergic projections.

4.2. *Subacute (Subcortical) VaD*

Subacute VaD follows a slowly progressive course seen mainly in patients with nonocclusive small-vessel disease affecting periventricular white matter (Binswanger's disease), usually accompanied by clinically asymptomatic lacunes; a stepwise worsening may occur when small-vessel occlusion leads to recurrent lacunar strokes *(2)*. This pattern of clinical onset and progression is the same one observed in patients with CADASIL *(80–82)*. Most subcortical VaD cases have a subacute presentation and result from the combination of nonocclusive small-vessel disease and lacunes *(2)*. The temporal profile of presentation of these forms of VaD is typically subacute with a chronic course marked by fluctuations and slowly progressive worsening that resembles that of AD. Patients present clinically with frontal lobe deficits, executive dysfunction, slow information processing, impaired memory, inattention, depressive mood changes, motor involvement, parkinsonian features, urinary disturbances, and pseudobulbar palsy. Frontal executive functions control volition, planning, programming, and monitoring of complex goal-directed activities, such as cooking, shopping, and housework *(2,5)*. Loss of executive function is a major component of cognitive disability and dementia resulting from the loss of planning capacity, working memory, attention and concentration, stimuli discrimination, abstraction, conceptual flexibility, and self-control *(39–42)*. Patients with executive dysfunction are often capable of performing individual steps of a complex problem but are unable to provide a correct strategy to solve it.

As mentioned, this is one of the most common forms of VaD and results from small-vessel disease with lacunes and white matter lesions that damage structures (caudate nucleus, globus pallidus, thalamus, and connecting fibers) of the prefrontal-subcortical circuits *(37–40)*. The main forms of subacute subcortical VaD are lacunar state *(état lacunaire)*, Binswanger's disease, CADASIL, and some forms of cerebral amyloid angiopathy. Diagnostic criteria for subcortical VaD have been recently proposed *(83)*.

4.2.1. *Lacunar State* (État Lacunaire)

This clinical syndrome of the elderly results from the presence of multiple brain lacunes. Occlusion of the arterial lumen of small arterioles, including deep thalamoperforating and long medullary arterioles, leads to lacunar strokes. Lacunes are small areas of ischemic necrosis and liquefaction less than 15 mm in diameter, typically located in the basal ganglia, internal capsule, thalamus, pons, corona radiata, and centrum semiovale, and usually seen in the chronic cavitated stage *(84)*. White matter lacunes may overlap with nonconfluent focal areas of ischemic leukoencephalopathy. Lacunes must be distinguished from dilated perivascular spaces (*état criblé*). Microscopically, these cavities show no evidence of necrosis, macrophages, or tissue debris and have a small vessel within the lacuna. In addition to lacunes, ventricular dilatation and white matter lesions resulting from recurrent ischemia-hypoxia frequently coexist. Patients may have a history of repeated small strokes with transient motor deficits or minimal residuum or the subacute presentation of Binswanger's disease. Cognitive deficits in patients with subcortical lacunes correlate better with the extent of white matter lesions than with the number of lacunes.

As mentioned, approximately one-fourth of the 3660 participants in the CHS had one or more lacunes demonstrated by cranial MRI *(23)*. The CHS is a population-based random sample of the elderly US population that includes African Americans age 65 and older. In most of these participants (89%), lacunes were clinically silent; however, gait problems and subtle cognitive impairments—not recognized as stroke—were found more often in those with silent lacunes than in subjects with normal MRI *(23)*. Similar results, with frequencies of silent lacunes ranging from 11 to 24%, have been found in other population-based studies, as well as in patient cohorts of initial stroke.

4.2.2. *Binswanger's Disease*

In 1894, Binswanger described the presence of an ischemic periventricular leukoencephalopathy that typically spares the arcuate subcortical U fibers as the hallmark of this condition *(85)*. Small-vessel disease and multiple lacunes often coexist in Binswanger's disease, and it has been postulated that this condition and the so-called "lacunar dementia" of patients with lacunar state may represent a single entity *(86)*.

Their clinical manifestations are similar and consist of a cognitive and motor syndrome, with characteristics of subcortical dementia, including executive dysfunction, loss of verbal fluency, slowing of motor function with perseveration, impersistence, inattention, difficulties with set shifting, and abnormal Luria's kinetic melody tests. Memory loss is characterized by poor retrieval and intact recognition. Apathy, depression, and behavioral problems are common. Mild residual hemiparesis or other discrete focal findings are often found. There is a peculiar short-stepped gait *(marche à petits pas)*, dysarthria, pseudobulbar palsy, and, in some cases, astasia-abasia. Extrapyramidal features, such as inexpressive facies, slowness of movement, axial rigidity, loss of postural reflexes, frequent falls, increased urinary frequency, and nocturia, are also common findings *(85)*. The differential diagnosis is with the clinical triad of dementia, abnormal gait, and urinary incontinence typical of normal pressure hydrocephalus.

4.2.3. Cerebral Autosomal Dominant Arteriopathy With Subcortical Infarcts and Leukoencephalopathy

One of the most important recent developments in the field of VaD has been the clinical and genetic description of CADASIL *(80)*. Originally called familial Binswanger's disease, this condition offers a natural model for the study of subcortical-subacute forms of VaD, particularly Binswanger's disease. Numerous pedigrees have been described in Europe and North America.

CADASIL is an autosomal dominant disorder of cerebral small vessels mapped to chromosome 19q12 *(81,82)*. Clinical manifestations include TIAs and strokes (80%), cognitive deficits and VaD (50%), migraine with focal deficits (40%), mood disorders (30%), and epilepsy (10%). Onset is usually in early adulthood (mean age 46 yr) in the absence of risk factors for VaD, culminating in dementia and death usually approximately 20 yr after symptom onset. The dementia is slow in onset, subcortical and frontal in type, accompanied by gait and urinary disturbances, and pseudobulbar palsy clinically identical to that of sporadic Binswanger's disease. MRI reveals a combination of small lacunar lesions and diffuse white matter abnormalities; these are often present in asymptomatic relatives. Also, cerebral blood flow reactivity to inhaled carbon dioxide is impaired.

The underlying vascular lesion is a unique nonamyloid nonatherosclerotic microangiopathy involving arterioles (100–400 μ in diameter) and capillaries, primarily in the brain but also in other organs. The diagnosis may be established by skin biopsy *(87)* confirmed by immunostaining with a *Notch3* monoclonal antibody *(88)*.

The vessels show deposits of eosinophilic, PAS-positive material in the arterial media that on electron microscopy consists of granular osmiophilic deposits and accumulation of the ectodomain of the *Notch3* receptor in the basal lamina of degenerated smooth muscle cells *(87)*. The brain lesions are ischemic infarcts, mainly lacunar strokes, localized in basal ganglia, thalamus, centrum ovale, and pons and associated with extensive, confluent areas of frontal ischemic leukoencephalopathy, particularly in periventricular regions.

4.2.4. Cerebral Amyloid Angiopathy

Cerebral amyloid angiopathy (CAA) is a heterogeneous group of disorders characterized by deposition of amyloid in the walls of leptomeningeal and cerebral cortical blood vessels, characterized clinically by recurrent or multiple lobar hemorrhages, cognitive deterioration, and ischemic strokes. MRI displays diffuse white matter abnormalities, along with ischemic or hemorrhagic focal brain lesions. On histology, the vessels show amyloid deposition, microaneurysms, and fibrinoid necrosis. There are several autosomal dominant forms of CAA with differences in their clinical, genetic, biochemical, and pathologic findings. Aβ, the major amyloid component in the Dutch-, Flemish-, and Iowa-type of familial CAA, is also the major amyloid component in sporadic CAA and in AD. However, at least in the Dutch-type, the severity of the dementia correlates better with the degree of vascular lesions than with the amount of amyloid deposition *(89)*. Familial British dementia (FBD) with amyloid angiopathy is an autosomal dominant condition characterized by VaD, progressive spastic paraparesis, and cerebellar ataxia, with onset in the sixth decade *(90)*. A point mutation in the BRI gene on chromosome 13 is the genetic abnormality. On brain MRI, Binswanger-type deep white-matter hyperintensities and lacunar infarcts are seen, but no intracerebral hemorrhages are seen. The corpus callosum is severely affected and atrophic. Plaques and tangles are present, but the amyloid subunit (ABri) found in FBD brains is entirely different and unrelated to other amyloid proteins. FBD combines neurodegeneration and dementia with systemic amyloid deposition *(91,92)*.

5. DIAGNOSIS OF VAD

Although numerous diagnostic criteria for VaD have been proposed, the NINDS-AIREN criteria *(54)* (*see* Table 4) have been used in most controlled clinical trials and offer an operative approach to the basic elements needed to reach a diagnosis of VaD. These are: (1) *cognitive loss*, (2) *cerebrovas-*

Table 4
NINDS-AIREN Diagnostic Criteria for Vascular Dementia*

I. The criteria for the diagnosis of *probable* VaD include *all* of the following:

1. Dementia: Impairment of memory and two or more cognitive domains (including executive function), interfering with ADLs and not resulting from effects of stroke alone.
   Exclusion criteria: Alterations of consciousness, delirium, psychoses, severe aphasia or deficits preclud ing testing, systemic disorders, *Alzheimer's disease,* or other forms of dementia.
2. Cerebrovascular disease: Focal signs on neurological examination (hemiparesis, lower facial weakness, Babinski sign, sensory deficit, hemianopia, dysarthria) consistent with stroke (with or without history of stroke, *and* evidence of relevant CVD by brain CT or MRI including *multiple large-vessel infarcts* or a *single strategically placed infarct* (angular gyrus, thalamus, basal forebrain, or PCA or ACA territories), as well as *multiple basal ganglia* and *white-matter lacunes* or *extensive periventricular white-matter lesions,* or combinations thereof.
   Exclusion criteria: Absence of cerebrovascular lesions on CT or MRI.
3. A relationship between the above two disorders: Manifested or inferred by the presence of one or more of the following:
   a. onset of dementia within 3 mo after a recognized stroke,
   b. abrupt deterioration in cognitive functions; or fluctuating, stepwise progression of cognitive deficits.

II. Clinical features *consistent* with the diagnosis of *probable* VaD include the following:

1. Early presence of gait disturbances (small step gait or marche à petits pas, or magnetic, apraxic-ataxic, or parkinsonian gait).
2. History of unsteadiness and frequent, unprovoked falls.
3. Early urinary frequency, urgency, and other urinary symptoms not explained by urologic disease.
4. Pseudobulbar palsy.
5. Personality and mood changes, abulia, depression, emotional incontinence, or other deficits, including psychomotor retardation and abnormal executive function.

III. Features that make the diagnosis of VaD uncertain or unlikely include:

1. Early onset of memory deficit and progressive worsening of memory and other cognitive functions, such as language (transcortical sensory aphasia), motor skills (apraxia), and perception (agnosia), in the absence of corresponding focal lesions on brain imaging.
2. Absence of focal neurological signs, other than cognitive disturbances.
3. Absence of CVD on CT or MRI.

Abbr: ACA, anterior cerebral artery; ADLs, activities of daily living; CT, computerized tomography; CVD, cerebrovascular disease; MRI, magnetic resonance imaging; PCA, posterior cerebral artery; VaD, vascular dementia.
From G. Román et al *(56).*

cular lesions demonstrated by brain imaging (CT, MRI), (3) a *temporal link* between stroke and cognitive loss, and (4) *exclusion of other causes of dementia,* such as AD. A temporal relationship, i.e., development of dementia within 3 mo after stroke, has proved to be more difficult to fulfill, particularly in patients with silent strokes.

The NINDS-AIREN criteria require objective proof of dementia, validated by neuropsychological tests. In practical terms, tests for subcortical dysfunction, including executive function testing, should be used *(93).* Demonstration of the presence of vascular lesions by brain imaging MRI or CT is needed. Lesions range from a single strategic lacunar stroke to multiple cortical-subcortical strokes to periventricular ischemia. Mungas et al. *(94)* determined by MRI that hippocampal atrophy, volume of cortical gray matter, and volume of white mater lesions—but not lacunes—were strong and independent predictors of vascular cognitive impairment. The neuropathological substrate of the lesions mentioned in patients with VaD is widespread ischemia from microvascular disease, including ischemic hippocampal injury pathologically resembling mesial temporal lobe sclerosis *(95,96)*. By definition, absence of vascular lesions by brain imaging excludes VaD.

5.1. Separating AD From VaD

A practical problem that frequently confronts the internist is the elderly patient with cognitive and behavioral decline, presenting with abnormal score in the MMSE and presence of vascular lesions on brain imaging. The *ischemic score* may provide elements for the diagnosis of VaD *(97)*. A score of 7 or more is consistent with MID, a score of 4 or less with AD, and a score of 5 to 6 is suggestive of AD plus CVD. In a recent meta-analysis *(98)*, the following features were found more often in VaD than in AD: stepwise deterioration, fluctuating course, history of hypertension, history of stroke, and focal neurological symptoms.

Careful interview of relatives and caregivers should provide elements for the diagnosis of prestroke dementia *(16,17)*. In most instances, probable AD is a likely etiology for the progressive memory loss occurring before the ictus. The amnestic form of MCI is easily identifiable and carries a risk of conversion to clinically probable AD at a rate of 10 to 15% per year, compared with 1 to 2% per year in healthy age-matched control subjects *(99)*. However, the frequency and severity of CVD in older patients with AD point to the possibility that vascular risk factors may predispose not only to VaD but also to the AD development *(100)*. Population-based epidemiological data have shown that vascular risk factors, such as hypertension, carotid artery wall thickness, cholesterol, and peripheral vascular disease often occur in patients who develop AD *(14)*. The vascular role of the apolipoprotein E ε4 allele, which is a risk factor for AD, may explain, in part, this interaction. Early treatment and control of vascular risk factors are one of the most promising avenues for the prevention of dementia in the elderly.

6. CONCLUSIONS

In summary, the diagnosis of VaD is relatively straightforward in most patients who have significant vascular risk factors and acute development of cognitive deficits and dementia after a clinically eloquent stroke. The diagnosis of VaD should also be entertained when these manifestations occur in patients after a cardiovascular episode, such as MI or CHF, in elderly patients recovering from laborious surgical procedures, in particular hip- or knee-replacement, and more often after a CABG surgery.

REFERENCES

1. Román GC. Vascular dementia revisited: diagnosis, pathogenesis, treatment, and prevention. Med Clin N Am 2002;86: 477–499.
2. Román GC, Erkinjuntti T, Wallin A, Pantoni L, Chui HC. Subcortical ischaemic vascular dementia. Lancet Neurol 2002;1:426–436.
3. Folstein MF, Folstein SE, McHugh PR. A practical method for grading the cognitive state of patients for the clinician. J Psychiatr Res 1975;12:189–198.
4. Huppert FA, Brayne C, Gill C, Paykel ES, Beardsall L. CAMCOG—a concise neuropsychological test to assist dementia diagnosis: sociodemographic characteristics in an elderly population sample. Br J Clin Psychol 1995;34: 529–541.
5. Román GC, Royall DR. Executive control function: a rational basis for the diagnosis of vascular dementia. Alzheimer Dis Assoc Disord 1999;13 (Suppl):S69–S80.
6. Dubois MF, Herbert R. The incidence of vascular dementia in Canada: a comparison with Europe and East Asia. Neuroepidemiology 2001;20:179–187.
7. Murray CJ, Lopez AD. Global mortality, disability, and the contribution of risk factors: global burden of disease study. Lancet 1997;349:1436–1442.
8. Román GC. Stroke, cognitive decline and vascular dementia: the silent epidemic of the 21st century. Neuroepidemiology 2003;22:161–164.
9. Erkinjuntti T, Gauthier S, eds. Vascular cognitive impairment. London, UK: Martin Dunitz, 2002.

10. Bowler JV, Hachinski V, eds. Vascular Cognitive Impairment: Preventable dementia. Oxford, UK: Oxford University Press, 2003.
11. Petersen RC, ed. Mild cognitive impairment: aging to Alzheimer's disease. Oxford, UK: Oxford University Press, 2003.
12. Wentzel C, Rockwood K, MacKnight C, et al. Progression of impairment in patients with vascular cognitive impairment without dementia. Neurology 2001;57:714–716.
13. Ingles JL, Wentzel C, Fisk JD, Rockwood K. Neuropsychological predictors of incident dementia in patients with vascular cognitive impairment, without dementia. Stroke 2002;33:1999–2002.
14. O'Brien JT, Erkinjuntti T, Reisberg B, et al. Vascular cognitive impairment. Lancet Neurol 2003;2:89–98.
15. Polvikowski T, Sulkava R, Myllykangas L, et al. Prevalence of Alzheimer's disease in very old people: a prospective neuropathological study. Neurology 2001;56:1690–1696.
16. Hénon H, Pasquier F, Durieu I, et al. Pre-existing dementia in stroke patients: baseline frequency, associated factors and outcome. Stroke 1997;28:2429–2436.
17. Hénon H, Durieu I, Guerouaou D, et al. Post-stroke dementia: incidence and relationship to pre-stroke cognitive decline. Neurology 2001;57:1216–1222.
18. Snowdon DA, Grenier LH, Mortimer JA, Riley KP, Markesbery WR. Brain infarction and the clinical expression of Alzheimer disease. The Nun study. J Am Med Assoc 1997;277:813–817.
19. Zekry D, Duyckaerts C, Belmin J, et al. The vascular lesions in vascular and mixed dementia: the weight of functional neuroanatomy. Neurobiol Aging 2003;24:213–219.
20. Zekry D, Duyckaerts C, Moulias R, et al. Degenerative and vascular lesions of the brain have synergistic effects in dementia of the elderly. Acta Neuropathol 2002;103:481–487.
21. Zekry D, Hauw J-J, Gold G. Mixed dementia: epidemiology, diagnosis, and treatment. JAGS 2002;50:1431–1438.
22. Goulding JM, Signorini DF, Chatterjee S, et al. Inverse relation between Braak stage and cerebrovascular pathology in Alzheimer predominant dementia. J Neurol Neurosurg Psychiatry 1999;67:654–657.
23. Longstreth WT Jr, Bernick C, Manolio T, et al. Lacunar infarcts defined by magnetic resonance imaging of 3660 elderly people: the Cardiovascular Health Study. Arch Neurol 1998;55:1217–1225.
24. Vermeer SE, Prins ND, den Heijer T, et al. Silent brain infarcts and the risk of dementia and cognitive decline. N Engl J Med 2003;348:1215–1222.
25. Rocca WA, Hofman A, Brayne C, et al. The prevalence of vascular dementia in Europe: facts and fragments from 1980–1990 studies. Ann Neurol 1991;30: 817–824.
26. de la Torre JC. Alzheimer disease as a vascular disorder: nosological evidence. Stroke 2002;33:1152–1162.
27. Nolan KA, Lino MM, Seligmann AW, Blass JP. Absence of vascular dementia in an autopsy series from a dementia clinic. J Am Geriatr Soc 1998;46:567–604.
28. Barclay LL, Weiss EM, Mattis S, Bond O, Blass JP. Unrecognized cognitive impairment in cardiac rehabilitation patients. J Am Geriatr Soc 1988;36:22–28.
29. Abildstrom H, Rasmussen LS, Rentowl P, et al. Cognitive dysfunction 1-2 years after non-cardiac surgery in the elderly: International Study of Post-Operative Cognitive Dysfunction. Acta Anaesthesiol Scand 2000;44:1246–1251.
30. Pullicino P, Mifsud V, Wong E, Graham S, Ali I, Smajlovic D. Hypoperfusion-related cerebral ischemia and cardiac left ventricular systolic dysfunction. J Stroke Cerebrovasc Dis 2001;10:178–182.
31. McKhann GM, Goldsborough MA, Borowicz LM Jr, et al. Cognitive outcome after coronary artery bypass: a one-year prospective study. Ann Thorac Surgery 1997;63:510–515.
32. Newman MF, Kirchner JL, Phillips-Bute B, et al. Longitudinal assessment of neurocognitive function after coronary artery bypass surgery. N Engl J Med 2001;344:395–402.
33. Restrepo L, Wityk RJ, Grega MA, et al. Diffusion- and perfusion-weighted magnetic resonance imaging of the brain before and after coronary artery bypass graft surgery. Stroke 2002;33:2909–2915
34. Alexopoulos GS, Kiosses DN, Klimstra S, Kalayam B, Bruce ML. Clinical presentation of the 'depression-executive dysfunction syndrome' of late life. Am J Geriatr Psychiatry 2002;10:98–106.
35. Pugh KG, Lipsitz LA. The microvascular frontal-subcortical syndrome of aging. Neurobiol Aging 2002;23:421–431.
36. Verghese J, Lipton RB, Hall CB, et al. Abnormal gait as a predictor of non-Alzheimer's dementia. N Engl J Med 2002; 347:1761–1768.
37. Alexander GE, DeLong MR, Strick PL. Parallel organization of functionally segregated circuits linking basal ganglia and cortex. Ann Rev Neurosci 1986;9:137–181.
38. Cummings JL. Frontal-subcortical circuits and human behavior. Arch Neurol 1993;50:873–880.
39. Mega MS, Cummings JL. Frontal-subcortical circuits and neuropsychiatric disorders. J Neuropsychiatry Clin Neurosci 1994;6:358–370.
40. Masterman DL, Cummings JL. Frontal-subcortical circuits: the anatomic basis of executive, social and motivated behaviors. J Psychopharmacol 1997;11:107–114.
41. Fuster JM. Executive frontal functions. Exp Brain Res 2000;133:66–70.
42. Royall DR, Lauterbach EC, Cummings JL, et al., and the Committee on Research of the American Neuropsychiatric Association. Executive Control Function: a review of its promise and challenges to clinical research. J Neuropsy Clin Neurosci 2002;14:377–405.

43. Luria AR. Higher Cortical Functions in Man. New York, NY: Basic Books, 1966.
44. Royall DR, Cordes JA, Polk M. CLOX: an executive drawing task. J Neurol Neurosurg Psychiatry 1998;64:588–594.
45. Reitan RM, Davidson LA. Clinical Neuropsychology: Current Status and Applications. Washington, DC: Hemisphere, 1974.
46. Teng EL, Chui HC. The Modified Mini-Mental State (3MS) examination. J Clin Psychiatry 1987;48:314–318.
47. Teng EL, Hasegawa K, Homma A, et al. The Cognitive Abilities Screening Instrument (CASI): a practical test for cross-cultural epidemiological studies of dementia. Int Psychogeriatr 1994;6:45–56.
48. Román GC. Vascular dementia today. Rev Neurol (Paris) 1999;155(Suppl):S64–S72.
49. Pohjasvaara T, Erkinjuntti T, Vataja R, Kaste M. Dementia three months after stroke. Baseline frequency and effect of different definitions of dementia in the Helsinki Stroke Aging Memory Study (SAM) cohort. Stroke 1997;28:785–792.
50. Tatemichi TK, Desmont DW, Paik M, et al. Clinical determinants of dementia related to stroke. Ann Neurol 1993;33: 568–575.
51. Barba R, Martinez-Espinosa S, Rodriguez-Garcia E, Pondal M, Vivancos J, Del Ser T. Poststroke dementia: clinical features and risk factors. Stroke 2000;31:1494–501.
52. Leys D, Erkinjuntti T, Desmond DW, et al. Vascular dementia: the role of cerebral infarcts. Alzheimer Dis Assoc Disord 1999;13(Suppl):S38–S48.
53. Ferro JM. Hyperacute cognitive stroke syndromes. J Neurol 2001;248:841–849.
54. Román GC, Tatemichi TK, Erkinjuntti T, et al. Vascular dementia: diagnostic criteria for research studies. Report of the NINDS-AIREN International Workshop. Neurology 1993;43: 250–60.
55. Desmond DW. Vascular dementia: a construct in evolution. Cerebrovasc Brain Metab Res 1996;8:296–325.
56. Delay J, Brion S. Les Démences Tardives. Paris, France: Masson et Cie, 1962.
57. Kopelman MD. Disorders of memory. Brain 2002;125:2152–2190.
58. Brandt T, Steinke W, Thie A, Pessin MS. Posterior cerebral artery territory infarcts: clinical features, infarct topography, causes and outcome. Multicenter results and a review of the literature. Cerebrovasc Dis 2000;10:170–82.
59. Servan J, Verstichel P, Catala M, Rancurel G. Syndromes amnésiques et fabulations au cours d'infarctus du territoire de l'artère cérébrale postérieure. Rev Neurol (Paris) 1994;150: 201–208.
60. Swartz RH, Sahlas DJ, Black SE, et al. Strategic involvement of cholinergic pathways and executive dysfunction: does location of white matter signal hyperintensity matter? J Stroke Cerebrovasc Dis 2003;12:29–36.
61. Mann DM, Yates PO, Marcyniuk B. The nucleus basalis of Meynert in multi-infarct (vascular) dementia. Acta Neuropathol (Berl) 1986;71:332–337.
62. Richardson JT. Cognitive performance following rupture and repair of intracranial aneurysms. Acta Neurol Scand 1991;83:110–122.
63. von Cramon DY, Markowitsch HJ. Human memory dysfunctions due to septal lesions. In: Numan R, ed. The behavioral neuroscience of the septal region. New York, NY: Springer, 2000, pp. 380–413.
64. Phillips S, Sangalang V, Sterns G. Basal forebrain infarction. A clinicopathologic correlation. Arch Neurol 1987;44: 1134–1138.
65. Looi JCL, Sachdev PS. Differentiation of vascular dementia from AD on neuropsychological tests. Neurology 1999;53: 670–678.
66. Castaigne P, Buge A, Cambier J, Escourolle R, Brunet P, Degos JD. Démence thalamique d'origine vasculaire par ramollissement bilatéral, limité au territoire du péduncule retromamillaire. A propos de deux observations anatomo-cliniques. Rev Neurol (Paris) 1966;114:89–107.
67. Castaigne P, Lhermitte F, Buge A, et al. Paramedian thalamic and midbrain infarcts: clinical and neuropathological study. Ann Neurol 1981;10:127–148.
68. Katz DI, Alexander MP, Mandell AM. Dementia following strokes in the mesencephalon and diencephalon. Arch Neurol 1987;44:1127–1133.
69. von Cramon DY, Hebel N, Schuri U. A contribution to the anatomical basis of thalamic amnesia. Brain 1985;108:993–1008.
70. Van der Werf Y, Witter MP, Uylings HB, Jolles J. Neuropsychology of infarctions in the thalamus: a review. Neuropsychologia 2000;38:613–627.
71. Ghika-Schimid F, Bogousslavsky J. The acute behavioral syndrome of anterior thalamic infarction: a prospective study of 12 cases. Ann Neurol 2000;48:220–227.
72. Tatemichi TK, Desmont DW, Prohovnik I, et al. Confusion and memory loss from capsular genu infarction: a thalamocortical disconnection syndrome? Neurology 1992;42:1966–1979.
73. Tatemichi TK, Desmont DW, Prohovnik I, et al. Strategic infarcts in vascular dementia. A clinical and imaging experience. Arzneimittel-Forschung/Drug Res 1995;45:371–385.
74. Madureira S, Guerreiro M, Ferro JM. A follow-up study of cognitive impairment due to inferior capsular genu infarction. J Neurol 1999;246:764–769.
75. Pantoni L, Basile AM, Romanelli M, et al. Abulia and cognitive impairment in two patients with capsular genu infarct. Acta Neurol Scand 2001;104:185–190.
76. Ghika J, Bogousslavsky J, Regli F. Infarcts in the territory of the deep perforators from the carotid system. Neurology 1989;39:507–512.

77. Chukwudelunzu FE, Meschia JF, Graff-Radford NR, Lucas JA. Extensive metabolic and neuropsychological abnormalities associated with discrete infarction of the genu of the internal capsule. J Neurol Neurosurg Psychiatry 2001;71: 658–662.
78. Caplan LR, Schmahmann JD, Kase CS, et al. Caudate infarcts. Arch Neurol 1990;47:133–143.
79. Kumral E, Evyapan D, Balkir K. Acute caudate vascular lesions. Stroke 1999;30:100–108.
80. Tournier-Lasserve E, Joutel A, Melki J, et al. Cerebral autosomal dominant arteriopathy with subcortical infarcts and leukoencephalopathy maps to chromosome 19q12. Nat Genet 1993;3:256–259.
81. Joutel A, Vahedi K, Corpechor C, et al. Strong clustering and stereotyped nature of mutations in CADASIL patients. Lancet 1997;350:1511–1515.
82. Dichgans M, Herzog J, Gasser T. *Notch3* mutation involving three cysteine residues in a family with typical CADASIL. Neurology 2001;57:1714–1717.
83. Erkinjuntti T, Inzitari D, Pantoni L, et al. Research criteria for subcortical vascular dementia in clinical trials. J Neural Transmission 2000;59(Suppl):23–30.
84. Fisher CM. Lacunes: small deep cerebral infarcts. *Neurology* 1965;15:774–784.
85. Román GC. Senile dementia of the Binswanger type: a vascular form of dementia in the elderly. JAMA 1987;258: 1782–1788.
86. Román GC. The identity of lacunar dementia and Binswanger disease. Med Hypotheses 1985;16:389–391.
87. Ruchoux MM, Guerouaou D, Vandenhaute B, et al. Systemic vascular smooth muscle impairment in cerebral autosomal dominant arteriopathy with subcortical infarcts and leukoencephalopathy. Acta Neuropathol (Berl) 1995;89:500–512.
88. Joutel A, Favrole P, Labauge P, et al. Skin biopsy immunostaining with a Notch3 monoclonal antibody for CADASIL diagnosis. Lancet 2001;358:2049–2051.
89. Natte R, Maaat-Schieman ML, Haan J, et al. Dementia in hereditary cerebral hemorrhage with amyloidosis-Dutch type is associated with cerebral amyloid angiopathy but is independent of plaques and neurofibrillary tangles. Ann Neurol 2001;50:765–772.
90. Mead S, James-Galton M, Revesz T, et al. Familial British dementia with amyloid angiopathy: early clinical, neuropsychological and imaging findings. Brain 2000;123:975–991.
91. Ghiso J, Revesz T, Holton J, et al. Chromosome 13 dementia syndromes as models of neurodegeneration. Amyloid 2001;8:277–284.
92. Ghiso JA, Holton J, Miravalle L, et al. Systemic amyloid deposits in familial British dementia. J Biol Chem 2001;276: 43,909–43,914.
93. Kramer JH, Reed BR, Mungas D, Weiner MW, Chui HC. Executive dysfunction in subcortical ischaemic vascular disease. J Neurol Neurosurg Psychiatry 2002;72:217–220.
94. Mungas D, Jagust WJ, Reed BR, et al. MRI predictors in subcortical ischemic vascular disease and Alzheimer's disease. Neurology 2001;57:2229–2235.
95. Fein G, Di Sclafani V, Tanabe J, et al. Hippocampal and cortical atrophy predict dementia in subcortical ischemic vascular disease. Neurology 2000;55:1626–1635.
96. Vinters HV, Ellis WG, Zarow C, et al. Neuropathologic substrates of ischemic vascular dementia. J Neuropathol Exper Neurol 2000;59:931–945.
97. Hachinski VC, Iliff LD, Zilkha E, et al. Cerebral blood flow in dementia. Arch Neurol 1975;32:632–637.
98. Moroney JT, Bagiella E, Desmond DW, et al. Meta-analysis of the Hachinski ischemic score in pathologically verified dementias. Neurology 1997;49:1096–1105.
99. Petersen RC, Doody R, Kurz A, et al. Current concepts in mild cognitive impairment. Arch Neurol 2001;58:1985–1992.
100. Skoog I. Status of risk factors for vascular dementia. Neuroepidemiology 1998;17:2–9.

3

The Neuropathologic Substrates of Vascular-Ischemic Dementia

Kurt A. Jellinger

1. INTRODUCTION

1.1. Historical Background and Synonyms

Although Alzheimer's disease (AD) has become widely accepted as the most common cause of dementia in advanced age *(1)*, the role of cerebrovascular disease (CVD) and ischemic brain lesions in cognitive decline remains controversial and confusing *(2–5)*. Until the 1950 and 1960s, dementia in elderly subjects was usually labeled "atherosclerotic dementia," although in 1919, Mingazzini *(6)* stated that this was the result of cerebral infarctions, similar to the concept stressed by Fisher *(7)*. Tomlinson et al. *(8)* described the relationship between the volume of infarcted tissue and cognitive impairment, suggesting that destruction of large volumes of cortex may be necessarily followed by dementia, whereas subtle cerebrovascular lesions (CVLs) may or may not contribute to dementia, probably depending on their location. Hachinsky et al. *(9)* criticized the term "arteriosclerotic dementia" as both inaccurate and misleading and coined the term "multi-infarct dementia" (MID). Because MID constitutes only a small subdivision of all dementias of vascular etiology, the terms "vascular dementia" (VaD) *(4,10–13)*, "cerebrovascular dementia" *(14)*, "dementia associated with stroke" *(15)*, or, more recently, "ischemic-vascular dementia" *(16,17)* "vascular-ischemic dementia" or "vascular cognitive impairment" (ViD) *(18)* were chosen.

Although considerable progress has been made in understanding ViD, many questions remain, particularly regarding what pathologic lesion produces cognitive impairment and by what mechanisms. Many authors consider ViD to be a multifactorial disorder or an ill-defined entity *(19)*, and causal relationships between CVD and dementia are difficult to prove. Even though some authors *(20,21)* provided strong reasons for the use of "vascular cognitive impairment," the term ViD will be used in this chapter. It refers to cognitive dysfunction caused by cerebral lesions secondary to a spectrum of vascular/ischemic pathology.

1.2. Neuropathologic Classification

In contrast to recently refined morphologic criteria for the diagnosis of AD and other degenerative dementias *(22,23)*, no validated neuropathologic criteria have been established for ViD. The California's Alzheimer's Disease Diagnostic and Treatment Centers (ADDTC) *(24)* did not suggest specific details for the postmortem VaD diagnosis but indicated that histopathologic examination of the brain with clinical evidence of dementia was necessary to confirm the presence of multiple infarcts. The National Institute of Neurological Disorders and Stroke-Association Internationale pour la Recherche et l'Enseignement en Neurosciences (NINDS-AIREN) criteria emphasized the hetero-

From: *Current Clinical Neurology*
Vascular Dementia: Cerebrovascular Mechanisms and Clinical Management
Edited by: R. H. Paul, R. Cohen, B. R. Ott, and S. Salloway © Humana Press Inc., Totowa, NJ

geneity of the VaD syndrome and its pathologic subtypes *(25)*. For a diagnosis of "definite" VaD, criteria required that the clinical probability be completed by histopathologic evidence of CVD and absence of AD-type lesions exceeding those expected for age and other conditions causing dementia. Other investigators have emphasized the importance of clinicopathologic correlations *(2,11,24,26)* and the inverse relation between Braak stage and cerebrovascular pathology *(27,28)* or have used variable criteria *(26,29–32)*. Notwithstanding, controversies concerning the validity and liability of diagnostic criteria for ViD continue *(29)*.

Fundamental pathological lesions in ViD consist of atherosclerosis with or without thrombosis/thromboembolism of extracerebral and intracerebral arteries, intracerebral microangiopathies—arteriosclerotic, hyalinotic, inflammatory, and amyloid-related—often combined with systemic factors that may produce small and large infarcts and several forms of white matter degeneration. The extent and location of cerebrovascular lesions (CVLs) and destroyed tissues, which differ considerably from case to case, multiplicity, and bilateral occurrence, are the most important factors underlying cognitive impairment *(3–5,10–20,26,33)*.

One of the most controversial and incompletely understood issues is the degree to which vascular pathology contributes to dementia. Complicating the postmortem ViD diagnosis are other pathologic entities coexisting with vascular lesions that could lead to cognitive decline. Many of these can be found at postmortem examination, particularly in multimorbid elderly subjects. However, it should be emphasized that the presence of CVLs at autopsy does not prove that they cause cognitive decline *(4,12–14,33)*, underscoring that thorough clinicopathologic correlation is essential to establish a definite diagnosis.

Although several class I and II studies that compared clinical diagnosis and neuropathologic findings in reference cohorts, which are similar to population-based studies, reported low sensitivity and specificity for the currently used clinical diagnostic ViD criteria *(12,29,34–39)* with variable interrater reliability *(12,40–42)*. According to recent clinicopathologic studies, The Mayo Clinic criteria (temporal relationship between stroke and dementia or worsening or bilateral infarctions in specified locations) had 75% sensitivity and 81% specificity for pure VaD *(26)*. Because the criteria chosen to diagnose VaD will influence estimates on its incidence and prevalence, as well as its recognition and treatment, new research criteria (e.g., for subcortical VaD) have been proposed *(14,29,43,44)*, and the need for prospective clinicopathologic correlation studies has been emphasized *(45,46)*. These criteria can only be established at autopsy in patients who have been thoroughly and longitudinally evaluated before death and who do not have other causes of dementia. ViD is related to a variety of pathologic lesions *(4,12–14,17–20)*, the clinical significance of which and their relation to AD and other age-related changes of the brain (e.g., subcortical white matter lesions [WMLs]) remain controversial *(10–18,29,34,47–50)*. However, we are not aware of any validation study of the neuropathologic ViD criteria.

1.3. Questionnaire for Vascular Lesions in Routine Pathological Examination

Based on a proposal by Pantoni and others *(13,51)*, a group of international neuroscientists is currently preparing a questionnaire for a standardized examination of CVLs in routine neuropathology programs. On April 4, 2003, this questionnaire (*see* Table 1) has been sent to several investigators throughout the world to prepare a position paper. It is intended to standardize the neuropathologic examination of CVLs and may present a basis for further establishment of standardized morphologic ViD criteria.

1.4. Prevalence and Epidemiology

There is considerable lack of agreement about ViD epidemiology and prevalence. Given the difficulties in diagnosing the disorder *(10,12–20,24,26,34,46)*, epidemiologic studies must be interpreted cautiously. Although ViD previously was considered the second most common type of dementia after AD *(11,52–56)* and is the second leading cause of death worldwide *(57)*, in the Western world it follows AD (60–70%), dementia with Lewy bodies (DLB) (10–25%), and other non-Alzheimer's dementias (8–10%) at place 3 or 4 *(17,58)*. A review of clinical studies showed a frequency of ViD ranging from 4.5% to 39% *(59)*, but in most Western memory clinic-based series, it is diagnosed in no more than 8–10% *(14)*.

Evaluation of 11 pooled European population-based clinical studies of persons over 65 yr of age revealed an age-standardized prevalence of 6.4% for all causes of dementia, 4.4% for AD, and 1.6% for ViD *(60)*; ViD accounted for 15.8% of all dementia cases. In Canadian clinical studies of demented individuals, 12.1% had ViD and 12.8% mixed AD/ViD *(61)*, with an incidence of 6–12 cases per 1000 persons over 70 yr of age *(62)*. In the Finnish "Kuopio 75+ study," ViD accounted for 23% vs 22% for DLB, 47% for AD, and 8% for other dementias in people aged 75 yr or older *(58)*. Even though studies from Japan revealed that the prevalence of ViD was more than double that of AD *(63–67)*, in other reports, AD was two times more frequent than ViD *(68)*. Roman *(57)* recently suggested that ViD may be the most underdiagnosed and underestimated form of dementia in the elderly, because most individuals with dementia after a stroke probably are not included in the data cited *(69)*. This is important because "silent" cerebral infarcts increase with advancing age and are considered a major contributor to the increasing incidence of dementia *(70,71)*. Dementia is common after stroke, occurring in 25 to 30% of patients *(15)*, and cerebral infarctions are associated with a twofold increase in odds of dementia *(72)*.

Therefore, a review of pathologic studies on the prevalence of ViD is difficult, because most studies may contain referral bias because they are weighted with patients from clinical centers, where AD predominates (e.g., in the Consortium to Establish a Registry for Alzheimer's Disease [CERAD] group) *(73,74)*. The divergence in estimates of prevalence *(26,60,70)* and incidence of ViD *(67,75)* suggests that the concept of ViD needs further investigation and validation.

A review of autopsy studies of patients with dementia from 1962 to 1995 revealed an overall mean risk of 17.3% *(4)*, whereas others classified 15–19% as pure VaD *(76)* or showed an even wider range from 0 to 85.2%, with a mean of 17.9%, but reasonable values, based on comparable diagnostic criteria, are between 2 and 11% *(59)*. Reports since 1988 have an overall lower prevalence (mean of 12 studies since 1989 was10.8%) (*see* Table 2). Although several recent studies have reported prevalence rates of 2–9%, others suggest that in very old subjects (85 yr plus), ViD may be more frequent than AD *(77)*. In contrast, among 1929 autopsies of subjects with dementia collected by 10 US centers participating in the CERAD neuropathology program, autopsy revealed CVLs without morphologic features of AD or other disorders in only six cases (0.03%) *(73)*. The Nun study revealed only three pure ViD cases among 118 old-age subjects with dementia (2.5%) at autopsy *(78)*.

For comparison, in recent autopsy series of subjects with dementia from Japanese geriatric hospitals, the incidence rates for AD, ViD, and mixed and other dementias were 34, 35, 11, and 20%, respectively, in one series *(95)* and 47, 22, 6, and 26%, respectively, in the other series *(96)*. A recent community-based population study in England in 209 autopsies of elderly subjects, of whom 48% had dementia, showed CVLs in 78% and AD-pathology in 70%. The proportion of multiple vascular pathology was higher in the group with dementia (46 vs 33%), indicating that most patients had mixed disease *(97)*. In a personal consecutive autopsy series of 1000 aged individuals with dementia in Vienna, Austria, ViD was seen in 8.5% but in only 2.8% of 600 patients with the clinical diagnosis of probable AD. Alzheimer-type pathology was present in 83.5 and 91.7%, respectively, but "pure" AD in only 40 and 47%, respectively, whereas the other brains showed different coexisting pathologies (Lewy bodies, CVDs, etc.); 4.5 to 7% had dementia disorders of other etiologies (neurodegenerations, prion diseases, tumors, etc.) *(17,18)*. The prevalence of CVLs in a large series of autopsy-proven AD cases was significantly higher than in age-matched controls (48.1 vs 32.6%, $p < 0.01$), with minor to moderate CVLs (lacunes and cerebral amyloid angiopathy [CAA] with and without vascular lesions) in 31.9 vs 27.1%. Severe vascular pathology (old and recent infarcts or hemorrhages) in AD was also significantly higher than in controls (16.0 vs 5.5%; $p < 0.01$) *(98)*.

Table 1
Questionnaire for Vascular Lesions in Routine Pathological Examination

VASCULAR LESIONS IN ROUTINE PATHOLOGICAL EXAMINATION
FORM

General issues

In your center, is the neuropathological examination performed by one person or by several individuals?
One □ Several (please, list how many) □ ______________

Is your center involved in specific research studies leading to the fact that some cases are differently processed?
yes □ no □

Examination of large vessels and other organs

On a routine basis, do you examine?

carotid arteries in the neck yes □ no □
if yes, **do you quantitate the extent of the lesions?** yes □ no □

vertebral arteries in the neck yes □ no □
if yes, **do you quantitate the extent of the lesions?** yes □ no □

Willis circle vessels yes □ no □
if yes, **do you quantitate the extent of the lesions?** yes □ no □

heart yes □ no □

kidneys yes □ no □

Brain cutting, sampling, and examination of slices

Do you slice the entire brain? yes □ no □

Do you use only one half of the brain (the other half being frozen or something else)?
yes □ no □

How do you cut the brain? Coronal □ Transverse □ Saggital □

Where do you sample for microscopic examination (tick more than 1 if needed)?
□ Middle frontal gyrus
□ Superior and middle temporal gyri
□ Inferior parietal lobule
□ Occipital cortex
□ Hippocampus with entorhinal cortex
□ White matter
If yes, from what structures (please, specify, e.g. subcortical white matter, internal capsule, corpus callosum, etc.)?
____
□ Basal ganglia
□ Thalami
□ Cerebellar hemisphere incl. the dentate nucleus
□ Midbrain including substantia nigra
□ Pons
□ Medulla oblongata
□ Basal structures including the nucleus of Meynert
□ Any lesion (if exists)

Do you examine the presence of lesions in the fresh brain? yes □ no □
or **in stained coronal sections only?** yes □ no □

Continued on next page

Histology assessment: staining

Do you stain? coronal sections ☐
whole hemibrain ☐
entire lobes ☐
small blocks only☐

Do you apply on a routine basis staining for the myelin? yes ☐ no ☐
If yes, please specify which: ....

Do you apply on a routine basis staining for the nerve fibers? yes ☐ no ☐
If yes, please specify which: ....

Do you apply on a routine base silver staining? yes ☐ no ☐
If yes, please specify which: ....

Do you apply on a routine basis immunohistochemical methods for gliosis (e.g., GFAP)? yes ☐ no ☐
If yes, please specify which: ....

Histological evaluation

Parenchyma alterations

Which of these lesions do you consider as "vascular" (tick more than 1 if needed)?

☐ Cerebral infarcts [including territorial; superficial borderzone (cortico-subcortical at the border ACA-MCA or MCA-PCA; deep borderzone (watershed) infarcts]
☐ Lacunar infarcts
☐ Cortical micro-infarcts associated with amyloid angiopathy
☐ Multiple large infarcts associated with amyloid angiopathy
☐ Enlarged perivascular spaces (including cribriform state)
☐ White matter rarefaction (any degree)
☐ White matter rarefaction (only of a certain severity, please specify the degree) ______________________________
☐ A ventricular enlargement associated with white matter atrophy
☐ Hippocampal sclerosis
☐ Cortical granular atrophy
☐ Laminar necrosis of the cortex
☐ Incomplete grey matter infarction (defined as selective neuronal necrosis, i.e., irreversible neuronal damage limited to specific cellular types)

Comments:

....

How do you define a lacunar infarct?

Any infarct with ∅ < 15 mm? yes ☐ no ☐

Any infarct with ∅ < 15 mm located in basal ganglia, thalamus, pons, hemispheric white matter?
yes ☐ no ☐

Any infarct with ∅ < 15 mm associated with arteriolosclerosis? yes ☐ no ☐

How do you define an enlarged perivascular space? (open question)

Continued on next page

Do you make a distinction between lacunar infarcts and micro-infarcts? yes ☐ no ☐
If yes, how? (open question): ....

In case of brain infarcts, do you record?
the bilaterality? yes ☐ no ☐
the location? yes ☐ no ☐
the total volume of the lesions? yes ☐ no ☐
the multiplicity? yes ☐ no ☐

On a routine basis, do you look for the presence of incomplete grey matter infarction? yes ☐ no ☐
If yes, **how do you define incomplete gray matter infarction?** (open question): ....

How do you define the rarefaction of white matter? (multiple choices allowed)
Paler appearance in comparison with white matter considered as normal? yes ☐ no ☐
A looser appearance of myelinated fibers? yes ☐ no ☐
White matter with decreased number of oligodendrocytes? yes ☐ no ☐
White matter with axonal loss? yes ☐ no ☐
Gliosis of the white matter? yes ☐ no ☐
Combination of the above (please, specify): ....

Do you quantitate the severity of white matter changes? yes ☐ no ☐
If yes, by what scale or method (please, give details): ....

Do you consider a diagnosis of Wallerian degeneration? yes ☐ no ☐
If yes, how do you define from the histological viewpoint Wallerian degeneration and how do you differentiate it from "vascular rarefaction" (i.e., related to angiopathy) of white matter (open questions)? ....

On a routine basis, do you evaluate the presence of gliosis
in the white matter? yes ☐ no ☐
in the gray matter? yes ☐ no ☐
everywhere? yes ☐ no ☐

If yes, **do you quantitate it?** yes ☐ no ☐
If yes, **please specify by what method** (open question): ....

Small vessel disease

What do you mean for small vessels?
All the vessels with ∅ < 500 μ yes ☐ no ☐
All the vessels with a ∅ < of a certain amount yes ☐ no ☐
If yes, please, specify the ∅: ......
Only arterioles yes ☐ no ☐
All the vessels deeper than cortex yes ☐ no ☐
Other (please, specify): ______________________________

Do you examine small vessel appearance on a routine basis? yes ☐ no ☐
If yes, **in what regions?**
Cortex yes ☐ no ☐ in how many samples? _____
white matter yes ☐ no ☐ in how many samples? _____
basal ganglia yes ☐ no ☐
thalami yes ☐ no ☐
brainstem yes ☐ no ☐

If yes, **by applying what staining** (multiple choice allowed)?
H&E yes ☐ no ☐
Masson's trichrome yes ☐ no ☐
Van Gieson's elastica yes ☐ no ☐
Other (please specify): ____________________

Continued on next page

What do you consider as small vessel disease?

- Hyaline degeneration of tunica media ☐
- Loss of smooth muscle cells in the tunica media ☐
- Thickening of vessel wall and lumen narrowing ☐
- Lypohyalinosis ☐
- Necrotic aspects in the vessel wall ☐
- Combination of the above (please, specify) ☐

On a routine basis, do you assess mean vessel density per unit area? yes ☐ no ☐

Do you look for amyloid angiopathy on a routine basis?

- ☐ yes, in all autopsy cases
- ☐ yes, but only in patients with a history of cognitive decline
- ☐ Only if suggested on inspection of H&E stained sections
- ☐ no

If yes, **by what method?**

H&E	yes ☐	no ☐
Congo red	yes ☐	no ☐
Thioflavine S	yes ☐	no ☐
Beta amyloid antibodies	yes ☐	no ☐
Other (please, specify): ______________		

If yes, **do you quantitate it?** yes ☐ no ☐

If yes, **by what method?** (please, specify): ________________

If yes, **in what brain regions?** (please, specify): ________________

On a routine basis, do you look for inflammatory aspects of small vessels (e.g., leukocyte and/or macrophage infiltration, necrotic aspects, granulomata?) yes ☐ no ☐

<u>Interpretation of findings</u>

When do you consider a patient as having vascular alterations in the brain?

When he/she has any amount of any the above reported lesions (either affecting the parenchyma or the vessels)
yes ☐ no ☐

When he/she has a certain amount of any of the above reported lesions (either affecting the parenchyma or the vessels) yes ☐ no ☐ please, try to specify a "certain amount" ....

Only in the case he/she has lesions affecting the parenchyma
yes ☐ no ☐

In what cases do you consider that the cognitive deterioration was <u>exclusively</u> caused by a vascular process (please, specify)? ....

In what cases do you consider that the cognitive deterioration was <u>primarily</u> caused by a vascular process (please, specify)? ....

In what cases do you consider that the cognitive deterioration was caused by a vascular process <u>in combination with other causes</u> (please, specify)? ....

What criteria do you use on a routine basis for the pathological diagnosis of Alzheimer's disease?

CERAD	☐	Braak & Braak	☐
Kachaturian	☐	Other (please, specify)	☐ ....

What criteria do you use on a routine basis for the pathological diagnosis of fronto-temporal dementia? (please, specify)

What criteria do you use on a routine basis for the pathological diagnosis of Lewy body dementia? (please, specify)

Table 2
Autopsy Series Showing Prevalence of ViD (Compliment to ref. 4)

Year	Location	Authors	No. of cases	ViD	%
1962	England	Corsellis *(79)*	167	46	27
1970	England	Tomlinson et al. *(8)*	50	9	18
1972	United States	Birkett *(80)*	24	14	58
1975	Switzerland	Todorov et al. *(81)*	776	132	22
1977	Sweden	Sourander et al. *(82)*	258	72	28
1982	Belgium	De Reuck et al. *(83)*	312	21	6.7
1985	Finland	Mölsä et al. *(84)*	58	11	19
1986	Switzerland	Ulrich et al. *(32)*	54	9	17
1987	Sweden	Alafuzoff et al. *(85)*	74	13	17.6
1987	Canada	Wade et al. *(86)*	65	6	9
1988	United States	Joachim et al. *(87)*	150	3	2
1988	Finland	Erkinjuntti et al. *(30)*	27	23	85.2
1989	United States	Boller et al. *(88)*	54	4	7
1990	Spain	Jellinger et al. *(31)*	675	106	16
1990	Austria	Del Ser et al. *(89)*	40	28	70
1994	Sweden	Brun *(90)*	175	59	34
1995	Norway	Ince et al. *(91)*	69	4	5
1995	United States	Markesbery *(4)*	557	13	2
1997	United States (CERAD)	Hulette et al. *(73)*	1929	6	0.03
1997	Canada	Bowler et al. *(92)*	122	4/5 [a]	3/4 [a]
1998	Different countries (1962–1995)	Markesbery *(4)*	?	?	11.3
1999	United States (Nun study)	Snowdon and Markesbery *(93)*	118	3	1.3
1999	United States	Nolan et al. *(94)*	87	0	0
1999	Japan	Seno et al. *(95)*	122	42	35
2001	Japan	Akatsu et al. *(96)*	270	60	22
2003	Rochester, MN, US	Knopman et al. *(26)*	89	12	13
2003	Austria	Jellinger (dementias/probable AD)	1000/600	85/17	8.5/2.8

[a] Reexamination.

Abbr: ViD, vascular-ischemic dementia; CERAD, Consortium to Establish a Registry for Alzheimer's Disease; AD, Alzheimer's disease.

2. MAJOR CEREBROVASCULAR LESIONS ASSOCIATED WITH ViD

The major CVD subtypes in VaD have been summarized by Romano in the previous chapter and by others *(2,4,10,11,13,16–18,33,69,99)*. Although causal relationships between certain CVLs and dementia evade strict classifications *(2,15,18,29,49)* and no classification of brain lesions causing cognitive impairment is ideal, the major CVLs associated with cognitive impairment are summarized in Tables 3 and 4.

2.1. *Classical Multiinfarct Encephalopathy (MIE)/Large Vessel Disease*

Single or multiple infarctions involving the areas of major cerebral arteries commonly result from atherosclerosis affecting intracranial or extracranial blood vessels, giving rise to local thromboembolism or hypoperfusion. These infarcts may be large, involving much of a cerebral hemisphere, or may be multiple small lesions in the cortex and/or adjacent white matter, mainly in the medial cerebral artery (MCA) territories and less frequently in other supply areas, involving the left or both hemispheres *(10,11,56,72,99)*. Stroke patients with dementia had infarcts in the left that were eight times larger than those in the right hemisphere, with a strong correlation between dementia and infarctions in the left posterior cerebral artery (PCA), anterior cerebral artery (ACA), and

Table 3
Major Morphological Types of Vascular Dementia

1. Classical multiinfarct encephalopathy (MIE) Multiple large (sub/territorial) infarcts in cortex and white matter/basal ganglia in territories of large cerebral arteries, MCA, MCA plus PCA; involving left or both hemispheres
2. Strategic infarct dementia (SID) Small or medium-sized infarcts/ischemic scars in functionally important brain regions: thalamus; hippocampus (PCA), basal forebrain angular gyrus (ACA), bilaterally or dominant hemispheres
3. Microangiopathic (small vessel infarct) dementia (SMVA)
   a. Subcortical arteriosclerotic leukoencephalopathy Binswanger (SAE) Multiple small infarcts in basal ganglia plus white matter with preservation of cortex
   b. Multilacunar state Multiple microinfarcts (scars up to 1.5 cm Ø); basal ganglia, hemispheral white matter, pontine basis Multiple cortico-subcortical microinfarctions (mixed encephalopathies)
   c. Granular cortical atrophy Multiple small scars within border zones ACA MCA in one/both hemispheres
4. Subcortical microvascular leukoencephalopathy (acquired/genetically determined)
5. Gliosis or hippocampal sclerosis
6. Inflammatory angiopathy and other mechanisms

Abbr: MCA, middle cerebral artery; PCA, posterior cerebral artery; ACA, anterior cerebral artery.
Modified from refs. *2,25,55.*

Table 4
Dementia Associated With Cerebrovascular Disease

A. Multifocal/diffuse disease
   1. Multiple atherosclerotic/watershed infarcts (large artery/border zone territories)
   2. Anti-PL-related ischemia
   3. "Granular atrophy" of cortex (multifocal cortical microinfarcts)
   4. Multiple lacunar infarcts (resulting from microvascular disease or microatheroma)
   5. Binswanger subcortical leukoencephalopathy (BSLE) [? linked to #4]
   6. CADASIL
   7. Angiitis (PCNSA, granulomatous angiitis; some cases linked to CAA)
   8. Cerebral amyloid angiopathy (CAA) plus/minus infarcts, hemorrhages (AD variant?)—Familial forms, including Dutch, Icelandic, British
   9. Miscellaneous angiopathies (FMD, Moyamoya)
   10. Cortical laminar necrosis (post-cardiac arrest, hypotension)
   11. Extreme dilatation/enlargement of brain parenchymal perivascular spaces
B. Focal disease/strategically placed infarcts
   1. Mesial temporal (including hippocampal) infarcts/ischemia/sclerosis
   2. Caudate and thalamic infarcts (especially DM nucleus, bilateral damage)
   3. Fronto-cingulate infarcts (ACA territory)
   4. Angular gyrus infarct (dominant cerebral hemisphere)

Abbr: ACA, anterior cerebral artery; Anti-PL, anti-phospholipid; CADASIL, cerebral autosomal dominant arteriopathy with subcortical infarcts and leukoencephalopathy; DM, dorsomedial; FMD, fibromuscular dysplasia; PCNSA, primary angiitis/arteritis of the central nervous system.
From ref. *16.*

parietal areas *(100)*. In addition, cardiac disorders, such as atrial fibrillation and myocardial infarction (MI), provide a source for cerebral emboli, whereas most other causes, such as hematological conditions, inflammatory angiopathies, Sneddon's disease *(101)*, and familial CVD (e.g., cerebral autosomal dominant arteriopathy with subcortical infarcts and leukoencephalopathy [CADASIL] or cerebral amyloid angiopathy [CAA]), usually cause multiple subcortical and/or cortical vascular lesions (*see* Chapter 6).

2.2. *Microangiopathic Small Vessel Infarct Lesions*

The most prominent features of small vessel infarct lesions (SMVAs) are lacunar infarcts that Pierre Marie *(102)* already described as small miliary softenings, from 0.5 to 1.5 cm or less in diameter, or small cavitations that may have more than one pathologic substrate, the most significant representing small infarcts and, less frequently, healed or reabsorbed tiny hemorrhages *(2,103)*.

Their most common sites are the periventricular white matter around the lateral ventricles, basal ganglia, thalamus, internal capsule, pons, and cerebellar white matter *(104,105)*. A neuropathologic classification that remains useful *(106,107)* distinguishes lacunes as follows: Type I lacunes as irregular cavities containing lipid-laden macrophages and blood vessels surrounded by a rim of gliotic, rarified brain. They represent small foci of ischemic necrosis resulting from narrowing or occlusion of short penetrating arteries branching directly from larger cerebral arteries. This type of lacune is the most significant and has been reported in 6–11% of selected brain autopsy series *(103,108)*. A variant type—incomplete lacunar infarct—characterized by loss of only selectively vulnerable cellular elements without cavitation, suggests a common underlying cause (i.e., arterial obstruction) but perhaps of shorter duration or lesser severity *(109)*, or it may represent the sequelae of edema or edema-related gliosis *(110)*. Type II lacunes are smaller in size and distribution and contain numerous hemosiderin-laden macrophages, representing old, small hemorrhages or old hemorrhagic microinfarcts resulting from fibrinoid vascular necrosis, but are rare *(111,112)*. Type III lacunes are dilatations of perivascular spaces surrounded by a single layer of epithelial-like cells and by compressed or mildly gliotic brain, often with corpora amylacea. They usually contain one or more segments of a normal artery and have been ascribed variously to small vessel wall permeability, interstitial fluid drainage disorders *(113,114)*, cerebral atrophy, mechanical stress from pulsating arterioles *(115)*, perivascular inflammation, or other nonspecific factors.

Roman *(116)* found lacunar infarcts in 36% of the patients studied, whereas a recent Japanese ViD study reported multiple lacunar infarcts in 42% of the patients studied, representing the most frequent type of CVLs *(66)*. In a personal study of 750 autopsy-proved AD brains and 562 age-matched controls, lacunar lesions were found in 32 vs 27% *(98)*.

The majority of lacunes, as found by the meticulous work of Fisher *(103,104)*, are caused by intracranial atherosclerosis, "lipohyalinosis," or segmental fibrinoid necrosis affecting small arteries, with subsequent occlusion of single deep perforating vessels, whereas in one-fifth of patients, no thrombosis can be found. However, most perforating branches have multiple stenoses and poststenotic dilatations, suggesting that hemodynamic events might also play a role in the pathogenesis of lacunar state *(117)*. These lesions are usually caused by hypertension, diabetes mellitus, etc. Other mechanisms are cerebral microembolism of vascular or cardiac origin, such as atrial fibrillation *(2,14,69)*, CADASIL, or inflammatory angiopathies. The type of vascular lesions underlying lacunes and their causes have been recently reviewed *(111,112,118)*. According to the predominant location of SMVA, the following types of ViD can be distinguished.

2.2.1. *Strategic Infarct Dementia (SID)*

Infarcts or ischemic scars, often involving isolated strategically important brain regions, despite relatively small losses of cerebral parenchyma, may cause mental deterioration, culminating in dementia. Such strategic areas include the following: *(2,4,10,16,18)*.

1. *Watershed Infarcts*: Watershed infarcts in circulatory border zones between the deep or superficial branches of ACA, MCA, and PCA may result from hypotension with "misery perfusion" or showers of microemboli, causing laminar necrosis between small superficial branches of the ACA and ACM or in bilateral hippocampal or thalamic softening *(2,4,10,16–18)*. These infarcts usually occur in patients with extracranial carotid stenosis or occlusion and are often associated with decrease in blood pressure *(119)*.
2. *Angular Gyrus*: Angular gyrus are present in the supply area of the ACA of the dominant hemisphere or bilaterally *(120)*.

3. *Frontocingulate Infarcts*: Frontocingulate infarcts involve the orbital and medial frontal cortex, the territory of frontopolar and callosal marginal arteries *(121)*.
4. *Dorsal-Paramedian, Dorsomedial, and Polar Areas of the Thalamus*: Dorsal-paramedian, dorsomedial, and polar areas of thalamus are unilateral and often bilateral lesions resulting from occlusion of the thalamoperforate artery *(122–124)*.
5. *Mesial Temporal Area of the Hippocampus*: Bilateral infarcts in these areas result from circulation disorders in the supply area of the PCA *(4,18,121,125–127)*.
6. *Caudate Nucleus*: Caudate nucleus lesions result from obstruction of the lateral lenticulostriate arteries and may include the anterior portion of putamen and anterior limb of internal capsule *(128)*.
   Strategically situated small lesions that may represent a mixture of large and small vessel disease rather than an isolated entity, may destruct thalamocortical and striatocortical pathways involving cognition, memory, and behavior *(2,4,10,99,112,119–129)*, but their relative contribution to the severity of dementia is poorly understood.

2.2.2. White Matter Lesions

Recent studies have placed emphasis on deep white matter lesions (WMLs) and their relation to CVD and ViD.

2.2.2.1. Pathology of White Matter Lesions

For this type of lesions that has been increasingly detected *intra vitam* by modern neuroimaging methods *(130–134)*, synonyms include subcortical arteriosclerosis (leuko)encephalopathy or Binswanger's disease *(135)*, diffuse white matter disease, WMLs, leukoariosis *(136)*, periventricular arteriosclerotic leukoencephalopathy or leukomalacia, (progressive) subcortical vascular encephalopathy, and periventricular lucency *(134)*.

Using computed cranial tomography (CCT) and magnetic resonance imaging (MRI), WMLs have been found in 22% of patients under age 40 and in 27–60% of subjects over 65 yr of age *(130)*, whereas in patients with AD and ViD, they are detected by MRI in nearly 100% of patients *(131)* and enable the diagnosis of ViD with a sensitivity of 88% and a specificity of approximately 95% *(133)*. The true meaning of these lesions is controversial, and WMLs can be found in normal-aged individuals and in individuals with AD, ViD, multiple sclerosis, posttraumatic encephalopathies, obstructive and communicating hydrocephalus, progressive multifocal leukoencephalopathy, lymphoma, tumor edema, HIV encephalopathy, leukodystrophies, or other metabolic disorders *(134)*.

The neuropathologic lesions underlying radiologically observed WMLs include several morphologic alterations *(130–134)*. In general, a morphologic triad of demyelination, axonal loss, and lacunar infarcts are found mainly in the frontal, parietal, and occipital white matter of the centrum semiovale. Myelin degeneration usually has a patchy confluent form sparing the subcortical U-fibers. There may be multiple, often asymmetrical, cavitary or noncavitary infarctions or areas of incomplete infarction with vacuolation; loss or pallor of myelin, axon, and oligodendroglia; reactive astrocytosis; and sparse macrophage reaction. Silver stains demonstrate that myelin pallor is secondary to fiber loss. Lacunes are often scattered in the hemispheric white matter, at the centers of areas of pallor. Vascular abnormalities include atherosclerosis of the large arterioles on the base and convexity of the brain, and several types of microangiopathy of the penetrating arteries, with thickened fibrotic or hyalinized arterioles in white matter and deep grey matter with or without occlusions *(16,50,128,132,134,137–143)*. Microangiopathy with focal fibrinoid necrosis of vascular walls is found in the penetrating arterioles of cortex and deep gray matter, associated with small infarcts, microaneurysms, and fibrotic or thrombotic vessel occlusion. Other lesions may include small arteriovenous malformations, isolated central white matter infarcts, small foci of gliosis, dilated perivascular spaces, vascular ectasia *(134)*, or microvascular convolute formations *(143)*. Punctate hyperintensive lesions on MRI, corresponding to dilated perivascular spaces, are to be distinguished from extensive WMLs, the histologic correlate of which are confluent patches of white matter pallor without cavitation *(132)*. Under high-power histology, these areas show vacuolation and decreased numbers of oligodendroglia. Perivascular vacuolation may represent an early stage of these changes. Comparative studies of postmortem MRI and histology showed that periventricular lesions on MRI correlated well with the severity of demyelination and astrogliosis, which are often associated with small lacunar infarcts in both the white matter and the basal ganglia *(132,144,145)*. Pathologic studies have shown a close association between diffuse WMLs and lacunes *(89,134,137,139)*, suggesting a common pathophysiology, particularly arteriosclerosis of the penetrating arteries. Erkinjuntti et al. *(44)* suggested a subclassification of subcortical ViD in which lacunar infarcts and ischemic WMLs related to small vessel disease are the major pathologic features. Correlative positron emission tomography (PET) and MRI studies showed that in patients without cortical infarctions, anterior periventricular hyperintensities reduced ipsilateral metabolic function *(44)*.

2.2.2.2. Pathogenetic Features of White Matter Lesions

The suggestion that WML pathogenesis is a chronic ischemic disorder of heterogenous pathophysiology and causes, with hypoperfusion of the penetrating arteries supplying the deep white matter resulting from hypotension and narrowing of arterioles rather than by occlusion of the arterioles *(90)*, was recently confirmed by experimental studies *(146,147)*.

Structural changes of small intraparenchymal cerebral arteries and arterioles related to hypertension and other stroke risk factors, altered cerebral blood flow (CBF) autoregulation, and the conditions created by the unique arterial blood supply of the hemispheral white matter contribute to WML development *(142)*. Prospective MRI studies showed increased rates of subcortical and periventricular WMLs in subjects with hypertension. This relationship was influenced by age and duration of hypertension, whereas treatment of hypertension may reduce the risk of both lesion types *(131)*. WMLs are associated with reduced white matter CBF, although their severity correlated better with the reduction in regional CBF in the cortex *(148)*. Others reported impaired vasodilatatory capacity in the deep white matter *(149,150)*. PET studies demonstrated that periventricular and deep white matter hyperintensities and lacunar infarcts in basal ganglia and thalamus correlated with both a decline in mean global cortical metabolism and lowered cognitive function *(151)*. The cortical global metabolic rates were lower in patients with subcortical strokes and cognitive impairment than in those without dementia *(152)*, whereas others stressed the heterogeneity of CBF in ViD *(153,154)*.

A striking feature of WMLs is that the changes spare the subcortical U-fibers, which may be related to the specific pattern of vascular supply. The periventricular regions and central white matter are supplied by long penetrating arteries coming from the pial vessels on the surface of the cortex, whereas the peripheral parts of the centrum semiovale are supplied from penetrating vessels from the cortical surface. Periventricular border/watershed zones between the long ventriculoseptal and ventriculofugal branches of the choroid and lateral striatal arteries *(155)*, resulting from lowered perfusion pressure, are particularly vulnerable to hypotensive episodes *(156)*. This concept has recently been rejected by those who believe that the ventriculofugal branches are veins rather than arteries *(157)*.

The distribution of WMLs with conspicuous sparing of the subcortical U-fibers also points to the pattern of cerebral edema *(158)*. The histologic findings—spongiosis and loss of oligodendrocytes—which are also comparable to edema induced by ischemia and other mechanisms, were confirmed by experimental studies *(159)*. Diffuse extravasation of serum proteins throughout the white matter owing to enhanced pinocytotic activity by endothelial cells is observed without accompanying infarction in the stroke-prone spontaneously hypertensive rat. Extravasated serum proteins diffuse over large areas of the white matter. Even a brief opening of the blood-brain barrier (BBB) may result in the persistent presence of serum proteins in the white matter, including fibronectin and fibrinogen, which are capable of exerting biologic effects *(160)*. The edema hypothesis is consistent with the clinical observation that patients with Binswanger's disease deteriorate during periods of sustained hypertension *(141)*.

Selective infarction in periventricular border zones in patients with carotid stenosis and superimposed hemodynamic failure *(161)* and ischemic leukoencephalopathies, irrespective of the cause (e.g., CO intoxication, acute hypoxia, arteriovenous [AV] malformations, delayed radiation encephalopathy, CAA, and CADASIL *[161–165]*), share widespread demyelination of the deep white matter and selective necrosis of the periventricular regions, sparing the cerebral cortex and U-fibers. In AD, WMLs do not always parallel the severity of AD-related gray matter pathology and, thus, may be caused by various factors *(48)*. In contrast to meningeal and cortical arteries, CAA in white matter is rare, whereas fibrohyalinosis of the white matter arteries is closely correlated with WMLs in AD, indicating their etiologic heterogeneity *(166)*.

The molecular mechanisms of subcortical vascular WMLs concern a higher susceptibility of white matter axons to the effects of abnormal influxes of calcium that travel through several routes, including reverse Na^+–Ca^{2+} exchange triggered by persistent Na^+ channels and by a parallel pathway involving Ca^{2+} channels. Oligodendrocytes and/or myelin sheaths are more vulnerable to glutamate-triggered injury, resulting from reverse Na^+-dependent glutamate transport. Some of the steps involved in these destructive events are subject to modifications by neurotransmitters, such as γ-aminobutyric acid (GABA), and by neuromodulators, such as adenosine *(167)*. Recent demonstration of increased apoptosis of oligodendrocytes has been proposed as a major histologic correlate of WMLs *(167a)*.

2.2.2.3. Subcortical Arteriosclerotic (Leuko)Encephalopathy

Binswanger's disease *(135)* has been the subject of much controversy and reassessment, and some authors concluded that it should not be considered a distinct entity *(4,128,142,168–170)*. In addition to the histologic lesions described, there may be many microbleeds *(168)*. Activated microglia is 3.1 times more immunoreactive for major histocompatability complex (MHC) class II antigen *(171,172)*. The number of oligodendrocytes in the deep white matter is reduced by approximately 50% *(173)*, indicating that loss of oligodendroglia may be involved in the reduction of nerve fibers. Cortical and/or white matter reactive astrocytosis and fibrillary gliosis are common *(171)*. The numbers of astrocytes with light metallothionein (MT) I-II immunoreactivity in the deep white matter are reduced in contrast to normal numbers of astrocytes with strong immunoreactivity for glial fibrillary acifd protein (GFAP) and MT-I-II in subcortical white matter and cortex, suggesting topographic and biochemical differences in their dynamic plasticity. MT expression is to regeneration, repair, and/or reaction to neural lesions, with metal ion metabolic processing, buffering, and detoxification or neuroprotection against free radicals *(174)*. In SAE pathogenesis, arteriosclerotic ischemia and, alternatively, recurrent edema resulting from severe disturbances of the BBB have been discussed *(139)*, but its exact etiology is unclear. It has been suggested that SAE represents an end-stage pathology of lacunar state *(26)*.

The exact pathologic substrate of dementia to be associated with WMLs remains uncertain. Although periventricular WMLs predict the rate of cognitive decline *(130)*, they are often associated with decline in executive functioning and visual memory, even in patients without dementia *(175)*. Synaptophysin immunoreactivity of the neuropil as a measure of synapse density in the cortex in SAE was almost as severely reduced as in AD, suggesting that the loss of synapses is a factor of dementia *(143,176)*. Although some authors have suggested that cognitive impairment associated with subcortical ischemic vascular disease is particularly the result of associated hippocampal and cortical changes *(177,178)*, others showed significant correlation between WML scores of the right frontal regions *(133)* and dementia.

2.3. *Multilacunar State*

The pathologic changes of lacunar state, in basal ganglia, thalamus, hemispheral white matter, and brainstem, have been reviewed *(111,112,179,180)*. People with dementia are more likely to have such lesions than patients without dementia. The pattern of cognitive impairment is consistent with models of disturbances of subcortical neuronal circuits *(175)*.

2.4. Hypoperfusion in "Border Zones" and Granular Cortical Atrophy

Hypoperfusion leads to diminished flow or stagnation of flow in distal vessels. It results in laminar necrosis of the cortex, multiple cortical and subcortical microinfarcts, or incomplete infarction of the white matter. Size and extent of these "watershed" or "border zone" infarcts in the end-field territories of the distal branches of cerebral arteries depend on the amount of leptomeningeal anastomoses between the main cerebral arteries *(181)* and the degree of arteriosclerotic stenosis of meningeal arterial branches. The superior frontal area, between the distal supply of the ACA and MCA, and the posterior parietooccipital junction, among ACA, MCA, and PCA, are involved more often. Hypoxia also causes alterations in the hippocampal sectors CA 1 and CA 4, the outer half of the caudate nucleus and putamen, and the anterior and dorsomedial nucleus of the thalamus. Bilateral internal carotid artery occlusive disease causing such lesions is frequently associated with impaired intellectual function *(182)*.

Granular cortical atrophy, which is characterized by multiple small cortical microinfarcts and scars most often in the boundary zone between ACA and MCA in one or both hemispheres, is usually caused by hypoperfusion owing to stenosis of the internal carotid arteries, cerebral microembolism to the cortex *(183)*, or CAA, but they are a rare cause of dementia *(4)*.

2.4.1. Mixed Cortico-Subcortical Encephalopathies

In some cases, multiple cortical and subcortical microinfarcts may occur, resulting from several of the reasons listed, and may be associated with ViD (*see* Table 5).

2.5. Postischemic Encephalopathy

The sequelae of local or diffuse hypoxia and ischemia resulting from different causes can be separated into three major groups according to their predominant distribution pattern.

2.5.1. Cortical Laminar Necrosis

Damage to the cerebral cortex with laminar necroses and their sequelae may arise from cardiac or respiratory arrest (hypotension, anesthesia accidents, cardiac, and/or respiratory failure). They are often associated with diffuse white matter damage and cerebellar atrophy.

2.5.2. Multiple Postischemic Lesions

These occur in case of dramatic systemic blood flow failure, combined with focal narrowing of large and small brain-feeding vessels, leading to disseminated or systemic postischemic lesions in the cortex, subcortical white matter, and basal ganglia.

2.5.3. Hippocampal Sclerosis

This specific form of ViD related to age-associated microcirculation disorders and hypoperfusion has been detected in 8–25% of very old subjects with dementia (>65 and often >89 yr of age) in some series *(77,184–186)*. Damage to the hippocampus ranges from selective neuronal loss and gliosis to frank infarction. It is often accompanied by multiple small infarcts in other brain regions, leukoencephalopathy, or both, whereas severe Alzheimer-type pathology is rare. Cognitive decline is often featured by marked memory impairment. It has been occasionally observed in elderly individuals after receiving general anesthesia. Age-associated and other disease-related processes, such as atherosclerosis and arteriosclerosis, explain why the elderly cannot tolerate hypoperfusion like younger adults.

Table 5
Types of Brain Injury in Ischemic-Vascular Encephalopathy

Category	MMSE (mean)	*N* patients (female/male)	Mean age	Cystic infarcts (mean age)	Lacunes (mean age)	Microinfarcts (mean age)	Hippocampal sclerosis
Dementia	10 ± 4	91 (37/54)	81.3	27 (80.3)	52 (80.5)[a]	8 (82.1)[b]	4 (84.5)[c]
Cognitively impaired	approximately 20	19 (7/12)	79.6	6 (86.0)[d]	11 (77.0)	2 (76.5)	—
Cognitively normal	>20	20 (11/9)	83.0	13 (79.4)	6 (81.6)	1 (88.0)	—
Total		130 (55/75)		46	69	11	4

[a] Two cases associated with hippocampal sclerosis, one with subcortical microinfarcts.
[b] One combined with multiple subcortical lacunes, one with cystic infarcts in left posterior cerebral artery area.
[c] Two combined with lacunes in striatum and thalamus.
[d] One with incidental Lewy body disease.
Abbr: MMSE, Mini-Mental State Examination.

3. FACTORS INVOLVED IN ViD

3.1. *Volume of Brain Destruction*

Although it is understandable that patients with large infarcts might experience intellectual decline, the idea that the diagnosis of MID requires a brain tissue loss exceeding 100 mL is a persistent component of neuromythology. In fact, Tomlinson et al. *(8)* showed that although all patients with brain tissue losses of more than 100 mL suffered from dementia and that infarct volumes between 50 and 100 mL produced dementia less consistently, they observed several patients with dementia with infarcts of lesser volumes. Those totaling over 20 mL were significantly more frequent in subjects with dementia than in controls, and a marked difference between the two groups was present at 50 mL tissue loss cut-off. According to their study, which has never been replicated, a relatively small aggregate volume of brain infarct may or may not contribute to dementia, probably depending on its location, whereas destruction of a larger volume of cortex is usually followed by dementia. Therefore, Tomlinson et al. proposed the concept of strategic sites of infarcts. A quantitative MRI study demonstrated that total cerebral infarct area and cortical involvement were significantly larger in stroke patients with dementia than those without dementia *(100)*. PET studies also showed a correlation between metabolic impairment of frontal and temporomedial cortex and the total volume of hypometabolic regions to dementia severity in both ViD and AD, whereas ViD cases showed also metabolic impairment in subcortical regions not present in AD *(187)*. Studies measuring the volume of macroscopic infarcts from photographs or drawings in ViD revealed mean volumes of infarcted brain of 39 mL (range 1–229 mL) in one study *(121)* and of 40.7 mL with a range of 6.9 to 220 mL in another study *(188)*, whereas patients with AD and AD plus VAD had infarct volumes of less than 10 mL. In patients who showed only vascular lesions on histologic examination with senile plaques below the level necessary for diagnosis of AD, the total volume of infarcted brain was more than twofold greater in subjects with dementia than in subjects without dementia *(88)*; only 3 patients had brain lesions larger than 100 g, and 17 had smaller volumes within the range of patients without dementia, suggesting that dementia is not directly and consistently related to the volume of infarction. These data were confirmed by recent studies that found only a nonsignificant trend for lobar infarcts to occupy more cerebral hemispheral volume in ViD than in patients without dementia *(16–18,69)*.

3.2. *Location of Vascular Lesions*

The location of CVLs is probably more important than the volume of tissue destruction. Multiple brain regions have been implicated in ViD (*see* Subheading 2.2.1.). Infarction in the left hemisphere and bilateral infarcts with more involvement of the dominant hemisphere increase the risk of dementia after stroke *(30,89,100)*. Vascular lesions in the angular gyrus in the dominant hemisphere showed clinical similarities to AD *(189,190)*. Cognitive impairment after stroke was more frequently associated with lesions in the left ACA and PCA territories *(100,191)* and after left or bilateral PCA occlusion *(190)*. Bilateral (paramedian) thalamic infarction is often associated with memory deficit and "subcortical" dementia *(122–124,190)* as are lacunar infarcts in basal ganglia, especially in the head of the caudate nucleus *(192,193)* and in the inferior genu of the anterior capsule, interrupting corticothalamic and thalamocortical pathways *(194,195)*. However, whether selective lesions of the thalamus constitute a distinct dementia entity remains uncertain *(5)*. In patients with ViD, infarcts in hippocampus were observed in 48%, in temporal lobe in 91%, and in basal ganglia in 83% *(30)*, and both hippocampal infarcts and sclerosis, either alone or in conjunction with other vascular lesions, are related to dementia *(4,185)*. Although the entorhinal cortex and hippocampus are less affected by subcortical CVLs than by AD *(196)*, ViD resulting from microvascular pathology showed significant hippocampal neuronal loss *(197)*, and hippocampal atrophy may increase the development of poststroke dementia *(198)*.

3.3. Number of CVLs

One of the concepts discussed in ViD is that multiple small infarcts, irrespective of their volume, can lead to intellectual decline. However, few studies address the important problem of the number of lesions in ViD and whether several large infarcts are more likely to cause dementia than multiple small lesions. Erkinjuntti et al. *(30)* found that the mean number of infarcts in ViD was 5.8, compared with 0.2 in mixed AD plus ViD, whereas Del Ser et al. *(89)* reported a mean number of 6.7 CVLs in patients with dementia, compared with 3.2. in patients without dementia. This significance reached statistiscal significance in ACA and MCA territory. Although infarct location, size, and number are important, other factors, such as age, systemic disease, other brain lesions, the degree of aging changes, the extent of WMLs, medial temporal lobe atrophy, and level of education are involved in determining intellectual decline *(34)*.

4. IMPORTANCE OF SMALL VASCULAR LESIONS

Esiri et al. *(69)* compared the neuropathologic findings in elderly subjects without dementia and CVD and subjects with dementia and CVD, and no other pathology accounting for dementia, including Alzheimer-type pathology. Microvascular brain damage was correlated with a history of dementia. Severe lacunar state and microinfarcts were more common in patients with dementia and CVD than in patients without dementia. CAA had a greater prevalence in the dementia group with dementia, which lacked evidence of macroscopic infarction more often than in patients without dementia. There was a nonsignificant trend for the ratio of infarcted vs noninfarcted tissue in one cerebral hemisphere to be higher in the group with dementia.

Vinters et al. *(16)* also emphasized the correlation of dementia with widespread small ischemic lesions distributed throughout the central nervous system (CNS). They observed cystic infarcts greater than 1 cm in diameter in three lacunes and microinfarcts in 12 brains each and hippocampal injury in 11 cases. Many brains showed more than one type of CVLs, most being associated with severe atherosclerosis and arteriolosclerosis. However, in two cognitively normal controls, similar multiple ischemic CVLs were seen. These data indicating that lacunar infarcts and microinfarcts are the most common neuropathologic features of ViD were confirmed by personal findings from a consecutive autopsy series. None except for a single brain showed severe Alzheimer pathology *(199)*, all had Braak stages 0–4, none fulfilled the criteria for DLB *(200)*, and only one single brain showed incidental Lewy body disease *(201,202)*. Among the 91 demented subjects, almost 20% showed old large infarcts of more than 1 cm^3 volume; the majority (57%) revealed multiple lacunes in striatum and thalamus, most frequently on both sides; 2 with hippocampal sclerosis; 9 brains showed multiple microinfarcts in cortical and subcortical areas, 4.5% hippocampal sclerosis. Of the cognitively impaired subjects, 31% showed larger cystic infarcts, 52% had multiple lacunes in basal ganglia, thalamus and/or white matter; multiple microinfarcts were observed in 2 brains, but hippocampal sclerosis in none. Of the 20 cognitively unimpaired subjects, almost two-thirds revealed cystic infarcts, 30% had multiple small subcortical lacunes with preserved thalamus and only one showed multiple old microinfarcts (*see* Table 5).

5. HEMORRHAGIC DEMENTIA

Primary intracerebral hypertensive hemorrhages are an uncommon cause of dementia. Most occur in the basal ganglia and thalamus, although a few are located in the cerebral cortex and white matter. These hemorrhages vary in size. Massive basal ganglia bleeds with rupture into the ventricles or brainstem compression are often fatal. Multiple small or slit-like hemorrhages in the cortex or white matter could lead to cognitive impairment *(4,10)*.

5.1. Cerebral Amyloid Angiopathy

The majority of dementing disorders related to cerebral hemorrhages and/or hemorrhagic infarcts occur in sporadic and familial conditions associated with CAA *(203)*.

Table 6
Incidence of Cerebral Amyloid Angiopathy in Alzheimer Disease (AD)

Author, year	Ref.	%
Yamada et al., 1987	*214*	88.2
Bergeron et al., 1987	*215*	88–90
Ellis et al., 1996 (CERAD)	*216*	83
Moderate-severe CAA		25.6
Cerebral hemorrhage in AD		18
Jellinger (1988–2000)		
AD with CAA 650/660		97.6
Cerebral hemorrhage (n = 47)		7.4
CAA plus hypertensive angiopathy; n = 20		
Hemorrhage owing to CAA without AD (14/28)		50
Esiri et al., 1986	*217*	
Vonsattel et al., 1991 (n = 300)	*218*	98
Kalaria and Ballard, 1999	*219*	

Abbr: CAA, cerebral amyloid angiopathy; CERAD, Consortium to Establish a Registry for Alzheimer Disease.

5.1.1. Sporadic Cerebral Amyloid Angiopathy

CAA is defined as deposition of Aβ peptide in the walls of meningeal and intracerebral vessels, with thickening of vessel walls and degeneration of smooth muscle cells (SMC). Current concepts of CAA formation are that SMCs synthesize Aβ-40 intracellularly, which aggregates extracellularly into fibrils that may induce complete replacement of medial SMCs bv fibrillary Aβ, with perivascular leakage of amyloid into the surrounding neuropil, fibrinoid necrosis, ensuing blood vessel rupture, and hemodynamic changes *(203)*. Injury to arteriolar SMCs may be one mechanism by which CAA and other angiopathies progress and become symptomatic *(204)*. Two types of CAA have been distinguished: type 1, showing Aβ deposits in meningeal and cortical arterioles, capillaries, veins, and venules associated with increased frequency of (apolipoprotein) (apo) E ε4 allele, and type 2, with Aβ deposits in meningeal and cortical vessels, except for cortical capillaries, which are associated with increased frequency of apo Eε2. The allele ε4 is a risk factor for CAA type 1 and neurophil-associated deposition in capillaries, whereas ε2 is not. Thus, both apo E alleles may support SMC-associated Aβ deposition *(205)*.

CAA is a common neuropathologic finding in the brains of elderly individuals with and without AD, and both its incidence and severity steadily increase with age *(206–213)* (Table 6); CAA is present in more than 80% of AD cases (Table 6).

Many vascular abnormalities are associated with CAA in nonhypertensive, nonatherosclerotic patients *(4,220)* that lead to a broad spectrum of CVLs, including large lobar and small cortical hemorrhages, small cortical and subcortical infarcts, and WMLs resulting from severe narrowing or occlusion of vessel lumina. One autopsy series of AD showed 48% CVLs with 32% microinfarction, 12.5% large infarcts, and 13.5% hemorrhages *(221)*. Another autopsy series, with CAA in 98%, showed 100% microvascular degeneration, 31% infarcts, and 7% intracerebral hemorrhages *(222)*. In a personal autopsy series of 750 AD cases, CAA was observed in 97.6% and CVLs in 48%, including cerebral hemorrhages in 4.3% *(98)*.

The most serious consequence of CAA is cerebral hemorrhage, and 3.8% to approximately 20% of all spontaneous (nontraumatic) cerebral bleeds in elderly subjects are of this type (*see* Table 7). Both acute and recurrent CAA-related cerebral hemorrhages are mainly located in the frontoparietal (35%),

Table 7
Incidence of Cerebral Amyloid Angiopathy in Spontaneous (Nontraumatic) Cerebral Hemorrhages

Author, year	Ref.	%
Lee and Stemmerman, 1978	*223*	10.0
Ishii et al., 1984	*224*	11.7
Tomonaga, 1985 (lobar hemorrhages)	*211*	20.0
Nadeau, 1989, quoted by >60 yr	*17*	15.0
>70 yr		ca. 20.0
Vonsattel et al., 1991	*218*	20.0
Feldman, 1994	*225*	12.0
Itoh et al., 1995	*207*	10.9
Ellis et al., 1996 (CERAD)	*216*	5.1
Jellinger, 1977–1997 >60 yr (94/482)		19.3

parietal (11–26%), temporal (15%), and occipital regions (5–18%); in basal ganglia (5–10%), with multiple bleeds in approximately 10%; and less frequently in cerebellum (1–2%) *(208)*. Several studies described multiple simultaneous intracerebral hemorrhages related to CAA *(226)*.

CAA is also associated with ischemic infarctions, the frequency of which increases with the severity of CAA. In autopsy-proved AD, increased overall frequency of CVLs was associated with severe CAA (SCAA) as opposed to mild CAA (MCAA) (40 vs 18% and 33 vs 19%). The combination of CAA and hypertension was highly associated with cerebral infarcts, suggesting a additive injury to blood vessels *(221,227)*. CAA as a risk factor for ischemic brain lesions was also observed in brain biopsies, where 13.1% of cases with cerebral or cerebellar infarcts showed CAA, mainly in large and less frequently in meningeal vessels, compared to 3.7% CAA and 13.1% plaques in controls *(228)*. These data indicate that CAA, not Aβ plaque formation, is significantly more common in elderly patients with cerebral infarcts than in those without CVLs, thus confirming that CAA is a major risk factor for both cerebral hemorrhages and infarcts.

The lack of correlation between the AD stage and the alterations of cerebral microvessels suggests that the changes in vasculature are not a consequence of AD pathology. Although the progress of AD may provoke early cerebrovascular damage *(27)*, significances in the incidence of CVD between low and high Braak stages were not found *(28)*.

CAA may be a cause of WMLs frequently found in AD, which may be a cause of dementia *(16,165,206,208,229)*, although the severity of WMLs in the frontal lobe in AD was less than in Binswanger's SAE but more severe than in age-matched controls *(166)*. The severity of WML in AD was significantly correlated with fibrohyalinosis, but neither with the age at onset nor the scores of CAA, which was present in 82%, but mainly in small meningocortical vessels. These data suggest that although CAA is an independent risk factor for WMLs in AD, its role is limited in comparison to that of fibrohyalinosis of white matter microvessels, which may or may not be associated with CAA, thus indicating the pathogenetic heterogeneity of WMLs in AD *(166)*. In any case, coexistent AD pathology is a much more common cause of dementia in sporadic CAA, which is explained by the closely related biologies of the two conditions *(217)*.

5.1.2. Inherited ViD and Familial Cerebral Amyloid Angiopathies

A comparatively small proportion of ViD is related to genetic disorders. These genetic disorders include familial CAA *(203)*, CADASIL *(162–164)*, and mitochondrial myopathy, encephalopathy, lactic acidosis, and stroke-like episodes (MELAS) syndrome.

5.1.3. *Familial Disorders With CAA—Hereditary CAA*

Most of these disorders that are associated with dementia combine vascular amyloid deposition with multiple cerebral hemorrhages or infarcts.

5.1.3.1. Hereditary Cerebral Hemorrhage With Amyloidosis (HCHWA)

The Dutch form (HCHWA-D) and the Islandic type (HCHWA-I) of HCHWA, which are both inherited as autosomal dominant traits, are morphologically featured by multiple recurrent hemorrhages and hemorrhagic infarcts associated with amyloid deposition in meningeal and cerebral vessels. Most of the hemorrhagic infarcts occur in the subcortical white matter, complemented by diffuse plaques *(230,231)*.

HCHWAD-D is caused by a point mutation on codon 693 of the amyloid precursor protein (APP) gene on chromosome 20 *(232)*. The clinical phenotypes of the A692G Flemish mutation *(233)* and of E693K (Italian mutation) *(234)* are also characterized by dementia and cerebral hemorrhages, whereas dementia is typical for the Arctic E693G mutation *(235)*. The D694N mutation in Antarctic patients is associated with dementia and leukodystrophy resulting from severe CAA *(236)*. In contrast, HCHWA-I or cysteine C-related familial CAA is associated with a point mutation in exon 2 of the cysteine C gene on chromosome 20, encoding the casein protease inhibitor cystin C *(237)*. Dementia in both forms is independent from tangles and plaques but has been attributed to multiple CAA-related CVLs *(238)*.

5.1.3.2. CAA and Transthyrein (Meningovascular) Amyloidosis

CAA and transthyretin (meningovascular) amyloidosis resulting from mutation of the *TTR* gene located on chromosome 18 is clinically featured by peripheral sensorimotor and autonomic neuropathies *(239)*. A large kindred with oculoleptomeningeal amyloidosis owing to a new transthyretin variant Tyr69His was described recently *(240)*.

5.1.3.3. Gelsolin-Related Amyloidosis (Familial Amyloidosis, Finnish Type)

This rare autosomal dominant disorder occurring in kindreds carrying a G654A or G6654T point mutation in the gelsolin gene on chromosome 9 *(241,242)* is clinically featured by facial palsy, peripheral neuropathy, corneal lattice dystrophy, gait ataxia, bulbar palsy, and mild cognitive impairment *(243,244)*. Neuropathology shows widespread CAA, with deposition of gelsolin-related amyloid in almost all organs and diffuse loss of myelin in centrum semiovale *(242)*.

5.1.3.4. Familial British Dementia (FBD)

This autosomal dominant condition associated with a point mutation in the *BRI1* gene located on chromosome 13 *(245)* is characterized by dementia, progressive spastic tetraparesis, and cerebellar ataxia. Neuropathology, in addition to neurofibrillary tangles and neuropil threads in the hippocampus, and nonneuritic, often perivascular plaques, shows widespread vascular amyloid in small cerebral and spinal arteries and Binswanger type WMLs but only rare cerebral hemorrhages *(203)*.

5.1.3.5. Familial Danish Dementia (FDD)

This autosomal dominant condition, also known as heredopathia ophthalmica-oto-encephalitica, is associated with a 10-nucleotide duplication between codons 265 and 266 of the *BRI2* gene *(246)* and is clinically characterized by cataracts, deafness, progressive ataxia, and dementia. Neuropathology includes CAA involving almost all CNS regions and hippocampal and perivascular amyloid plaques and tangles. Vascular pathology and parenchymal damage are more severe in FDD than in BFD *(247)*. Both conditions mimic pathologic aspects of AD, suggesting that Aβ peptide may be of primary importance in these disorders *(203)*.

5.2 Other Types of Familial ViD

5.2.1. Hereditary MID

In a Swedish family in which hereditary MID affected young adults with a disease onset between 29 and 38 yr of age, autopsy revealed multiple cystic infarcts in central gray and white matter and pons with cerebral cortical atrophy resulting from occlusion of small intracerebral and meningeal arteries and arterioles *(82)*. Because no CADASIL-type genetics or immunohistochemistry have been detected in this family *(164)*, its etiology is unknown.

5.2.2. CADASIL

CADASIL with clinical onset in midadult life and a history of small strokes, migraine, progressive dementia, and pseudobulbar palsy, is caused by a single mutation or small deletions in the Notch 3 gene on chromosome 19q12. Neuropathology shows multiple small, deep infarcts, diffuse leukoencephalopathy, and widespread vasculopathy similar to hypertensive lesions causing obliteration of small arteries *(162,164)*. The vascular lesions in the brain consisting of granular osmiophilic material (GOM) in smooth muscle cells are also seen (with electron microscopy) in other organs (e.g., vessels in spleen, liver, kidney, muscle and skin) allowing confirmation of diagnosis by skin biopsies *(243)*, but the composition of GOMs has not been definitely identified *(164)*. Some ViD cases showed decreased cholinergic markers in the brain *(248)*, and in the case of CADASIL with pure white matter infarcts, cholinergic denervation was seen in the posterior parietal, dorsal frontal, and occipital region, whereas the entorhinal region and temporal neocortex were conserved, which differs from the pattern in AD *(249)*.

5.2.3. MELAS Syndrome

MELAS, which was first described in 1984 *(250)* and is associated with mtDNA point mutations affecting tRNA genes with heteroplasmic A3243G mutation in the tRNA leucine gene in approximately 80% *(251)*, is clinically characterized by stroke-like episodes, seizures, and dementia with onset before 40 yr of age. Pathology reveals generalized mitochondrial microangiopathy without paracrystalline aggregates *(252)*. Gross findings are diffuse cerebral and cerebellar atrophy, with infarct-like lesions of the cortex and subcortical white matter. They are multifocal and asymmetric, favor the posterior cerebrum, and do not usually fall within the vascular territory of a major cerebral artery or border zones; they rarely involve the brainstem *(253)*. Cortical lesions are distributed in pseudolaminar, pancortical, and cortico-subcortical white matter patterns; the deep cortex is a major site of increased vascularity. Occasionally, the crests of gyri are predominantly affected. There may also be small foci of cortical necrosis, spongy changes in white matter, and, rarely, small infarcts in the basal ganglia. The meningeal and cortical arteries and arterioles are patent *(251)*, whereas myocytes and, rarely, the endothelium of surface arterioles and small arteries show degenerative changes with increased numbers of mitochondria. These data indicate that the mitochondrial vasculopathy is responsible for the CVLs in MELAS *(254)*; however, other authors questioned the hypothesis that defective mitochondria are responsible for the infarct-like lesions *(255)*.

6. THE PROBLEM OF MIXED DEMENTIA (ViD AND AD)

Mixed dementia (MD) is characterized by the pathologic alterations of both AD and ViD, but the distinction among AD, ViD, and MD remains controversial and is one of the most difficult clinical and pathologic challenges *(208,256,257)*. Few pathologic reports describe the criteria used to reach the diagnosis. The authors applied accepted histopathologic criteria for AD in conjunction with multiple lacunes and CVLs of the neocortex, basal ganglia, and hippocampus, or at least 30–50 mL of infarcted brain *(31,208)*, but definite criteria for the neuropathologic diagnosis of MD have not been developed. This is illustrated by the diversity in the prevalence rates of MD in autopsy studies, showing a range from 2 to 36%, with a mean of 17.7% (*see* Table 8). This cannot result only from

Table 8
Prevalence of Mixed Dementia (AD Plus VaD) in Autopsy Studies

Study, year	Ref.	No. of cases examined	Mixed cases	%
Tomlinson et al., 1970	*8*	50	9	18.0
Todorov et al., 1975	*81*	776	250	32.0
Mölsä et al., 1985	*84*	58	6	10.3
Ulrich et al., 1986	*32*	54	6	11.0
Alafuzoff et al., 1987	*85*	55	15	27.0
Joachim et al., 1988	*87*	150	10	7.0
Katzman et al., 1988	*260*	3 series	(<70 yr)	0.6
			(>70 yr)	15.2
Boller et al., 1989	*88*	54	2	3.7
O'Brien, 1988	*265*	?	?	10.0
Jellinger et al., 1990	*31*	675	53	7.9
Brun, 1994	*90*	175	63	36.0
Ince et al., 1995	*91*	69	4	5.9
Markesbery, 1998	*4*	Mixed series		mean 17.7
Knopman et al., 2003	*26*	81	10	12.2
Jellinger, 2003 (dementias/clinical AD)	*266*	950/600	34/9	3.6/1.5

recruitment biases or geographic factors and is, at least in part, related to differences in diagnostic criteria.

According to some authors, MD should be diagnosed only if there are sufficient vascular and degenerative lesions to make each diagnosis independently *(8,31)*, whereas other authors suggest the diagnosis of AD in addition to ischemic vascular lesions *(258)* and believe in an interaction between the two types of lesion, each of them alone being insufficient to account for dementia which, however, arises from their association *(78,256–262)*. The CERAD classification does not consider MD, and the presence or absence of other pathologic lesions likely to cause dementia does not interfere with the AD diagnosis *(199)*, whereas in the ADDTC criteria *(24)*, a second cerebrovascular disorder in addition to AD must be shown in order to be causally related to dementia. In the NINDS-AIREN criteria *(25)*, the term *AD with CVD* is reserved to patients fulfilling the clinical criteria of possible AD who have also clinical or imaging signs of relevant CVD, but the term *MD* should be avoided. It has even been questioned whether MD exists as an entity, and some authors have recommended reevaluation and more detailed redefinition of this term *(263,264)*.

It is well established that patients with AD frequently have other concomitant pathologic lesions *(208,267)*. Because strokes are common in elderly patients and increase with age, in most clinicopathologic series of demented subjects, 18–60% have AD with CVLs *(35,97,98,208,261,268)*. In a recent autopsy series of AD and age-matched controls *(98)*, the incidence of vascular pathology (48.1%) was significantly less than in previously smaller cohorts (82.3 and 56.5%, respectively) *(269,270)*. In centenarians, the prevalence of cerebral infarcts ranged from 30 to 55% *(271–273)*. These lesions, which were mainly in the MCA and PCA regions, were more frequent in subjects with dementia than in subjects who were cognitively normal or only mildly impaired. Vascular pathology has been discussed as a factor contributing to the pathogenesis of AD *(222,274–276)*. The association of vascular disease and AD is further supported by the finding that subjects dying from cardiovascular disease show more AD-type pathology than controls *(277,278)*, although more recent studies suggest that this association results from apo E ε4 and not cardiovascular disease *per se (279)*.

The contribution of CVLs to the development of dementia in AD patients remains unclear, but recent studies suggest that concomitant cerebral infarctions, in particularly strategic CVLs, but also

Table 9
Relation Between Cognitive State and Vascular Lesions in AD

Disorder	*n* (Male/female)	Age at death	Braak stage (mean)	Final MMSE (*n*)	History of stroke (%)
"Pure" AD	390 (155/235)	80.2 PM 8.9	5.2	1.1 (77) [c]	9.8
AD with lacunar state	132 (36/96)	83.2 PM 6.2	5.0	4.9 (19)	21.0 [a]
AD with old infarcts (<10 cm^3)	36 (12/24)	84.6 PM 6.7	4.8	7.0 (5)	33.0 [a]
AD with hippocampal sclerosis	16 (9/7)	86.1 PM 6.7 [b]	4.7	5.0 (5)	NG
Mix (AD plus CVD) >10	31 (7/24)	82.7 PM 5.9	4.8	7.3 (4)	94.0 [a]

[a] $p < 0.01$ vs "pure" AD.
[b] $p < 0.05$ vs "pure" AD.
[c] $p < 0.01$ vs other groups.
Abbr: kAD, Alzheimer's disease; CVD, cerebrovascular disease; NG, not given

cortical microinfarcts and demyelination have synergistic effects and, thus, may aggravate the severity of dementia *(78,279–281)*. CVLs may magnify the effect of mild AD pathology and result in earlier and more severe expression of dementia *(214,267)*. On the other hand, in patients with AD and other CNS pathologies, the densities of plaques and neuritic AD lesions were significantly lower than in those with AD and no other pathology for every given level of cognitive defect. In a recent prospective study in elderly patients, the severity of cognitive impairment was significantly correlated with the total volume of infarcts with effect on lesions in limbic and medial association areas, including the frontal cortex and white matter *(280)*. These findings are consistent with those in the Nun study *(78)*, in which patients with autopsy-confirmed AD and CVLs had a higher prevalence of dementia than those without infarcts, whereas in the OPTIMA study *(259)*, CVD significantly worsened cognitive performance in the earliest stages of AD. On the other hand, recent comparative studies of autopsy cases of AD with and without CVLs showed no differences in baseline, final, and change in Mini-Mental State Examination scores between groups *(208,281)* and could not detect any influence of the extent of cerebrovascular pathology on the age of death, clinical expression, and severity of AD pathology *(269)*.

Few studies have examined the contribution of small concomitant infarcts with a volume of less than 10 mL, which is generally considered insufficient to produce dementia. A recent study in 227 longitudinally autopsy cases of definite AD that were followed-up, 36 with concomitant small infarcts revealed significantly higher age with lower Braak stages in patients with MD compared to those with histologically "pure" AD *(261)*. These data, which varied from others that suggested a contribution to cognitive impairment in AD of CVLs even with volumes as low as 1 mL *(256,280)*, were largely confirmed in a personal autopsy series (*see* Table 9). The history of stroke was higher in MD than in AD plus minimal CVD and lowest in pure AD. In AD with minor CVD, the majority of lesions were lacunes in the basal ganglia and multiple microinfarcts, whereas in MD, large lobar infarcts were more frequent than small CVLs (*see* Table 10), suggesting different pathogenic mechanisms. These data suggest that coexistent small CVLs with a total volume of less than 10 mL do not significantly influence the overall rate of progression of cognitive impairment in patients with AD; although a concomitant pathology can modulate both cognitive and noncognitive features *(282)*. It is possible that elderly patients with subclinical AD and little functional brain reserve (with frequent entorhinal and hippocampal NFTs and modest numbers of neocortical neuritic plaques), who suffer from critically located CVLs, could demonstrate symptoms of intellectual decline. Similarly, subjects with early or midstage AD who develop cerebral infarcts could experience a marked decline in cognitive function by further depleting residual brain reserve, whereas in progressed or full-blown stages of AD with small CVLs that are frequently observed with modern neuroimaging methods, cognitive decline is mainly related to the severity and extent of AD pathology. This indicates that

Table 10
Types of Cerebrovascular Lesions in Mixed-Type Dementia [a]

1. AD plus multiple infarcts	25
MCA bilateral	6
MCA left	7
MCA plus PCA left	5
MCA plus PCA right	2
Multiple bilateral	2
Multiple left hemisphere	3
2. SID (strategic infarcts)	8
Thalamus plus hippocampus	1
Thalamus bilateral	2
3. SAE (subcortical type)	
Lacunes striatum, white matter	5
	Total 33

[a] 26 Female, 7 male, age 72–94, mean age = 82.7.
Abbr: MCA, medial central artery; PCA, posterior central artery; SAE, subcortical arteriosclerotic (leuko-) encephalopathy; SID, strategic infarct dementia; AD = Braak stages 4–6 (mean 4.8).

the combination of two or more pathologic processes may influence the severity of the cognitive deficit. CVD and other pathologies can "unmask" preclinical dementia resulting from relatively mild AD lesions; they may cause dementia of their own or by "summation" effects *(283)*, but the effect and pathogenetic role of each of these pathologic parameters is unknown.

7. CONCLUSION AND FUTURE ASPECTS

Recent autopsy data confirm that (1) ViD is a nonfrequent entity, in the course of which multiple ischemic or vascular brain lesion of variable etiology and pathogenesis result in progressive cognitive and memory impairment. No validated or reproducible morphologic classification of ViD and MD is currently available. The incidence and pathophysiologic effect of CVLs that may progress to ViD are not known exactly. "Pure" ViD without other coexisting pathology related to cognitive decline is rare, but ischemic/vascular brain lesion even of smaller volume, particularly in strategic brain areas, may aggravate the neuropsychologic deficit in aging brain and AD; (2) The concept that ViD is being determined primarily by the volume of infarcted brain is oversimplistic and cannot be confirmed in the majority of autopsy cases; (3) Although fairly unusual as an isolated nosologic entity, ViD is correlated with widespread ischemic and/or vascular lesions throughout the CNS with particular involvement of subcortical areas (basal ganglia and hemispheral white matter) and strategically important brain regions (limbic system, thalamus, and frontobasal area) associated with arteriosclerotic, hypertensive, other forms of microangiopathy, or both acute and chronic ischemic insults; (4) Sporadic and genetic/familial CAA frequently causes cerebral hemorrhages and other CVLs, which may result in dementia; (5) MD resulting from combined AD and ViD is a diagnostic challenge for which neither definite neuropathologic criteria nor epidemiologic data are available; (6) The histologic lesion pattern in "pure" ViD differs considerably from than in MD (AD plus ViD) that more often shows larger hemispheral infarcts than small subcortical lesions, suggesting different pathogenetic mechanisms; (7) Another form of ViD that is not infrequent in very old subjects is hippocampal sclerosis, a selective damage to the hippocampus that is often accompanied by multiple other CVLs; (8) Both mild Alzheimer-type pathology and small vessel disease-associated subcortical lesions are common and may interact in causing cognitive decline; AD-related pathology may be significantly less severe in the presence of CVLs. However, the effect of CVLs and their interrelationship to AD pathology on cognitive impairment need further elucidation.

REFERENCES

1. Jorm AF. Epidemiology: meta-analysis. In: Chiu E, Gustafson L, Ames D, Folstein M, eds. Cerebrovascular Disease and Dementia. Pathology, Neuropsychiatry and Management. London, UK: Martin Dunitz Publishers, 2000, pp. 85–97.
2. Garcia JH, Brown GG. Vascular dementia: neuropathologic alterations and metabolic brain changes. J Neurol Sci 1992;109:121–131.
3. Munoz DG. The pathological basis of multi-infarct dementia. Alzheimer Dis Assoc Disord 1991;5:77–90.
4. Markesbery WR. Vascular dementia. In: Markesbery W, ed. Neuropathology of Dementing Disorders. London, UK: Arnold Publishers, 1998, pp. 293–311.
5. Mirra SS, Hyman BT. Vascular dementia. In: Graham D, Lantos P, eds. Greenfield's Neuropathology. 7th Ed. London, UK: Arnold Publishing, 2002, pp. 241–245.
6. Mingazzini G. Anatomia clinica di centri nervosi. UTET, Torino 1913;548–573.
7. Fisher CM. Dementia in cerebral vascular disease. In: Toole J, Siekert R, Whisnant J, eds. Cerebral Vascular Disease. Sixth Princeton Conference. New York, NY: Greene and Stratton, 1968, pp. 232–236.
8. Tomlinson BE, Blessed G, Roth M. Observations on the brains of demented old people. J Neurol Sci 1970;11:205–242.
9. Hachinski VC, Lassen NA, Marshall J. Multi-infarct dementia. A cause of mental deterioration in the elderly. Lancet 1974;2:207–210.
10. Mikol J. Vascular dementia. In: Duckett S, De la Torre JC, eds. Pathology of the Aging Human Nervous System, 2nd ed. New York, Oxford Univ. Press, 2001, pp. 101–122.
11. Esiri MM, Hyman BT, Beyreuther K, Masters CL. Vascular dementia. In: Graham D, Lantos P, eds. Greenfield's Neuropathology. 6th Ed. London, UK: Arnold Publishing, 1997, pp. 204–210.
12. Leys D, Englund E, Erkinjuntti T. Vascular dementia. In: Qizilbash N, Schneider L, Brodaty H, Tariot P, Kaye J, Chui H, Erkinjuntti T, eds. Evidence Based Dementia Practice. Oxford, UK: Blackwell Science Publishing, 2002, pp. 260–287.
13. Markesbery WR. Overview of vascular dementia. In: Iqbal K, Sisodia S, Winblad B, eds. Alzheimer Disease: Advances in Etiology, Pathogenetics and Therapy. Paris, France: John Wiley & Sons, 2001, pp. 205–220.
14. Erkinjuntti T. Cerebrovascular dementia: pathophysiology, diagnosis and treatment. CNS Drugs 1999;12:35–48.
15. Gorelick PB. Status of risk factors for dementia associated with stroke. Stroke 1997;28:459–463.
16. Vinters HV, Ellis WG, Zarow C, et al. Neuropathologic substrates of ischemic vascular dementia. J Neuropathol Exp Neurol 2000;59:931–945.
17. Jellinger KA. The pathology of ischemic-vascular dementia: an update. J Neurol Sci 2002;203-204:153–157.
18. Jellinger KA. Vascular-ischemic dementia: an update. J Neural Transm 2002;(Suppl):1–23.
19. Moncayo J, Bogousslavski J. Vascular dementia: persisting controversies and questions. Eur J Neurol 1996;3:299–308.
20. Bowler JV, Hachinski V. Current criteria for vascular dementia—a critical appraisal. In: Bowler JV, Hachinski V, eds. Vascular Cognitive Impairment: Preventable Dementia. Oxford, Oxford Univ. Press, 2003, pp. 1–11.
21. Arvanitakis Z, Hachinski V. Vascular cognitive impairment: what else do we need to learn? In: Terry R, Katzman R, Bick K, Sisodia S, eds. Alzheimer Disease. 2nd Ed. Philadelphia, PA: Lippincott Williams & Wilkins, 1999, pp. 147–160.
22. Hyman BT. New neuropathological criteria for Alzheimer disease. Arch Neurol 1998;55:1174–1176.
23. Jellinger KA. What is new in degenerative dementia disorders? Wien Klin Wochenschr 1999;111:682–704.
24. Chui HC, Victoroff JI, Margolin D, Jagust W, Shankle R, Katzman R. Criteria for the diagnosis of ischemic vascular dementia proposed by the State of California Alzheimer's Disease Diagnostic and Treatment Centers. Neurology 1992;42:473–480.
25. Roman GC, Tatemichi TK, Erkinjuntti T, et al. Vascular dementia: diagnostic criteria for research studies. Report of the NINDS-AIREN International Workshop. Neurology 1993;43:250–260.
26. Knopman DS, Parisi JE, Boeve BF, et al. Vascular dementia in a population-based autopsy study. Arch Neurol 2003;60:569–575.
27. Goulding J, Signorini D, Chatterjee S, et al. Inverse relation between Braak stage and cerebrovascular pathology in Alzheimer predominant dementia. J Neurol Neurosurg Psychiatry 1999;67:654–657.
28. Jellinger KA. Inverse correlation between cerebrovascular lesions and Braak stage (letter). J Neurol Neurosurg Psychiatry 2000;68:799–800.
29. Erkinjuntti T. Classification and criteria. In: Chiu E, Gustafson L, Ames D, Folstein M, eds. Cerebrovascular Disease and Dementia. Pathology, Neuropsychiatry and Management. London, UK: Martin Dunitz Publishers, 2000, pp. 99–113.
30. Erkinjuntti T, Haltia M, Palo J, Sulkava R, Paetau A. Accuracy of the clinical diagnosis of vascular dementia: a prospective clinical and post-mortem neuropathological study. J Neurol Neurosurg Psychiatry 1988;51:1037–1044.
31. Jellinger K, Danielczyk W, Fischer P, Gabriel E. Clinicopathological analysis of dementia disorders in the elderly. J Neurol Sci 1990;95:239–258.
32. Ulrich J, Probst A, Wuest M. The brain diseases causing senile dementia. A morphological study on 54 consecutive autopsy cases. J Neurol 1986;233:118–122.
33. Olsson Y, Brun A, Englund E. Fundamental pathological lesions in vascular dementia. Acta Neurol Scand Suppl 1996;168:31–38.

34. Pohjasvaara T, Mantyla R, Salonen O, et al. How complex interactions of ischemic brain infarcts, white matter lesions, and atrophy relate to poststroke dementia. Arch Neurol 2000;57:1295–1300.
35. Galasko D, Hansen LA, Katzman R, et al. Clinical-neuropathological correlations in Alzheimer's disease and related dementias. Arch Neurol 1994;51:888–895.
36. Victoroff J, Mack WJ, Lyness SA, Chui HC. Multicenter clinicopathological correlation in dementia. Am J Psychiatry 1995;152:1476–1484.
37. Moroney JT, Bagiella E, Desmond DW, et al. Meta-analysis of the Hachinski Ischemic Score in pathologically verified dementias. Neurology 1997;49:1096–1105.
38. Wetterling T, Kanitz RD, Borgis KJ. Comparison of different diagnostic criteria for vascular dementia (ADDTC, DSM-IV, ICD-10, NINDS-AIREN). Stroke 1996;27:30–36.
39. Gertz HJ, Wolf H, Arendt T. [Vascular dementia]. Nervenarzt 2002;73:393–404.
40. Bowler JV, Munoz DG, Merskey H, Hachinski V. Fallacies in the pathological confirmation of the diagnosis of Alzheimer's disease. J Neurol Neurosurg Psychiatry 1998;64:18–24.
41. Chui HC, Mack W, Jackson JE, et al. Clinical criteria for the diagnosis of vascular dementia: a multicenter study of comparability and interrater reliability. Arch Neurol 2000;57:191–196.
42. Gold G, Giannakopoulos P, Montes-Paixao Junior C, et al. Sensitivity and specificity of newly proposed clinical criteria for possible vascular dementia. Neurology 1997;49:690–694.
43. O'Brien MD. How does cerebrovascular disease cause dementia. Dementia 1994;5:133–136.
44. Erkinjuntti T, Inzitari D, Pantoni L, et al. Research criteria for subcortical vascular dementia in clinical trials. J Neural Transm 2000;59(Suppl):23–30.
45. Gustafson I, Passant U. Clinical pathological correlates. In: Chiu E, Gustafson L, Ames D, Folstein M, eds. Cerebrovascular Disease and Dementia. Pathology, Neuropsychiatry and Management. London, UK: Martin Dunitz Publishers, 2000, pp. 85–97.
46. Knopman DS, DeKosky ST, Cummings JL, et al. Practice parameter: diagnosis of dementia (an evidence-based review). Report of the Quality Standards Subcommittee of the American Academy of Neurology. Neurology 2001;56: 1143–1153.
47. Englund E. White matter pathology in vascular dementia. In: Chiu E, Gustafson L, Ames D, Folstein M, eds. Cerebrovascular Disease and Dementia. Pathology, Neuropsychiatry and Management. London, UK: Martin Dunitz Publishers, 2000, pp. 77–84.
48. Englund E. Neuropathology of white matter lesions in vascular cognitive impairment. Cerebrovasc Dis 2002;13(Suppl): 11–15.
49. Esiri MM. Which vascular lesions are of importance in vascular dementia? Ann N Y Acad Sci 2000;903:239–243.
50. Janota I, Mirsen TR, Hachinski VC, Lee DH, Merskey H. Neuropathologic correlates of leuko-arabinosis. Arch Neurol 1989;46:1124–1128.
51. Pantoni L, Palumbo V, Sarti C. Pathological lesions in vascular dementia. Ann N Y Acad Sci 2002;977:279–291.
52. Rocca WA, Hofman A, Brayne C, et al. The prevalence of vascular dementia in Europe: facts and fragments from 1980-1990 studies. EURODEM-Prevalence Research Group. Ann Neurol 1991;30:817–824.
53. Fratiglioni L, Grut M, Forsell Y, et al. Prevalence of Alzheimer's disease and other dementias in an elderly urban population: relationship with age, sex, and education. Neurology 1991;41:1886–1892.
54. Hebert R, Brayne C. Epidemiology of vascular dementia. Neuroepidemiology 1995;14:240–257.
55. Meyer JS, Rauch GM, Lechner H, Loeb C. Vascular Dementia. Armonk, NY: Futura Publishing, 2001, pp. 320.
56. Reed BR. Vascular dementia. Arch Neurol 2004;61:433–435.
57. Roman GC. Vascular dementia may be the most common form of dementia in the elderly. J Neurol Sci 2002;203-204:7–10.
58. Rahkonen T, Eloniemi-Sulkava U, Rissanen S, Vatanen A, Viramo P, Sulkava R. Dementia with Lewy bodies according to the consensus criteria in a general population aged 75 years or older. J Neurol Neurosurg Psychiatry 2003;74:720–724.
59. Kase CS. Epidemiology of multi-infarct dementia. Alzheimer Dis Assoc Disord 1991;5:71–76.
60. Lobo A, Launer LJ, Fratiglioni L, et al. Prevalence of dementia and major subtypes in Europe: a collaborative study of population-based cohorts. Neurologic Diseases in the Elderly Research Group. Neurology 2000;54:S4–S9.
61. Rockwood K, Wentzel C, Hachinski V, Hogan DB, MacKnight C, McDowell I. Prevalence and outcomes of vascular cognitive impairment. Vascular Cognitive Impairment Investigators of the Canadian Study of Health and Aging. Neurology 2000;54:447–451.
62. Hebert R, Lindsay J, Verreault R, Rockwood K, Hill G, Dubois MF. Vascular dementia: incidence and risk factors in the Canadian study of health and aging. Stroke 2000;31:1487–1493.
63. Hasegawa K, Homma A, Imai Y. An epidemiological study of age-related dementia in the community. Int J Geriatr Psychiatry 1986;1:94–105.
64. Li G, Shen YC, Chen CH, Zhau YW, Li SR, Lu M. A three-year follow-up study of age-related dementia in an urban area of Beijing. Acta Psychiatr Scand 1991;83:99–104.

65. Ueda K, Kawano H, Hasuo Y, Fujishima M. Prevalence and etiology of dementia in a Japanese community. Stroke 1992;23:798–803.
66. Yoshitake T, Kiyohara Y, Kato I, et al. Incidence and risk factors of vascular dementia and Alzheimer's disease in a defined elderly Japanese population: the Hisayama Study. Neurology 1995;45:1161–1168.
67. Ikeda M, Hokoishi K, Maki N, et al. Increased prevalence of vascular dementia in Japan: a community-based epidemiological study. Neurology 2001;57:839–844.
68. Chiu HF, Lam LC, Chi I, et al. Prevalence of dementia in Chinese elderly in Hong Kong. Neurology 1998;50:1002–1009.
69. Esiri MM, Wilcock GK, Morris JH. Neuropathological assessment of the lesions of significance in vascular dementia. J Neurol Neurosurg Psychiatry 1997;63:749–753.
70. Vermeer SE, Prins ND, den Heijer T, Hofman A, Koudstaal PJ, Breteler MM. Silent brain infarcts and the risk of dementia and cognitive decline. N Engl J Med 2003;348:1215–1222.
71. Knopman DS, Rocca WA, Cha RH, Edland SD, Kokmen E. Incidence of vascular dementia in Rochester, MN, 1985–1989. Arch Neurol 2002;59:1605–1610.
72. Schneider JA, Wilson RS, Cochran EJ, et al. Relation of cerebral infarctions to dementia and cognitive function in older persons. Neurology 2003;60:1082–1088.
73. Hulette C, Nochlin D, McKeel D, et al. Clinical-neuropathologic findings in multi-infarct dementia: a report of six autopsied cases. Neurology 1997;48:668–672.
74. Skoog I, Nilsson L, Palmertz B, Andreasson LA, Svanborg A. A population-based study of dementia in 85-year-olds. N Engl J Med 1993;328:153–158.
75. Desmond DW, Moroney JT, Sano M, Stern Y. Incidence of dementia after ischemic stroke: results of a longitudinal study. Stroke 2002;33:2254–2260.
76. Mirsen T, Hachinski V. The epidemiology and classification of vascular and multi-infarct dementia. In: Meyer J, Lechner H, Marshall J, Toole J, eds. Vascular and Multi-infarct Dementia. Mount Kisco, NY: Futura Publishing, 1988, pp. 61–76.
77. Crystal HA, Dickson D, Davies P, Masur D, Grober E, Lipton RB. The relative frequency of "dementia of unknown etiology" increases with age and is nearly 50% in nonagenarians. Arch Neurol 2000;57:713–719.
78. Snowdon DA, Greiner LH, Mortimer JA, Riley KP, Greiner PA, Markesbery WR. Brain infarction and the clinical expression of Alzheimer disease. The Nun Study. JAMA 1997;277:813–817.
79. Corsellis JAN. Mental Illness and the Ageing Brain. London, UK: University Press, 1962.
80. Birkett DP. The psychiatric differentiation of senility and arteriosclerosis. Br J Psychiatry 1972;120:321–325.
81. Todorov AB, Go RC, Constantinidis J, Elston RC. Specificity of the clinical diagnosis of dementia. J Neurol Sci 1975; 26:81–98.
82. Sourander P, Walinder J. Hereditary multi-infarct dementia. Morphological and clinical studies of a new disease. Acta Neuropathol (Berl) 1977;39:247–254.
83. de Reuck J, Sieben G, de Coster W, vander Eecken H. Dementia and confusional state in patients with cerebral infarcts. A clinicopathological study. Eur Neurol 1982;21:94–97.
84. Mölsä PK, Paljarvi L, Rinne JO, Rinne UK, Sako E. Validity of clinical diagnosis in dementia: a prospective clinicopathological study. J Neurol Neurosurg Psychiatry 1985;48:1085–1090.
85. Alafuzoff I, Iqbal K, Friden H, Adolfsson R, Winblad B. Histopathological criteria for progressive dementia disorders: clinical-pathological correlation and classification by multivariate data analysis. Acta Neuropathol (Berl) 1987; 74:209–225.
86. Wade JP, Mirsen TR, Hachinski VC, Fisman M, Lau C, Merskey H. The clinical diagnosis of Alzheimer's disease. Arch Neurol 1987;44:24–29.
87. Joachim CL, Morris JH, Selkoe DJ. Clinically diagnosed Alzheimer's disease: autopsy results in 150 cases. Ann Neurol 1988;24:50–56.
88. Boller F, Lopez OL, Moossy J. Diagnosis of dementia: clinicopathologic correlations. Neurology 1989;39:76–79.
89. del Ser T, Bermejo F, Portera A, Arredondo JM, Bouras C, Constantinidis J. Vascular dementia. A clinicopathological study. J Neurol Sci 1990;96:1–17.
90. Brun A. Pathology and pathophysiology of cerebrovascular dementia: pure subgroups of obstructive and hypoperfusive etiology. Dementia 1994;5:145–147.
91. Ince PG, McArthur FK, Bjertness E, Torvik A, Candy JM, Edwardson JA. Neuropathological diagnoses in elderly patients in Oslo: Alzheimer's disease, Lewy body disease, vascular lesions. Dementia 1995;6:162–168.
92. Bowler JV, Eliasziw M, Steenhuis R, et al. Comparative evolution of Alzheimer disease, vascular dementia, and mixed dementia. Arch Neurol 1997;54:697–703.
93. Snowdon DA, Markesbery WR. The prevalence of neuropathologically confirmed vascular dementia: findings from the Nun study 1st Intern Congr on Vascular Dementia, Geneva, Switzerland, October 1999. Bologna, Italy: Monduzzi Editore S.p.A, 1999, pp. 19–24.
94. Nolan KA, Lino MM, Seligmann AW, Blass JP. Absence of vascular dementia in an autopsy series from a dementia clinic. J Am Geriatr Soc 1998;46:597–604.

95. Seno H, Ishino H, Inagaki T, Iijima M, Kaku K, Inata T. A neuropathological study of dementia in nursing homes over a 17-year period, in Shimane Prefecture, Japan. Gerontology 1999;45:44–48.
96. Akatsu H, Takahashi M, Matsukawa N, et al. Subtype analysis of neuropathologically diagnosed patients in a Japanese geriatric hospital. J Neurol Sci 2002;196:63–69.
97. Neuropathology G. Neuropathology Group of the Medical Research Council Cognitive Function and Ageing Study (MRC CFAS). Pathological correlates of late-onset dementia in a multicentre, community-based population in England and Wales. Lancet 2001;357:169–175.
98. Jellinger K, Mitter-Ferstl E. The impact of cerebrovascular lesions in Alzheimer disease. A comparative autopsy study. J Neurol 2003;250:1050–1055.
99. Loeb C. Neuropathological correlates of vascular dementia. In: Meyer J, Rauch G, Lechner H, Loeb C, Toole J, eds. Vascular Dementia. Armonk, NY: Futura Publishing, 2001, pp. 59–75.
100. Liu CK, Miller BL, Cummings JL, et al. A quantitative MRI study of vascular dementia. Neurology 1992;42:138–143.
101. De Reuck J, De Reus R, De Koninck J. Sneddon's syndrome. A not unusual cause of stroke in young women. In: Meyer J, Lechner H, Reivich M, Ott E, eds. Cerebral Vascular Disease. Amsterdam, The Netherlands: Excerpta Medica 6, 1987, pp. 171–174.
102. Marie P. Des foyers lacunaires de désintégration et de différents autres états cavitaires du cerveau. Rev Med 1901;21:281–3298.
103. Fisher CM. Lacunes: small, deep cerebral infarcts. 1965. Neurology 1998;50:841–852.
104. Fisher CM. Lacunar strokes and infarcts: a review. Neurology 1982;32:871–876.
105. Garcia JH, Lassen NA, Weiller C, Sperling B, Nakagawa J. Ischemic stroke and incomplete infarction. Stroke 1995;27:761–765.
106. Poirier J, Derouesne C. Cerebral lacunae. A proposed new classification. Clin Neuropathol 1984;3:266.
107. Poirier J, Derouesne C. [The concept of cerebral lacunae from 1838 to the present]. Rev Neurol (Paris) 1985;141:3–17.
108. Tuszynski MH, Petito CK, Levy DE. Risk factors and clinical manifestations of pathologically verified lacunar infarctions. Stroke 1989;20:990–999.
109. Lassen NA. Incomplete cerebral infarction—focal incomplete ischemic tissue necrosis not leading to emollision. Stroke 1982;13:522–523.
110. Ma CK, Olsson Y. The role of chronic brain edema in the formation of lacunes in Binswanger's encephalopathy. Histopathology and immunohistochemical observations. Cerebrovasc Dis 1997;7:324–331.
111. Lammie GA. Pathology of lacunar infarction. In: Donnan G, Norrving B, Bamford J, Bogousslavsky J, eds. Subcortical Stroke. Oxford, UK: Oxford University Press, 2002, pp. 38–46.
112. Lammie GA. Hypertensive cerebral small vessel disease and stroke. Brain Pathol 2002;12:358–370.
113. Derouesne C, Gray F, Escourelle R, Castaigne P. 'Expanding cerebral lacunae' in a hypertensive patient with normal pressure hydrocephalus. Neuropathol Appl Neurobiol 1987;13:309–320.
114. Pollock H, Hutchings M, Weller RO, Zhang ET. Perivascular spaces in the basal ganglia of the human brain: their relationship to lacunes. J Anat 1997;191:337–346.
115. Hughes W. Hypothesis—origin of lacunes. Lancet 1965;2:19–21.
116. Roman GC. Lagunas cerebrales. Estudio clínico y neurópatológico de 100 cases fatales. Rev Facultad Ciencias Medicas/Univ Nac Córdoba 1981;39:115–129.
117. De Reuck J, Van der Eecken H. The topography of infarcts in the lacunar state. In: Meyer J, Lechner H, Reivich M, eds. Cerebral Vascular Disease 7. Stuttgart, Germany: Thieme, 1976, pp. 162–165.
118. Pullicino PM. Pathogenesis of lacunar infarcts and small deep infarcts. Adv Neurol 1993;62:125–140.
119. Leys D, Bogousslavsky J. Mechanisms of vascular dementia. In: Leys D, Scheltens P, eds. Current Issues in Neurodegenerative Diseases. Vol. 6: Vascular Dementia. Amsterdam, The Netherlands: ICG, 1994, pp. 121–132.
120. Benson DF, Cummings JL. Angular gyrus syndrome simulating Alzheimer's disease. Arch Neurol 1982;39:616–620.
121. Zekry D, Duyckaerts C, Belmin J, et al. The vascular lesions in vascular and mixed dementia: the weight of functional neuroanatomy. Neurobiol Aging 2003;24:213–219.
122. Castaigne P, Lhermitte F, Buge A, Escourolle R, Hauw JJ, Lyon-Caen O. Paramedian thalamic and midbrain infarct: clinical and neuropathological study. Ann Neurol 1981;10:127–148.
123. de Freitas GR, Bogousslavsky J. Thalamic infarcts. In: Donnan G, Norrving B, Bamford J, Bogousslavsky J, eds. Subcortical Stroke. 2nd Ed. Oxford, UK: Oxford University Press, 2002, pp. 255–285.
124. Szirmai I, Vastagh I, Szombathelyi E, Kamondi A. Strategic infarcts of the thalamus in vascular dementia. J Neurol Sci 2002;203-204:91–97.
125. Brion S, Pragier G, Guerin R, Teitgen M. Syndrome de Korsakoff par ramollissement bilateral du fornix. Rev Neurol 1969;120:255–262.
126. Escourolle R, Gray F. Les accidents vasculaires du systeme limbique 7th Congr Neuropathol Budapest. Amsterdam, The Netherlands: Excerpta Medica, 1975.
127. Glees P, Griffith GH. Bilateral destruction of the hippocampus in case of dementia. Monatsschr Psych Neurol 1953;123:193–204.

128. Caplan LR. Binswanger's disease—revisited. Neurology 1995;45:626–633.
129. Caplan LR, Helgason CM. Caudate infarcts. In: Donnan G, Norrving B, Bamford J, Bogousslavsky J, eds. Lacunar and Other Subcortical Infarctions. Oxford, UK: Oxford University Press, 1995, pp. 117–130.
130. de Groot JC, de Leeuw FE, Oudkerk M, et al. Cerebral white matter lesions and cognitive function: the Rotterdam Scan Study. Ann Neurol 2000;47:145–151.
131. de Leeuw FE, de Groot JC, Oudkerk M, et al. Hypertension and cerebral white matter lesions in a prospective cohort study. Brain 2002;125:765–772.
132. Fazekas F, Schmidt R, Kleinert R, Kapeller P, Roob G, Flooh E. The spectrum of age-associated brain abnormalities: their measurement and histopathological correlates. J Neural Transm Suppl 1998;53:31–39.
133. Hentschel F, Kreis M, Damian M, Krumm B. [Microangiopathic lesions of white matter. Quantitation of cerebral MRI findings and correlation with psychological tests]. Nervenarzt 2003;74:355–361.
134. Ward NS, Brown MM. Leukoariosis. In: Cummings JL, ed. Subcortical Dementia. Oxford, UK: Oxford University Press, 1990, pp. 47–68.
135. Binswanger O. Die Abgrenzung der allgemeinen progressiven Paralyse. Berliner Klin Wochenschr 1894;31:1103–1105, 1137–1139, 1180–1186.
136. Hachinski VC, Potter P, Merskey H. Leuko-araiosis. Arch Neurol 1987;44:21–23.
137. Babikian V, Ropper AH. Binswanger's disease: a review. Stroke 1987;18:2–12.
138. Blass JP, Hoyer S, Nitsch R. A translation of Otto Binswanger's article, 'The delineation of the generalized progressive paralyses'. 1894. Arch Neurol 1991;48:961–972.
139. Brun A, Fredriksson K, Gustafson L. Pure subcortical arteriosclerotic encephalopathy (Binswanger's disease): a clinicopathological study. Part I: pathological features. Cerebrovasc Dis 1992;2:87–92.
140. Fisher CM. Binswanger's encephalopathy: a review. J Neurol 1989;236:65–79.
141. Jellinger K, Neumayer E. Progressive subcortical Encephalopathie Binswanger. Eine klinisch-neuropathologische Studie. Arch Psych Z Ges Neurologie 1964;205:523–554.
142. Pantoni L, Garcia JH. The significance of cerebral white matter abnormalities 100 years after Binswanger's report. A review. Stroke 1995;26:1293–1301.
143. Van de Nes JAP, Zimmer R, Janzen RWC, Turowski B, Hürtle E, Schlote W. Mini-infarct encephalopathy associated with uncommon microvessel convolute formation presenting with presenile dementia. Clin Neuropathol 2003;22:101–109.
144. Grafton ST, Sumi SM, Stimac GK, Alvord EC, Jr., Shaw CM, Nochlin D. Comparison of postmortem magnetic resonance imaging and neuropathologic findings in the cerebral white matter. Arch Neurol 1991;48:293–298.
145. van Swieten JC, Geyskes GG, Derix MM, et al. Hypertension in the elderly is associated with white matter lesions and cognitive decline. Ann Neurol 1991;30:825–830.
146. Pantoni L. Pathophysiology of age-related cerebral white matter changes. Cerebrovasc Dis 2002;13:7–10.
147. Wakita H, Tomimoto H, Akiguchi I, et al. Axonal damage and demyelination in the white matter after chronic cerebral hypoperfusion in the rat. Brain Res 2002;924:63–70.
148. Kobari M, Meyer JS, Ichijo M, Oravez WT. Leukoariosis: correlation of MR and CT findings with blood flow, atrophy, and cognition. AJNR Am J Neuroradiol 1990;11:273–281.
149. Brown MM, Pelz DM, Hachinski VC. White matter vasodilatory reserve is impaired in patients with cerebrovascular disease and diffuse periventricular lacunes. J Neurol 1990;237:157.
150. Isaka Y, Okamoto M, Ashida K, Imaizumi M. Decreased cerebrovascular dilatory capacity in subjects with asymptomatic periventricular hyperintensities. Stroke 1994;25:375–381.
151. Sultzer DL, Mahler ME, Cummings JL, Van Gorp WG, Hinkin CH, Brown C. Cortical abnormalities associated with subcortical lesions in vascular dementia. Clinical and position emission tomographic findings. Arch Neurol 1995;52:773–780.
152. Kwan LT, Reed BR, Eberling JL, et al. Effects of subcortical cerebral infarction on cortical glucose metabolism and cognitive function. Arch Neurol 1999;56:809–814.
153. Yoshikawa T, Murase K, Oku N, et al. Quantification of the heterogeneity of cerebral blood flow in vascular dementia. J Neurol 2003;250:194–200.
154. Yoshikawa T, Murase K, Oku N, et al. Statistical image analysis of cerebral blood flow in vascular dementia with small-vessel disease. J Nucl Med 2003;44:505–511.
155. DeReuck J, Schaumburg HH. Periventricular atherosclerotic leukoencephalopathy. Neurology 1972;22:1094–1097.
156. Moody DM, Bell MA, Challa VR. Features of the cerebral vascular pattern that predict vulnerability to perfusion or oxygenation deficiency: an anatomic study. AJNR Am J Neuroradiol 1990;11:431–439.
157. Mayer PL, Kier EL. The controversy of the periventricular white matter circulation: a review of the anatomic literature. AJNR Am J Neuroradiol 1991;12:223–228.
158. Feigin L, Poport N. Neuropathological changes late in cerebral edema. The relationship to trauma, hypertensive disease and Binswanger's encephalopathy. J Neuropathol Exp Neurol 1963;22:500–511.
159. Kirkpatrick JB, Hayman LA. White-matter lesions in MR imaging of clinically healthy brains of elderly subjects: possible pathologic basis. Radiology 1987;162:509–511.

160. Salahuddin TS, Johansson BB, Kalimo H, Olsson Y. Structural changes in the rat brain after carotid infusions of hyperosmolar solutions: a light microscopic and immunohistochemical study. Neuropathol Appl Neurobiol 1988;14: 467–482.
161. De Reuck J. Neuropathology of vascular dementia. In: Leys D, Scheltens P, eds. Current Issues in Neurodegenerative Diseases. Vol. 6: Amsterdam, The Netherlands: Vascular Dementia. ICG, 1994, pp. 9–15.
162. Chabriat H, Bousser MG. Cerebral autosomal dominant arteriopathy with subcortical infarcts and leukoencephalopathy. In: Donnan G, Norrving B, Bamford J, Bogousslavsky J, eds. Subcortical Stroke. 2nd Ed. Oxford, UK: Oxford University Press, 2002, pp. 116–126.
163. Filley CM, Thompson LL, Sze CI, Simon JA, Paskavitz JF, Kleinschmidt-DeMasters BK. White matter dementia in CADASIL. J Neurol Sci 1999;163:163–167.
164. Kalimo H, Ruchoux MM, Viitanen M, Kalaria RN. CADASIL: a common form of hereditary arteriopathy causing brain infarcts and dementia. Brain Pathol 2002;12:371–384.
165. Gray F, Dubas F, Roullet E, Escourolle R. Leukoencephalopathy in diffuse hemorrhagic cerebral amyloid angiopathy. Ann Neurol 1985;18:54–59.
166. Tomimoto H, Akiguchi I, Akiyama H, et al. Vascular changes in white matter lesions of Alzheimer's disease. Acta Neuropathol (Berl) 1999;97:629–634.
167. Waxman SG. Molecular mechanisms of subcortical versus cortical infarction. In: Donnan G, Norrving B, Bamford J, Bogousslavsky J, eds. Subcortical Stroke. Oxford, UK: Oxford University Press, 2002, pp. 67–83.
167a. Brown WR, Moody DM, Thore CR, Challa VR. Apoptosis in leukoaraiosis. AJNR Am J Neuroradiol 2000;21:79–82.
168. Hanyu H, Tanaka Y, Shimizu S, et al. Cerebral microbleeds in Binswanger's disease: a gradient-echo T2*-weighted magnetic resonance imaging study. Neurosci Lett 2003;340:213–216.
169. Loeb C. Binswanger's disease is not a single entity. Neurol Sci 2000;21:343–348.
170. Tanoi Y, Okeda R, Budka H. Binswanger's encephalopathy: serial sections and morphometry of the cerebral arteries. Acta Neuropathol (Berl) 2000;100:347–355.
171. Tomimoto H, Akiguchi I, Wakita H, Kimura J. [Changes in glial cells in Binswanger-type infarction]. No To Shinkei 1994;46:771–779.
172. Zhang WW, Badonic T, Hoog A, et al. Structural and vasoactive factors influencing intracerebral arterioles in cases of vascular dementia and other cerebrovascular disease: a review. Immunohistochemical studies on expression of collagens, basal lamina components and endothelin-1. Dementia 1994;5:153–162.
173. Yamanouchi H. Loss of white matter oligodendrocytes and astrocytes in progressive subcortical vascular encephalopathy of Binswanger type. Acta Neurol Scand 1991;83:301–305.
174. Zambenedetti P, Schmitt HP, Zatta P. Metallothionein I-II immunocytochemical reactivity in Binswanger's encephalopathy. J Alzheimers Dis 2002;4:459–466.
175. Kramer JH, Reed BR, Mungas D, Weiner MW, Chui HC. Executive dysfunction in subcortical ischaemic vascular disease. J Neurol Neurosurg Psychiatry 2002;72:217–220.
176. Zhan SS, Beyreuther K, Schmitt HP. Synaptophysin immunoreactivity of the cortical neuropil in vascular dementia of Binswanger type compared with the dementia of Alzheimer type and nondemented controls. Dementia 1994;5:79–87.
177. Fein G, Di Sclafani V, Tanabe J, et al. Hippocampal and cortical atrophy predict dementia in subcortical ischemic vascular disease. Neurology 2000;55:1626–1635.
178. Mungas D, Jagust WJ, Reed BR, et al. MRI predictors of cognition in subcortical ischemic vascular disease and Alzheimer's disease. Neurology 2001;57:2229–2235.
179. Fisher CM. Capsular infarcts: the underlying vascular lesions. Arch Neurol 1979;36:65–73.
180. Wardlaw JM, Dennis MS, Warlow CP, Sandercock PA. Imaging appearance of the symptomatic perforating artery in patients with lacunar infarction: occlusion or other vascular pathology? Ann Neurol 2001;50:208–215.
181. Van der Eecken H. Anastomoses between the leptomeningeal arteries of the brain. Springfield, IL: Charles C. Thomas, 1959.
182. Paulson GW, Kapp J, Cook W. Dementia associated with bilateral carotid artery disease. Geriatrics 1966;21:159–166.
183. Torvik A. The pathogenesis of watershed infarcts in the brain. Stroke 1984;15:221–223.
184. Dickson DW. Neuropathology of Alzheimer's disease and other dementias. Clin Geriatr Med 2001;17:209–228.
185. Dickson DW, Davies P, Bevona C, et al. Hippocampal sclerosis: a common pathological feature of dementia in very old (>or = 80 years of age) humans. Acta Neuropathol (Berl) 1994;88:212–221.
186. Jellinger KA. Hippocampal sclerosis: a common pathological feature of dementia in very old humans. Acta Neuropathol (Berl) 1994;88:599.
187. Mielke R, Herholz K, Grond M, Kessler J, Heiss WD. Severity of vascular dementia is related to volume of metabolically impaired tissue. Arch Neurol 1992;49:909–913.
188. Erkinjuntti T, Benavente O, Eliasziw M, et al. Diffuse vacuolization (spongiosis) and arteriolosclerosis in the frontal white matter occurs in vascular dementia. Arch Neurol 1996;53:325–332.
189. Basso A, Capitani E, Luzzatti C, Spinnler H. Intelligence and left hemisphere disease. The role of aphasia, apraxia and size of lesion. Brain 1981;104:721–734.

190. Cummings JL, Benson DF. Psychological dysfunction accompanying subcortical dementias. Annu Rev Med 1988;39:53–61.
191. Tatemichi TK, Sacktor N, Mayeux R. Dementia associated with cerebrovascular disease, other degenerative diseases, and metabolic disorders. In: Terr RD, Katzman R, Bick KL, eds. Alzheimer's Disease. New York, NY: Raven Press, 1994, pp. 123–166.
192. Bhatia KP, Marsden CD. The behavioural and motor consequences of focal lesions of the basal ganglia in man. Brain 1994;117:859–876.
193. Caplan LR. Caudate infarcts. In: Donnan G, Norrving B, Bamford J, Bogousslavsky J, eds. Subcortical Stroke. 2nd Ed. Oxford, UK: Oxford University Press, 2002, pp. 208–223.
194. Tatemichi TK, Desmond DW, Prohovnik I. Strategic infarcts in vascular dementia. A clinical and brain imaging experience. Arzneimittelforschung 1995;45:371–385.
195. Tatemichi TK, Desmond DW, Prohovnik I, et al. Confusion and memory loss from capsular genu infarction: a thalamocortical disconnection syndrome? Neurology 1992;42:1966–1979.
196. Du AT, Schuff N, Laakso MP, et al. Effects of subcortical ischemic vascular dementia and AD on entorhinal cortex and hippocampus. Neurology 2002;58:1635–1641.
197. Kril JJ, Patel S, Harding AJ, Halliday GM. Patients with vascular dementia due to microvascular pathology have significant hippocampal neuronal loss. J Neurol Neurosurg Psychiatry 2002;72:747–751.
198. Cordoliani-Mackowiak MA, Henon H, Pruvo JP, Pasquier F, Leys D. Poststroke dementia: influence of hippocampal atrophy. Arch Neurol 2003;60:585–590.
199. Mirra SS, Heyman A, McKeel D, et al. The Consortium to Establish a Registry for Alzheimer's Disease (CERAD). Part II. Standardization of the neuropathologic assessment of Alzheimer's disease. Neurology 1991;41:479–486.
200. McKeith IG, Galasko D, Kosaka K, et al. Consensus guidelines for the clinical and pathologic diagnosis of dementia with Lewy bodies (DLB): report of the consortium on DLB international workshop. Neurology 1996;47:1113–1124.
201. Del Tredici K, Rub U, De Vos RA, Bohl JR, Braak H. Where does Parkinson disease pathology begin in the brain? J Neuropathol Exp Neurol 2002;61:413–426.
202. Fearnley JM, Lees AJ. Pathology of Parkinson disease. In: Calne D, ed. Neurodegenerative Diseases. Philadelphia, PA: WB Saunders, 1994, pp. 545–554.
203. Revesz T, Ghiso J, Lashley T, Plant G, Rostagno A, Frangione B, Holton JL. Cerebral amyloid angiopathies: a pathologic, biochemical, and genetic view. J Neuropathol Exp Neurol 2003;62:885–898.
204. Vinters HV, Farag ES. Amyloidosis of cerebral arteries. In: Barnett HJM, Bogousslavsky J, Meldrum H, eds. Ischemic Stroke: Advances in Neurology, Vol. 92. Philadelphia, PA: Lippincott Williams & Wilkins, 2003, pp. 105–120.
205. Thal DR, Ghebremedhin E, Rub U, Yamaguchi H, Tredici KD, Braak H. Two types of sporadic cerebral amyloid angiopathy. J Neuropathol Exp Neurol 2002;61:282–293.
206. Greenberg SM, Vonsattel JP, Segal AZ, et al. Association of apolipoprotein E e2 and vasculopathy in cerebral amyloid angiopathy. Neurology 1998;50:961–965.
207. Itoh Y, Yamada M, Hayakawa M, Otomo E, Miyatake T. Cerebral amyloid angiopathy: a significant cause of cerebellar as well as lobar cerebral hemorrhage in the elderly. J Neurol Sci 1993;116:135–141.
208. Jellinger KA. Alzheimer disease and cerebrovascular pathology: an update. J Neural Transm 2002;109:813–836.
209. Masuda J, Tanaka K, Ueda K, Omae T. Autopsy study of incidence and distribution of cerebral amyloid angiopathy in Hisayama, Japan. Stroke 1988;19:205–210.
210. Scholz W. Studien zur Pathologie der Hirngefässe II: Die drusige Entartung der Hirnarterien und Capillaren. Z Ges Neurol Psychiat 1938;162:694–715.
211. Tomonaga M. Cerebral amyloid angiopathy in the elderly. J Am Geriatr Soc 1981;29:151–157.
212. Vinters HV, Gilbert JJ. Cerebral amyloid angiopathy: incidence and complications in the aging brain. II. The distribution of amyloid vascular changes. Stroke 1983;14:924–928.
213. Yoshimura M, Yamanouchi H, Kuzuhara S, et al. Dementia in cerebral amyloid angiopathy: a clinicopathological study. J Neurol 1992;239:441–450.
214. Yamada M, Tsukagoshi H, Otomo E, Hayakawa M. Cerebral amyloid angiopathy in the aged. J Neurol 1987;234:371–376.
215. Bergeron C, Ranalli PJ, Miceli PN. Amyloid angiopathy in Alzheimer's disease. Can J Neurol Sci 1987;14:564–569.
216. Ellis RJ, Olichney JM, Thal LJ, et al. Cerebral amyloid angiopathy in the brains of patients with Alzheimer's disease: the CERAD experience, Part XV. Neurology 1996;46:1592–1596.
217. Esiri MM, Wilcock GK. Cerebral amyloid angiopathy in dementia and old age. J Neurol Neurosurg Psychiatry 1986;49: 1221–1226.
218. Vonsattel JP, Myers RH, Hedley-Whyte ET, Ropper AH, Bird ED, Richardson EP, Jr. Cerebral amyloid angiopathy without and with cerebral hemorrhages: a comparative histological study. Ann Neurol 1991;30:637–649.
219. Kalaria RN, Ballard C. Overlap between pathology of Alzheimer disease and vascular dementia. Alzheimer Dis Assoc Disord 1999;13(Suppl 3):S115–S123.
220. Farkas E, Luiten PG. Cerebral microvascular pathology in aging and Alzheimer's disease. Prog Neurobiol 2001;64:575–611.

221. Olichney JM, Ellis RJ, Katzman R, Sabbagh MN, Hansen L. Types of cerebrovascular lesions associated with severe cerebral amyloid angiopathy in Alzheimer's disease. Ann N Y Acad Sci 1997;826:493–497.
222. Kalaria RN. The role of cerebral ischemia in Alzheimer's disease. Neurobiol Aging 2000;21:321–330.
223. Lee SS, Stemmermann GN. Congophilic angiopathy and cerebral hemorrhage. Arch Pathol Lab Med 1978;102:317–321.
224. Ishii N, Nishihara Y, Horie A. Amyloid angiopathy and lobar cerebral haemorrhage. J Neurol Neurosurg Psychiatry 1984;47:1203–1210.
225. Feldmann E, Tornabene J. Diagnosis and treatment of cerebral amyloid angiopathy. Clin Geriatr Med 1991;7: 617–630.
226. Hill MD, Silver FL, Austin PC, Tu JV. Rate of stroke recurrence in patients with primary intracerebral hemorrhage. Stroke 2000;31:123–127.
227. Olichney JM, Hansen LA, Hofstetter CR, Lee JH, Katzman R, Thal LJ. Association between severe cerebral amyloid angiopathy and cerebrovascular lesions in Alzheimer disease is not a spurious one attributable to apolipoprotein E epsilon4. Arch Neurol 2000;57:869–874.
228. Cadavid D, Mena H, Koeller K, Frommelt RA. Cerebral beta amyloid angiopathy is a risk factor for cerebral ischemic infarction. A case control study in human brain biopsies. J Neuropathol Exp Neurol 2000;59:768–773.
229. Tabaton M, Caponnetto C, Mancardi G, Loeb C. Amyloid beta protein deposition in brains from elderly subjects with leukoariosis. J Neurol Sci 1991;106:123–127.
230. Wattendorff AR, Frangione B, Luyendijk W, Bots GT. Hereditary cerebral haemorrhage with amyloidosis, Dutch type (HCHWA-D): clinicopathological studies. J Neurol Neurosurg Psychiatry 1995;58:699–705.
231. Grabowski TJ, Cho HS, Vonsattel JP, Rebeck GW, Greenberg SM. Novel amyloid precursor protein mutation in an Iowa family with dementia and severe cerebral amyloid angiopathy. Ann Neurol 2001;49:697–705.
232. Abrahamson M, Jonsdottir S, Olafsson I, Jensson O, Grubb A. Hereditary cystatin C amyloid angiopathy: identification of the disease-causing mutation and specific diagnosis by polymerase chain reaction based analysis. Hum Genet 1992; 89:377–380.
233. Hendriks L, van Duijn CM, Cras P, et al. Presenile dementia and cerebral haemorrhage linked to a mutation at codon 692 of the beta-amyloid precursor protein gene. Nat Genet 1992;1:218–221.
234. Tagliavini F, Rossi G, Padovani A, et al. A new βPP mutationrelated to hereditary cerebral hemorrhage. Alz Reports 1999;2:S28.
235. Nilsberth C, Westlind-Danielsson A, Eckman CB, et al. The 'Arctic' APP mutation (E693G) causes Alzheimer's disease by enhanced Abeta protofibril formation. Nat Neurosci 2001;4:887–893.
236. Wang Z, Natte R, Berliner JA, van Duinen SG, Vinters HV. Toxicity of Dutch (E22Q) and Flemish (A21G) mutant amyloid beta proteins to human cerebral microvessel and aortic smooth muscle cells. Stroke 2000;31:534–538.
237. Levy E, Sastre M, Kumar A, et al. Codeposition of cystatin C with amyloid-beta protein in the brain of Alzheimer disease patients. J Neuropathol Exp Neurol 2001;60:94–104.
238. Natté R, Maat-Schieman ML, Haan J, Bornebroek M, Roos RA, van Duinen SG. Dementia in hereditary cerebral hemorrhage with amyloidosis—Dutch type is associated with cerebral amyloid angiopathy but is independent of plaques and neurofibrillary tangles. Ann Neurol 2001;50:765–772.
239. Benson MD. Leptomeningeal amyloid and variant transthyretins. Am J Pathol 1996;148:351–354.
240. Blevins G, Macaulay R, Harder S, et al. Oculoleptomeningeal amyloidosis in a large kindred with a new transthyretin variant Tyr69His. Neurology 2003;60:1625–1630.
241. Haltia M, Ghiso J, Prelli F, et al. Amyloid in familial amyloidosis, Finnish type, is antigenically and structurally related to gelsolin. Am J Pathol 1990;136:1223–1228.
242. Kiuru S, Salonen O, Haltia M. Gelsolin-related spinal and cerebral amyloid angiopathy. Ann Neurol 1999;45: 305–311.
243. Mayer M, Straube A, Bruening R, et al. Muscle and skin biopsies are a sensitive diagnostic tool in the diagnosis of CADASIL. J Neurol 1999;246:526–532.
244. Yousry TA, Seelos K, Mayer M, et al. Characteristic MR lesion pattern and correlation of T1 and T2 lesion volume with neurologic and neuropsychological findings in cerebral autosomal dominant arteriopathy with subcortical infarcts and leukoencephalopathy (CADASIL). AJNR Am J Neuroradiol 1999;20:91–100.
245. Vidal R, Frangione B, Rostagno A, et al. A stop-codon mutation in the BRI gene associated with familial British dementia. Nature 1999;399:776–781.
246. Vidal R, Revesz T, Rostagno A, et al. A decamer duplication in the 3' region of the BRI gene originates an amyloid peptide that is associated with dementia in a Danish kindred. Proc Natl Acad Sci USA 2000;97:4920–4925.
247. Holton JL, Lashley T, Ghiso J, et al. Familial Danish dementia: a novel form of cerebral amyloidosis associated with deposition of both amyloid-Dan and amyloid-beta. J Neuropathol Exp Neurol 2002;61:254–267.
248. Tohgi H, Abe T, Kimura M, Saheki M, Takahashi S. Cerebrospinal fluid acetylcholine and choline in vascular dementia of Binswanger and multiple small infarct types as compared with Alzheimer-type dementia. J Neural Transm 1996;103: 1211–1220.
249. Mesulam M, Siddique T, Cohen B. Cholinergic denervation in a pure multi-infarct state: observations on CADASIL. Neurology 2003;60.

250. Oldfors A, Fyhr IM, Holme E, Larsson NG, Tulinius M. Neuropathology in Kearns-Sayre syndrome. Acta Neuropathol (Berl) 1990;80:541–546.
251. Powers JM, DeVivo DC. Peroxismal and mitochondrial disorders. In: Graham D, Lantos P, eds. Greenfield's Neuropathology. 7th Ed. London, UK: Arnold Publishing, 2002, pp. 737–797.
252. Muller-Hocker J, Hubner G, Bise K, et al. Generalized mitochondrial microangiopathy and vascular cytochrome c oxidase deficiency. Occurrence in a case of MELAS syndrome with mitochondrial cardiomyopathy-myopathy and combined complex I/IV deficiency. Arch Pathol Lab Med 1993;117:202–210.
253. Sparaco M, Bonilla E, DiMauro S, Powers JM. Neuropathology of mitochondrial encephalomyopathies due to mitochondrial DNA defects. J Neuropathol Exp Neurol 1993;52:1–10.
254. Ohama E, Ohara S, Ikuta F, Tanaka K, Nishizawa M, Miyatake T. Mitochondrial angiopathy in cerebral blood vessels of mitochondrial encephalomyopathy. Acta Neuropathol (Berl) 1987;74:226–233.
255. Love S, Hilton DA. Assessment of the distribution of mitochondrial ribosomal RNA in melas and in thrombotic cerebral infarcts by in situ hybridization. J Pathol 1996;178:182–189.
256. Bowler J, Hachinski V. Vascular dementia. In: Ginsberg M, Bogousslavsky J, eds. Cerebrovascular disease. II: Pathophysiology, Diagnosis and Management. Oxford, UK: Blackwell Science, 1998, pp. 1126–1144.
257. Kaye JA. Diagnostic challenges in dementia. Neurology 1998;51:S45–S52; discussion S65-7.
258. Mendez MF, Mastri AR, Sung JH, Frey WH. Clinically diagnosed Alzheimer disease: neuropathologic findings in 650 cases. Alzheimer Dis Assoc Disord 1992;6:35–43.
259. Esiri MM, Nagy Z, Smith MZ, Barnetson L, Smith AD. Cerebrovascular disease and threshold for dementia in the early stages of Alzheimer's disease. Lancet 1999;354:919–920.
260. Katzman R, Brown T, Thal LJ, et al. Comparison of rate of annual change of mental status score in four independent studies of patients with Alzheimer's disease. Ann Neurol 1988;24:384–389.
261. Lee JH, Olichney JM, Hansen LA, Hofstetter CR, Thal LJ. Small concomitant vascular lesions do not influence rates of cognitive decline in patients with Alzheimer disease. Arch Neurol 2000;57:1474–1479.
262. O'Brien KD, Olin KL, Alpers CE, et al. Comparison of apolipoprotein and proteoglycan deposits in human coronary atherosclerotic plaques: colocalization of biglycan with apolipoproteins. Circulation 1998;98:519–527.
263. Cohen CI, Araujo L, Guerrier R, Henry KA. "Mixed dementia": adequate or antiquated? A critical review. Am J Geriatr Psychiatry 1997;5:279–283.
264. Rockwood K. Lessons from mixed dementia. Int Psychogeriatr 1997;9:245–249.
265. O'Brien MD. Vascular dementia is underdiagnosed. Arch Neurol 1988;45:797–798.
266. Jellinger KA, Attems J. Incidence of cerebrovascular lesions in Alzheimer disease: a postmortem study. Acta Neuropathol 2003;105:14–17.
267. Nagy Z, Esiri MM, Jobst KA, et al. The effects of additional pathology on the cognitive deficit in Alzheimer Disease. J Neuropathol Exp Neurol 1997;56:165–170.
268. Gearing M, Mirra SS, Hedreen JC, Sumi SM, Hansen LA, Heyman A. The Consortium to Establish a Registry for Alzheimer's Disease (CERAD), Part X: Neuropathology confirmation of the clinical diagnosis of Alzheimer's disease. Neurology 1995;45:461–466.
269. Crystal H, Dickson D. Cerebral infarcts in patients with autopsy proven Alzheimer's disease (abstract). Neurobiol Aging 2002;23:207.
270. Jellinger KA, Attems J. Incidence of cerebrovascular lesions in Alzheimer's disease: a postmortem study. Acta Neuropathol (Berl) 2003;105:14–17.
271. Fayet G, Hauw JJ, Delaere P, et al. Neuropathology of 20 centenarians. I: Clinical data. Rev Neurol 1994;150:16–21.
272. Giannakopoulos P, Hof PR, Surini M, Michel JP, Bouras C. Quantitative immunohistochemical analysis of the distribution of neurofibrillary tangles and senile plaques in the cerebral cortex of nonagenarians and centenarians. Acta Neuropathol 1993;85:602–610.
273. Mizutani T, Shimada H. Neuropathological background of twenty-seven centenarian brains. J Neurol Sci 1992;108:168–177.
274. Aliev G, Smith MA, Seyidov D, et al. The role of oxidative stress in the pathophysiology of cerebrovascular lesions in Alzheimer's disease. Brain Pathol 2002;12:21–35.
275. De La Torre JC. Alzheimer disease as a vascular disorder: nosological evidence. Stroke 2002;33:1152–1162.
276. Grammas P, Moore P, Weigel PH. Microvessels from Alzheimer's disease brains kill neurons in vitro. Am J Pathol 1999;154:337–342.
277. Sparks DL. Coronary artery disease: hypertension, ApoE, and cholesterol: a link to Alzheimer's disease? Ann NY Acad Sci 1997;826:128–146.
278. Sparks DL, Hunsaker JC, 3rd, Scheff SW, Kryscio RJ, Henson JL, Markesbery WR. Cortical senile plaques in coronary artery disease, aging and Alzheimer's disease. Neurobiol Aging 1990;11:601–607.
279. Kovari E, Gold G, Herrmann FR, et al. Cortical microinfarcts and demyelination significantly affect cognition in brain aging. Stroke 2004;35:410–414.
280. Corbett A, Bennett H, Kos S. Cognitive dysfunction following subcortical infarction. Arch Neurol 1994;51:999–1007.

281. Heyman A, Fillenbaum G, Welsh-Bohmer K, et al. Cerebral infarcts in patients with autopsy-proven Alzheimer's disease, CERAD, Part XVIII (abstract). Neurology 1998;51:159–162.
282. Frisoni GB, Geroldi C. Cerebrovascular disease affects noncognitive symptoms in Alzheimer disease. Arch Neurol 2001;58:1939–1940.
283. Brun A. Neuropathology of cerebrovascular lesions in dementia. Seventh International Conference on Alzheimer's Disease and Related Disorders. Neurobiol Aging 2000;21:S7.

4

Diagnosis of Vascular Dementia

Conceptual Challenges

José G. Merino and Vladimir Hachinski

Before I build a wall I'd ask to know
What I was walling in or walling out.

Robert Frost

1. INTRODUCTION

Vascular dementia (VaD) is diagnosed when a syndrome of dementia or cognitive impairment is found concurrently with evidence of cerebrovascular disease (CVD). There are no pathognomonic neuropathological lesions of vascular dementia—no individual pathological feature has any value in relation to an individual case—because subjects with and without dementia can have similar changes *(1)*. This means that VaD is a theoretical construct *(2)*; therefore, diagnosis relies on criteria defined in terms of clinically identifiable features. The validity of the criteria depends on whether they satisfy the requirements of construct, content, and criterion validity *(2)*.

Several groups have put forth diagnostic criteria for vascular dementia. Their characteristics, strengths, and shortcomings are discussed below. The features that comprise each set of criteria reflect the features that their authors consider essential and are shaped by theoretical notions of what constitutes VaD. To be useful, diagnostic systems and criteria must fulfill two roles: enhance clinical care and promote productive scientific research *(3)*. The first objective is met when diagnostic criteria "reduce the clinical uncertainty and contribute to an understanding of clinical problems that results in the design, implementation, and assessment of useful intervention strategies" *(3)*. Criteria promote scientific research when they lead to the design and implementation of high-quality studies whose results provide an understanding of the pathophysiology of the disease and when they facilitate communication among scientists about epidemiology, clinical features, etiology, prognosis, and effects of treatment *(3)*. As we discuss in this chapter, the current criteria fulfill these requirements only partially. They are of limited value in clinical care because they focus on patients who have severe cognitive impairment in whom strategies to prevent or modify the course of dementia are no longer useful and they are restricted to patients with prominent memory loss, excluding patients whose major cognitive decline is in other domains. They hamper research efforts because they are not interchangeable *(4–6)*, have poor sensitivity *(7)*, do not allow for mixed states, and make comparison between studies difficult.

2. DIAGNOSTIC CRITERIA

The criteria for VaD that are most frequently used for research, clinical care, and health planning are the *Diagnostic and Statistical Manual of Mental Disorders*, 4th ed. (DSM-IV) *(8)*; the *Interna-*

From: *Current Clinical Neurology*
Vascular Dementia: Cerebrovascular Mechanisms and Clinical Management
Edited by: R. H. Paul, R. Cohen, B. R. Ott, and S. Salloway © Humana Press Inc., Totowa, NJ

tional Classification of Diseases, 10th ed. (ICD-10) *(9,10)*; the State of California Alzheimer Disease Diagnostic and Treatment Centers (SCADDTC) criteria *(11)*; and the criteria of the National Institute of Neurological Disorders and Stroke–Association Internationale pour la Recherche et l'Enseignement en Neurosciences (NINDS-AIREN) *(12)*. The first two are categorical diagnostic systems that classify patients with dementia into several exclusive diagnostic groups; patients with the same or similar symptom patterns belong to a given category that summarizes the basic information about that patient, and VaD is one of the categories within the system. They provide general guidelines for diagnosis. The SCADDTC and NINDS-AIREN criteria are not part of a diagnostic system but operationalize the requirements for diagnosis and list clinical and radiological features that support or are required for establishing the diagnosis. They classify patients as having or not having VaD but do not provide criteria for alternative diagnoses. All the criteria place patients into exclusionary groups: patients within a category or group have a unique set of features that is both sufficient and necessary for membership in the diagnostic category *(13)*. Recently, other criteria have been proposed (DSM-IV text revision [TR] *[14]* and the Mayo Clinic Criteria *[15])*, but they have not been widely used.

All the current criteria were established by consensual agreement among experts and are not derived from prospective population studies or based on detailed natural histories *(16,17)*. To diagnose VaD dementia the current criteria require the presence of a syndrome (dementia) and an association with a pathophysiological mechanism (CVD) *(18)*. However, they differ in the specifics of how the dementia syndrome is defined, the clinical and radiological features that are required to consider CVD as pathophysiologically significant, and what constitutes an etiologic relationship between both processes. Table 1 lists the features of the criteria.

Differences in the elements that comprise these criteria mean that they are not interchangeable. According to the set of criteria used, different patients are diagnosed with the syndrome of dementia *(4,19)* and VaD *(5,6,20,21)*, as detailed in Table 2 (the differences between studies result from differences in the population under study). The lack of comparability is a barrier to research and clinical care and has a significant effect on health care policy *(6)*.

There are several criteria for the pathological diagnosis of Alzheimer's disease (AD) *(22,23)*, but none for vascular dementia. Very few studies that validate the clinical criteria with neuropathological examination have been conducted *(7,24)*; these have used *ad hoc* criteria that reflect the multiinfarct dementia (MID) model, thus the studies only evaluate the validity of diagnostic criteria for the detection of MID. Given the heterogeneity of stroke and the variety of possible lesions of vascular origin in the brain, these definitions are too narrow. None of the criteria are sensitive, but some have relatively high specificity, as shown in Table 3.

The reliability of a diagnostic system refers to the consistency with which subjects are classified as having a given condition. The current criteria are not interchangeable and are neither sensitive nor specific; therefore, they are unreliable. As Spitzer and Fleiss highlight, there is no guarantee that a reliable system is valid, but assuredly an unreliable system must be invalid *(25)*. The construct of VaD, as currently understood and operationalized in these criteria, has significant flaws. Before new criteria are written, several conceptual issues regarding the vascular pathology and the severity, course, and nature of cognitive impairment that characterize patients with VaD must be clarified.

3. THE COGNITIVE SYNDROME IN VASCULAR DEMENTIA

The criteria for VaD were written at a time when the Alzheimer's paradigm was dominant and, therefore, require early prominent memory loss, impairment of normal daily activities, and a progressive and irreversible course *(17)*. However, the cognitive impairment in patients with CVD or vascular risk factors does not always share these features *(26)*, but this is not reflected in the current criteria.

Table 1
Diagnostic Criteria for Vascular Dementia

Criteria		SCADDTC *(11)* [a]	NINDS-AIREN *(12)* [a]	ICD-10 (Research) *(10)*	DSM-IV *(144)*
Dementia syndrome	Cognitive domains	Deterioration in more than one category of intellectual performance, independent of level of consciousness	Memory and two or more cognitive domains	Unequal distribution of deficits in higher cognitive functions (requires memory impairment, which must be present for 6 mo, executive dysfunction, and emotional control)	Memory impairment AND one or more of the following: aphasia, apraxia, agnosia, disturbance in executive function
	Severity	Deterioration form a known or estimated prior level of intellectual function sufficient to interfere broadly with the conduct of the patient's customary affairs of life	Decline from a previously higher level of functioning; deficits sufficiently severe to interfere with activities of daily living (ADLs) not resulting from physical effects of stroke alone	Impairments of ADLs must result from cognitive deficits and not from physical dysfunction	The cognitive criteria cause significant impair ment in social or occupational functioning and epresent a significant decline from a previous level of functioning
	Documentation	Must be supported by historical evidence and documented by bedside mental status testing or neuropsychological examination	Clinical examination and neuropsychological testing	Must be objectively verifiable by history and neuropsychological testing	Not specified
CVD	Deficits on physical examination	Evidence of two or more ischemic strokes by history, neurologic signs, and/or neuroimaging studies (CT or T1-weighted MRI) OR occurrence of single stroke with clearly documented temporal relationship to the onset of dementia	Focal signs on neurological examination consistent with stroke (with or without history of stroke) and evidence of relevant CVD on brain imaging	Evidence of focal brain damage: unilateral spastic weakness of limbs, unilateral increased tendon reflexes, extensor plantar response, and pseudobulbar palsy	Focal neurological signs and symptoms that are judged to be etiologically related to the disturbance

Continued on next page

Table 1 *(continued)*
Diagnostic Criteria for Vascular Dementia

Criteria		SCADDTC *(11)*[a]	NINDS-AIREN *(12)*[a]	ICD-10 (Research) *(10)*	DSM-IV *(144)*
	Imaging	Required: evidence of at least one infarct outside the cerebellum by CT or MRI	Required: large-vessel infarcts or a single strategically placed infarct, as well as multiple ganglia and white matter basal lacunes, or extensive periventricular white matter lesions, or combinations thereof	Not required (VERIFY!)	Not required
	Etiologic relationship between CVD and dementia	Temporal relationship required if only a single stroke is documented	A relationship is inferred by onset of dementia within 3 mo of stroke, abrupt deterioration or fluctuating, stepwise progression	Not specified clearly, a relationship must be "reasonably judged" to exist	
Subtypes		Yes: cortical, subcortical, Binswanger's disease, and thalamic dementia	Do not specify but recommend description of stroke features for research purposes	Allows subtypes—6 with only superficial clinical description: acute onset, MID, subcortical, mixed cortical and subcortical, other, and unspecified	None
Levels of certainty		Yes. also has mixed dementia category	Yes, probable, possible, definite		
WML		WML do not qualify as imaging evidence of CVD for probable diagnosis but may support possible IVD			
Mixed dementia?		Mixed dementia to be diagnosed in the presence of one or more systemic or brain disorders that are believed to be causally related to the dementia	AD with CVD—patients who fulfill criteria for possible AD and who also present clinical or imaging evidence of relevant vascular brain lesions. Include dementias resulting from hypoperfusion from cardiac dysrhythmias and pump failure		

[a] Probable vascular dementia
Abbr: AD, Alzheimer's disease; CVD, cerebrovascular disease; CT, computed tomography; MID, multiinfarct dementia; MRI, magnetic resonance imaging; WML, white matter lesion.

Table 2
Agreement in Patient Classification Resulting From Various Criteria

Criteria	Chui et al., 2000 *(5)* $n = 25$	Pohjasvaara et al., 2000 *(6)* $n = 107$	Amar et al., 1996 *(20)* [a] $n = 20$	Amar et al., 1996 *(20)* [b] $n = 20$	Wetterling et al., 1996 *(21)* $n = 167$	Verhey et al., 1996 *(145)* $n = 124$
DSM-IV	25.7%	91.6%			27%	
SCADDTC probable	10.3%	86.9%	40%	20%	13%	12%
SCADDTC possible	14.3%		55%	35%		
SCADDTC probable and possible	20.6%		95%	55%		
NINDS-AIREN probable	5.1%	32.7%	40%	5%	7%	6%
NINDS-AIREN possible	6.3%		40%	20%		
NINDS-AIREN probable and possible	6.3%		80%	25%		
DSM-III		36.4%				
ICD-10		36.4%			13%	

[a] Hachinski Ischemic score > = 7.
[b] Hachinski Ischemic score = 4–6.
Abbr: DSM-IV, *Diagnostic and Statistical Manual of Mental Disorders*, 4th Ed.; SCADDTC, State of California Alzheimer Disease Diagnostic and Treatment Centers; NINDS-AIREN, National Institute of Neurological Disorders and Stroke-Association Internationale pour la Recherche et l'Enseignement en Neurosciences.

Data regarding the severity, nature, and course of cognitive impairment in patients with CVD must be collected, preferably through the prospective study of population cohorts *(27)*. Issues to consider when drafting these criteria are the threshold of cognitive impairment that will identify cases at a point when therapeutic and preventive strategies are possible, the cognitive domains that must be affected to qualify as a case, and the course of cognitive impairment in patients with VaD.

3.1. *Severity of Cognitive Impairment After Stroke*

Current criteria focus on patients with significant functional impairment and, therefore, identify patients with end-stage VaD *(28)*. This is a tragic shortcoming because in many patients, CVD is preventable *(29)*. Research and clinical efforts must identify patients who are at risk of developing dementia—those with vascular risk factors or CVD *(1)*. Focusing on the broad concept of vascular cognitive impairment instead of VaD can help us identify subjects who are at risk of dementia in whom vascular risk factors have an etiopathogenetic role *(30,31)*. The criteria should be set at a sensitive rather than specific level *(32)*.

3.2. *Cognitive Deficits in Patients With Vascular Disease*

In patients with CVD, other cognitive functions are affected as least as often as memory *(33–43)*. Pohjasvaara and coworkers found that, 3 mo after a stroke, 62, 35, and 27% of patients had cognitive decline in 1, 2, and 3 or more domains, respectively, *(44)*. In a separate series, Desmond et al. *(43)* found that patients with stroke and memory impairment at 3 mo always have deficits in one or more additional cognitive domains and that most patients have deficits in two or more. The domains

Table 3
Sensitivity and Specificity of Diagnostic Criteria

	Gold et al., 2002 *(7)* $n = 89$		Knopman et al., 2003 *(24)* $n = 89$			
	Vascular dementia		Pure vascular dementia		Broad vascular dementia	
	Sensitivity, %	Specificity, %	Sensitivity, %	Specificity, %	Sensitivity, %	Specificity, %
NINDS-AIREN probable, excluding WMLs	20	93	17	97	13	98
NINDS-AIREN possible, excluding WMLs			25	96	22	98
NINDS-AIREN possible	55	88				
DSM-IV, excluding WMLs	50	84	67	69	70	76
DSM-IV, including MLs			75	64	74	70
ICD-10	20	94	75	74	70	80
SCADDTC possible	70	78				
SCADDTC probable	25	94	67	79	57	83
Mayo criteria, excluding WMLs			75	81	65	86
Mayo criteria, including WMLs			75	73	70	79

Abbr: DSM-IV, *Diagnostic and Statistical Manual of Mental Disorders*, 4th Ed.; ICD-10, *International Classification of Diseases*, 10th Ed.; NINDS-AIREN, National Institute of Neurological Disorders and Stroke-Association Internationale pour la Recherche et l'Enseignement en Neurosciences; SCADDTC, State of California Alzheimer Disease Diagnostic and Treatment Centers; WMLs, white matter lesions.

that were affected most often in these cohorts were construction and visuospatial skills, memory, executive function, orientation, and attention *(41,44)*. Patients with vascular risk factors in midlife have cognitive impairment, particularly of executive function, later in life *(45)*. If the diagnostic criteria for VaD require memory impairment for diagnosis, then they will prove in a circular argument that memory is the major impairment *(17)*. It also means that a large number of patients who have primary decline in other cognitive domains are not diagnosed with VaD *(17,46,47)*. The domains that are affected in an individual patient depend on the nature, severity, and location of the vascular insults and on the coexistence of other pathologies. The relationship between neuropsychological deficits and specific vascular pathologies must be researched further so that meaningful subgroups can be identified clinically for routine care and research purposes.

3.3. *The Prognosis of Cognitive Impairment*

AD is an unrelenting progressive illness, but patients with VaD have a more variable course. Among 53 patients with minor stroke or TIA and cognitive impairment recruited from a stroke clinic, Bowler and colleagues found that only 24 had abrupt onset, and symptoms improved over time in all *(48)*. Gradual evolution of cognitive decline is also found in some patients with stroke-related dementia *(42,49,50)*, and it is clear that individuals can have a slowly progressive dementing illness caused by CVD *(51,52)*. Some patients with cognitive impairment after a stroke can get better *(34,53)*. Desmond and colleagues found that almost 15% of 151 patients who had cognitive impairment 3 mo after a stroke had improvement by the time of the 1-yr examination *(54)*, and when only those who met prespecified criteria for cognitive impairment were considered, 36% had improvement. The course of the deficits in the various subgroups needs further clarification.

4. VASCULAR DISEASE LEADING TO DEMENTIA

VaD is a syndrome that is as heterogeneous as CVD itself. However, traditional criteria treat it as a homogenous condition associated with a specific etiopathogenetic mechanism *(55)*. Unless the heterogeneity is incorporated into the concept of VaD, the construct will be too narrow. In addition, lack of recognition of the heterogeneity means that it will not be addressed in clinical trials and prospective studies, potentially leading to the rejection of therapeutic interventions that may be useful for a subgroup of patients with CVD and cognitive decline.

4.1. *Heterogeneity of Lesions*

Cognitive decline in patients with CVD results from the stroke itself, when a large volume of brain is affected by ischemia or hemorrhage *(44,45)* or when the lesion, because of its strategic location *(46)*, interrupts brain circuits that are critical for cognition *(47)*. Diseases of the large arteries and the heart can lead to cerebral hypoperfusion *(56,57)*, and a variety of conditions that predispose to cerebral hypoxia have been associated with the development of dementia after stroke *(58,59)*. The NINDS-AIREN criteria specify the vascular lesions that support the diagnosis of vascular dementia but do not describe specific subgroups *(12)*. These lesions include multiple large-vessel and single strategically placed infarcts, multiple basal ganglia and white matter lacunes, and extensive periventricular white matter lesions, or combinations thereof.

4.2. *Volume and Location of Lesions*

The radiological and pathological features of the lesions that cause cognitive impairment are not well understood. Tomlinson et al. postulated that there is "an upper limit or threshold of cerebral degeneration beyond which some degree of intellectual deterioration usually occurs," and concluded that in the case of "cerebral softening this is apparently around 100 mL" *(60)*. More recent studies suggest that smaller volumes can lead to dementia, but a threshold has not been identified *(26,61–63)*. Furthermore, there are data to suggest that the level of functional tissue loss resulting from cortical deafferentation, rather than the total volume, is critical for the development of dementia *(64,65)*.

Location is at least as important as size. Strategically placed lesions lead to intellectual decline when specific cortical or subcortical areas that are important for cognition are damaged and when critical frontal-subcortical pathways are interrupted *(37,66–68)*. However, the association between strategic lesions and cognitive deficits is based on case reports that relied on computed tomography (CT) scanning and had short follow-up *(66,67,69–81)*. As a result, the contribution of cortical lesions and concurrent Alzheimer-type pathology cannot be excluded *(82)*. Further research on the location of lesions that lead to dementia, using modern neuroimaging techniques and prolonged follow-up, is warranted.

Lacunar strokes are independent predictors of dementia *(83)*, and microvascular damage, but not macroscopic infarcts, may distinguish cases of VaD from cases of stroke without dementia *(84)*. There is controversy about the role of small strokes when white matter lesion changes and atrophy are considered *(51)*. Small-vessel disease leads to lacunar infarctions and subcortical ischemic white matter changes *(85)* and, when widespread, produces a distinct syndrome characterized by cognitive impairment, personality changes, gait disturbance, motor deficits, and urinary incontinence *(85–87)*. This may constitute a clinically meaningful subgroup that may be the target of specific interventions *(87)*.

4.3. *Silent Infarcts*

Silent cerebral infarcts are common, 15–25% of individuals aged 65 or older have them *(88–94)*. Patients with clinically apparent strokes generally have larger, cortically based infarcts *(88–90,94)* or multiple infarcts *(92)*, and patients with subcortical disease often lack such a history *(52)*. The burden of recurrent silent strokes can lead to an insidious dementia *(24,93,95,96)*. Patients with silent infarcts may have symptoms of pure AD (Medical Research Council [MRC], NUN, Consortium to Establish a Registry for Alzheimer's Disease [CERAD], etc.). Silent hypoperfusion can produce hippocampal neuronal loss *(51)* or severe white matter changes *(97)*, and concurrent AD is likely important to the genesis of dementia in many individuals with asymptomatic CVD and dementia. In the Cardiovascular Health Study, there was a significant increase in the number of individuals with a history of memory loss among those with silent cerebral infarction *(98)* and a significant association between silent cerebral infarcts and decreased performance on the Mini-Mental State Examination (MMSE) and the Digit-Symbol Substitution Test *(93)*.

If silent strokes and white matter changes are important, then the requirement that clinical stroke be present is inappropriate. In a neuropathological series, the need for a temporal requirement was the main limiting factor that lead to the low sensitivity and the high rate of false negatives associated with the SCADDTC and NINDS-AIREN criteria for probable VaD *(7)*. In a separate series, the temporal relationship between stroke and dementia was the best clinical predictor of pure vascular neuropathology, but this feature had poor sensitivity because one-third of patients with pure VaD lacked a temporal relationship between a clinical stroke event and dementia *(24)*. The relationship was missing in a higher proportion of patients with mixed dementia, and a few cases with pure vascular pathology lacked a history of clinical stroke temporarily related to the onset of the dementia. Based on these findings, Knopman postulates that there are two types of VaD: one emerges from a clinical stroke event, the other more insidiously without clinically apparent stroke *(24)*. This hypothesis merits further evaluation.

4.4. *White Matter Lesions*

Changes in the white matter are related to cerebrovascular risk factors *(99–101)*. They predict future stroke *(102)* and mortality *(103)*. White matter pathology is not invariably linked with dementia, but even patients without dementia have selective cognitive deficits: attention, visuospatial memory, and frontal-executive skills are preferentially affected *(99,104,105)*. Defects in sustained mental concentration and attention, difficulty in organizing material to be learned, lack of consistency of recall, difficulties in spontaneous recalling, reduced speed of information procession *(106)*, and slowness of thought *(107)* are most often found. In the Helsinki Aging Brain Study, for example, neurologically healthy individuals who had white matter changes performed worse on the Trailmaking test part A and in the Stroop test *(108)*. The majority of studies using CT imaging in patients with dementia found an association of white matter changes with poorer cognitive performance, especially of those mediated by the frontal lobes. MRI studies have not consistently found this association *(109)*.

The association between white matter changes and cognitive impairment must be clarified. The NINDS-AIREN criteria accept changes involving more than 25% of the white matter as supportive radiological evidence for VaD, but it is not clear how that threshold was selected. The issue of white matter changes is further confounded because they are common in the brains of patients with AD. The precise relationship between white matter lesions (volume and location) and the clinical features of cognitive impairment has received little attention, but this is an important issue if subgroups, including possibly mixed AD plus CVD, are to be made based on radiological features. There is insufficient data to propose a firm cutoff for the extent of white matter abnormalities or for the extent of infarction that is required *(110)*. Future studies should be prospective, use standardized methods for structural brain imaging, and administer comprehensive neuropsychological assessments to investigate more rigorously the relationship between evolving white matter lesions and declining cognitive functions *(111)*.

4.5. *Vascular Dementia Without Stroke*

There is growing awareness that underlying vascular factors other than cerebral infarction can cause dementia (noninfarct vascular dementia) *(55,112–114)*. The brains of individuals without dementia and hypertension have more senile plaques and neurofibrillary tangles, lower weight *(115,116)*, and more radiographic white matter changes *(117)* than those of people with normal blood pressure. It is unknown if risk factors act directly by leading to stroke or whether they have a direct effect on the brain *(118)*, but there is compelling evidence to suggest the latter possibility *(96)*.

5. MIXED STATES

AD and VaD are considered diagnoses of exclusion, but recent evidence suggests that this dichotomy is artificial *(47)*. Data from population *(119,120)* and cohort studies *(121)* show that the brains of the elderly often have mixed Alzheimer-type and vascular pathology *(122)*. Among 80 subjects from the Camberwell Dementia Case Register, 33.8% had mixed pathology *(119)*, and in a large multicenter, community-based study vascular and Alzheimer-type pathology were seen in a majority of patients, and most patients had features of both *(120)*. The effect of these processes in cognition are additive *(97,121,123,124)* or even multiplicative *(32)*.

Concurrent CVD may be seen in patients with a slowly progressing illness most consistent with AD *(125)*, and a large proportion of patients with dementia after a stroke may have had cognitive impairment before the stroke. In the Framingham Study, half the people who developed cognitive impairment after stroke had preexisting difficulties *(126)*. In stroke cohorts evaluated with a standardized questionnaire that assesses cognitive function in the preceding 10 yr, cognitive decline preceded the stroke in up to 20% of patients *(127,128)*, and two-thirds of patients had a course suggestive of AD *(127)*. In a stroke cohort from New York, functional and cognitive deficits preceded the index stroke in 40% of patients who had dementia after stroke *(129,130)*. After excluding patients with prestroke dementia, 30% of patients with poststroke dementia meet criteria for AD *(58)*, and in population series, the incidence of AD among patients with stroke is 50% higher than expected *(131)*.

VaD and AD have common risk factors *(132–134)* and may share etiologic pathways *(132)*. AD is characterized by a slowly progressive capillary dysfunction in the absence of widespread focal infarction *(135)*. Vascular factors may participate in the development of cytoskeletal alterations and amyloid deposits. Large population-based epidemiological studies that began in the 1980s and early 1990s have shown that vascular risk factors contribute to the clinical and pathological presentation of AD, and experimental and pathological studies support this view *(133,136)*. Medial temporal lobe atrophy is strongly associated with AD *(137)* and is more common in stroke patients with prestroke dementia than those without *(138)*. It is a predictor of dementia after stroke *(61)*, and hippocampal and cerebral atrophy may be critical factors in determining dementia after stroke *(51)*. Patients with subcortical ischemic vascular dementia have smaller volumes of the entorhinal cortex and hippocampus than normal controls, but for similar degrees of dementia, the volumes are smaller in patients with AD than VaD *(139)*. A fundamental issue in each patient is whether the vascular changes seen in a particular patient are solely responsible for the dementia, contribute to it, or are coincidental. In addition, it is possible that the vascular and neurodegenerative changes have a common etiology or precipitating mechanism. The border between AD and VaD has become blurred as shared pathophysiological processes have been identified *(96,134,140)*. Recognizing this fact, Kalaria and Ballard propose a continuum of dementia with pure AD at one extreme, pure VaD at the other, and a wide intermediate area *(141)*; most cases of dementia may actually have mixed origin *(96)*. The burden of vascular risk factors and CVD goes beyond the traditional boundaries of the concept of VaD. Because these can be prevented, the concept of mixed etiology must be incorporated, perhaps as a specific subgroup, into the construct of VaD.

6. FUTURE PERSPECTIVES

The major obstacle to the diagnosis of VaD is that this complex nosological concept encompasses many clinical syndromes that result from a variety of pathogenic mechanisms that lead to different cognitive syndromes with varying evolution and progression *(142)*. This fact must be incorporated into the theoretical construct. Emery has suggested that one way to recognize this heterogeneity is to place the nosologic concept of VaD at a superordinate level with a number of subtypes comprising the lower categories of this hierarchical level *(55)*. These subtypes must be clinically meaningful and fulfill the criteria for a disease: the presence of a distinct pattern of clinical features that matches a distinct pathological picture *(143)*. The classification may be based on: (1) primary vascular etiology, (2) primary type of ischemic brain lesions, (3) primary location of the brain lesions, and (4) primary clinical syndrome *(87)*. Subcortical ischemic VaD is an example of such a subgroup *(85)*. Other subgroups include poststroke dementia and mixed AD plus CVD.

Only after data on the cognitive, radiological, and clinical features of patients with CVD and vascular risk factors are collected can criteria be established based on knowledge—building on the experience of large population-based epidemiological studies—and not supposition *(17)*. All investigators should use the same minimal set of standardized, validated measures and record key demographic characteristics, so that patients can be reclassified and the findings reinterpreted in light of the emerging knowledge *(1)*. Data collection must be done without the use of criteria originally to avoid proving them in a circular argument *(30)*. The focus should be the spectrum of cognitive impairment caused by vascular disease (cerebral and cardiac) and by vascular risk factors, even in the absence of frank strokes. The label "dementia" should even be abandoned. The criteria could group individuals according to a large number of shared characteristics but not require a single feature as essential to group membership (thus avoiding, for example, *sine qua non* requirement of impairment in a specific cognitive domain. This nonexclusionary approach helps classify borderline cases and addresses the heterogeneity of VaD.

The source of the patients will be important. The development and validation of diagnostic criteria for VaD cannot be done in the setting of a memory clinic, because patients with CVD may not be referred to it *(17)*. Patients may come from vascular clinics or, ideally, the study should be population based *(24)*.

REFERENCES

1. Hachinski V. Preventable senility: a call for action against the vascular dementias. Lancet 1992;340:645–648.
2. A Dictionary of Epidemiology. 3rd Ed. New York, NY: Oxford University Press,1995.
3. Poland J, von Eckardt B, Spaulding W. Problems with the DSM approach to classifying psychopathology. In: Graham G, Stephens G, ed. Philosophical Psychopathology. Cambridge, MA: MIT Press, 1994, pp. 235–260.
4. Erkinjuntti T, Ostbye T, Steenhuis R, Hachinski V. The effect of different diagnostic criteria on the prevalence of dementia. N Engl J Med 1997;337:1667–1674.
5. Chui HC, Mack W, Jackson JE, et al. Clinical criteria for the diagnosis of vascular dementia: a multicenter study of comparability and interrater reliability. Arch Neurol 2000;57:191–196.
6. Pohjasvaara T, Mantyla R, Ylikoski R, Kaste M, Erkinjuntti T. Comparison of different clinical criteria (DSM-III, ADDTC, ICD-10, NINDS-AIREN, DSM-IV) for the diagnosis of vascular dementia. National Institute of Neurological Disorders and Stroke-Association Internationale pour la Recherche et l'Enseignement en Neurosciences. Stroke 2000;31:2952–2957.
7. Gold G, Bouras C, Canuto A, et al. Clinicopathological validation study of four sets of clinical criteria for vascular dementia. Am J Psychiatry 2002;159:82–87.
8. American Psychiatric Association. Diagnostic and Statistical Manual of Mental Disorders. 4th Ed. Washington, DC: American Psychiatric Association, 1994.
9. World Health Organization. The International Classification of Diseases. 10th Ed. Geneva, Switzerland: World Health Organization, 1993.
10. World Health Organization. ICD-10 Classification of Mental and Behavioural Disorders: Diagnostic Criteria for Research. Geneva, Switzerland: World Health Organization, 1993.
11. Chui HC, Victoroff JI, Margolin D, Jagust W, Shankle R, Katzman R. Criteria for the diagnosis of ischemic vascular dementia proposed by the State of California Alzheimer's Disease Diagnostic and Treatment Centers. Neurology 1992; 42:473–480.
12. Roman GC, Tatemichi TK, Erkinjuntti T, et al. Vascular dementia: diagnostic criteria for research studies. Report of the NINDS-AIREN International Workshop. Neurology 1993;43:250–260.
13. Cantor N, Smith EE, French RS, Mezzich J. Psychiatric diagnosis as prototype categorization. J Abnorm Psychol 1980; 89:181–193.
14. American Psychiatric Association. Diagnostic and Statistical Manual of Mental Disorders. 4th Ed., text revision. Washington, DC: American Psychiatric Association, 2000.
15. Knopman DS, Rocca WA, Cha RH, Edland SD, Kokmen E. Incidence of vascular dementia in Rochester, Minn, 1985–1989. Arch Neurol 2002;59:1605–1610.
16. Drachman DA. New criteria for the diagnosis of vascular dementia: do we know enough yet? Neurology 1993;432:243–245.
17. Bowler JV. Criteria for vascular dementia: replacing dogma with data. Arch Neurol 2000;572:170–171.
18. Scheltens P, Hijdra AH. Diagnostic criteria for vascular dementia. Haemostasis 1998;28:151–157.
19. Pohjasvaara T, Erkinjuntti T, Vataja R, Kaste M. Dementia three months after stroke. Baseline frequency and effect of different definitions of dementia in the Helsinki Stroke Aging Memory Study (SAM) cohort. Stroke 1997;28:785–792.
20. Amar K, Wilcock GK, Scott M. The diagnosis of vascular dementia in the light of the new criteria. Age Ageing 1996;25:51–55.
21. Wetterling T, Kanitz RD, Borgis KJ. Comparison of different diagnostic criteria for vascular dementia (ADDTC, DSM-IV, ICD-10, NINDS-AIREN). Stroke 1996;27:30–36.
22. Mirra SS, Heyman A, McKeel D, et al. The Consortium to Establish a Registry for Alzheimer's Disease (CERAD). Part II. Standardization of the neuropathologic assessment of Alzheimer's disease. Neurology 1991;41:479–486.
23. Braak H, Braak E. Neuropathological staging of Alzheimer-related changes. Acta Neuropathol (Berl) 1991;82:239–259.
24. Knopman DS, Parisi JE, Boeve BF, et al. Vascular dementia in a population-based autopsy study. Arch Neurol 2003; 60:569–575.
25. Spitzer RL, Fleiss JL. A re-analysis of the reliability of psychiatric diagnosis. Br J Psychiatry 1974;125:341–347.
26. Del Ser T, Bermejo F, Portera A, Arredondo JM, Bouras C, Constantinidis J. Vascular dementia. A clinicopathological study. J Neurol Sci 1990;96:1–17.
27. Tatemichi TK. How acute brain failure becomes chronic: a view of the mechanisms of dementia related to stroke. Neurology 1990;40:1652–1659.
28. Bowler JV, Eliasziw M, Steenhuis R, et al. Comparative evolution of Alzheimer disease, vascular dementia, and mixed dementia. Arch Neurol 1997;54:697–703.
29. Straus SE, Majumdar SR, McAlister FA. New evidence for stroke prevention: scientific review. JAMA 2002;288: 1388–1395.
30. Bowler JV, Steenhuis R, Hachinski V. Conceptual background to vascular cognitive impairment. Alzheimer Dis Assoc Disord 1999;13(Suppl):S30–S37.
31. O'Brien JT, Erkinjuntti T, Reisberg B, et al. Vascular cognitive impairment. Lancet Neurol 2003;2:89–98.
32. Hachinski VC, Bowler JV. Vascular dementia. Neurology 1993;43:2159–2160.

33. Perez FI, Rivera VM, Meyer JS, Gay JR, Taylor RL, Mathew NT. Analysis of intellectual and cognitive performance in patients with multi-infarct dementia, vertebrobasilar insufficiency with dementia, and Alzheimer's disease. J Neurol Neurosurg Psychiatry 1975;38:533–540.
34. Wade DT, Parker V, Langton HR. Memory disturbance after stroke: frequency and associated losses. Int Rehabil Med 1986;8:60–64.
35. Babikian VL, Wolfe N, Linn R, Knoefel JE, Albert ML. Cognitive changes in patients with multiple cerebral infarcts. Stroke 1990;21:1013–1018.
36. Hom J, Reitan RM. Generalized cognitive function after stroke. J Clin Exp Neuropsychol 1990;12:644–654.
37. Wolfe N, Linn R, Babikian VL, Knoefel JE, Albert ML. Frontal systems impairment following multiple lacunar infarcts. Arch Neurol 1990;47:129–132.
38. Villardita C. Alzheimer's disease compared with cerebrovascular dementia. Neuropsychological similarities and differences. Acta Neurol Scand 1993;87:299–308.
39. Bowler JV, Hadar U, Wade JP. Cognition in stroke. Acta Neurol Scand 1994;90:424–429.
40. Breteler MM, van Swieten JC, Bots ML, et al. Cerebral white matter lesions, vascular risk factors, and cognitive function in a population-based study: the Rotterdam Study. Neurology 1994;44:1246–1252.
41. Tatemichi TK, Desmond DW, Stern Y, Paik M, Sano M, Bagiella E. Cognitive impairment after stroke: frequency, patterns, and relationship to functional abilities. J Neurol Neurosurg Psychiatry 1994;57:202–207.
42. Pohjasvaara T, Erkinjuntti T, Ylikoski R, Hietanen M, Vataja R, Kaste M. Clinical determinants of poststroke dementia. Stroke 1998;29:75–81.
43. Desmond DW, Moroney JT, Bagiella E, Sano M, Stern Y. Dementia as a predictor of adverse outcomes following stroke: an evaluation of diagnostic methods. Stroke 1998;29:69–74.
44. Pohjasvaara T, Erkinjuntti T, Vataja R, Kaste M. Dementia three months after stroke. Baseline frequency and effect of different definitions of dementia in the Helsinki Stroke Aging Memory Study (SAM) cohort. Stroke 1997;28:785–792.
45. Swan GE, DeCarli C, Miller BL, Reed T, Wolf PA, Carmelli D. Biobehavioral characteristics of nondemented older adults with subclinical brain atrophy. Neurology 2000;54:2108–2114.
46. Bowler JV. The concept of vascular cognitive impairment. J Neurol Sci 2002;203-204:11–15.
47. Roman GC. Defining dementia: clinical criteria for the diagnosis of vascular dementia. Acta Neurol Scand 2002; 178(Suppl):6–9.
48. Bowler JV, Hachinski V, Steenhuis R, Lee D. Vascular cognitive impairment; clinical, neuropsychological and imaging findings in early vascular dementia. Lancet 1998;352(Suppl 4):63.
49. Censori B, Manara O, Agostinis C, et al. Dementia after first stroke. Stroke 1996;27:1205–1210.
50. Bowirrat A, Friedland RP, Korczyn AD. Vascular dementia among elderly Arabs in Wadi Ara. J Neurol Sci 2002;203-204:73–76.
51. Fein G, Di S, V, Tanabe J, et al. Hippocampal and cortical atrophy predict dementia in subcortical ischemic vascular disease. Neurology 2000;55:1626–1635.
52. Pantoni L, Inzitari D. Pathological examination in vascular dementia. Am J Psychiatry 2002;159:1439–1440.
53. Kotila M, Waltimo O, Niemi ML, Laaksonen R, Lempinen M. The profile of recovery from stroke and factors influencing outcome. Stroke 1984;15:1039–1044.
54. Desmond DW, Moroney JT, Sano M, Stern Y. Recovery of cognitive function after stroke. Stroke 1996;27:1798–1803.
55. Emery VOB, Gillie EX, Smith JA. Noninfarct vascular dementia. The spectrum of vascular dementia and Alzheimer syndrome. In: Emery VOB, Oxman TE, eds. Dementia. Presentation, differential diagnosis and nosology. Baltimore, MD: Johns Hopkins University Press, 2003, pp. 263–290.
56. Sulkava R, Erkinjuntti T. Vascular dementia due to cardiac arrhythmias and systemic hypotension. Acta Neurol Scand 1987;76:123–128.
57. Meyer JS, Rauch G, Rauch RA, Haque A. Risk factors for cerebral hypoperfusion, mild cognitive impairment, and dementia. Neurobiol Aging 2000;21:161–169.
58. Henon H, Durieu I, Guerouaou D, Lebert F, Pasquier F, Leys D. Poststroke dementia: incidence and relationship to prestroke cognitive decline. Neurology 2001;57:1216–1222.
59. Desmond DW, Moroney JT, Sano M, Stern Y. Incidence of dementia after ischemic stroke: results of a longitudinal study. Stroke 2002;33:2254–2262.
60. Tomlinson BE, Blessed G, Roth M. Observations on the brains of demented old people. J Neurol Sci 1970;11:205–242.
61. Pohjasvaara T, Mantyla R, Salonen O, et al. MRI correlates of dementia after first clinical ischemic stroke. J Neurol Sci 2000;181:111–117.
62. Liu CK, Miller BL, Cummings JL, et al. A quantitative MRI study of vascular dementia. Neurology 1992;42:138–143.
63. Gorelick PB, Chatterjee A, Patel D, et al. Cranial computed tomographic observations in multi-infarct dementia. A controlled study. Stroke 1992;23:804–811.
64. Mielke R, Herholz K, Grond M, Kessler J, Heiss WD. Severity of vascular dementia is related to volume of metabolically impaired tissue. Arch Neurol 1992;49:909–913.
65. Kwan LT, Reed BR, Eberling JL, et al. Effects of subcortical cerebral infarction on cortical glucose metabolism and cognitive function. Arch Neurol 1999;56:809–814.

66. Tatemichi TK, Desmond DW, Prohovnik I, et al. Confusion and memory loss from capsular genu infarction: a thalamocortical disconnection syndrome? Neurology 1992;42:1966–1979.
67. Tatemichi TK, Desmond DW, Prohovnik I. Strategic infarcts in vascular dementia. A clinical and brain imaging experience. Arzneimittelforschung 1995;45:371–385.
68. Lafosse JM, Reed BR, Mungas D, Sterling SB, Wahbeh H, Jagust WJ. Fluency and memory differences between ischemic vascular dementia and Alzheimer's disease. Neuropsychology 1997;11:514–522.
69. Benson DF, Cummings JL. Angular gyrus syndrome simulating Alzheimer's disease. Arch Neurol 1982;39:616–620.
70. Caplan LR, Hedley-Whyte T. Cuing and memory dysfunction in alexia without agraphia. A case report. Brain 1974; 97:251–262.
71. Ott BR, Saver JL. Unilateral amnesic stroke. Six new cases and a review of the literature. Stroke 1993;24:1033–1042.
72. Alexander MP, Freedman M. Amnesia after anterior communicating artery aneurysm rupture. Neurology 1984;34:752–757.
73. Damasio AR, Graff-Radford NR, Eslinger PJ, Damasio H, Kassell N. Amnesia following basal forebrain lesions. Arch Neurol 1985;42:263–271.
74. Castaigne P, Lhermitte F, Buge A, Escourolle R, Hauw JJ, Lyon-Caen O. Paramedian thalamic and midbrain infarct: clinical and neuropathological study. Ann Neurol 1981;10:127–148.
75. Michel D, Laurent B, Foyatier N, Blanc A, Portafaix M. [Left paramedian thalamic infarct. Memory and language study]. Rev Neurol (Paris) 1982;138:533–550.
76. Guberman A, Stuss D. The syndrome of bilateral paramedian thalamic infarction. Neurology 1983;33:540–546.
77. Choi D, Sudarsky L, Schachter S, Biber M, Burke P. Medial thalamic hemorrhage with amnesia. Arch Neurol 1983; 40:611–613.
78. Mendez MF, Adams NL, Lewandowski KS. Neurobehavioral changes associated with caudate lesions. Neurology 1989; 39:349–354.
79. Caplan LR, Schmahmann JD, Kase CS, et al. Caudate infarcts. Arch Neurol 1990;47:133–143.
80. Trimble MR, Cummings JL. Neuropsychiatric disturbances following brainstem lesions. Br J Psychiatry 1981;138:56–59.
81. Katz DI, Alexander MP, Mandell AM. Dementia following strokes in the mesencephalon and diencephalon. Arch Neurol 1987;44:1127–1133.
82. Leys D, Erkinjuntti T, Desmond DW, et al. Vascular dementia: the role of cerebral infarcts. Alzheimer Dis Assoc Disord 1999;13(Suppl 3):S38–S48.
83. Tatemichi TK, Desmond DW, Paik M, et al. Clinical determinants of dementia related to stroke. Ann Neurol 1993; 33:568–575.
84. Esiri MM. Which vascular lesions are of importance in vascular dementia? Ann N Y Acad Sci 2000;903:239–243.
85. Roman GC, Erkinjuntti T, Wallin A, Pantoni L, Chui HC. Subcortical ischaemic vascular dementia. Lancet 2002;1:426–436.
86. Inzitari D, Erkinjuntti T, Wallin A, Del Ser T, Pantoni L. Is subcortical vascular dementia a clinical entity for clinical drug trials? Alzheimer Dis Assoc Disord 1999;13(Suppl 3):S66–S68.
87. Erkinjuntti T, Inzitari D, Pantoni L, et al. Limitations of clinical criteria for the diagnosis of vascular dementia in clinical trials. Is a focus on subcortical vascular dementia a solution? Ann N Y Acad Sci 2000;903:262–272.
88. Kase CS, Wolf PA, Chodosh EH, et al. Prevalence of silent stroke in patients presenting with initial stroke: the Framingham Study. Stroke 1989;20:850–852.
89. Boon A, Lodder J, Heuts-van Raak L, Kessels F. Silent brain infarcts in 755 consecutive patients with a first-ever supratentorial ischemic stroke. Relationship with index-stroke subtype, vascular risk factors, and mortality. Stroke 1994;25:2384–2390.
90. Brott T, Tomsick T, Feinberg W, et al. Baseline silent cerebral infarction in the Asymptomatic Carotid Atherosclerosis Study. Stroke 1994;25:1122–1129.
91. Ezekowitz MD, James KE, Nazarian SM, et al. Silent cerebral infarction in patients with nonrheumatic atrial fibrillation. The Veterans Affairs Stroke Prevention in Nonrheumatic Atrial Fibrillation Investigators. Circulation 1995;92: 2178–2182.
92. Shinkawa A, Ueda K, Kiyohara Y, et al. Silent cerebral infarction in a community-based autopsy series in Japan. The Hisayama Study. Stroke 1995;26:380–385.
93. Longstreth WT, Jr., Bernick C, Manolio TA, Bryan N, Jungreis CA, Price TR. Lacunar infarcts defined by magnetic resonance imaging of 3660 elderly people: the Cardiovascular Health Study. Arch Neurol 1998;55:1217–1225.
94. Jorgensen HS, Nakayama H, Raaschou HO, Gam J, Olsen TS. Silent infarction in acute stroke patients. Prevalence, localization, risk factors, and clinical significance: the Copenhagen Stroke Study. Stroke 1994;25:97–104.
95. Vermeer SE, Prins ND, den Heijer T, Hofman A, Koudstaal PJ, Breteler MM. Silent brain infarcts and the risk of dementia and cognitive decline. N Engl J Med 2003;348:1215–1222.
96. DeCarli C. The role of cerebrovascular disease in dementia. Neurology 2003;9:123–136.
97. Esiri MM, Wilcock GK, Morris JH. Neuropathological assessment of the lesions of significance in vascular dementia. J Neurol Neurosurg Psychiatry 1997;63:749–753.
98. Price TR, Manolio TA, Kronmal RA, et al. et al. Silent brain infarction on magnetic resonance imaging and neurological abnormalities in community-dwelling older adults. The Cardiovascular Health Study. CHS Collaborative Research Group. Stroke 1997;28:1158–1164.

99. Steingart A, Hachinski VC, Lau C, et al. Cognitive and neurologic findings in subjects with diffuse white matter lucencies on computed tomographic scan (leukoaraiosis). Arch Neurol 1987;44:32–35.
100. Merino JG, Hachinski V. Leukoaraiosis: reifying rarefaction. Arch Neurol 2000;57:925–926.
101. Schmid R, Roob G, Kapeller P, et al. Longitudinal change of white matter abnormalities. J Neural Transm 2000;59 (Suppl):9–14.
102. Miyao S, Takano A, Teramoto J, Takahashi A. Leukoaraiosis in relation to prognosis for patients with lacunar infarction. Stroke 1992;23:1434–1438.
103. Streifler JY, Eliasziw M, Benavente OR, et al. Development and progression of leukoaraiosis in patients with brain ischemia and carotid artery disease. Stroke 2003;34:1913–1916.
104. Skoog I, Nilsson L, Palmertz B, Andreasson LA, Svanborg A. A population-based study of dementia in 85-year-olds. N Engl J Med 1993;328:153–158.
105. de Groot JC, de Leeuw FE, Oudkerk M, et al. Cerebral white matter lesions and cognitive function: the Rotterdam Scan Study. Ann Neurol 2000;47:145–151.
106. Gupta SR, Naheedy MH, Young JC, Ghobrial M, Rubino FA, Hindo W. Periventricular white matter changes and dementia. Clinical, neuropsychological, radiological, and pathological correlation. Arch Neurol 1988;45:637–641.
107. Junque C, Pujol J, Vendrell P, et al. Leuko-araiosis on magnetic resonance imaging and speed of mental processing. Arch Neurol 1990;47:151–156.
108. Ylikoski R, Ylikoski A, Erkinjuntti T, Sulkava R, Raininko R, Tilvis R. White matter changes in healthy elderly persons correlate with attention and speed of mental processing. Arch Neurol 1993;50:818–824.
109. Inzitari D. Age-related white matter changes and cognitive impairment. Ann Neurol 2000;47:141–143.
110. Bowler JV. The concept of vascular cognitive impairment. J Neurol Sci 2002;203-204:11–15.
111. Desmond DW. Cognition and white matter lesions. Cerebrovasc Dis 2002;13(Suppl 2):53–57.
112. Emery VO, Gillie EX, Smith JA. 1995 IPA/Bayer Research Awards in Psychogeriatrics. Reclassification of the vascular dementias: comparisons of infarct and noninfarct vascular dementias. Int Psychogeriatr 1996;8:33–61.
113. Emery VO, Gillie EX, Smith JA. Interface between vascular dementia and Alzheimer syndrome. Nosologic redefinition. Ann N Y Acad Sci 2000;903:229–238.
114. Roman GC, Erkinjuntti T, Wallin A, Pantoni L, Chui HC. Subcortical ischaemic vascular dementia. Lancet Neurology 2003;1:426.
115. Sparks DL, Scheff SW, Liu H, Landers TM, Coyne CM, Hunsaker JC, III. Increased incidence of neurofibrillary tangles (NFT) in non-demented individuals with hypertension. J Neurol Sci 1995;131:162–169.
116. Petrovitch H, White LR, Izmirilian G, et al. Midlife blood pressure and neuritic plaques, neurofibrillary tangles, and brain weight at death: the HAAS. Honolulu-Asia aging Study. Neurobiol Aging 2000;21:57–62.
117. van Swieten JC, Geyskes GG, Derix MM, et al. Hypertension in the elderly is associated with white matter lesions and cognitive decline. Ann Neurol 1991;30:825–830.
118. Desmond DW, Tatemichi TK, Paik M, Stern Y. Risk factors for cerebrovascular disease as correlates of cognitive function in a stroke-free cohort. Arch Neurol 1993;50:162–166.
119. Holmes C, Cairns N, Lantos P, Mann A. Validity of current clinical criteria for Alzheimer's disease, vascular dementia and dementia with Lewy bodies. Br J Psychiatry 1999;174:45–50.
120. Pathological correlates of late-onset dementia in a multicentre, community-based population in England and Wales. Neuropathology Group of the Medical Research Council Cognitive Function and Ageing Study (MRC CFAS). Lancet 2001;357:169–175.
121. Heyman A, Fillenbaum GG, Welsh-Bohmer KA, et al. Cerebral infarcts in patients with autopsy-proven Alzheimer's disease: CERAD, part XVIII. Consortium to Establish a Registry for Alzheimer's Disease. Neurology 1998;51:159–162.
122. Zekry D, Hauw JJ, Gold G. Mixed dementia: epidemiology, diagnosis, and treatment. J Am Geriatr Soc 2002;50:1431–1438.
123. Snowdon DA, Greiner LH, Mortimer JA, Riley KP, Greiner PA, Markesbery WR. Brain infarction and the clinical expression of Alzheimer disease. The Nun Study. JAMA 1997;277:813–817.
124. Nagy Z, Esiri MM, Jobst KA, et al. The effects of additional pathology on the cognitive deficit in Alzheimer disease. J Neuropathol Exp Neurol 1997;56:165–170.
125. Mungas D, Reed BR, Ellis WG, Jagust WJ. The effects of age on rate of progression of Alzheimer disease and dementia with associated cerebrovascular disease. Arch Neurol 2001;58:1243–1247.
126. Kase CS, Wolf PA, Kelly-Hayes M, Kannel WB, Beiser A, D'Agostino RB. Intellectual decline after stroke: the Framingham Study. Stroke 1998;29:805–812.
127. Henon H, Pasquier F, Durieu I, et al. Preexisting dementia in stroke patients. Baseline frequency, associated factors, and outcome. Stroke 1997;28:2429–2436.
128. Barba R, Martinez-Espinosa S, Rodriguez-Garcia E, Pondal M, Vivancos J, Del Ser T. Poststroke dementia: clinical features and risk factors. Stroke 2000;31:1494–1501.
129. Tatemichi TK, Desmond DW, Mayeux R, et al. Dementia after stroke: baseline frequency, risks, and clinical features in a hospitalized cohort. Neurology 1992;42:1185–1193.
130. Desmond DW, Moroney JT, Paik MC, Sano M, Mohr JP, Aboumatar S et al. Frequency and clinical determinants of dementia after ischemic stroke. Neurology 2000;54:1124–1131.

131. Kokmen E, Whisnant JP, O'Fallon WM, Chu CP, Beard CM. Dementia after ischemic stroke: a population-based study in Rochester, Minnesota (1960-1984). Neurology 1996;46:154–159.
132. Skoog I. Status of risk factors for vascular dementia. Neuroepidemiology 1998;17:2–9.
133. Breteler MM. Vascular risk factors for Alzheimer's disease: an epidemiologic perspective. Neurobiol Aging 2000;21: 153–160.
134. De La Torre JC. Alzheimer disease as a vascular disorder: nosological evidence. Stroke 2002;33:1152–1162.
135. Gold G, Giannakopoulos P, Bouras C. Re-evaluating the role of vascular changes in the differential diagnosis of Alzheimer's disease and vascular dementia. Eur Neurol 1998;40:121–129.
136. Launer LJ. Demonstrating the case that AD is a vascular disease: epidemiologic evidence. Ageing Res Rev 2002;1:61–77.
137. Jobst KA, Smith AD, Szatmari M, et al. Detection in life of confirmed Alzheimer's disease using a simple measurement of medial temporal lobe atrophy by computed tomography. Lancet 1992;340:1179–1183.
138. Henon H, Pasquier F, Durieu I, Pruvo JP, Leys D. Medial temporal lobe atrophy in stroke patients: relation to pre-existing dementia. J Neurol Neurosurg Psychiatry 1998;65:641–647.
139. Du AT, Schuff N, Laakso MP, et al. Effects of subcortical ischemic vascular dementia and AD on entorhinal cortex and hippocampus. Neurology 2002;58:1635–1641.
140. Gorelick PB, Nyenhuis DL, Garron DC, Cochran E. Is vascular dementia really Alzheimer's disease or mixed dementia? Neuroepidemiology 1996;15:286–290.
141. Kalaria RN, Ballard C. Overlap between pathology of Alzheimer disease and vascular dementia. Alzheimer Dis Assoc Disord 1999;13(Suppl 3):S115–S123.
142. Korczyn AD. The complex nosological concept of vascular dementia. J Neurol Sci 2002;203-204:3–6.
143. Patterson CJ, Clarfield AM. Diagnostic procedures for dementia. In: Emery VOB, Oxman TE, eds. Dementia. Presentation, differential diagnosis and nosology. Baltimore, MD: Johns Hopkins University Press, 2003, pp. 61–85.
144. American Psychiatric Association. Diagnostic and Statistical Manual of Mental Disorders. 4th Ed. Washington, DC: American Psychiatric Association, 1994.
145. Verhey FR, Lodder J, Rozendaal N, Jolles J. Comparison of seven sets of criteria used for the diagnosis of vascular dementia. Neuroepidemiology 1996;15:166–172.

II Basic Mechanisms of Vascular Dementia

5

Cerebral Hemodynamics in the Elderly

Jorge M. Serrador, William P. Milberg, and Lewis A. Lipsitz

1. INTRODUCTION

Regulation of cerebral blood flow (CBF) is critical for proper neural function. Therefore, alterations in CBF regulation resulting from aging or age-related disease may have important clinical consequences, including cognitive impairment, gait disorders, falls, and syncope. This chapter reviews mechanisms of CBF regulation, their changes with aging, and their clinical implications, including the frontal subcortical dysfunction in cognition and gait that is commonly observed in elderly people, reductions in global CBF with Alzheimer's disease (AD), and local cerebral hypoperfusion associated with Alzheimer's dementia and vascular dementia (VaD).

The regulation of CBF involves several interacting mechanisms *(1,2)*. In 1914, Barcroft proposed that CBF was matched to metabolic demands *(1)*. This has since been validated in both animal and human studies. Cognitive activation in humans increases both global and local blood flow to the brain *(3–5)*. The ability to augment flow is critical; for example, cognitive deficits with cerebral ischaemia are reversed by increases in global CBF *(6)*. Although metabolic vasodilation augments regional brain blood flow during cognitive activation, this vasodilation may be insufficient if flow is already limited. To ensure sufficient CBF is available, the cerebrovasculature must dilate or constrict in response to prevailing perfusion pressure. The ability to maintain brain blood flow over a range of perfusion pressures is termed cerebral autoregulation *(2)*. Thus, impairment of either metabolic cerebral vasodilation or cerebral autoregulation could adversely affect cognitive function in the elderly, possibly leading to cerebrovascular disease (CVD) and/or dementia.

2. AUTOREGULATION OF CEREBRAL BLOOD FLOW

Cerebral autoregulation maintains relatively constant blood flow across a range of cerebral perfusion pressures (CPPs). CBF is determined by CPP and cerebrovascular resistance, with the relationship between these variables being defined as CBF = CPP/CVR. Thus, to maintain CBF constant in the face of changing perfusion pressure, the vascular resistance must be adjusted. For example, to maintain flow during increases in pressure, resistance must increase. The pial arteries constrict in response to increased CPP, causing an increase in cerebrovascular resistance *(2)*. Figure 1 demonstrates that within a normal pressure range, cerebrovascular resistance adjusts to the prevailing CPP to maintain a relatively constant flow. When pressure becomes sufficiently low to result in maximal vasodilation, resistance will no longer be able to adjust to decreasing perfusion pressures and CBF will fall. In contrast, when pressures become sufficiently high, the pial arterioles will be forced open by the driving pressure, and, thus, resistance will decrease, resulting in an increase in CBF. This condition is termed autoregulatory breakthrough.

From: *Current Clinical Neurology*
Vascular Dementia: Cerebrovascular Mechanisms and Clinical Management
Edited by: R. H. Paul, R. Cohen, B. R. Ott, and S. Salloway © Humana Press Inc., Totowa, NJ

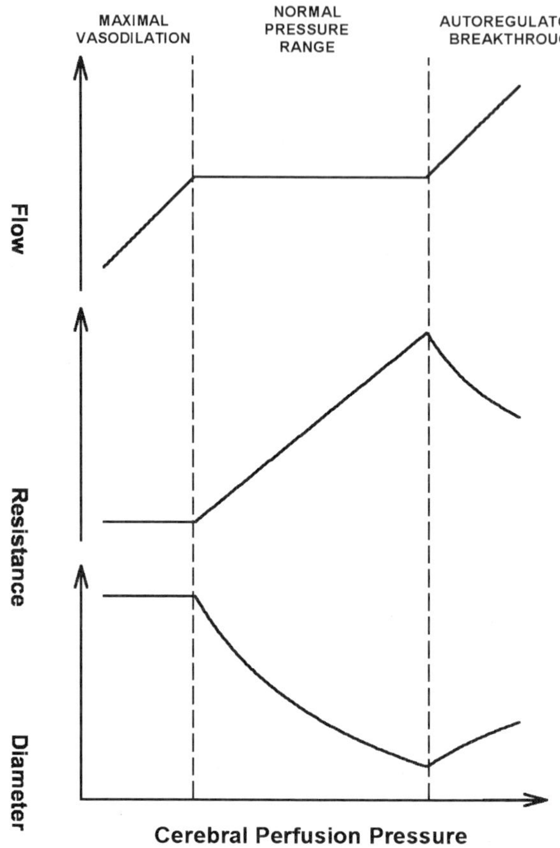

Fig. 1. Representation of autoregulatory response to changes in cerebral perfusion pressure (CPP). Cerebral blood flow (CBF) is maintained constant over a range of perfusion pressures by adjusting cerebrovascular resistance via dilating or constricting pial arterioles. Once pial arterioles are maximally dilated, further reductions in perfusion pressure result in decreases in CBF (lower limit of autoregulation). If perfusion pressure is sufficiently high, pial arterioles are forced open and CBF increases with increasing perfusion pressure (autoregulatory breakthrough).

Previous research has demonstrated that the autoregulatory curve is not static and is affected by numerous conditions. It is well known that changing arterial carbon dioxide levels will result in changes in CBF without affecting cerebral autoregulation (*see* Fig. 2) *(2)*. For example, a decrease in arterial CO_2 will cause an overall cerebral vasoconstriction, which will reduce global CBF; however, the inherent ability of the cerebrovasculature to respond to pressure changes will remain intact. Thus, CBF will now be autoregulated around this new lower level of CBF (i.e., this can be described as a shift down in the curve). Similarly, stimulation of the fastigial nucleus in primates results in vasodilatation, which increases CBF *(7,8)*, without a loss of autoregulation (i.e., an upward shift in the autoregulation curve) *(8)*. This vasodilatation may be mediated by parasympathetic pathways *(9)*. Another example of a shift in the curve is the observation that CBF is maintained during hypotension in both chronic local cerebral hypoperfusion *(1,10)* and orthostatic hypotension *(11,12)*. Thus, individuals with these conditions are able to maintain CBF at pressures that would be expected to cause maximal vasodilation and thus impair the ability of the cerebral vessels to adjust to perfusion pressure. This increased ability to vasodilate at lower perfusion pressures can be described as a leftward shift in the autoregulation curve.

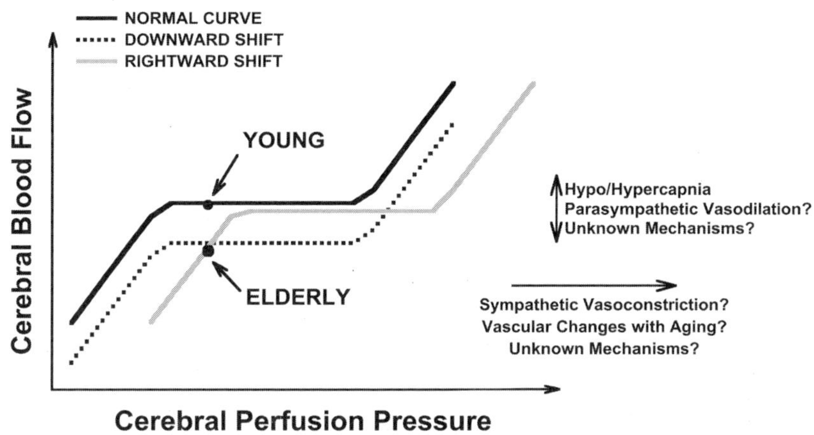

Fig. 2. Theoretical shifts in the cerebral autoregulation curve associated with changes in arterial carbon dioxide and sympathetic nervous system activity. Elderly subjects are known to have reduced global cerebral blood flow (CBF) at the same perfusion pressure. One possible explanation is a rightward shift in the curve resulting from diminished vasodilatory capacity. In this case, elderly subjects are no longer able to autoregulate in response to perfusion pressure and, thus, CBF falls. Another explanation is that a downward shift in the curve occurs so that overall cerebrovascular resistance increases, decreasing flow without affecting cerebral autoregulation. The underlying mechanism of this aging-related cerebral hypoperfusion remains unclear.

It is possible that leftward/rightward shifts in the curve are mediated by changes in sympathetic activity. For example, sympathectomized baboons demonstrate a leftward shift in the curve *(8)*, presumably because the sympathetically mediated vasoconstriction of cerebral vessels is no longer present and thus greater cerebral vasodilation is possible. Although the role of sympathetic tone in humans is still under debate *(2,13)*, studies have suggested that interruption of cerebral sympathetic pathways through the superior cervical ganglia in spinal cord injured patients may shift autoregulation to a lower pressure zone. Similar to the sympathectomized baboons, a reduction in vasoconstrictive inputs would allow for greater dilation, and thus explain the ability of these patients to tolerate lower CPPs *(12)*. However, the authors recently found that patients with spinal cord injuries with high cervical lesions demonstrated similar decreases in CBF as controls, suggesting they have not shifted their curve leftward *(14)*.

There are also data suggesting that acute changes in sympathetic outflow can shift the autoregulation curve. Levine et al. *(15)* have proposed that a rightward shift of the autoregulation curve during lower body negative pressure results from sympathetic activation (i.e., increased sympathetic cerebral vasoconstriction). This derives from the finding that decreases in CBF occur without any appreciable alteration in arterial pressure *(15,16)*. This could occur if there is a rightward shift in the autoregulation curve such that the current CPP perfusion pressure falls onto the downward slope of the curve, decreasing CBF without drops in pressure (*see* Fig. 2). Moreover, recent work has found evidence of decreased ability to regulate against fluctuations in pressure during higher levels of lower body negative pressure *(17)* or upright tilt *(18)*. Because autoregulation works to maintain CBF constant in the face of changing perfusion pressure, this decreased ability to regulate against fluctuations in pressure suggests that autoregulation is impaired, and, thus, these subjects may be on the linear portion of the curve associated with maximal vasodilation.

In contrast, the authors previously found that sympathetic activation caused by upright tilt in healthy subjects did not impair the ability to regulate against pressure fluctuations *(19)*, similar to the findings of Diehl et al. *(20)*. Because these subjects had similar decreases in CBF velocity to the previous studies using lower body negative pressure *(17,18)* but did not demonstrate alteration in their ability to regulate against perfusion pressure fluctuations (i.e., intact autoregulation), they demonstrated a downward rather than rightward shift in the curve.

Thus, although it remains unclear what mechanisms are involved in shifting the autoregulation curve, current data suggests that the curve does shift. Because autoregulation is critical to the maintenance of CBF, impaired autoregulation in the elderly could have detrimental effects, resulting in impaired cognition, orthostatic intolerance, and even permanent neuronal damage.

3. EFFECTS OF AGE ON CEREBRAL BLOOD FLOW

Aging is associated with a well-documented decrease in global CBF *(21–26)* and increase in cerebral vascular resistance *(21)*. One possible cause of this decrease could be a rightward shift in the cerebral autoregulation curve (*see* Fig. 2). A chronic rightward shift in the absence of increased perfusion pressure could result in the greatest risk for hypoperfusion, because elderly individuals would now be operating on the linear down sloping portion of the curve, resulting in a compromised ability to defend CBF against rises and falls in arterial pressure (i.e., impaired autoregulation). Couple that with impaired blood pressure regulation in elderly individuals *(27,28)* and one would expect large swings in CBF, resulting in repeated bouts of cerebral hypoperfusion.

Because aging is associated with increased sympathetic activity *(29)* and increased sympathetic activity has been suggested to cause a rightward shift in the curve *(15)*, it is logical that impaired autoregulation be considered as a possible cause of the global reduction in CBF with aging (i.e., a rightward shift in the curve). Evidence supporting this hypothesis can be found in previous work demonstrating that older rats are less able to tolerate hypotensive stimuli *(30,31)*, have reduced cerebrovascular reactivity to CO_2 (often used as an indicator of intact autoregulation), and have an increased lower limit of autoregulation *(32–34)*. These findings suggest a rightward shift in the autoregulation curve.

Studies of CBF in elderly humans have produced conflicting results. Examining the response to changes in arterial CO_2 levels, studies have reported that aging has either no effect on cerebrovascular reactivity *(35,36)* or is associated with reduced reactivity *(37–40)*. Myogenic tone in isolated human pial arteries was unaffected by age, suggesting intact autoregulatory capacity *(41)*. Furthermore, measures of cerebral autoregulation in elderly humans based on the response of CBF to spontaneous fluctuations in blood pressure have found that autoregulation remains intact *(38,42)*. Similarly, the authors found that during a sit-to-stand maneuver in which subjects experience transient hypotension, elderly subjects are able to maintain CBF velocity effectively *(38)* (*see* Fig. 3). In fact, during standing, elderly subjects demonstrated better attenuation of spontaneous blood pressure oscillations than younger subjects, suggesting improved autoregulation. Similarly, Oblak et al. *(40)* found that CBF velocity was better maintained in the elderly during head up tilt. These data suggest that autoregulation remains intact in healthy elderly individuals.

If impaired autoregulation is not involved in the reduction in CBF, could a direct sympathetically mediated vasoconstriction be the cause? Sympathetic innervation of cerebral vessels in animals originates in the superior cervical ganglion, stellate ganglion, and via several central pathways, including the locus ceruleus, fastigial nucleus, dorsal raphe nucleus, dorsal medullary reticular formation, and rostral ventrolateral medulla *(13)*. However, the role of sympathetic pathways in humans remains unclear. For example, blockade of sympathetic activity through the stellate ganglion increases CBF, as measured by single photon emission computed tomography (SPECT), presumably through the blockade of a sympathetic vasoconstrictor signal *(43)*. However, magnetic resonance imaging (MRI) measures of CBF using the same blocking technique found no change in internal carotid flow but did demonstrate an increase in common carotid flow, suggesting vasodilatation in the extracerebral beds *(44)*. Therefore, it is possible that the increase in CBF observed with SPECT *(43)* resulted in part from increased scalp and facial blood flow. In contrast, direct stimulation of the cervical ganglia and presumably sympathetic pathways during surgery caused an increase in CBF and arterial pressure *(45)*. However, patients in this study were anesthetized with isoflurane, which ablates autoregulation

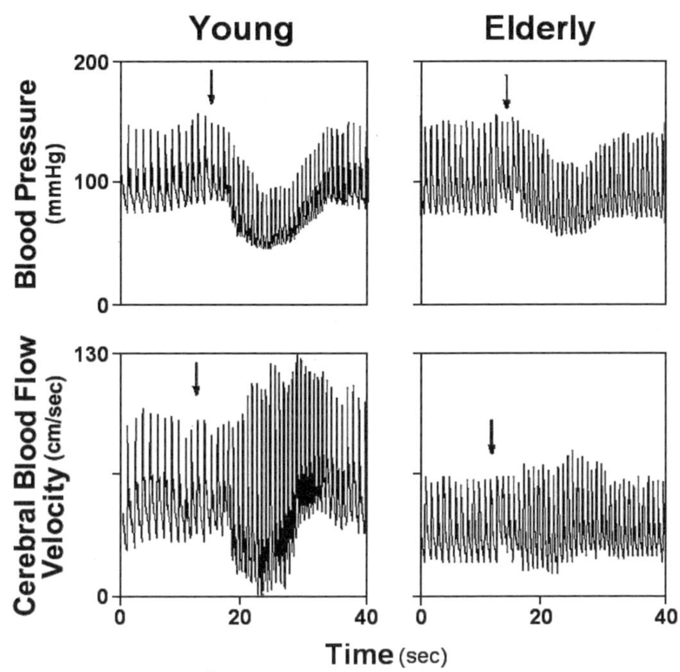

Fig. 3. Response of a healthy young and elderly subject to a sit-to-stand maneuver. Arrow indicates initiation of the stand. Both the young and the elderly subjects maintained cerebral blood flow (CBF) velocity despite a decrease in blood pressure with standing. These data indicate that autoregulation remains intact with healthy aging.

(46), and nitrous oxide, which is a potent vasodilator, particularly when used in combination with isoflurane *(47)*. These considerations suggest that the elevated cerebral perfusion was the result of increased arterial pressure augmenting CBF through vessels with pharmacologically impaired autoregulation.

In primates, cerebral vasoconstriction has been found with stimulation of the locus ceruleus *(48)*. This vasoconstriction was unaffected by sectioning of the vagus nerve or sympathetic trunk, suggesting no peripheral sympathetic role. In humans, direct measures of middle cerebral artery diameter using MRI during sympathetic activation induced by lower body negative pressure did not demonstrate a vasoconstriction at the basal artery level, even though flow decreased, suggesting the constriction occurred at the peripheral resistance arteries *(49)*. Direct intrathecal infusion of the locus ceruleus with clonidine, an α2-agonist, which at low doses inhibits central sympathetic activity, in one patient resulted in a reduction in CBF velocity, presumably through a downstream vasoconstriction *(50)*. In healthy individuals, clonidine attenuates the decrease in CBF velocity during sympathetic activation by the cold pressor test *(50,51)*. Furthermore, the use of α-blockers improved autoregulation during hypotension in stroke patients *(52)* and attenuated the decrease in CBF velocity of patients with orthostatic intolerance during head-up tilt testing *(53)*. In all these studies it was proposed that the observed changes in CBF resulted from a decrease in cerebrovascular resistance as a result of reduced cerebral sympathetic activity. In contrast, Lee et al. *(54)* found that inhibition of sympathetic activity with clonidine caused a reduction in CBF velocity, suggesting a cerebral vasoconstriction, even when pressure was maintained at control levels with phenylephrine. Furthermore, direct infusions of norepinephrine in both anesthetized *(55)* and conscious patients *(56,57)* do not affect CBF or vascular resistance. Therefore, the role of sympathetic activation on cerebrovascular tone is as yet unclear.

If direct sympathetic vasoconstriction is not responsible, other mechanisms may be involved in the age-related decline in CBF. In animals, infusion of adenosine, a vasodilator, produces an attenuated vasodilatory response in aged rats *(58)*. Similarly, endothelium-dependent vasodilation is attenuated in aged animals *(59,60)*. In addition, cholinergic vasodilator systems are impaired in older rats *(61,62)*. In contrast, application of a high dose of intravascular serotonin, a dose-dependent vasoconstrictor, produced augmented vasoconstriction in aged rats *(63)*. These data suggest that in older animals, vasoconstrictor stimuli may dominate. Extrapolating these mechanisms to aged humans may prove difficult because there are inherent differences in the cerebrovascular systems of aged animals and humans. For example, as mentioned, myogenic tone remains intact with age in isolated human pial arteries *(41)* but is reduced in older rat cerebral arteries, reducing their ability to dilate or constrict in response to pressure changes *(59)*.

Finally, aging is associated with a general cerebral atrophy that includes the loss of gray matter *(25)*. Thus, reductions in CBF may just be the result of reduced metabolic demand because of the reduced volume of neural tissue. Yoshii et al. *(64)* found that age-related reductions in global cerebral metabolic rate were eliminated when metabolic rate was normalized to brain volume. However, use of advanced imaging techniques during the last decade suggest that reductions in cerebral metabolic rate with aging, especially in the frontal lobes, are independent of brain atrophy *(25)*.

Although current data do not provide a clear mechanism for the reduction in CBF with aging, the fact that older individuals have reduced CBF but are still able to attenuate fluctuations in pressure (i.e., cerebral autoregulation is intact) suggests that a rightward shift in the cerebral autoregulation curve is not involved. Regardless of the mechanism, it is possible that reductions in CBF with aging may result in chronic hypoperfusion and ischemic damage to watershed areas, particularly in frontal subcortical regions. For example, older adults have a high prevalence of orthostatic and postprandial hypotension, which not only are risk factors for falls and syncope but also threaten cerebral perfusion during everyday activities. In fact, older adults demonstrate a paradoxical cerebral vasoconstriction during postprandial hypotension, which likely threatens cerebral perfusion *(65)*. With near-infrared spectroscopy, it has been shown that healthy older adults frequently develop decreased cortical oxygenation levels in the frontal lobes when assuming an upright posture *(66,67)*. Because humans spend a majority of their time in the upright posture, these data raise the question of what effect do repeated bouts of cerebral hypoperfusion have on cerebral function.

4. CEREBRAL HYPOPERFUSION: CAUSE OR CONSEQUENCE?

The human frontal lobe is necessary to plan and execute goals, coordinate complex motor functions, make decisions, express creativity, and navigate through complex social situations. Aging is associated with loss of frontal lobe volume, changes in frontal subcortical white matter, and the familiar geriatric syndrome of gait impairment, falls, executive cognitive dysfunction, and depression, which are common manifestations of frontal subcortical dysfunction *(68)*. The pathogenesis of age-related white matter abnormalities, which are seen with increasing frequency as multifocal, as well as diffuse areas of white matter hyperintensity on T2-weighted brain MRIs of older people *(69)*, is still a matter of rigorous investigation. The strong association of these white matter hyperintensities (WMH) with cardiovascular risk factors *(70,71)* supports a vascular basis for the development of white matter abnormalities and age-related frontal lobe dysfunction. These WMHs have been related pathologically to cerebral microangiopathy *(69,72,73)* and clinically to hypoperfusion in affected areas *(74,75)*. However, it is not known whether hypoperfusion causes damage to subcortical white matter with the subsequent development of symptoms or whether hypoperfusion simply results from loss of brain tissue.

Chronic hypoperfusion in animals is related to reductions in cerebral metabolism *(76)*, impaired cognitive function *(76,77)*, and white matter degeneration *(78)*. These data suggest that white matter degeneration caused by cerebrovascular dysfunction may constitute a major determinant of common neurological symptoms in older persons with risk factors for CVD *(68)*.

5. EVIDENCE LINKING HYPOPERFUSION TO FRONTAL LOBE DYSFUNCTION

The notion that hypoperfusion plays a role in the pathogenesis of white matter abnormalities is supported by xenon contrast computed tomography (CT) *(79)* and MRI (80) studies showing reduced cerebral blood flow in regions with high WMH concentrations. Using a new quantitative MRI perfusion technique, O'Sullivan et al. *(75)* have shown reduced CBF in the white matter but not gray matter of older adults with white matter abnormalities. This study also demonstrates a reduction of CBF in normal-appearing periventricular white matter in patients with WMHs compared with controls, providing evidence that hypoperfusion may precede the appearance of new lesions on T2-weighted images.

Further evidence linking hypoperfusion to frontal lobe dysfunction comes from a limited, but emerging, set of data, which shows that abnormalities of blood pressure regulation may lead to perfusion abnormalities in the frontal lobes and contribute to functional frontal-subcortical deficits. With near-infrared spectroscopy, it was shown that healthy elderly persons frequently develop decreased cortical oxygenation levels in the frontal lobes when assuming an upright posture, even in the absence of clinical symptoms of orthostasis *(66)*. Both orthostatic hypotension and postprandial hypotension are associated with cognitive abnormalities and WMH *(81–83)*. Because the subcortical white matter is supplied by terminal vessels with scarce anastomoses, it represents a "watershed" region in the cerebral circulation, and, thus, it is particularly vulnerable to ischemic injury during periods of hypotension *(84)*. Increased blood pressure variability is also associated with WMHs of the brain *(85,86)*. In patients with Binswanger's disease with diffuse white matter abnormalities, Tohgi et al. *(87)* reported greater 24-h systolic blood pressure standard deviations and a larger difference between the maximum and minimum systolic blood pressure compared to normal controls. Although it is not known whether frequent daily pressure declines in older patients increase the risk of developing white matter abnormalities and its clinical consequences, there is some evidence that lower standing blood pressure increases the risk of falls during 1 yr of follow-up among community-dwelling older adults over age 65 *(88)*. In a study of a nursing home population, the authors found that increased orthostatic blood pressure variability is a risk factor for stroke *(89)*.

These data suggest that elderly subjects with white matter abnormalities may have impaired frontal blood flow regulation, resulting in repeated hypoperfusion during periods of hypotension. Previous work demonstrating intact cerebral autoregulation in healthy elderly subjects has examined flow velocity in the middle cerebral artery, which primarily feeds the temporal and parietal cortex *(38,42)*. It is possible that abnormal regulation to the frontal lobes was present but undetected. Further work is necessary to examine cerebral autoregulation in the frontal lobes of these individuals.

6. CEREBRAL BLOOD FLOW AND DEMENTIA

AD is associated with numerous markers, including neuritic plaques, neurofibrillary tangles, granulovacuolar degeneration, and atrophy *(90)*. The onset of the disease is marked by the appearance of these markers primarily in the medial temporal lobe and hippocampus *(91)*. As the disease advances, these pathological changes may be found throughout the neocortex, particularly in the association areas of the temporal, frontal, and parietal lobes.

There is recent intriguing evidence that cardiovascular risk factors may also be associated with increased risk for AD. In a survey-based study conducted in 1449 older adults in Finland, Kivipelto et al. *(92)* found that systolic blood pressure and hypertension in middle-age were predictive of later diagnoses of AD. Unfortunately, the interpretability of these data was clouded because the participants who received the diagnosis of AD (i.e., met most of the *Diagnostic and Statistical Manual of Mental Disorders*, 4th Edition [DSM-IV] clinical criteria for AD) were not excluded if they showed evidence of lacunar infarcts or periventricular white matter disease. Consequently, it is not known how many of the 57 participants who were diagnosed as having dementia were affected by the early signs of microvascular disease. Particularly interesting from a clinical perspective is the apparent association between cholesterol level and the diagnosis of AD *(92)*. Simons et al. *(93)* have proposed a link between neuritic plaques and cholesterol, thus cholesterol-lowering drugs may also reduce the prevalence of AD.

There is now increasing evidence that the cognitive deficits associated with vascular disease may be different from those of AD, despite the fact that current clinical diagnostic criteria for both of these disorders focuses on the presence of a memory disorder (*see* DSM-IV-TR and National Institute of Neurological Disorders and Stroke-Association Internationale pour la Recherche et l'Enseignement en Neurosciences [NINDS-AIREN]). There is now reason to believe that the pathological substrates of these disorders are quite different, at least in the early stages of disease, and adults who are at risk of either disorder may show subtle but disease-specific deficits in performance on neuropsychological tests. Furthermore, these preclinical deficits may be accompanied by distinct changes in neural structure and function, as well as CBF.

Increasingly, vascular causes of cognitive impairment that do not fully meet the established criteria for dementia are being recognized. Executive dysfunction is the primary cognitive abnormality that characterizes both VaD and lesser forms of vascular cognitive impairment. This is quite different from AD, which, in its earliest preclinical stages, may be characterized by changes in memory performance and reductions in the volume of such structures as the hippocampus and entorhinal cortex *(91)*. However, this underlying dissociation in the pattern of neuropsychological deficits between AD and VaD may be clouded because there is now increasing evidence that the risk factors for CVD may also be risk factors for AD *(94–97)*. Recent reports also suggest that executive function deficits may mark the onset of both disorders *(98)*. Currently, there are little or no data on the relationship between risk for AD, risk for CVD, and the association of these risk patterns with underlying changes in brain structure and function.

Both Alzheimer's dementia and VaD are associated with reduced CBF *(99–106)*. Although decreases in temporal and parietal regional flow have been consistently found in AD *(102,104,106)*, decreases in frontal lobe blood flow have only been found in VaD *(99,100,103)*. In fact, frontal hypoperfusion has been suggested as a method to differentiate AD and VaD *(100,103)*.

7. SUMMARY

Aging is associated with numerous physiological changes that affect CBF and possibly cerebrovascular blood flow regulation. These changes may result in both global reductions in CBF, as well as regional cerebral hypoperfusion in the frontal lobes. Sustained or intermittent cerebral hypoperfusion could be involved in the development of subcortical and periventricular white matter abnormalities. Atrophy of the frontal lobes may be responsible for impairment of executive function in elderly individuals and may underlie the development of VaD. Future work needs to focus prospectively on age-related structural and functional changes in the brain and how they may lead to common geriatric symptoms affecting cognition.

REFERENCES

1. Lassen NA. Cerebral blood flow and oxygen consumption in man. Physiol Rev 1959;39:183–238.
2. Paulson OB, Strandgaard S, Edvinsson L. Cerebral autoregulation. Cerebrovasc Brain Metab Rev 1990;2:161–192.
3. Gur RC, Jaggi JL, Ragland JD, et al. Effects of memory processing on regional brain activation: cerebral blood flow in normal subjects. Int J Neurosci 1993;72:31–44.
4. Perani D, Gilardi MC, Cappa SF, Fazio F. PET studies of cognitive functions: a review. J Nucl Biol Med 1992;36:324–36.
5. Ramsay SC, Adams L, Murphy K, et al. Regional cerebral blood flow during volitional expiration in man: a comparison with volitional inspiration. 1993;461:101.
6. Nunn J, Hodges H. Cognitive deficits induced by global cerebral ischaemia: relationship to brain damage and reversal by transplants. Behav Brain Res 1994;65:1–31.
7. Goadsby PJ, Lambert GA. Electrical stimulation of the fastigial nucleus increases total cerebral blood flow in the monkey. Neurosci Lett 1989;107:141–144.

8. McKee JC, Denn MJ, Stone HL. Neurogenic cerebral vasodilation from electrical stimulation of the cerebellum in the monkey. Stroke 1976;7:179–186.
9. Toda N, Tanaka T, Ayajiki K, Okamura T. Cerebral vasodilatation induced by stimulation of the pterygopalatine ganglion and greater petrosal nerve in anesthetized monkeys. Neuroscience 2000;96:393–398.
10. Keunen RW, Eikelboom BC, Stegeman DF, Ackerstaff RG. Chronic cerebral hypotension induces a downward shift of the cerebral autoregulation: a hypothesis based on TCD and OPG-GEE studies in ambulatory patients with occlusive cerebrovascular disease. Neurol Res 1994;16:413–416.
11. Novak V, Novak P, Spies JM, Low PA. Autoregulation of cerebral blood flow in orthostatic hypotension. Stroke 1998;29:104–111.
12. Nanda RN, Wyper DJ, Harper AM, Johnson RH. Cerebral blood flow in paraplegia. Paraplegia 1974;12:212–218.
13. Sandor P. Nervous control of the cerebrovascular system: doubts and facts. Neurochem Intl 1999;35:237–259.
14. Houtman S, Serrador JM, Colier WN, Strijbos DW, Shoemaker K, Hopman MT. Changes in cerebral oxygenation and blood flow during LBNP in spinal cord-injured individuals. J Appl Physiol 2001;91:2199–2204.
15. Levine BD, Giller CA, Lane LD, Buckey JC, Blomqvist CG. Cerebral versus systemic hemodynamics during graded orthostatic stress in humans. Circulation 1994;90:298–306.
16. Bondar RL, Kassam MS, Stein F, Dunphy PT, Fortney S, Riedesel ML. Simultaneous cerebrovascular and cardiovascular responses during presyncope. Stroke 1995;26:1794–800.
17. Zhang R, Zuckerman JH, Giller CA, Levine BD. Transfer function analysis of dynamic cerebral autoregulation in humans. Amer J Physiol 1998;274:H233–H241.
18. Carey BJ, Manktelow BN, Panerai RB, Potter JF. Cerebral autoregulatory responses to head-up tilt in normal subjects and patients with recurrent vasovagal syncope. Circulation 2001;104:898–902.
19. Serrador JM, Shoemaker JK, Brown TE, Kassam MS, Bondar RL, Schlegel TT. Cerebral vasoconstriction precedes orthostatic intolerance after parabolic flight. Brain Res Bull 2000;53:113–120.
20. Diehl RR, Linden D, Chalkiadaki A, Diehl A. Cerebrovascular mechanisms in neurocardiogenic syncope with and without postural tachycardia syndrome. J Auton Nerv Syst 1999;76:159–166.
21. Krejza J, Mariak Z, Walecki J, Szydlik P, Lewko J, Ustymowicz A. Transcranial color Doppler sonography of basal cerebral arteries in 182 healthy subjects: age and sex variability and normal reference values for blood flow parameters. AJR Am J Roentgenol 1999;172:213–218.
22. Marchal G, Rioux P, Petit-Taboue MC, et al. Regional cerebral oxygen consumption, blood flow, and blood volume in healthy human aging. Arch Neurol 1992;49:1013–1020.
23. Catafau AM, Lomena FJ, Pavia J, et al. Regional cerebral blood flow pattern in normal young and aged volunteers: a 99mTc-HMPAO SPET study. Eur J Nucl Med 1996;23:1329–137.
24. Krausz Y, Bonne O, Gorfine M, Karger H, Lerer B, Chisin R. Age-related changes in brain perfusion of normal subjects detected by 99mTc-HMPAO SPECT. Neuroradiology 1998;40:428–434.
25. Nobler MS, Mann JJ, Sackeim HA. Serotonin, cerebral blood flow, and cerebral metabolic rate in geriatric major depression and normal aging. Brain Res Brain Res Rev 1999;30:250–263.
26. Schultz SK, O'Leary DS, Boles Ponto LL, Watkins GL, Hichwa RD, Andreasen NC. Age-related changes in regional cerebral blood flow among young to mid-life adults. Neuroreport 1999;10:2493–2496.
27. Lipsitz LA. Orthostatic hypotension in the elderly. N Engl J Med 1989;321:952–957.
28. Lipsitz LA, Marks ER, Koestner J, Jonsson PV, Wei JY. Reduced susceptibility to syncope during postural tilt in old age. Is beta-blockade protective? Arch Intern Med 1989;149:2709–2712.
29. Seals DR, Esler MD. Human ageing and the sympathoadrenal system. J Physiol 2000;528:407–417.
30. Larsen FS, Olsen KS, Hansen BA, Paulson OB, Knudsen GM. Transcranial Doppler is valid for determination of the lower limit of cerebral blood flow autoregulation. Stroke 1994;25:1985–1988.
31. Hoffman WE, Miletich DJ, Albrecht RF. The influence of antihypertensive therapy on cerebral autoregulation in aged hypertensive rats. Stroke 1982;13:701–704.
32. Hoffman WE, Albrecht RF, Miletich DJ. The influence of aging and hypertension on cerebral autoregulation. Brain Res 1981;214:196–199.
33. Fujishima M, Sadoshima S, Ogata J, et al. Autoregulation of cerebral blood flow in young and aged spontaneously hypertensive rats (SHR). Gerontology 1984;30:30–36.
34. Toyoda K, Fujii K, Takata Y, Ibayashi S, Fujikawa M, Fujishima M. Effect of aging on regulation of brain stem circulation during hypotension. J Cereb Blood Flow Metab 1997;17:680–685.
35. Kastrup A, Dichgans J, Niemeier M, Schabet M. Changes of cerebrovascular CO2 reactivity during normal aging. Stroke 1998;29:1311–1314.
36. Ito H, Kanno I, Ibaraki M, Hatazawa J. Effect of aging on cerebral vascular response to PaCo2 changes in humans as measured by positron emission tomography. J Cereb Blood Flow Metab 2002;22:997–1003.
37. Lartaud I, Bray-des-Boscs L, Chillon JM, Atkinson J, Capdeville-Atkinson C. In vivo cerebrovascular reactivity in Wistar and Fischer 344 rat strains during aging. Amer J Physiol 1993;264:H851–H858.
38. Lipsitz LA, Mukai S, Hamner J, Gagnon M, Babikian V. Dynamic regulation of middle cerebral artery blood flow velocity in aging and hypertension. Stroke 2000;31:1897–1903.

39. Matteis M, Troisi E, Monaldo BC, Caltagirone C, Silvestrini M. Age and sex differences in cerebral hemodynamics: a transcranial Doppler study. Stroke 1998;29:963–967.
40. Oblak JP, Zaletel M, Zvan B, Kiauta T, Pogacnik T. The effect of age on cerebrovascular reactivity to cold pressor test and head-up tilt. Acta Neurol Scand 2002;106:30–33.
41. Thorin-Trescases N, Bartolotta T, Hyman N, et al. Diameter dependence of myogenic tone of human pial arteries. Possible relation to distensibility. Stroke 1997;28:2486–2492.
42. Carey BJ, Eames PJ, Blake MJ, Panerai RB, Potter JF. Dynamic cerebral autoregulation is unaffected by aging. Stroke 2000;31:2895–2900.
43. Umeyama T, Kugimiya T, Ogawa T, Kandori Y, Ishizuka A, Hanaoka K. Changes in cerebral blood flow estimated after stellate ganglion block by single photon emission computed tomography. J Auton Nerv Syst 1995;50:339–346.
44. Nitahara K, Dan K. Blood flow velocity changes in carotid and vertebral arteries with stellate ganglion block: measurement by magnetic resonance imaging using a direct bolus tracking method. Reg Anesth Pain Med 1998;23:600–604.
45. Wahlgren NG, Hellstrom G, Lindquist C, Rudehill A. Sympathetic nerve stimulation in humans increases middle cerebral artery blood flow velocity. Cerebrovasc Dis 1992;2:359–364.
46. Strebel S, Lam AM, Matta B, Mayberg TS, Aaslid R, Newell DW. Dynamic and static cerebral autoregulation during isoflurane, desflurane, and propofol anesthesia. Anesthesiology 1995;83:66–76.
47. Strebel S, Kaufmann M, Anselmi L, Schaefer HG. Nitrous oxide is a potent cerebrovasodilator in humans when added to isoflurane. A transcranial Doppler study. Acta Anaesthesiol Scand 1995;39:653–658.
48. Goadsby PJ, Duckworth JW. Low frequency stimulation of the locus coeruleus reduces regional cerebral blood flow in the spinalized cat. Brain Res 1989;476:71–77.
49. Serrador JM, Picot PA, Rutt BK, Shoemaker JK, Bondar RL. MRI measures of middle cerebral artery diameter in conscious humans during simulated orthostasis. Stroke 2000;31:1672–1678.
50. Bramanti P, Mariani CA, D'Aleo G, Malara A. The first in vivo experience of the effects of the continuous intrathecal infusion of clonidine on the locus ceruleus in the regulation of cerebral blood flow: a TCD study. Ital J Neurol Sci 1997; 18:139–144.
51. Micieli G, Tassorelli C, Bosone D, Cavallini A, Viotti E, Nappi G. Intracerebral vascular changes induced by cold pressor test: a model of sympathetic activation. Neurol Res 1994;16:163–167.
52. Meyer JS, Shimazu K, Okamoto S, et al. Effects of alpha adrenergic blockade on autoregulation and chemical vasomotor control of CBF in stroke. Stroke 1973;4:187–200.
53. Jordan J, Shannon JR, Black BK, Paranjape SY, Barwise J, Robertson D. Raised cerebrovascular resistance in idiopathic orthostatic intolerance: evidence for sympathetic vasoconstriction. Hypertension 1998;32:699–704.
54. Lee HW, Caldwell JE, Dodson B, Talke P, Howley J. The effect of clonidine on cerebral blood flow velocity, carbon dioxide cerebral vasoreactivity, and response to increased arterial pressure in human volunteers. Anesthesiology 1997; 87:553–558.
55. Strebel SP, Kindler C, Bissonnette B, Tschaler G, Deanovic D. The impact of systemic vasoconstrictors on the cerebral circulation of anesthetized patients. Anesthesiology 1998;89:67–72.
56. Olesen J. The effect of intracarotid epinephrine, norepinephrine, and angiotensin on the regional cerebral blood flow in man. Neurology 1972;22:978–987.
57. Kimmerly DS, Tutungi E, Wilson TD, et al. Circulating norepinephrine and cerebrovascular control in conscious humans. Clin Physiol Funct Imaging 2003;23:314–319.
58. Jiang HX, Chen PC, Sobin SS, Giannotta SL. Age related alterations in the response of the pial arterioles to adenosine in the rat. Mech Ageing Dev 1992;65:257–276.
59. Geary GG, Buchholz JN. Selected contribution: effects of aging on cerebrovascular tone and [Ca2+]i. J Appl Physiol 2003;95:1746–1754.
60. Geary GG, Buchholz JN, Pearce WJ. Maturation depresses mouse cerebrovascular tone through endothelium-dependent mechanisms. Am J Physiol Regul Integr Comp Physiol 2003;284:R734–R741.
61. Sato A, Sato Y, Uchida S. Regulation of cerebral cortical blood flow by the basal forebrain cholinergic fibers and aging. Auton Neurosci 2002;96:13–19.
62. Uchida S, Suzuki A, Kagitani F, Hotta H. Effects of age on cholinergic vasodilation of cortical cerebral blood vessels in rats. Neurosci Lett 2000;294:109–112.
63. Hajdu MA, McElmurry RT, Heistad DD, Baumbach GL. Effects of aging on cerebral vascular responses to serotonin in rats. Amer J Physiol 1993;264:H2136–H2140.
64. Yoshii F, Barker WW, Chang JY, et al. Sensitivity of cerebral glucose metabolism to age, gender, brain volume, brain atrophy, and cerebrovascular risk factors. J Cereb Blood Flow Metab 1988;8:654–661.
65. Krajewski A, Freeman R, Ruthazer R, Kelley M, Lipsitz LA. Transcranial Doppler assessment of the cerebral circulation during postprandial hypotension in the elderly. J Am Geriatr Soc 1993;41:19–24.
66. Mehagnoul-Schipper DJ, Vloet LC, Colier WN, Hoefnagels WH, Jansen RW. Cerebral oxygenation declines in healthy elderly subjects in response to assuming the upright position. Stroke 2000;31:1615–1620.
67. Mehagnoul-Schipper DJ, Colier WN, Jansen RW. Reproducibility of orthostatic changes in cerebral oxygenation in healthy subjects aged 70 years or older. Clin Physiol 2001;21:77–84.

68. Geroldi C, Ferrucci L, Bandinelli S, et al. Mild cognitive deterioration with subcortical features: prevalence, clinical characteristics, and association with cardiovascular risk factors in community-dwelling older persons (The InCHIANTI Study). J Am Geriatr Soc 2003;51:1064–1071.
69. van Swieten JC, van den Hout JH, van Ketel BA, Hijdra A, Wokke JH, van Gijn J. Periventricular lesions in the white matter on magnetic resonance imaging in the elderly. A morphometric correlation with arteriolosclerosis and dilated perivascular spaces. Brain 1991;114:761–774.
70. Pantoni L, Garcia JH. Cognitive impairment and cellular/vascular changes in the cerebral white matter. Ann N Y Acad Sci 1997;826:92–102.
71. Yamauchi H, Fukuyama H, Nagahama Y, et al. Brain arteriolosclerosis and hemodynamic disturbance may induce leukoaraiosis. Neurology 1999;53:1833–1838.
72. Takao M, Koto A, Tanahashi N, Fukuuchi Y, Takagi M, Morinaga S. Pathologic findings of silent hyperintense white matter lesions on MRI. J Neurol Sci 1999;167:127–131.
73. Fazekas F, Schmidt R, Scheltens P. Pathophysiologic mechanisms in the development of age-related white matter changes of the brain. Dement Geriatr Cogn Disord 1998;9(Suppl):2–5.
74. Meyer JS, Rauch G, Rauch RA, Haque A. Risk factors for cerebral hypoperfusion, mild cognitive impairment, and dementia. Neurobiol Aging 2000;21:161–169.
75. O'Sullivan M, Lythgoe DJ, Pereira AC, et al. Patterns of cerebral blood flow reduction in patients with ischemic leukoaraiosis. Neurology 2002;59:321–326.
76. Cada A, de la Torre JC, Gonzalez-Lima F. Chronic cerebrovascular ischemia in aged rats: effects on brain metabolic capacity and behavior. Neurobiol Aging 2000;21:225–233.
77. Sopala M, Danysz W. Chronic cerebral hypoperfusion in the rat enhances age-related deficits in spatial memory. J Neural Transm 2001;108:1445–1456.
78. Tomimoto H, Ihara M, Wakita H, et al. Chronic cerebral hypoperfusion induces white matter lesions and loss of oligodendroglia with DNA fragmentation in the rat. Acta Neuropathol (Berl) 2003;106:527–534.
79. Miyazawa N, Satoh T, Hashizume K, Fukamachi A. Xenon contrast CT-CBF measurements in high-intensity foci on T2-weighted MR images in centrum semiovale of asymptomatic individuals. Stroke 1997;28:984–987.
80. Hatazawa J, Shimosegawa E, Satoh T, Toyoshima H, Okudera T. Subcortical hypoperfusion associated with asymptomatic white matter lesions on magnetic resonance imaging. Stroke 1997;28:1944–1947.
81. Perlmuter LC, Greenberg JJ. Do you mind standing? Cognitive changes in orthostasis. Exp Aging Res 1996;22: 325–341.
82. Matsubayashi K, Okumiya K, Wada T, et al. Postural dysregulation in systolic blood pressure is associated with worsened scoring on neurobehavioral function tests and leukoaraiosis in the older elderly living in a community. Stroke 1997;28:2169–2173.
83. Kohara K, Jiang Y, Igase M, et al. Postprandial hypotension is associated with asymptomatic cerebrovascular damage in essential hypertensive patients. Hypertension 1999;33:565–568.
84. De Reuck J. The human periventricular arterial blood supply and the anatomy of cerebral infarctions. Eur Neurol 1971; 5:321–334.
85. Raiha I, Tarvonen S, Kurki T, Rajala T, Sourander L. Relationship between vascular factors and white matter low attenuation of the brain. Acta Neurol Scand 1993;87:286–289.
86. Puisieux F, Monaca P, Deplanque D, et al. Relationship between leuko-araiosis and blood pressure variability in the elderly. Eur Neurol 2001;46:115–120.
87. Tohgi H, Chiba K, Kimura M. Twenty-four-hour variation of blood pressure in vascular dementia of the Binswanger type. Stroke 1991;22:603–608.
88. Kario K, Tobin JN, Wolfson LI, et al. Lower standing systolic blood pressure as a predictor of falls in the elderly: a community-based prospective study. J Am Coll Cardiol 2001;38:246–252.
89. Hossain M, Ooi WL, Lipsitz LA. Intra-individual postural blood pressure variability and stroke in elderly nursing home residents. J Clin Epidemiol 2001;54:488–494.
90. Tomlinson BE, Blessed G, Roth M. Observations on the brains of demented old people. J Neurol Sci 1970;11:205–242.
91. Killiany RJ, Gomez-Isla T, Moss M, et al. Use of structural magnetic resonance imaging to predict who will get Alzheimer's disease. Ann Neurol 2000;47:430–439.
92. Kivipelto M, Helkala EL, Laakso MP, et al. Midlife vascular risk factors and Alzheimer's disease in later life: longitudinal, population based study. Br Med J 2001;322:1447–1451.
93. Simons M, Keller P, Dichgans J, Schulz JB. Cholesterol and Alzheimer's disease: is there a link? Neurology 2001;57:1089–1093.
94. Hofman A, Ott A, Breteler MM, et al. Atherosclerosis, apolipoprotein E, and prevalence of dementia and Alzheimer's disease in the Rotterdam Study. Lancet 1997;349:151–154.
95. Skoog I, Lernfelt B, Landahl S, et al. 15-year longitudinal study of blood pressure and dementia. Lancet 1996;347:1141–1145.
96. Snowdon DA, Greiner LH, Mortimer JA, Riley KP, Greiner PA, Markesbery WR. Brain infarction and the clinical expression of Alzheimer disease. The Nun Study. JAMA 1997;277:813–817.

97. van Kooten F, Bots ML, Breteler MM, et al. The Dutch Vascular Factors in Dementia Study: rationale and design. J Neurol 1998;245:32–39.
98. Albert MS, Moss MB, Tanzi R, Jones K. Preclinical prediction of AD using neuropsychological tests. J Int Neuropsychol Soc 2001;7:631–639.
99. Kuwabara Y, Ichiya Y, Otsuka M, Masuda K, Ichimiya A, Fujishima M. Cerebrovascular responsiveness to hypercapnia in Alzheimer's dementia and vascular dementia of the Binswanger type. Stroke 1992;23:594–598.
100. Nagata K, Maruya H, Yuya H, et al. Can PET data differentiate Alzheimer's disease from vascular dementia? Ann N Y Acad Sci 2000;903:252–261.
101. O'Brien JT, Eagger S, Syed GM, Sahakian BJ, Levy R. A study of regional cerebral blood flow and cognitive performance in Alzheimer's disease. J Neurol Neurosurg Psychiatry 1992;55:1182–1187.
102. Soininen H, Helkala EL, Kuikka J, Hartikainen P, Lehtovirta M, Riekkinen PJ, Sr. Regional cerebral blood flow measured by 99mTc-HMPAO SPECT differs in subgroups of Alzheimer's disease. J Neural Transm Park Dis Dement Sect 1995;9:95–109.
103. Starkstein SE, Sabe L, Vazquez S, et al. Neuropsychological, psychiatric, and cerebral blood flow findings in vascular dementia and Alzheimer's disease. Stroke 1996;27:408–414.
104. Syed GM, Eagger S, O'Brien J, Barrett JJ, Levy R. Patterns of regional cerebral blood flow in Alzheimer's disease. Nucl Med Commun 1992;13:656–663.
105. Wyper D, Teasdale E, Patterson J, et al. Abnormalities in rCBF and computed tomography in patients with Alzheimer's disease and in controls. Br J Radiol 1993;66:23–27.
106. Zimmer R, Leucht S, Radler T, Schmauss F, Gebhardt U, Lauter H. Variability of cerebral blood flow deficits in 99mTc-HMPAO SPECT in patients with Alzheimer's disease. J Neural Transm 1997;104:689–701.

6

The CADASIL Syndrome and Other Genetic Causes of Stroke and Vascular Dementia

Stephen Salloway and Sophie Desbiens

1. INTRODUCTION

Genetic factors play an important role in the etiology of stroke and vascular dementia (VaD). Genetic influences are primarily polygenic, although several monogenic disorders causing stroke have recently been identified. The clearest example of a monogenic disorder causing small artery stroke and vascular dementia is the cerebral autosomal dominant arteriopathy with subcortical infarcts and leukoencephalopathy (CADASIL) syndrome. CADASIL is a useful model for studying the pathogenesis of small artery disease and the correlation between imaging changes and the evolution of clinical symptoms in VaD. CADASIL is a nonatherosclerotic, nonamyloid angiopathy caused by mutations in the Notch-3 gene on chromosome 19. Affected individuals develop subcortical strokes, cognitive deficits, migraines with aura, mood disorders, pseudobulbar palsy, and physical disability in their 50s and 60s *(1)*. Brain magnetic resonance imaging (MRI) reveals large areas of leukoencephalopathy and multiple subcortical lacunar infarctions. More than 500 families have been identified worldwide *(2)*, but the disease is underdiagnosed and its prevalence is unknown. The first transgenic model expressing a notch3 mutation has been developed and considerable progress has been made in understanding the physiology of notch3 signaling and the sequence of arterial degeneration in CADASIL. This chapter concludes with a review of the recent advances in identifying gene candidates of other monogenic and polygenic disorders associated with stroke.

2. CADASIL

In 1977, Sourander and Walinder described a syndrome of "hereditary multi-infarct dementia" *(1)*. In this family, the disease was transmitted in an autosomal dominant mode and characterized by multiple infarcts starting between 30 and 40 yr of age, followed by a progressive evolution toward dementia. This multifaceted condition was given several names in the literature, such as familial Binswanger's syndrome, familial disorder with subcortical ischaemic strokes, dementia and leukoencephalopathy, and chronic familial vascular encephalopathy. In 1993, Joutel et al. proposed the currently accepted and more complete name for this illness: cerebral autosomal dominant arteriopathy with subcortical infarcts and leukoencephalopathy, with the acronym CADASIL *(3,4)*.

CADASIL cases have been reported throughout the world, predominantly in Europe *(1)*. Joutel and colleagues first mapped the disease to chromosome 19 in a group of French families *(5,6)* and later identified the Notch-3 gene at locus 19p13.1-13.2 6. In a subsequent article *(7)*, the group published a list of the specific mutations found in these families. Ultrastructural and immunohistochemical analysis of skin biopsies *(8,9)* have also been employed to develop a more extensive profile of the disease.

From: *Current Clinical Neurology*
Vascular Dementia: Cerebrovascular Mechanisms and Clinical Management
Edited by: R. H. Paul, R. Cohen, B. R. Ott, and S. Salloway © Humana Press Inc., Totowa, NJ

Retrospective analysis and tests of living family members showed that the first description of CADASIL was likely given by Bogaert et al. in 1955 as a familial form of Binswanger's disease *(1)*. It is also interesting to note that recent examinations performed on material from the family described by Sourander and Walinder showed that they do not have the immunohistochemical and pathological abnormalities present in other CADASIL patients. Hence, they must suffer from a different form of VaD.

2.1. Clinical Presentation

There are four principal clinical symptoms of CADASIL: migraine with aura, ischemic strokes, psychiatric disturbances, and cognitive decline leading to dementia. The evolution of the disease is progressive, lasting from 10 to 30 yr from the first stroke to death *(10)*. Although the oldest known individual with CADASIL is a 94-yr-old woman *(1)*, the mean age at death is 64.5 yr *(11)*. The pattern of cardiovascular risk factors, such as hypertension, is usually absent or mild.

Approximately 38% of patients with CADASIL suffer from migraine with or without aura *(12,13)*. The headaches begin in the mid-20s to late 30s and are generally the first symptom to appear. The aura is frequently visual or sensorial but often atypical, extremely strong, and/or long lasting. In some cases, the aura may even appear as hemiplegia. This could be explained by the proximity of the CADASIL gene on chromosome 19p13.1-13.2 6 to the gene for familial hemiplegic migraine, also on chromosome 19p13.1 5. *(5)*. The severity of the migraines decreases after the first stroke.

For most of the patients suffering from CADASIL, the first symptom is a transient ischemic attack (TIA) or an ischemic stroke. Approximately 85% of the patients report episodes of TIA or stroke in their lifetimes. These attacks usually start between 40 and 50 yr of age, although some reports have described patients experiencing their first TIA as early as 28 yr old *(14)* and as late as 70 yr old *(15)*. The strokes are primarily lacunar, usually producing sensory or motor symptoms. The strokes are almost always subcortical, occurring in the periventricular and deep white matter as well as in the basal ganglia (*see* Fig. 1). They can sometimes occur in the brainstem and are rarely seen in the spinal cord. As more strokes occur, other deficits, such as pseudobulbar palsy and gait disturbances, appear, with immobility and mutism occurring late in the illness. For the other 10–15% of CADASIL cases without a documented stroke or TIA, ischemic lesions can be seen by imaging but are clinically silent.

Mood disorders are the most frequently reported psychiatric disturbance, affecting approx 30% of patients. Depression is most common, whereas manic depressive disorders and panic attacks are less frequent. Schizophrenia has been reported in one CADASIL patient *(16)*. In addition to mood disorders, seizures are observed in 6–10% of cases.

Cognitive decline can be seen in early stages of the disease, especially in the frontal lobe-related tasks, such as concentration, organization, and executive functions. Patients perform relatively well at first on the Mini-Mental State Examination (MMSE); however, scores generally decline as the disease progresses. Memory impairment and slowing of psychomotor speed occur because of progressive ischemic injury involving frontal-subcortical systems. Patients perform poorly on tests of psychomotor speed, such as the Trailmaking test. The progressive decline in cognitive functions eventually leads to subcortical vascular dementia and by the age of 65, 80% of the patients develop dementia *(12)*.

2.2. Imaging

Patients with CADASIL show evidence of signal hyperintensities (SH) on T2-weighted magnetic resonance imaging (MRI) scans beginning in their early 20s. Fluid attenuated inversion recovery (FLAIR) MRI is the most sensitive sequence for detecting the SH in CADASIL. In the early stages of the illness, punctate and early confluent areas of SH are present in the deep white matter and periventricular regions in a pattern that resembles early multiple sclerosis. As the disease progresses, the hyperintensities become more confluent and involve large areas of the deep white matter involving the anterior temporal lobes, external capsule, basal ganglia, and extending out to

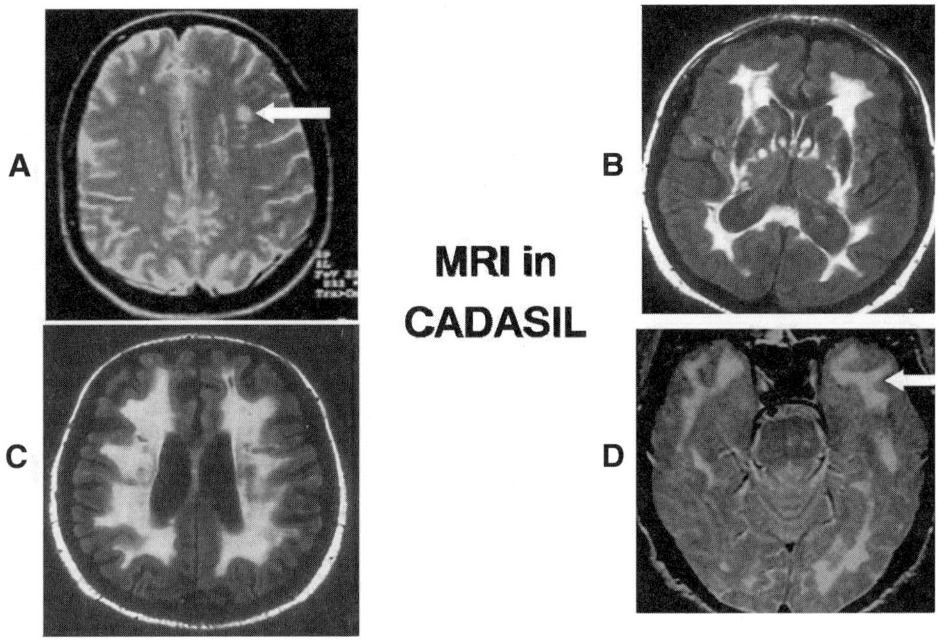

Fig. 1. Magnetic resonance imaging (MRI) in cerebral autosomal dominant arteriopathy with subcortical infarcts and leukoencephalopathy (CADASIL). **(A)** Early/presymptomatic CADASIL. A 29-yr-old woman with a history of one episode of migraine with aura and no cognitive symptoms or ischemic events. T2-weighted MRI shows areas of beginning confluence in the deep white matter on the left (arrow). **(B)** Early ischemic phase. A 58-yr-old man with mild cognitive difficulty and two transient ischemic attack (TIA) episodes. Fluid attenuated inversion recovery sequence (FLAIR) shows large confluent areas of high signal in the white matter anterior and posterior to the lateral ventricles. **(C)** Late-stage CADASIL. A 63-yr-old woman with multiple stroke-like events and gradually progressive subcortical dementia. FLAIR sequence shows a large area of confluent high signal occupying most of the white matter. Low-density areas in the white matter represent lacunar infarctions. **(D)** Areas of high signal in the anterior temporal lobe white matter on T2-weighted scans (arrow) are characteristic MRI findings in later stage CADASIL.

the cortical U-fibers (*see* Fig. 1). Subcortical brain areas are more affected than the brainstem. Over time single, multiple or numerous small lacunar infarctions develop within the areas of confluent SH in the white matter and basal ganglia and can be seen as areas of well-circumscribed hypointensity on T1-weighted MRI sequences and computed tomography (CT). The addition of contrast does not usually demonstrate evidence of contrast enhancement. Punctate areas of microhemorrhage on gradient echo MRI sequences have been reported in approximately one-third of CADASIL patients *(17,18)*. Larger territorial infarctions are rare and the cerebral cortex is usually unaffected.

Diffusion tensor MRI, a new MRI technique that maps diffusion of water in specific directions in white matter tracts, has revealed a significant increase in water diffusivity and a loss of anisotropy, meaning the water diffuses with less restraint in any direction in areas of confluent SH in CADASIL *(19)*. Similar changes in diffusion and anisotropy in normal-appearing white matter in patients with CADASIL may be a good predictor of later functional decline.

Investigators using single photon emission computed tomography (SPECT) *(20)* and positron emission tomography (PET) *(13)* have reported a reduction in cerebral blood flow (CBF) in CADASIL. The PET study indicated that the decrease in CBF precedes tissue destruction because the

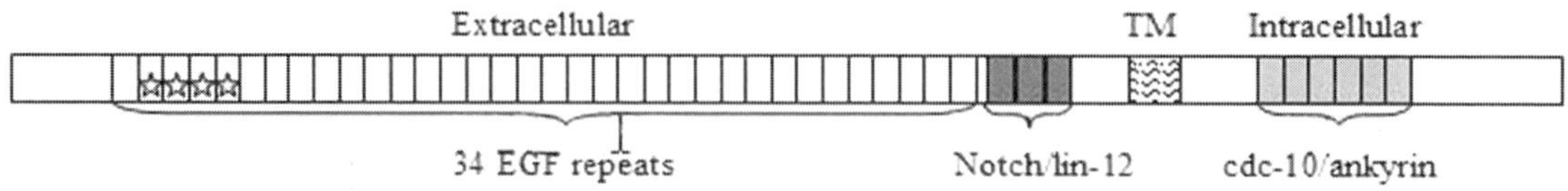

Fig. 2. Notch 3 receptor. The Notch-3 protein comprises 34 epidermal growth factor (EGF)-like repeats and 3 Notch/lin-12 repeats on the extracellular side and 6 cdc-10/ankyrin repeats on the intracellular side. The stars indicate the EGF repeats most often mutated in patients with cerebral autosomal dominant arteriopathy with subcortical infarcts and leukoencephalopathy.

oxygen extraction fraction is increased in asymptomatic patients with dementia, whereas oxygen consumption is decreased only in patients with dementia. This result suggests that the brain compensates for a decreased CBF by increasing the oxygen extraction fraction. Using MRI bolus tracking, Chabriat and colleagues *(21)* showed that both the basal perfusion and the hemodynamic reserve are decreased in the T2-weighted hyperintense areas. In addition, the group related the severity of the hypoperfusion to disease progression such that patients with CADASIL who also have dementia have a lower perfusion compared to symptomatic but patients without dementia.

2.3. Genetics

CADASIL is primarily caused by a mutation in the Notch3 gene, located on chromosome 19p13.1-13.2 6. Transmission is autosomal dominant with 100% penetrance. Rare sporadic mutations have been reported. The gene contains 33 exons and encodes a transmembrane protein of 2321 amino acids. The Notch-3 protein is a receptor comprising several functional domains (*see* Fig. 2). On its extracellular portion, it contains 34 epidermal growth factor-like (EGF) repeats followed by three notch/lin-12 repeats. The intracellular domain contains six cdc-10/ankyrin repeats. Interestingly, all the mutations found in patients with CADASIL involved the addition or removal of a cysteine (three cysteines in a rare deletion case) in one of the EGF repeats, leading to an odd number of cysteines (EGF repeats have 6 cysteines). Sixty percent of these mutations are caused by a single base pair change in exon 3 or 4, which code for the EGF repeats 2–5. To date, more than 65 point mutations and 4 deletions causing CADASIL have been reported *(1)*. Dichgans and colleagues *(22)* generated a three-dimensional model of the first 6 EGF repeats based on nuclear magnetic resonance (NMR) data from human fibrilin-1 *(22)*. For the addition or removal of a cysteine, the model predicted a protein misfolding. Several polymorphisms have also been reported in the Notch3 gene, which do not cause an amino acid substitution, do not cause CADASIL, and do not increase the risk for ischemic cerebrovascular disease (CVD) *(23)*.

2.4. Pathology and Pathogenesis

CADASIL is characterized by a nonatherosclerotic, nonamyloid angiopathy, primarily involving small arteries in the CNS but also seen to a lesser degree in medium and small arteries in other organs. Postmortem examination of the brains of patients with CADASIL reveals extensive demyelination and gliosis with scattered lacunar infarctions in the deep white matter and basal ganglia, as well as in the brainstem, with relative sparing of the cerebral cortex. The walls of the small and medium-sized leptomeningeal and penetrating arteries are thickened because of the accumulation of extracellular matrix proteins. Characteristic basophilic granular osmiophilic material (GOM) accumulates in the degenerating tunica media. This granular material stains positive for Notch3 ectodomain. The granular deposits are characteristic of CADASIL and may help to distinguish between other diseases, such as Binswanger's disease and hypertensive arteriosclerotic disease (*see* Fig. 3).

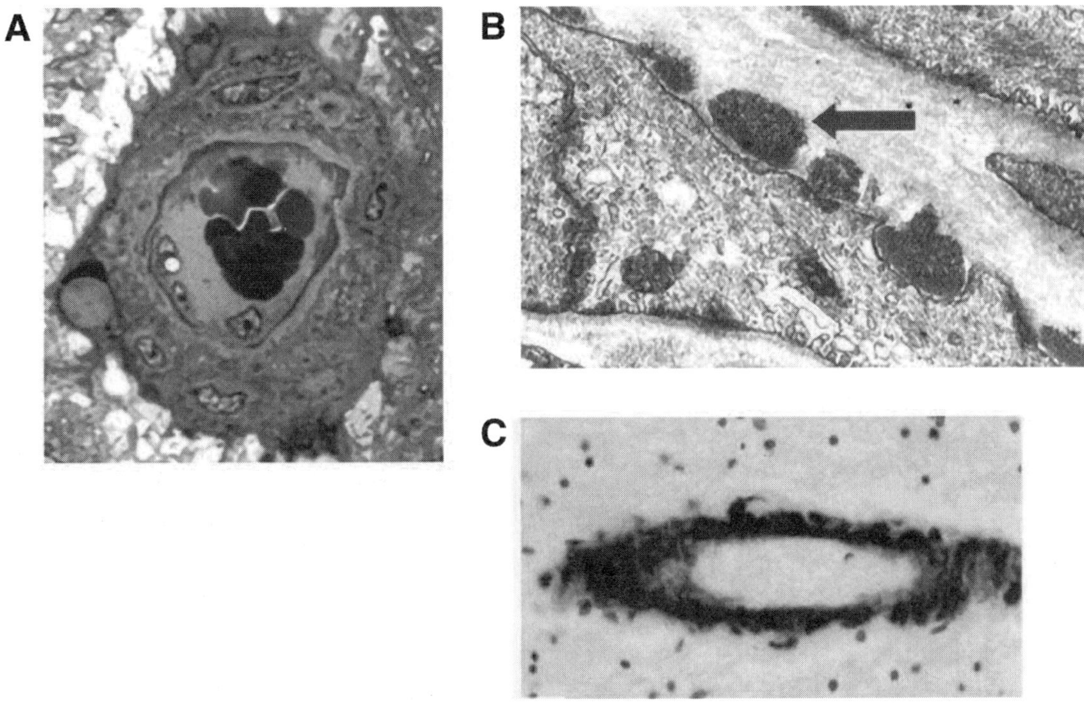

Fig. 3. Small artery changes in cerebral autosomal dominant arteriopathy with subcortical infarcts and leukoencephalopathy (CADASIL). **(A)** Semithin section from a 40-m diameter blood vessel from a deep white matter biopsy in a patient with CADASIL shows degeneration of the smooth muscle layer with replacement by diffuse granular material. **(B)** Electron micrograph of a small artery from the same biopsy in A (×38,000) shows dense core granules emanating from the smooth muscle layer, which is a characteristic feature of CADASIL. **(C)** Notch3 antibody staining of a small artery from a skin biopsy in a patient with CADASIL shows heavy staining of notch3 antibody denoting accumulation of notch3 protein in the smooth muscle layer.

Electron microscopic (EM) analysis of skin biopsies is an effective tool for both diagnosis and research, because skin samples are more easily obtained than brain tissue and provide useful information about mechanisms of disease. Originally, CADASIL was believed to decrease the luminal size of the arteries *(9)*. However, more recent analysis on 152 skin biopsy samples showed that the sclerotic index, defined as: 1-(internal diameter/external diameter), was the same for patients and controls *(24)*. Skin biopsies show degeneration and loss of smooth muscle cells (SMC), as well as the loss of the link between the SMC and endothelial cells, and the unusual presence of luminal electrolucent vacuoles in the endothelial cells. SMC secrete vascular endothelial growth factor (VEGF), which is an important permeability factor. A current hypothesis is that damage to the SMC would decrease the secretion of VEGF, which, in turn, would lead to a decrease in permeability and a loss of vessel wall tonicity *(24)*. A slight increase in the extracellular matrix, combined with the loss of SMC, contributes to preserve the sclerotic index in CADASIL patients. Moreover, GOM deposits are seen near the vascular smooth muscle cell (VSMC) indentations. All these changes can be observed in asymptomatic carriers as young as 20 yr old, even before MRI changes appear, and become stronger as the disease worsens.

GOM was described for the first time in 1991 *(24a)* and was associated with CADASIL in 1993 *(4)*. These electron-dense circular deposits are approx 0.5-1 μm in diameter *(25)* and their composition remains unknown (*see* Fig. 2). However, GOM can be stained using the periodic acid-Schiff stain (PAS), suggesting that it may contain acid polysaccharides. Several groups have shown that the deposits do not contain certain components, such as amyloid, elastin, chromatin, calcium, iron, and other metals and minerals. The number of GOM deposits varies with the patient's age *(24)*, increasing until a maximum at approx 50 yr and then decreasing. It is sometimes difficult to find GOM deposits in older patients.

Recently, Joutel and colleagues *(8)* developed a Notch3 monoclonal antibody and used it in immunostaining of skin biopsies. Staining was seen in approx 80% of the small arterioles and in a few veins and capillaries of the patients with CADASIL and was weak or absent in controls. Studies in adults have shown that Notch3 expression is restricted to vascular SMC of arteries and occasionally some veins and capillaries, which is in agreement with the pathological findings *(26,27)*. The mutant receptor can still be expressed on the cell surface and bind ligand *(28,29)*. According to Karlström and colleagues, the mutations impair intracellular trafficking and maturation of the receptor. In their HEK expression system, the mutated Notch3 receptors tend to form more intracellular aggregates than the wild type receptor. However, receptors reaching the surface had the correct molecular weight and could bind the ligand to trigger the expression of a reporter gene, indicating that Notch3 signaling was not affected by the mutation.

The Notch3 protein is cleaved in the Golgi, producing a 210 kDa extracellular and a 97 kDa intracellular fragment, which remain associated to form a heterodimer *(27)*. Protein extraction followed by western blot of brain samples from the control subjects showed no immunoreactivity to antibodies against the intracellular or extracellular fragments. However, for the patients with CADASIL, there was a strong signal near 210 kDa with the antibody against the extracellular fragment, suggesting that there is an accumulation of the Notch3 ectodomain. Because the amount of mRNA for Notch3 is identical in controls and patients, it was suggested that this accumulation most likely resulted from an impaired clearance of the protein and not from overproduction.

The first transgenic mouse model of CADASIL was recently reported *(30)*, which provides important clues about the steps involved in the arterial degeneration seen in CADASIL. This transgenic animal was created by inserting a human Notch3 Arg90Cys mutation, driven by a promoter insuring localized expression in arterial VSMCs. Mice did not show any signs of parenchymal brain damage but did show characteristic changes in small arteries, especially in the tail. The cytoarchitectural changes were first noted at 10 mo of age and consisted of enlargement of the subendothelial and intra-SMC spaces, which were filled with cellular debris. This was followed by blurring of the plasma membrane of VSMCs with development of vacuoles and accumulation of mitochondria in the VSMCs. The accumulation of notch3 protein and GOM, the pathological hallmarks of CADASIL, were noted after 14–16 mo of age, long after the endothelial and SMC changes noted.

2.5. Notch Signaling

Notch was first identified in *Drosophila* where a null allele or deletion causes a notch in the fly's wing. The Notch gene is involved in the development of several tissues and organs, such as the central nervous system (CNS), the eye, the sensory bristles, and the germ lines *(31)*. Notch homologues have been found in multiple species, including two in *Caenorhabditis elegans*, four in the mouse, and four in humans. In *Drosophila*, two ligands can bind to Notch in a calcium-dependent manner. The first, Delta, has one mammalian homologue named Delta-1, whereas the second, Serrate, and has two mammalian homologues called Jagged-1 and 2.

Notch is first translated as a 300 kD protein. During its passage through the Golgi, the protein is cleaved into a 200-kD extracellular fragment and a 100-kD transmembrane domain by a furin-like convertase. Both fragments remain noncovalently associated and are inserted into the membrane. When the ligand binds to the receptor, proteolytic cleavage occurs on the extracellular side by an ADAM/TACE family metalloprotease. A second cut occurs within the transmembrane segment by presenilin *(32)*. Interestingly, presinilin (PS) has been implicated in a similar intramembraneous cleavage of amyloid precursor protein (APP). In the case of Alzheimer's disease (AD), a mutation in PS1 or PS2 increases the production of the amyloidogenic $A\beta_{42}$ *(33)*.

The Notch intracellular domain (IC), which contains two nuclear localization signals, then enters the nucleus and binds to CBF-1, Suppressor of Hairless, Lag-1 (CSL) proteins. The Notch/CSL complex activates the transcription of genes that contain a CSL response element, including the Hairy, Enhancer of Split (Hes) family, which encode transcriptional repressors.

Studies have shown that the various Notch proteins found in mammals have evolved to different roles than those of the *Drosophila* Notch, and that they are not functionally redundant since knockout mice for Notch1 and Notch2 are embryonically lethal *(34,35)*. However, the general scheme described previously seems to hold with RBP-Jk, as the mammalian CSL protein, and the HES genes.

Initial studies done in vitro *(36,37)* revealed that Notch3 IC binds to RBP-Jk but is a poor activator of the HES-1 and HES-5 promoters, contrary to the Notch-1 IC/RBP-Jk complex, which is a strong activator. These studies were conducted in JEG cells, human chorion carcinoma, mouse myoblasts C2C12 cells, and monkey kidney epithelial COS-7 cells. However, more recent studies conducted by Wang et al. in VSMCs and rat carotid artery proposed a different picture for the Notch3 signaling transduction pathway *(38,39)*. In one of the papers, the group showed that Notch3 IC binds RBP-Jk and that the complex then activates the HRT-1 and -2 (Hairy-related transcription factor) genes, which are related to the HES genes39. The HRT family has been suggested as potential regulator of the VSMC terminal differentiation. In that same paper, Wang et al. also showed that Notch-3, HRT-1 and HRT-2 are all downregulated in response to arterial injury and that the time course for this decrease and recovery follows identical patterns for all three proteins. They showed that Notch-3 signaling can occur without RBP-Jk in VSMC. In this part of the pathway, Notch-3 upregulates c-FLIP via an ERK/MAPK-dependent pathway and prevents apoptosis. Apoptosis is believed to play an important role in vascular remodeling and atherogenesis and in the VSMC, this could occur through Fas. This protein is ubiquitously expressed in several tissues. When it binds its ligand, Fas induces apoptosis by recruiting caspase-8. c-FLIP inhibits the binding of caspase-8 to Fas, thus preventing apoptosis. When there is arterial injury both Notch-3 and c-FLIP are downregulated for approx 1 wk. A third study by the same group *(40)* showed that angiotensin II (Ang II) and platelet-derived growth factor (PDGF) down regulated the expression of Notch3 and of the ligand Jagged-1 and prevented glycosylation of Jagged-1. Ang II downregulation was mediated by an ERK-dependent pathway. They also showed that under low cell density, the Notch3 signaling pathway decreased cell growth, whereas under high cell confluence, the pathway perturbed the normal cell growth decrease. Therefore, the Notch3 signaling is regulated by an ensemble of cues from the cell's environment. However, more studies are required to uncover all the proteins implicated and their effects within the pathway. It is interesting to think that the interaction between Notch3 and Ang II could potentially provide a molecular explanation to the observation that blockade of Ang II synthesis is clinically effective in preventing strokes.

2.6. Diagnosis and Treatment of CADASIL

CADASIL should be considered for young patients without significant cardiovascular risk factors presenting with a history of migraines, depression, stroke-like symptoms, and/or cognitive impairments who demonstrate characteristic hyperintensities on MRI (*see* Fig. 4). In the majority of the cases, the disease is inherited, so there should be a familial history of strokes and dementia. However, there has been report of a case with a *de novo* mutation *(41)*, so absence of family history should not prevent further testing.

Genetic testing for notch3 mutations is commercially available, although the testing is often impractical because of the high cost and lack of third party reimbursement. DNA is extracted from peripheral blood and the Notch3 exons are sequenced, giving a high sensitivity. If a mutation has already been identified in the family, some testing centers will consider sequencing only the desig-

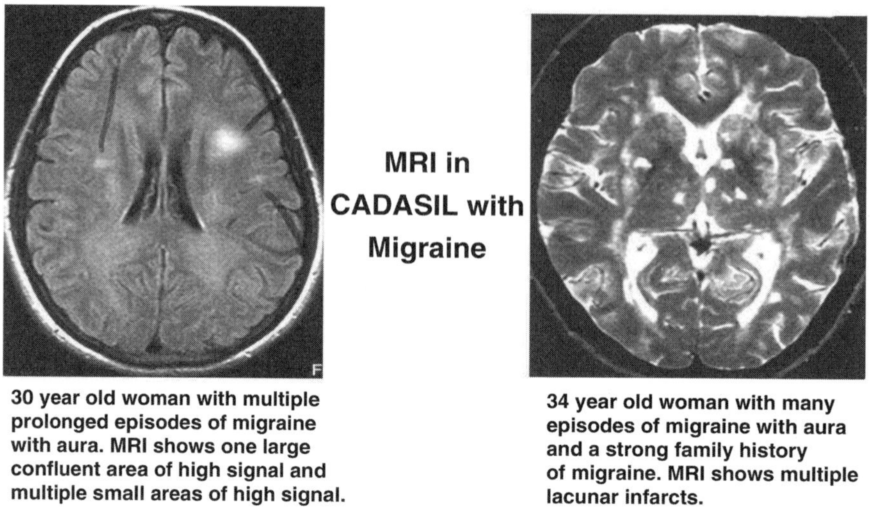

Fig. 4. Magnetic resonance imaging (MRI) in cerebral autosomal dominant arteriopathy with subcortical infarcts and leukoencephalopathy (CADASIL) with migraine. **(A)** A 30-yr-old woman with multiple prolonged episodes of migraine with aura. MRI shows one large confluent area of high signal and multiple small areas of high signal in the deep white matter. **(B)** A 34-yr-old woman with many episodes of migraine with aura and a strong family history of migraine. MRI shows multiple lacunar infarcts.

nated exon for other family members. Skin biopsy is sensitive but not specific and can be used for diagnosis. The presence of GOM on EM in small arteries in skin biopsies confirms the diagnosis, but its absence does not exclude a diagnosis of CADASIL. Also, the sensitivity of this method is highly dependent on sampling and the experience of the observer. Immunohistochemistry can also be performed on skin biopsies using the Notch3 monoclonal antibody. This technique, in combination with MRI changes, has a sensitivity of 96% and an accuracy of 100% *(8)* and is less costly than the EM studies but is still a research tool.

The MRI pattern first seen in asymptomatic CADASIL carriers is similar to that of demyelinating diseases, such as multiple sclerosis (MS). The differential diagnosis also includes other inflammatory disorders, such as sarcoidosis and vasculitis. For older patients with hypertension and other cardiovascular risk factors, Binswanger's disease or arteriosclerotic ischemic vascular disease should be considered. Amyloid angiopathy can also present with large areas of confluent SH on T2-weighted MRI sequences. The SH pattern can help distinguish between CADASIL and arteriosclerotic disease, which is much more common. Involvement of the anterior temporal lobe white matter, cortical U-fibers, and corpus callosum with milder SH in the brainstem is highly suggestive of CADASIL.

The impact of notch3 testing and MRI scanning in symptomatic and asymptomatic family members suspected of having CADASIL should be carefully considered. No treatment is currently available, and individuals may learn that they have a gene that will cause stroke and dementia. A positive test may induce a negative psychological reaction, may have important implications for family planning, and can adversely affect health insurance status. At the authors' institution, individuals who are strongly suspected of having a CADASIL mutation are encouraged to receive genetic counseling. Asymptomatic individuals from families with a known CADASIL mutation are required to complete a protocol, similar to the process involved in genetic testing for Huntington's disease, that includes genetic counseling, psychological counseling, and neurological assessment before being tested. Asymptomatic individuals from known CADASIL families who are tested as part of a research protocol may elect to receive or not receive the results of their MRI and notch3 testing.

Specific treatment for CADASIL is not currently available. Antiplatelet agents, although untested in CADASIL, should be prescribed empirically to prevent stroke. Cholinesterase inhibitors, which have shown some efficacy in improving cognition and activities in VaD should be tried as well *(42,43)*. New mechanism based therapies to slow vascular degeneration will hopefully be developed based on advances in our knowledge of the pathogenesis of CADASIL.

3. OTHER GENES IMPLICATED IN DISORDERS ASSOCIATED WITH STROKE

The cause of most common strokes is multifactorial, involving a combination of genetic and environmental factors. Studies of stroke risk in twins, siblings, and families consistently demonstrate a 1.5–2.5 increase in stroke risk among family members *(44)*. Common stroke is extremely heterogenous and most likely results from the additive or multiplicative effect of a spectrum of pathological alleles, each of which carries a small degree of risk. Some of these alleles may predispose individuals to specific subtypes of stroke, affect an intermediate factor, or be associated with specific risk factors, such as hypertension, diabetes mellitus, or hyperlipidemia *(45)*.

There have been important advances in identifying genetic mutations in a variety of monogenic and polygenic disorders associated with stroke. Some of the candidate genes are presented as follows.

Familial amyloid angiopathy usually presents with intracerebral hemorrhage rather than ischemic lesions. However, familial British dementia (FBD), a form of amyloid angiopathy, may present with extensive white matter lesions without hemorrhage with stroke-like episodes and a progressive dementia. Inheritance is autosomal dominant. A stop codon mutation has been found in the BRI gene in FBD *(46)*, and single base mutations (Glu693-Gly) in the amyloid precursor protein gene on chromosome 21 have been reported in the Dutch variant of cerebral amyloidosis *(47)*.

Familial hemiplegic migraine (FHM) is associated with ictal hemiparesis and, in some families, progressive cerebellar atrophy and episodic ataxia. In 1998, the gene for FHM was linked to chromosome 19p13, near the locus for the notch3 gene. The FHM gene codes for the calcium channel alpha 1A subunit, CACNL1A4 *(48)*.

Mitochondrial disorders, such as mitochondrial myopathy, encephalopathy, lactic acidosis, and stroke-like episodes (MELAS), exhibit a pattern of maternal inheritance. One MELAS subtype includes stroke-like episodes in people under age 40. Serial MRIs in patients with MELAS have shown a distinctive pattern, with stroke-like lesions spreading from temporal cortex to surrounding parietal-occipital cortex *(49)*. MELAS mutations are usually missense and lie within the tRNA-leu gene (UUR). MELAS demonstrates the phenomenon of heteroplasmy, with variation of DNA within different tissues, which may explain the phenotypic variation associated with mitochondrial mutations within the same family. The most frequent gene mutation in MELAS is A3243G. Mutations at 3243 may result in somatic mutations in mitochondrial DNA leading to progressive mitochondrial dysfunction *(44,47)*.

Using a genome-wide search for common forms of stroke in an extensive computerized Icelandic genealogy database clustering 476 individuals with stroke from 179 extended pedigrees, Gretarsdottir and colleagues found a susceptibility locus for stroke on chromosome 5q12 *(50)*. Fine mapping at this locus found a strong association with a gene encoding phosphodiesterase 4D (PDE4D), especially for carotid and cardiogenic stroke, forms closely associated with atherosclerosis *(51)*. They have classified the haplotypes into three groups; wild-type, at-risk, and protective.

Angiotensin has important effects on vascular tone, endothelial function, and smooth muscle proliferation, and the role of the angiotensin-converting enzyme (ACE) gene on chromosome 17q has been extensively investigated in ischemic stroke *(52)*. People with the angiotensin-1 converting enzyme genotype DD are at increased risk of myocardial infarction (MI) in some studies. In a meta-analysis, Sharma found that the D allele, acting recessively, is a modest (OR 1.31, CI 1.06-1.62) but independent risk factor for ischemic stroke *(52)*. Other studies have failed to find a significant association between the ACE gene and ischemic stroke.

4. CONCLUSION

CADASIL provides an excellent genetic model for studying the pathogenesis and clinical sequelae of small artery degeneration. Advances in understanding the microcellular events underlying the arteriopathy in CADASIL will lead to specific treatments and a better understanding of the more common forms microvascular disease seen in aging. Advances in molecular genetics have led to the identification of other candidate genes causing both monogenic and polygenic forms of stroke. The recent findings linking common stroke to chromosome 5q12 provide a valuable opportunity for studying the relationship between enzyme PDE4D and stroke associated with large-vessel atherosclerosis.

The coming decades will produce significant progress in our knowledge of the genetic basis of stroke, including complex interactions among risk factors that each carry a small genetic risk. Our technical advances in identifying risk through genetic testing in vulnerable populations will raise important ethical considerations requiring us to address the large effect that testing can have on the well-being of both affected and unaffected individuals.

ACKNOWLEDGMENTS

This work was supported in part by NIMH KO8 MH01487 and PZORR15578. The authors thank Philip Caffery for proofreading and making useful comments on the manuscript and Lisa Schultz, MD, for her suggestions regarding advances in the genetics of stroke.

REFERENCES

1. Kalimo H, Ruchoux MM, Viitanen M, Kalaria RN. CADASIL: a common form of hereditary arteriopathy causing brain infarcts and dementia. Brain Pathol 2002;12:371–384.
2. Sourander P, Walinder J. Hereditary multi-infarct dementia. Morphological and clinical studies of a new disease. Acta Neuropathol (Berl) 1977;39:247–254.
3. Tournier-Lasserve E, Joutel A, Melki J, et al. Cerebral autosomal dominant arteriopathy with subcortical infarcts and leukoencephalopathy maps to chromosome 19q12. Nat Genet 1993;3:256–259.
4. Baudrimont M, Dubas F, Joutel A, Tournier-Lasserve E, Bousser MG. Autosomal dominant leukoencephalopathy and subcortical ischemic stroke. A clinicopathological study. Stroke 1993;24:122–125.
5. Joutel A, Bousser MG, Biousse V, et al. A gene for familial hemiplegic migraine maps to chromosome 19. Nat Genet 1993;5:40–45.
6. Joutel A, Corpechot C, Ducros A, et al. Notch3 mutations in CADASIL, a hereditary adult-onset condition causing stroke and dementia. Nature 1996;383:707–710.
7. Joutel A, Vahedi K, Corpechot C, et al. Strong clustering and stereotyped nature of Notch3 mutations in CADASIL patients. Lancet 1997;350:1511–1515.
8. Joutel A, Favrole P, Labauge P, et al. Skin biopsy immunostaining with a Notch3 monoclonal antibody for CADASIL diagnosis. Lancet 2001;358:2049–2051.
9. Ruchoux MM, Maurage CA. Endothelial changes in muscle and skin biopsies in patients with CADASIL. Neuropathol Appl Neurobiol 1998;24:60–65.
10. Viitanen M, Kalimo H. CADASIL: hereditary arteriopathy leading to multiple brain infarcts and dementia. Ann N Y Acad Sci 2000;903:273–284.
11. Salloway S, Hong J. CADASIL syndrome: a genetic form of vascular dementia. J Geriatr Psychiatry Neurol 1998;11:71–77.
12. Dichgans M, Mayer M, Uttner I, et al. The phenotypic spectrum of CADASIL: clinical findings in 102 cases. Ann Neurol 1998;44:731–739.
13. Chabriat H, Vahedi K, Iba-Zizen MT, et al. Clinical spectrum of CADASIL: a study of 7 families. Cerebral autosomal dominant arteriopathy with subcortical infarcts and leukoencephalopathy. Lancet 1995;346:934–939.
14. Tuominen S, Juvonen V, Amberla K, et al. Phenotype of a homozygous CADASIL patient in comparison to 9 age-matched heterozygous patients with the same R133C Notch3 mutation. Stroke 2001;32:1767–1774.
15. Dichgans M. Cerebral autosomal dominant arteriopathy with subcortical infarcts and leukoencephalopathy: phenotypic and mutational spectrum. J Neurol Sci 2002;203-204:77–80.
16. Lagas PA, Juvonen V. Schizophrenia in a patient with cerebral autosomally dominant arteriopathy with subcortical infarcts and leucoencephalopathy (CADASIL disease). Nord J Psychiatry 2001;55:41–42.
17. Dichgans M, Holtmannspotter M, Herzog J, Peters N, Bergmann M, Yousry TA. Cerebral microbleeds in CADASIL: a gradient-echo magnetic resonance imaging and autopsy study. Stroke 2002;33:67–71.

18. Lesnik Oberstein SA, van den Boom R, van Buchem MA, et al. Cerebral microbleeds in CADASIL. Neurology 2001; 57:1066–1070.
19. Chabriat H, Pappata S, Poupon C, et al. Clinical severity in CADASIL related to ultrastructural damage in white matter: in vivo study with diffusion tensor MRI. Stroke 1999;30:2637–2643.
20. Mellies JK, Baumer T, Muller JA, et al. SPECT study of a German CADASIL family: a phenotype with migraine and progressive dementia only. Neurology 1998;50:1715–1721.
21. Chabriat H, Pappata S, Ostergaard L, et al. Cerebral hemodynamics in CADASIL before and after acetazolamide challenge assessed with MRI bolus tracking. Stroke 2000;31:1904–1912.
22. Dichgans M, Ludwig H, Muller-Hocker J, Messerschmidt A, Gasser T. Small in-frame deletions and missense mutations in CADASIL: 3D models predict misfolding of Notch3 EGF-like repeat domains. Eur J Hum Genet 2000;8:280–285.
23. Ito D, Tanahashi N, Murata M, et al. Notch3 gene polymorphism and ischaemic cerebrovascular disease. J Neurol Neurosurg Psychiatry 2002;72:382–384.
24. Brulin P, Godfraind C, Leteurtre E, Ruchoux MM. Morphometric analysis of ultrastructural vascular changes in CADASIL: analysis of 50 skin biopsy specimens and pathogenic implications. Acta Neuropathol (Berl) 2002;104: 241–248.
24a. Estes ML, Chimowitz MI, Awad IA, McMahon IT, Furlan AJ, Ratliff NB Sclerosing vasculopathy of the central nervous system in nonelderly demented patients. Arch Neurol 1991;48(6):631–636.
25. Kanitakis J, Thobois S, Claudy A, Broussolle E. CADASIL (cerebral autosomal dominant arteriopathy with subcortical infarcts and leukoencephalopathy): a neurovascular disease diagnosed by ultrastructural examination of the skin. J Cutan Pathol 2002;29:498–501.
26. Villa N, Walker L, Lindsell CE, Gasson J, Iruela-Arispe ML, Weinmaster G. Vascular expression of Notch pathway receptors and ligands is restricted to arterial vessels. Mech Dev 2001;108:161–164.
27. Joutel A, Andreux F, Gaulis S, et al. The ectodomain of the Notch3 receptor accumulates within the cerebrovasculature of CADASIL patients. J Clin Invest 2000;105:597–605.
28. Karlstrom H, Beatus P, Dannaeus K, Chapman G, Lendahl U, Lundkvist J. A CADASIL-mutated Notch 3 receptor exhibits impaired intracellular trafficking and maturation but normal ligand-induced signaling. Proc Natl Acad Sci USA 2002;99:17119–17124.
29. Haritunians T, Boulter J, Hicks C, et al. CADASIL Notch3 mutant proteins localize to the cell surface and bind ligand. Circ Res 2002;90:506–508.
30. Ruchoux MM, Domenga V, Brulin P, et al. Transgenic mice expressing mutant Notch3 develop vascular alterations characteristic of cerebral autosomal dominant arteriopathy with subcortical infarcts and leukoencephalopathy. Am J Pathol 2003;162:329–342.
31. Artavanis-Tsakonas S, Matsuno K, Fortini ME. Notch signaling. Science 1995;268:225–232.
32. Ray WJ, Yao M, Nowotny P, et al. Evidence for a physical interaction between presenilin and Notch. Proc Natl Acad Sci USA 1999;96:3263–3268.
33. Selkoe DJ. Presenilin, Notch, and the genesis and treatment of Alzheimer's disease. Proc Natl Acad Sci USA 2001;98: 11,039–11,041.
34. Swiatek PJ, Lindsell CE, del Amo FF, Weinmaster G, Gridley T. Notch1 is essential for postimplantation development in mice. Genes Dev 1994;8:707–719.
35. Lindsell CE, Boulter J, diSibio G, Gossler A, Weinmaster G. Expression patterns of Jagged, Delta1, Notch1, Notch2, and Notch3 genes identify ligand-receptor pairs that may function in neural development. Mol Cell Neurosci 1996;8:14–27.
36. Beatus P, Lundkvist J, Oberg C, Pedersen K, Lendahl U. The origin of the ankyrin repeat region in Notch intracellular domains is critical for regulation of HES promoter activity. Mech Dev 2001;104:3–20.
37. Beatus P, Lundkvist J, Oberg C, Lendahl U. The notch 3 intracellular domain represses notch 1-mediated activation through Hairy/Enhancer of split (HES) promoters. Development 1999;126:3925–3935.
38. Wang W, Campos AH, Prince CZ, Mou Y, Pollman MJ. Coordinate Notch3-hairy-related transcription factor pathway regulation in response to arterial injury. Mediator role of platelet-derived growth factor and ERK. J Biol Chem 2002; 277:23,165–23,171.
39. Wang W, Prince CZ, Mou Y, Pollman MJ. Notch3 signaling in vascular smooth muscle cells induces c-FLIP expression via ERK/MAPK activation. Resistance to Fas ligand-induced apoptosis. J Biol Chem 2002;277:21,723–21,729.
40. Campos AH, Wang W, Pollman MJ, Gibbons GH. Determinants of Notch-3 receptor expression and signaling in vascular smooth muscle cells: implications in cell-cycle regulation. Circ Res 2002;91:999–1006.
41. Joutel A, Dodick DD, Parisi JE, Cecillon M, Tournier-Lasserve E, Bousser MG. De novo mutation in the Notch3 gene causing CADASIL. Ann Neurol 2000;47:388–391.
42. Black S, Roman GC, Geldmacher DS, et al. Efficacy and tolerability of donepezil in vascular dementia: positive results of a 24-week, multicenter, international, randomized, placebo-controlled clinical trial. Stroke 2003;34:2323–2330.
43. Wilkinson D, Doody R, Helme R, et al. Donepezil in vascular dementia: A randomized, placebo-controlled study. Neurology 2003;61:479–486.
44. Hassan A, Markus HS. Genetics and ischaemic stroke. Brain 2000;123:1784–1812.
45. Tournier-Lasserve E. New players in the genetics of stroke. N Engl J Med 2002;347:1711–1712.

46. Vidal R, Frangione B, Rostagno A, et al. A stop-codon mutation in the BRI gene associated with familial British dementia. Nature 1999;399:776–781.
47. Hademenos GJ, Alberts MJ, Awad I, et al. Advances in the genetics of cerebrovascular disease and stroke. Neurology 2001;56:997–1008.
48. Ophoff RA, Terwindt GM, Vergouwe MN, et al. Familial hemiplegic migraine and episodic ataxia type-2 are caused by mutations in the Ca2+ channel gene CACNL1A4. Cell 1996;87:543–552.
49. Iizuka T, Sakai F, Kan S, Suzuki N. Slowly progressive spread of the stroke-like lesions in MELAS. Neurology 2003;61:1238–1244.
50. Gretarsdottir S, Sveinbjornsdottir S, Jonsson HH, et al. Localization of a susceptibility gene for common forms of stroke to 5q12. Am J Hum Genet 2002;70:593–603.
51. Gretarsdottir S, Thorleifsson G, Reynisdottir ST, et al. The gene encoding phosphodiesterase 4D confers risk of ischemic stroke. Nat Genet 2003;35:131–138.
52. Sharma P. Meta-analysis of the ACE gene in ischaemic stroke. J Neurol Neurosurg Psychiatry 1998;64:227–230.

7

Estrogen, the Cerebrovascular System, and Dementia

Sharon X. C. Yang and George A. Kuchel

1. INTRODUCTION

Dementia has been recognized as a major public health issue that will grow in prominence as life expectancy increases. It has been proposed that estrogen (E2) deficiency in postmenopausal women may predispose older women to increased vulnerability of developing neurodegenerative diseases, such as Alzheimer's disease (AD), and injury associated with cerebrovascular stroke. Indeed, some epidemiological data *(1–3)* indicate a higher incidence of dementia in women than in men, especially after the age of 85. Even though the gender differences in risk for dementia are generally shown for AD, not for vascular dementia (VaD), the longitudinal Bronx Aging Study reported that a history of myocardial infarction (MI) increased women's risk to develop dementia fivefold but had no effect on dementia risk in men *(3)*, suggesting the vascular effect on dementia in relationship to E2 status. In contrast, other studies report no gender differences in the age-adjusted incidence of dementia up to high age *(4–6)*. In fact, the longer life expectancy in women than in men seemingly exposes women to higher risk of cognitive impairment in their late life.

During the past decades, we have become increasingly aware that E2 exerts several biological effects on tissues other than the reproductive system, first in maintaining bone integrity and much later in its effects on the immune, cardiovascular, and nervous systems *(7–9)*. Osteoporosis, cerebrovascular disease (CVD), and dementia represent three of the most important causes of morbidity, lost independence, and death in older women. Ovarian production of E2 becomes negligible after menopause, and although serum E2 levels in postmenopausal women are highly variable, overall they decline markedly *(7,10)*. There is biological plausability that maintaining higher levels of E2 in postmenopausal women by means of E2 replacement therapy (ERT) could be protective against these diseases. On the basis of evidence mainly obtained from observational trials and biological studies, ERT had become one of the commonly recommended therapies with a presumed beneficial profile of cardiac protection, bone protection, and cognitive protection, as well as of well-being. However, studies from randomized controlled trials examining the risks and benefits of hormone therapy have produced conflicting results.

Beginning in 1998, results from a series of controlled clinical trials examining the effects of postmenopausal hormone therapy for the prevention of diseases have failed to show protection but instead demonstrated a slightly increased risk for cardiovascular events in women with established coronary disease *(11)* or in previously healthy women *(12)*. The same findings were apparent for increased risk of ischemic stroke *(13–15)*. In May 2002, the Women's Health Initiative (WHI) *(12)* trial of daily combined therapy with estrogen plus progestin was terminated early because the risks (e.g., four more cases of coronary heart disease and stroke, nine more venous thromboembolisms,

From: *Current Clinical Neurology*
Vascular Dementia: Cerebrovascular Mechanisms and Clinical Management
Edited by: R. H. Paul, R. Cohen, B. R. Ott, and S. Salloway © Humana Press Inc., Totowa, NJ

and four more invasive breast cancers per 1000 women followed) outweighed the benefits (e.g., two fewer hip fractures and three fewer colorectal cancers). As a result, the striking discrepancies in studies have raised considerable confusion for both patients and health-care professionals regarding the use of hormone therapy. On the other hand, the discrepancies have also brought out questions about the validity of observational data, about methodological differences (e.g., confounding bias of "healthy user," adherence bias, and incomplete capture of early clinical events). Questions have also been raised about biologic issues, including formulation and dose of the hormone regimen and the characteristics of study population (e.g., time since menopause, endogenous E2 level, and stage of atherosclerosis) *(16)*. Therefore, careful review of these studies and appropriate bridges between basic research findings with clinical relevance should not only enhance our understanding of the diverse actions of E2 but also facilitate the development of rational strategies that will promote overall health and cognitive function in older women.

In this chapter, clinical evidence from observational studies, which suggested a protective but inconsistent role for postmenopausal hormone therapy in cognitive function and dementia, is reviewed. In contrast, most recent controlled trials have failed to show the cognitive protection. On the other hand, there is a larger pool of biological evidence from in vivo animal modules and in vitro cellular studies suggesting the protective role of E2 on cerebral vascular and brain function. This chapter focuses mainly on the role of E2 on cerebral blood flow (CBF) and neuromodulatory effects in response to ischemic insults. Some of underlying mechanisms involving the modulation of CBF and neuronal survival will also be addressed. In viewing growing evidence of inflammatory theory in the pathogenesis of neurodegenerative diseases, the biphasic and complex of tissue-specific effects of E2 on inflammation and the interactions between E2 and proinflammatory cytokines are discussed. In summary, current concerns and recommendations regarding postmenopausal hormone therapy for the prevention and treatment of cognitive impairment and questions that need to be answered in future studies are briefly discussed.

2. EFFECTS OF ESTROGEN ON COGNITION AND DEMENTIA

Most research on postmenopausal hormone therapy and cognition and dementia has studied and focused on AD as opposed to all-cause dementia, while a few distinguished VaD. Nevertheless, recent studies have suggested overlap between AD and VaD in pathogenesis, clinical symptoms, and treatment strategies. AD and VaD share certain vascular risk factors, such as hypertension, hyperlipidemia, diabetes mellitus, and hyperhomocystinemia, which are mainly modifiable risks and should be the focus for early interventional strategies. Here, the data available in VaD, as well as in AD, are reviewed.

2.1. Estrogen Deficiency, Cognition, and Dementia

Ovarian E2 production essentially ceases with the menopause. In postmenopausal women, serum estradiol concentrations are often lower than 20 pg/mL, and most of the estradiol is formed via extragonadal conversion of testosterone by the aromatase enzyme, which is expressed in many nonovarian tissues, including adipose tissues and the nervous system *(7)*. Little is known about the regulation of E2 production in postmenopausal women. It is likely that body composition, polymorphisms in the genes coding for steroidogenic enzymes, and the expression and activity of aromatase influence the production of endogenous E2 in postmenopausal women, resulting in enormous interindividual variability *(7,10)*. Several observational studies have demonstrated that the presence of particularly low endogenous E2 levels during postmenopausal years may represent a risk factor for the development of dementia *(17,18)*. For example, Yaffe et al. *(18)* reported that in a cohort of 425 women (65 yr or older) who had not received E2 therapy, women with higher endogenous serum levels of free and bioavailable estradiol at baseline, but not testosterone, were less likely to develop cognitive impairment 6 yr later. Although these findings suggest that higher concentrations of endogenous E2s may prevent cognitive decline, these observations have recently been challenged methodologically *(19)*. E2 deficiency and cognitive aging remains an open area for future study.

2.2. Role of Estrogen Replacement Therapy in Preventing Cognitive Impairment

In addition to a possible relationship between low endogenous E2s and the risk of dementia, a series of observational and, to a lesser extent, interventional studies have suggested that the use of ERT could enhance cognitive function and reduce the risk for developing AD, such as improving working memory and verbal learning and memory. However, there is a significant heterogeneity in the findings from these studies (*see* Yaffe *[20]*, Fillit *[21]*, and Hogervorst *[22]* for reviews). Among the important studies is the Baltimore Longitudinal Study of Aging (BLSA), a prospective multidisciplinary study of normal aging conducted by the National Institute on Aging *(23)*. In BLSA, 472 postmenopausal or perimenopausal women were followed for up to 16 yr; approximately 45% of these women were using or had used ERT in the past. A total of 34 incident cases of AD (National Institute of Neurological and Communicative Diseases and Stroke/Alzheimer's Disease and Related Disorders Association [NINCDS/ADRDA] criteria) were diagnosed during follow-up, including 9 in ERT users. After adjusting for education, the relative risk for AD in ERT users as compared with nonusers was 0.46 (95% CI, 0.209–0.997), indicating an reduced risk of AD among ERT users. The Cache County study *(24)* represents another large prospective population-based cohort investigating the relationship between ERT use and AD development. Nearly 2000 women and 1357 men, both with a mean age of 75 yr, were followed for 3 yr, revealing a overall reduced risk of AD with ERT users (adjusted HR, 0.59; 95% CI, 0.36–0.96) *(25)*. Interestingly, only prior ERT use was associated with reduced risk in subgroup analysis, whereas among current users, ERT had to be used for more than 10 yr for a benefit to be apparent. These findings have raised the hypothesis that temporal factors are important: ERT may be beneficial only if administered in early stages of AD.

Yaffe et al. *(26)* had performed a meta-analysis estimating risks for developing any dementia (AD and other types of dementia) in E2 users as compared with nonusers. The results of eight case-control studies and two prospective cohort studies varied. Although some studies suggested the protective effects of ERT on developing dementia, others indicated an increased risk for developing dementia. The summary data suggested an overall 29% decreased risk for developing dementia in ERT users. In the subgroup analysis examining cognitively intact postmenopausal women, it was reported that the improved cognition in ERT users possibly resulted from improved menopausal symptoms, yet there was no clear benefit in totally asymptomatic women. These heterogeneous results may be attributed to the variable study design (e.g., case-control vs cohort), small sample size, and short study duration. In addition, substantial methodological issues also exist because the results were not adjusted for education or depression, both of which are important contributors to cognitive impairment in late life.

On the other hand, a recent meta-analysis of 15 randomized and controlled trials has failed to demonstrate overall protection of cognitive decline in healthy postmenopausal women *(27)*. The Heart and Estrogen/Progestin Replacement Study (HERS) *(28)* was a randomized, placebo-controlled trial involving 2763 women with coronary disease. In HERS, women were assigned randomly to conjugated equine estrogen (CEE) 0.625 mg plus medroxyprogesterone acetate (MPA) 2.5 mg per day or placebo, with a mean follow-up of 4.2 yr. Participants at one-half of the study centers were invited to enroll in a cognitive function substudy, which produced a group with a mean age of 71 and with 517 women in the hormone group and 546 in the placebo group. A battery of six standard cognitive measures (Modified Mini-Mental Status Examination [3MSE], Verbal Fluency, Boston Naming, Word List Memory, Word List Recall, and Trails B test) was administered to study subjects. No difference was observed in age-adjusted cognitive function test scores between the two groups. However, women assigned to the hormone group scored lower on the Verbal Fluency test than placebo controls (15.9 ± 4.8 vs 16.6 ± 4.8, $p = 0.02$). Results of HERS clearly indicate that 4 yr of treatment with postmenopausal hormone therapy did not improve cognitive function in older women with coronary disease. Whether these results also apply to elderly women without coronary disease cannot be determined from this study.

The Women's Health Initiative Memory Study (WHIMS) represents the largest and most ambitious trial of postmenopausal hormone therapy to date. Its cognitive arms, published this year, have examined the effects of CEEs plus progesterone on global cognitive function *(29)*, probable dementia, and mild cognitive impairment (MCI) *(30)* in postmenopausal women. In the dementia and MCI trial, a total of 4532 women, aged 65 yr or older, were followed for 4 yr. Overall, 61 women were diagnosed with probable dementia, with 40 of 2229 women in the ERT and 21 of 2303 women in the placebo group. The hazard ratio for probable dementia was 2.05 (95% CI 1.21–3.48; 45 vs 22 per 10,000 person-years). Although the total number of women developing dementia was small, it is striking that women taking E2 plus progestin had twice the risk of developing dementia than nonusers. The risk of developing MCI did not differ between groups. In the global cognitive study from WHIMS *(29)*, the 3MSE was used as a measurement of global cognitive function in 4381 women followed for 4 yr. Although hormone therapy did not cause an overall decrease in cognitive function, significantly more women in the hormone group had a substantial decline ($\geq$ 2 SD) in cognition. The WHIMS investigators concluded that the risks of using a standard dose of CEE (0.625 mg) in conjunction with progestin (2.5 mg) outweigh the benefits. Another WHIMS arm examining the benefits of CEEs (0.625 mg) without progestin on global cognitive function, MCI and probable dementia is still ongoing. Once completed, the study should provide important insights into the effects of unopposed E2 on cognitive status among postmenopausal women.

2.3. *Role of E2 in Treating Dementia*

Studies of the effects of E2 as therapy for women with dementia have even more equivocal results. Several randomized and placebo-controlled trials have failed to show beneficial effects of hormone therapy in women with mild to moderate AD *(31–33)*. Nevertheless, many of these trials were small, and short-term studies lasting from 12 wk to a maximum of 1 yr in one study *(31)*. In a meta-analysis of randomized trials, Hogervorst et al. *(34)* reported no overall meaningful cognitive improvement or stabilization in women with dementia, but interestingly, a 2-mo treatment using lower (0.625 mg/d), not higher (1.25 mg/d), doses of CEE resulted in a limited positive effect on the Mini-Mental State Examination (MMSE). Regarding memory, only transdermal estradiol had positive effects on delayed recall of a word list. These observations have raised the speculation that factors such as age, dosage and duration, mode of delivery (oral, transdermal, or intramuscular), type of treatment (E2 with or without progestin), or use of a particular preparation (CEE vs 17β-estradiol) could influence the effects of E2 on cognition. In addition, it remains to be seen whether the absence or presence of menopausal symptoms influences the cognitive effects.

In view of the results discussed, plus equivocal evidence from other earlier studies, it has been proposed that the E2 plus progestin regimen used in WHIMS may not be optimal because it increases the risk of cardiovascular events, possibly, at least partially, by inappropriate activation of inflammatory pathways. Thus, additional studies combining the rigorous research design of WHIMS with a choice of other, more physiologic and potentially safer regimens are urgently needed. Furthermore, the temporal aspect of hormone therapy has also been proposed. Results from the Cache County study suggest that hormone therapy may exert protective effects only during a critical early period in the pathogenesis of dementia *(25)*. The concept of a fixed and relatively early window of opportunity in terms of obtaining cognitive benefits from hormone therapy is biologically plausible given a widely held view of AD in which synaptic pathology followed by loss of specific axonal pathways represents an early stage in the pathogenesis of AD *(35,36)*. As noted, the results from WHI were criticized for such concerns as roughly 10% of women in the placebo group began taking hormone therapy during follow-up *(37)*. In light of the future, several ongoing large-scale and long-term trials studying hormone therapy on cognition and dementia *(38)* should assist in elucidating these crucial questions.

3. EFFECTS OF ESTROGEN ON CEREBROVASCULATURE AND NEUROPROTECTION

Cumulative evidence from basic science and clinical research indicates that E2 may play an important mediator role in the central nervous system (CNS). The numerous estrogenic effects in the brain have been reported, including modulation of CBF and neuronal synaptogenesis, interaction with neurotransmitters and hormones, mediating intracellular signaling pathways involving apoptosis and necrosis, and antioxidant and anti-atherogenesic properties *(7,9,39–41)*.

3.1. *Effects of Estrogen on Cerebrovasculature*

3.1.1. Cellular Evidence of the Effects of Estrogen on Cerebral Vascular Function

The cerebral vasculature has been identified as one of the important target tissues for E2. E2 receptors (ERs) are present in the cerebrovascular system and localized to both endothelial and smooth muscle cells (SMCs) *(42,43)*. Jesmin et al. *(44)* recently discovered significant reduction in the total capillary density in the frontal cortex, plus significantly reduced expression of both ER subtypes, ERα and ERβ, in cerebral vessels after ovariectomy (OVx) in middle-aged rats. These OVx-induced changes were completely prevented by E2. It has been well-known that E2 enhances the production and activity of endothelial-derived vasodilators, such as nitric oxide and prostacyclin in blood vessels, including cerebral arteries *(42,45)* (*see* Pelligrino for a review *[41]*) and other evidence of cytoprotectivity, such as blocking cytotoxicity in cultured cerebral endothelial cells *(46)*. Ospina et al. *(47)* reported that chronic in vivo 17β-estradiol treatment significantly induced cyclooxygenase (COX)-1 and prostacyclin synthase activities with enhanced production of prostacyclin in cerebral arteries of OVx rats and increased middle cerebral artery vasodilatation through these endothelium- and COX-dependent mechanisms *(48)*. It is likely that E2 exerts its various bioactivities on cerebral vascular both through direct effects on the cerebrovascular system regulated by genomic and/or nongenomic pathways and through systemic effects on circulating factors *(41)*. The biphasic effects of E2 on inflammation will be discussed in Section 4.2. of this chapter.

3.1.2. Evidence of the Effects of Estrogen on Cerebral Blood Flow in Animal Studies

The protective effects of E2 in the context of ischemic brain injury have now been observed in several in vivo animal studies (*see* Wise *[39,49]* and Hurn *[50]* for reviews). For example, in a study of the effects of E2 on the temporal evolution of focal ischemia by middle cerebral artery occlusion (MCAO) in OVx rats, a single dose of E2 (100 μg/kg) administered 2 h before the ischemic insult reduced the size of ischemic lesions by 50–60% as measured using sequential diffusion-weighted MRI *(51)*. The protective effects were evident during both the occlusion and the reperfusion phases of ischemia and were almost exclusively limited to cortical regions. Interestingly, there were no differences in CBF between E2 treatment and control group during occlusion, early reperfusion, or 1 d after reperfusion, suggesting that the neuroprotection of E2 was mediated independent of blood flow. In a similar experimental model of stroke (e.g., MCAO), but without OVx, McCullough et al. *(52)* reported that acute E2 therapy by intravenous infusion of a pharmacological E2 dose (1 mg/kg) during early reperfusion rapidly promoted CBF recovery and reduced hemispheric no-reflow zones, yet the protective effects of E2 appeared only if it was given during early reperfusion. It is important to note that the different effects of E2 on CBF in these studies may result from different endogenous E2 status, e.g., E2 depletion by OVx in the first study, not in the second one, and from different dosages of E2 used, e.g., a pharmacological dose of E2 resulting in a supraphysiologic E2 level in the second study but a rather lower dose of E2 in the first study.

3.1.3. Evidence of the Effects of Estrogen on Cerebral Blood Flow in Human Studies

Maki et al. *(53)* performed positron emission tomography (PET) in postmenopausal women in a small longitudinal study. They observed increased regional CBF in ERT users as compared with age-matched nonusers. Interestingly, the greatest differences in observed regional CBF were precisely in those regions (hippocampus, parahippocampal gyrus, and temporal lobe) known to be important in memory, to be involved in early stages of AD, and to be sensitive to E2 in animal studies. These changes in regional CBF were accompanied with higher scores on neuropsychological memory tests in ERT users as compared to nonusers, suggesting that E2 may modulate brain activity and enhance cognitive function, at least in part, through increases in blood flow, by which the brain is protected from the metabolic abnormalities. Greene et al. *(54)* reported similar findings in a short-term cohort in women taking CEE therapy. However, the evidence is inconsistent, even controversial. A randomized and controlled trial that reported that a short-term higher dose of E2 therapy (CEE 1.25 mg/d) did not produce meaningful changes on cerebral perfusion nor on cognitive performance in women with AD *(33)*.

3.2. Effects of Estrogen on Stroke

The role of ERT in altering stroke incidence and outcome in postmenopausal women is apparently unfavorable. The third study in the WHI series *(13)* reported the outcome of E2 plus progestin on risk of stroke among the 16,608 women. Women taking hormone therapy had a 31% increased risk of total stroke in comparison with women taking placebo. This increased risk was significant for ischemic, but not for hemorrhagic, stroke, and the increase in risk did not appear until after 1 yr of treatment. Extensive subgroup analyses based on baseline characteristics of the study participants and risk factors for stroke failed to identify any differences in the results.

The Women's Estrogen for Stroke Trial (WEST) *(15)* was another large randomized trial, but for the secondary prevention of stroke and death. In this high-risk population of postmenopausal women with a recent cerebrovascular event, estrogen therapy (17β-estradiol 1 mg/d) with or without a progestin (MPA 5 mg/d for 12 d) for 3 yr increased fatal stroke approximately threefold, primarily in the incidence of ischemic stroke with no difference in the incidence of nonfatal stroke. Another secondary prevention trial, HERS *(14)*, which tested a different regimen (CEE 0.625 mg plus MPA 2.5 mg/d) and enrolled slightly younger women with established coronary disease, demonstrated a slightly increased, not statistically significant, risk of stroke in the study population. In addition, data from the multiple risks analysis of stroke patients during aspirin therapy in the trial of the Stroke Prevention in Atrial Fibrillation (SPAF) *(55)* indicated that E2 therapy was independently associated with a higher risk of ischemic stroke.

Interestingly, the Nurses' Health Study *(56)*, a large prospective observational study, showed that the risk of stroke was significantly increased among women taking 0.625 mg or higher dose of CEE daily and those taking CEE plus progestin, but the risk was not increased in women taking 0.3mg CEE daily. As discussed above in Section 2.3. and later in Section 4.2., there is evidence suggesting that the use of lower doses of unopposed 17β-estradiol may result in an improved overall safety profile, and further studies are needed to examine the benefit of this approach in terms of cognition and cerebrovascular disease.

3.3. Effects of Estrogen on Neuroprotection

E2 plays a critical role in the developing brain. In adult and aging brains, E2 may exert effects on neuronal plasticity and survival, but the mechanism is rather complex and remains largely unknown. E2-mediated neuroprotection has been described in several neuronal culture systems with toxicities, including serum-deprivation, β-amyloid-induced toxicity, excitotoxicity, and oxidative stress. In animal models, E2 has attenuates neuronal death in rodent models from cerebral ischemia, traumatic injury, and Parkinson's disease (*see* Green and Simpkins *[57]* and Wise *[58]* for reviews). It should be noted that although the majority of basic research has demonstrated neurotrophic effects of E2, under certain conditions, E2 may exert neuronal effects that are not protective and are, at times, even deleterious *(58)*. As discussed in the Introductory section of this chapter, these discrepancies have raised questions in terms of the methodological differences and biologic factors.

E2 has a plethora of cellular effects, including activation of nuclear ERs, altered expression of antiapoptotic bcl-2 family proteins, interactions with second messenger cascades, alterations in glutaminergic activation, activation of cyclic adenosine monophosphate (cAMP) signal transduction pathways, maintenance of intracellular calcium homeostasis, and direct antioxidant activity *(21,57,59,60)*. These effects have been implicated as the mechanisms for the neuroprotective effects of E2.

The traditional view of E2 actions at the cellular level involved the binding of E2 to an ER (now known as ER-α or ER α), followed by the translocation of this steroid-receptor complex to the nucleus and the activation of specific transcriptional events *(7)*. Interestingly, several lines of evidence suggest that these neuroprotective effects of estradiol are not solely mediated by a classical nuclear ER-mediated mechanism. Studies using genetically-modified mice in which the ER α or the ER β genes have been deleted have demonstrated that ER α, but not ER β, is required for E2 to exert its neuroprotective effect *(61)*. In fact, deletion of the ER α gene completely abolished the protective actions of estradiol in all regions of the brain, whereas the neuroprotective effects of E2 remained intact in ER β gene knockout mice *(61)*. In contrast, other studies have suggested that the neuroprotective activity of E2 may be mediated independently of classical ERs *(62)*.

Recently, the view of E2 signaling has become more complex with the discoveries of ER βand its coactivators and corepressors *(37)* and with the realization that E2 signaling can also occur through pathways that are not receptor-mediated, with considerable cross-talk existing among these and other signaling pathways *(7)*. More recently, the findings of ER-independent ER activation, particularly in nonreproductive organs, including the brain *(63)*, and the identifications of several ER α polymorphisms and other gene mutants (such as presenilin-1) *(21)* have opened novel approaches for future studies. In addition, E2 analogs, e.g., selective ER modulators (SERMs), could potentially be useful to selectively express the desirable actions and selectively suppress the undesirable actions of E2 *(63,64)*.

4. ESTROGEN, CYTOKINES, AND INFLAMMATION

Systemic chronic inflammation has been associated with all-cause mortality risk in older persons *(65,66)*. The Women's Health and Aging Study *(67)* reported a strong, nonspecific association between levels of interleukin (IL)-6 (IL-6), a major proinflammatory cytokine, and subsequent risk of mortality among older women with CVD. Recently, the Women's Health Initiative Observational Study (WHI-OS) *(68)* demonstrated that increased baseline C-reactive protein (CRP) and IL-6 levels were independently associated with a twofold increased risk of developing CVD in initially healthy postmenopausal women. CRP is a sensitive but nonspecific inflammatory marker and a strong predictor of cardiovascular events in apparently healthy postmenopausal women *(69)*, as well as in women and men with established CVD *(70,71)*. Vascular inflammation plays an important role in the pathogenesis of atherosclerosis *(72,73)*. Similarly, postmortem studies *(74,75)* have demonstrated the presence of inflammatory changes even in the early stage of AD. The MacArthur Study of Successful Aging *(76)*, a longitudinal cohort study, showed an association between elevated baseline IL-6 and risk for a subsequent decline of cognitive function in initially high functioning older men and women. Moreover, because inflammatory mediators commonly possess neurotoxic properties *(77)* and the prevalence of AD is lower among individuals taking antiinflammatory medications *(78)*, it has been proposed that the presence of inflammation may contribute to the neurodegenerative changes seen in AD *(79)*.

4.1. Interactions Among Estrogen Deficiency, Inflammation, and Dementia

The decline in ovarian function with menopause has been associated with increases in the production of proinflammatory cytokines, even though the increases are subtle in comparison with the increases observed in response to infection or major tissue injury (*see* Pfeilschifter *[80]* for a review).

For example, studies indicated that women in both early and late menopause *(81–83)* have higher serum levels of tumor necrosis factor-α (TNF-α), another major proinflammatory cytokine, than do premenopausal women. Nevertheless, there are mixed results regarding changes in circulating levels of major inflammatory cytokines, e.g., IL-6, IL-1, and TNF-α, with menopause. It remains to be seen whether elevations in circulating levels of proinflammatory cytokines seen in older age result from chronic inflammation associated with specific diseases or aging itself or are the results of disrupted hormonal signaling balance, specifically E2 depletion, after menopause.

4.2. Interactions Among Estrogen Therapy, Cytokines, and Inflammation

Because of the increased proinflammatory cytokines with menopause, E2 administration might be expected to induce corresponding decreases in cytokine expressions. In fact, the existing literature is seemingly controversial regarding both the direction and the magnitude of the relationship between ERT and the levels of cytokines and other inflammatory biomarkers. Randomized controlled studies evaluating the effect of ERT on circulating IL-6 levels have yielded highly inconsistent results, suggesting that ERT increases *(84)*, decreases *(68,85,86)*, or does not influence IL-6 levels *(87,88)*. These discrepancies are not explained simply by differences in time after menopause, length of ERT, or other cardiovascular comorbidities, highlighting the complex nature of the relationship between E2 and inflammation, which may contribute, at least partially, to the metabolic syndrome associated with menopause.

Of note, numerous studies have now reported that CEE (0.625 mg) alone or combined with MPA (2.5 mg) induced several circulating markers of inflammation (*see* Koh *(73)* for a review). Both randomized trials *(88–90)*, as well as observational studies *(91,92)* have shown that CEE, with or without concomitant progestin, slightly but significantly increases serum CRP levels in postmenopausal women. In contrast, Stork et al. *(93)* reported that a combination therapy using 1 mg of natural 17 β-estradiol had a neutral effect on CRP levels and favorable effects on cell adhesion molecules, suggesting that the type of estrogen included in the ERT regimen affects the inflammatory response.

The Postmenopausal Estrogen/Progestin Interventions study's (PEPI) *(90)* recent randomized controlled trials *(85,93)* and several small prospective studies *(84,94)* have all consistently demonstrated the reduction of E-selectin and other vascular adhesion molecules by ERT. Interestingly, Kennedy et al. *(95)* reported the presence of significantly elevated plasma E-selectin levels in postmenopausal women, with ERT reducing these levels to premenopausal values. E-selectin, also known as endothelial-leukocyte adhesion molecule-1, is a biomarker of inflammation and endothelial dysfunction. E-selectin facilitates chemotaxis involving leukocyte subsets, and it is also a potent activator of leukocyte integrins, allowing their interaction with their endothelial count-receptors *(96)*, suggesting a favorable effect of ERT on vascular inflammation. The expression of E-selectin is restricted to the activated vascular endothelium *(94,97)*. In contrast, CRP is primarily synthesized and regulated in the liver, while its expression in injured vascular cells and degenerating neurons has also been reported *(75,98)*, suggesting that the inflammatory effects of E2 may be mediated via hepatic metabolic activation. In addition, because many types of inflammatory cells are responsive to E2 *(99)* and IL-6 is the major stimulant for hepatic CRP production, mechanisms independent of IL-6 have also been described *(100)*. Other inflammation-associated cytokines, including IL-1 β, TNF-α, IFN-γ, TGF-β, and IL-8, may exert additive, inhibitory or synergistic effects on hepatic CRP expression, which are likely mediated by a combination of cytokines, cytokine receptors, and hormones *(101)*. Bruun et al. *(102)* have reported results of animal studies indicating that OVx significantly increased IL-6 and IL-8 gene expression in rodent adipose tissue, with no apparent effects on TNF-α gene or protein level. Low-dose E2 replacement (9.5 μg 17β-estradiol/d) administered at the time of OVx and continued for 5 mo prevented these increases. However, no direct effects of E2 on these three adipose tissue-derived cytokines were observed in adipose tissue cultures after 24-h incubation. These findings suggest that that the effect of E2 on these cytokines may be more long-term or that the in vivo effects of E2 on cytokines are mediated indirectly through one or more intermediators.

Several clinical trials *(103–105)* have shown that lower doses of ERT (CEE 0.45, 0.3, or 0.25 mg/d alone or combined with MPA 1.5 mg/d) induce favorable changes in bone turnover, bone loss, serum lipids, and hemostatic factors, similar to those obtained using commonly prescribed regimens (CEE 0.625 mg/d or combined with MPA 2.5 mg/d). Additionally, these lower dose regimens are better tolerated and are associated with fewer side effects. Interestingly, a recent study *(106)* indicates that the biological effects of HRT are tissue specific and closely related to serum estradiol levels. For example, a very low serum level of estradiol (<15 pg/mL) was sufficient to suppress gonadotropins and to relieve vasomotor symptoms. Although the minimum level of estradiol needed to increase bone mineral density was 15 pg/mL, a higher level of estradiol was required to improve the lipid profile (>25 pg/mL). The effects of lower dose ERT on inflammatory markers and clinical outcomes are highly promising, yet more studies are clearly needed.

4.3. *Effects of Estrogen on Homocysteine and Other Inflammatory Mediators*

One of the established risk factors for dementia is hyperhomocystinemia. The Framingham study *(107)* and several population-based cohorts *(108,109)* have shown that plasma levels of homocysteine were positively associated with the risk of developing dementia and AD. It has been proposed that elevated homocysteine may reflect inflammation related to CVD and neurodegenerative disease. Thus, one of the neurophysiological mechanisms by which ERT could influence cognition may be a reduction of homocysteine levels, which, in turn, could lessen the extent of hippocampal neuronal damage *(109)*. The report from the Sacramento Area Latino Study on Aging (SALSA) cohort indicated that ERT users had significantly lower homocysteine levels in comparison with nonusers among postmenopausal women *(109)*. Furthermore, ERT users had modest but statistically significant higher global cognitive performance than controls *(109)*. Adjustments for lipids, CVD, and homocysteine levels did not confound the association, suggesting that ERT could exert its effect on cognition, at least in part, by influencing plasma homocysteine levels.

Although likely important, the effects of E2 deficiency or replacement on vascular inflammation have been difficult to establish, as have been the roles of any such relationships on cognitive impairments. In contrast, researchers addressing the pathogenesis of postmenopausal osteoporosis have been able to demonstrate a complex relationship among E2, bone, and immune cells, with osteoclasts sharing a common lineage to macrophages *(110)*. For example, the presence of localized inflammation has been implicated in the pathogenesis of postmenopausal osteoporosis *(110)*. In animal modules, OVx is a well-known signal for inducing osteoclast activation and subsequent bone loss in the presence of type I IL-1 receptors *(110,111)*. Macrophage migration inhibitory factor (MIF) has been known for a long time as one of the cytokines involved in the regulation of inflammation with unique and diverse functions *(112)*. Only recently has a study reported a possibly crucial role for this molecule as an integrator between E2 and inflammation *(113)*. In this in vivo study, excessive inflammation and delayed-cutaneous wound healing associated with markedly elevated MIF expression were found in mice rendered hypogonadal by OVx, whereas systemic replacement of E2 reversed these changes and restored normal wound-healing capacity. In contrast, OVx in mice rendered null for the MIF gene did not impair wound healing. Moreover, these investigators further demonstrated a striking E2-mediated decrease in MIF release by activated inflammatory cells in their in vitro study. Thus, it is suggested that E2 inhibits the local inflammatory response by downregulating MIF, providing a potential mechanism by which E2 could exert antiinflammatory effects.

5. SUMMARY

The hypothesis that ERT could be used to prevent, slow, or even reverse the development and progression of cognitive impairments in older women has attracted widespread interest. Although considerable progress has been made during the past decade in our understanding of the molecular and cellular mechanisms of E2 action on cerebral vascular and brain function, efforts to translate these findings into clinically relevant outcomes in human studies have been disappointing. Given the absence of supportive evidence from controlled trials and the overall higher risk than benefit, postmenopausal hormone therapy should not be recommended for the prevention of chronic disease, including CVDs and dementia *(16,114)*.

It has become apparent that the biological effects of E2 on cognitive aging are highly complex, and a deeper understanding of the important pathogenesis of cognitive decline and dementia in older women must be achieved. Future research examining the influence of multiple potential mediators of E2 action (e.g., coactivators, corepressors, and other unknown proteins) and of genetic makeup (e.g., polymorphisms), the temporal factors of hormone therapy (e.g., time since menopause, age, and duration of treatment) and the biologic aspects of the estrogens (e.g., the route of administration, the dose of physiologic vs pharmacologic, the form of conjugated estrogens vs estradiol, and opposed vs unopposed E2 and selective E2 analogs), in combination with sensitive neuropsychological measures, may provide more definitive information in these areas.

ACKNOWLEDGMENT

This work was supported in part by NIH Grant: The Center for Interdisciplinary Research in Women's Health (CIRWH) Scholar Award (to SY).

REFERENCES

1. Andersen K, Launer LJ, Dewey ME, Gender differences in the incidence of AD and vascular dementia: The EURODEM Studies. EURODEM Incidence Research Group. Neurology 1999;53:1992–1997.
2. Gao S, Hendrie HC, Hall KS, Hui S. The relationships between age, sex, and the incidence of dementia and Alzheimer disease: a meta-analysis. Arch Gen Psychiatry 1998;55:809–815.
3. Aronson MK, Ooi WL, Morgenstern H, et al. Women, myocardial infarction, and dementia in the very old. Neurology 1990;40:1102–1106.
4. Ruitenberg A, Ott A, Van Swieten JC, Hofman A, Breteler MM. Incidence of dementia: does gender make a difference? Neurobiol Aging 2001;22:575–580.
5. Ganguli M, Dodge HH, Chen P, Belle S, Dekosky ST. Ten-year incidence of dementia in a rural elderly US community population: the MoVIES Project. Neurology 2000;54:1109–1116.
6. Rocca WA, Cha RH, Waring SC, Kokmen E. Incidence of dementia and Alzheimer's disease: a reanalysis of data from Rochester, Minnesota, 1975–1984. Am J Epidemiol 1998;148:51–62.
7. Gruber CJ, Tschugguel W, Schneeberger C, Huber JC. Production and actions of estrogens. N Engl J Med 2002;346: 340–352.
8. Mendelsohn ME, Karas RH. The protective effects of estrogen on the cardiovascular system. N Engl J Med 1999;340: 1801–1811.
9. Behl C. Estrogen as a neuroprotective hormone. Nat Rev Neurosci 2002;3:433–442.
10. Kuchel GA, Tannenbaum C, Greenspan DS, Resnick NM. Can variability in the hormonal status of elderly women assist in the decision to administer estrogens? J Women Health Gend Based Med 2001;10:109–116.
11. Hulley S, Grady D, Bush T, et al. Randomized trial of estrogen plus progestin for secondary prevention of coronary heart disease in postmenopausal women. Heart and Estrogen/progestin Replacement Study (HERS) Research Group [see comments]. JAMA 1998;280:605–613.
12. Rossouw JE, Anderson GL, Prentice RL, et al. Risks and benefits of estrogen plus progestin in healthy postmenopausal women: principal results. From the Women's Health Initiative randomized controlled trial. JAMA 2002;288: 321–333.
13. Wassertheil-Smoller S, Hendrix SL, Limacher M, et al. Effect of estrogen plus progestin on stroke in postmenopausal women: the Women's Health Initiative: a randomized trial. JAMA 2003;289:2673–2684.
14. Simon JA, Hsia J, Cauley JA, et al. Postmenopausal hormone therapy and risk of stroke: the Heart and Estrogen-progestin Replacement Study (HERS). Circulation. 2001;103:638–642.
15. Viscoli CM, Brass LM, Kernan WN, Sarrel PM, Suissa S, Horwitz RI. A clinical trial of estrogen-replacement therapy after ischemic stroke. N Engl J Med 2001;345:1243–1249.
16. Grodstein F, Clarkson TB, Manson JE. Understanding the divergent data on postmenopausal hormone therapy. N Engl J Med 2003;348:645–650.
17. Manly JJ, Merchant CA, Jacobs DM, et al. Endogenous estrogen levels and Alzheimer's disease among postmenopausal women. Neurology 2000;54:833–837.

18. Yaffe K, Lui LY, Grady D, Cauley J, Kramer J, Cummings SR. Cognitive decline in women in relation to non-protein-bound oestradiol concentrations. Lancet 2000;356:708–712.
19. Hogervorst E, Williams J, Combrinck M, David SA. Measuring serum oestradiol in women with Alzheimer's disease: the importance of the sensitivity of the assay method. Eur J Endocrinol 2003;148:67–72.
20. Yaffe K, Haan M, Byers A, Tangen C, Kuller L. Estrogen use, APOE, and cognitive decline: evidence of gene-environment interaction. Neurology. 2000;54:1949–1954.
21. Fillit HM. The role of hormone replacement therapy in the prevention of Alzheimer disease. Arch Intern Med 2002;162: 1934–1942.
22. Hogervorst E, Williams J, Budge M, Riedel W, Jolles J. The nature of the effect of female gonadal hormone replacement therapy on cognitive function in post-menopausal women: a meta-analysis. Neuroscience 2000;101:485–512.
23. Kawas C, Resnick S, Morrison A, et al. A prospective study of estrogen replacement therapy and the risk of developing Alzheimer's disease: The Baltimore Longitudinal Study of Aging. Neurology 1997;48:1517–1521.
24. Carlson MC, Zandi PP, Plassman BL, et al. Hormone replacement therapy and reduced cognitive decline in older women: the Cache County Study. Neurology 2001;57:2210–2216.
25. Zandi PP, Carlson MC, Plassman BL, et al. Hormone replacement therapy and incidence of Alzheimer disease in older women: the Cache County Study. JAMA 2002;288:2123–2129.
26. Yaffe K, Sawaya G, Lieberburg I, Grady D. Estrogen therapy in postmenopausal women effects on cognitive function and dementia. JAMA 1998;279:688–695.
27. Hogervorst E, Yaffe K, Richards M, Huppert F. Hormone replacement therapy for cognitive function in postmenopausal women. Cochrane Database Syst Rev 2002;CD003122.
28. Grady D, Yaffe K, Kristof M, Lin F, Richards C, Barrett-Connor E. Effect of postmenopausal hormone therapy on cognitive function: the Heart and Estrogen/progestin Replacement Study. Am J Med 2002;113:543–548.
29. Rapp SR, Espeland MA, Shumaker SA, et al. Effect of estrogen plus progestin on global cognitive function in postmenopausal women: the Women's Health Initiative Memory Study: a randomized controlled trial. JAMA 2003;289: 2663–2672.
30. Shumaker SA, Legault C, Rapp SR, et al. Estrogen plus progestin and the incidence of dementia and mild cognitive impairment in postmenopausal women. The Women's Health Initiative Memory Study: A Randomized Controlled Trial. JAMA. 2003;2651:2651–2671.
31. Mulnard RA, Cotman CW, Kawas C, et al. Estrogen replacement therapy for treatment of mild to moderate Alzheimer disease: a randomized controlled trial. Alzheimer's Disease Cooperative Study. JAMA. 2000;283:1007–1015.
32. Henderson VW, Paganini-Hill A, Miller BL, et al. Estrogen for Alzheimer's disease in women: randomized, double-blind, placebo-controlled trial. Neurology 2000;54:295–301.
33. Wang PN, Liao SQ, Liu RS, et al. Effects of estrogen on cognition, mood, and cerebral blood flow in AD: a controlled study. Neurology 2000;54:2061–2066.
34. Hogervorst E, Yaffe K, Richards M, Huppert F. Hormone replacement therapy to maintain cognitive function in women with dementia. Cochrane Database Syst Rev. 2002;CD003799.
35. Masliah E, Mallory M, Alford M, et al. Altered expression of synaptic proteins occurs early during progression of Alzheimer's disease. Neurology 2001;56:127–129.
36. Selkoe DJ. Alzheimer's disease is a synaptic failure. Science 2002;298:789–791.
37. Herrington DM, Howard TD. From presumed benefit to potential harm—hormone therapy and heart disease. N Engl J Med 2003;349:519–521.
38. Zec RF, Trivedi MA. Effects of hormone replacement therapy on cognitive aging and dementia risk in postmenopausal women: a review of ongoing large-scale, long-term clinical trials. Climacteric 2002;5:122–134.
39. Wise P. Estradiol exerts neuroprotective actions against ischemic brain injury: insights derived from animal models. Endocrine 2003;21:11–15.
40. Cholerton B, Gleason CE, Baker LD, Asthana S. Estrogen and Alzheimer's disease: the story so far. Drugs Aging 2002; 19:405–427.
41. Pelligrino DA, Galea E. Estrogen and cerebrovascular physiology and pathophysiology. Jpn J Pharmacol 2001;86:137–158.
42. Stirone C, Duckles SP, Krause DN. Multiple forms of estrogen receptor-alpha in cerebral blood vessels: regulation by estrogen. Am J Physiol Endocrinol Metab 003;284:E184–E192.
43. Dan P, Cheung JC, Scriven DR, Moore ED. Epitope-dependent localization of estrogen receptor-alpha, but not -beta, in en face arterial endothelium. Am J Physiol Heart Circ Physiol 2003;284:H1295–H1306.
44. Jesmin S, Hattori Y, Sakuma I, Liu MY, Mowa CN, Kitabatake A. Estrogen deprivation and replacement modulate cerebral capillary density with vascular expression of angiogenic molecules in middle-aged female rats. J Cereb Blood Flow Metab 2003;23:181–189.
45. Geary GG, McNeill AM, Ospina JA, Krause DN, Korach KS, Duckles SP. Selected contribution: cerebrovascular nos and cyclooxygenase are unaffected by estrogen in mice lacking estrogen receptor-alpha. J Appl Physiol 2001;91: 2391–2399.
46. Mogami M, Hida H, Hayashi Y, et al. Estrogen blocks 3-nitropropionic acid-induced Ca2+i increase and cell damage in cultured rat cerebral endothelial cells. Brain Res 2002;956:116–125.

47. Ospina JA, Krause DN, Duckles SP. 17beta-estradiol increases rat cerebrovascular prostacyclin synthesis by elevating cyclooxygenase-1 and prostacyclin synthase. Stroke 2002;33:600–605.
48. Ospina JA, Duckles SP, Krause DN. 17beta-estradiol decreases vascular tone in cerebral arteries by shifting COX-dependent vasoconstriction to vasodilation. Am J Physiol Heart Circ Physiol. 2003;285:H241–H250.
49. Wise PM, Dubal DB, Wilson ME, Rau SW, Bottner M, Rosewell KL. Estradiol is a protective factor in the adult and aging brain: understanding of mechanisms derived from in vivo and in vitro studies. Brain Res Brain Res Rev 2001;37: 313–319.
50. Hurn PD, Macrae IM. Estrogen as a neuroprotectant in stroke. J Cereb Blood Flow Metab 2000;20:631–652.
51. Shi J, Bui JD, Yang SH, et al. Estrogens decrease reperfusion-associated cortical ischemic damage: an MRI analysis in a transient focal ischemia model. Stroke 2001;32:987–992.
52. McCullough LD, Alkayed NJ, Traystman RJ, Williams MJ, Hurn PD. Postischemic estrogen reduces hypoperfusion and secondary ischemia after experimental stroke. Stroke 2001;32:796–802.
53. Maki PM, Resnick SM. Longitudinal effects of estrogen replacement therapy on PET cerebral blood flow and cognition. Neurobiol Aging 2000;21:373–383.
54. Greene RA. Estrogen and cerebral blood flow: a mechanism to explain the impact of estrogen on the incidence and treatment of Alzheimer's disease. Int J Fertil Womens Med 2000;45:253–257.
55. Hart RG, Pearce LA, McBride R, Rothbart RM, Asinger RW. Factors associated with ischemic stroke during aspirin therapy in atrial fibrillation: analysis of 2012 participants in the SPAF I-III clinical trials. The Stroke Prevention in Atrial Fibrillation (SPAF) Investigators. Stroke 1999;30:1223–1229.
56. Grodstein F, Manson JE, Colditz GA, Willett WC, Speizer FE, Stampfer MJ. A prospective, observational study of postmenopausal hormone therapy and primary prevention of cardiovascular disease. Ann Intern Med 2000;133:933–941.
57. Green PS, Simpkins JW. Neuroprotective effects of estrogens: potential mechanisms of action. Int J Dev Neurosci 2000;18:347–358.
58. Wise PM. Estrogens: protective or risk factors in brain function? Prog Neurobiol 2003;69:181–191.
59. Bi R, Foy MR, Thompson RF, Baudry M. Effects of estrogen, age, and calpain on MAP kinase and NMDA receptors in female rat brain. Neurobiol Aging 2003;24:977–983.
60. Wise PM, Dubal DB, Wilson ME, Rau SW, Liu Y. Estrogens: trophic and protective factors in the adult brain. Front Neuroendocrinol 2001;22:33–66.
61. Dubal DB, Zhu H, Yu J, et al. Estrogen receptor alpha, not beta, is a critical link in estradiol-mediated protection against brain injury. Proc Natl Acad Sci USA 2001;98:1952–1957.
62. Liu R, Yang SH, Perez E, et al. Neuroprotective effects of a novel non-receptor-binding estrogen analogue: in vitro and in vivo analysis. Stroke 2002;33:2485–2491.
63. Ciana P, Raviscioni M, Mussi P, et al. In vivo imaging of transcriptionally active estrogen receptors. Nat Med 2003;9: 82–86.
64. Riggs BL, Hartmann LC. Selective estrogen-receptor modulators—mechanisms of action and application to clinical practice. N Engl J Med 2003;348:618–629.
65. Harris TB, Ferrucci L, Tracy RP, et al. Associations of elevated interleukin-6 and C-reactive protein levels with mortality in the elderly. Am J Med 1999;106:506–512.
66. Taaffe DR, Harris TB, Ferrucci L, Rowe J, Seeman TE. Cross-sectional and prospective relationships of interleukin-6 and C-reactive protein with physical performance in elderly persons: MacArthur studies of successful aging. J Gerontol A Biol Sci Med Sci 2000;55:M709–M715.
67. Volpato S, Guralnik JM, Ferrucci L, et al. Cardiovascular disease, interleukin-6, and risk of mortality in older women: the women's health and aging study. Circulation 2001;103:947–953.
68. Pradhan AD, Manson JE, Rossouw JE, et al. Inflammatory biomarkers, hormone replacement therapy, and incident coronary heart disease: prospective analysis from the Women's Health Initiative observational study. JAMA 2002;288: 980–987.
69. Ridker PM, Hennekens CH, Buring JE, Rifai N. C-reactive protein and other markers of inflammation in the prediction of cardiovascular disease in women. N Engl J Med 2000;342:836–843.
70. Tracy RP, Lemaitre RN, Psaty BM, et al. Relationship of C-reactive protein to risk of cardiovascular disease in the elderly. Results from the Cardiovascular Health Study and the Rural Health Promotion Project. Arterioscler Thromb Vasc Biol 1997;17:1121–1127.
71. Albert MA, Ridker PM. The role of C-reactive protein in cardiovascular disease risk. Curr Cardiol Rep 1999;1:99–104.
72. Ross R. Atherosclerosis—an inflammatory disease. N Engl J Med 1999;340:115–126.
73. Koh KK. Effects of estrogen on the vascular wall: vasomotor function and inflammation. Cardiovasc Res 2002;55: 714–726.
74. Rogers J, Shen Y. A perspective on inflammation in Alzheimer's disease. Ann N Y Acad Sci 2000;924:132–135.
75. Yasojima K, Schwab C, McGeer EG, McGeer PL. Generation of C-reactive protein and complement components in atherosclerotic plaques. Am J Pathol 2001;158:1039–1051.
76. Weaver JD, Huang MH, Albert M, Harris T, Rowe JW, Seeman TE. Interleukin-6 and risk of cognitive decline: MacArthur studies of successful aging. Neurology 2002;59:371–378.

77. Strohmeyer R, Rogers J. Molecular and cellular mediators of Alzheimer's disease inflammation. J Alzheimers Dis 2001;3:131–157.
78. Stewart WF, Kawas C, Corrada M, Metter EJ. Risk of Alzheimer's disease and duration of NSAID use. Neurology 1997;48:626–632.
79. McGeer PL, McGeer EG. Local neuroinflammation and the progression of Alzheimer's disease. J Neurovirol 2002;8: 529–538.
80. Pfeilschifter J, Koditz R, Pfohl M, Schatz H. Changes in proinflammatory cytokine activity after menopause. Endocr Rev 2002;23:90–119.
81. Sites CK, Toth MJ, Cushman M, et al. Menopause-related differences in inflammation markers and their relationship to body fat distribution and insulin-stimulated glucose disposal. Fertil Steril 2002;77:128–135.
82. Kamada M, Irahara M, Maegawa M, et al. Transient increase in the levels of T-helper 1 cytokines in postmenopausal women and the effects of hormone replacement therapy. Gynecol Obstet Invest 2001;52:82–88.
83. Kamada M, Irahara M, Maegawa M, et al. Postmenopausal changes in serum cytokine levels and hormone replacement therapy. Am J Obstet Gynecol 2001;184:309–314.
84. Herrington DM, Brosnihan KB, Pusser BE, et al. Differential effects of E and droloxifene on C-reactive protein and other markers of inflammation in healthy postmenopausal women. J Clin Endocrinol Metab 2001;86:4216–4222.
85. Silvestri A, Gebara O, Vitale C, et al. Increased levels of C-reactive protein after oral hormone replacement therapy may not be related to an increased inflammatory response. Circulation 2003;107:3165–3169.
86. Straub RH, Hense HW, Andus T, Scholmerich J, Riegger GA, Schunkert H. Hormone replacement therapy and interrelation between serum interleukin-6 and body mass index in postmenopausal women: a population-based study. J Clin Endocrinol Metab 2000;85:1340–1344.
87. Walsh BW, Cox DA, Sashegyi A, Dean RA, Tracy RP, Anderson PW. Role of tumor necrosis factor-alpha and interleukin-6 in the effects of hormone replacement therapy and raloxifene on C-reactive protein in postmenopausal women. Am J Cardiol 2001;88:825–828.
88. Lacut K, Oger E, Le Gal G, et al. Differential effects of oral and transdermal postmenopausal estrogen replacement therapies on C-reactive protein. Thromb Haemost 2003;90:124–131.
89. van Baal WM, Kenemans P, van der Mooren MJ, Kessel H, Emeis JJ, Stehouwer CD. Increased C-reactive protein levels during short-term hormone replacement therapy in healthy postmenopausal women. Thromb Haemost 1999;81: 925–928.
90. Cushman M, Legault C, Barrett-Connor E, et al. Effect of postmenopausal hormones on inflammation-sensitive proteins: the Postmenopausal Estrogen/Progestin Interventions (PEPI) Study. Circulation 1999;100:717–722.
91. Cushman M, Meilahn EN, Psaty BM, Kuller LH, Dobs AS, Tracy RP. Hormone replacement therapy, inflammation, and hemostasis in elderly women. Arterioscler Thromb Vasc Biol 1999;19:893–899.
92. Ridker PM, Hennekens CH, Rifai N, Buring JE, Manson JE. Hormone replacement therapy and increased plasma concentration of C-reactive protein. Circulation 1999;100:713–716.
93. Stork S, von Schacky C, Angerer P. The effect of 17beta-estradiol on endothelial and inflammatory markers in postmenopausal women: a randomized, controlled trial. Atherosclerosis 2002;165:301–307.
94. Koh KK, Blum A, Hathaway L, et al. Vascular effects of estrogen and vitamin E therapies in postmenopausal women. Circulation 1999;100:1851–1857.
95. Kennedy G, McLaren M, Belch JJ, Seed M. Elevated levels of sE-selectin in post-menopausal females are decreased by hormone replacement therapy to levels observed in pre-menopausal females. Thromb Haemost 1999;82:1433–1436.
96. Cid MC, Schnaper HW, Kleinman HK. Estrogens and the vascular endothelium. Ann N Y Acad Sci 2002;966:143–157.
97. Kaila N, Thomas BE. Design and synthesis of sialyl Lewis(x) mimics as E- and P-selectin inhibitors. Med Res Rev 2002;22:566–601.
98. Yasojima K, Schwab C, McGeer EG, McGeer PL. Human neurons generate C-reactive protein and amyloid P: upregulation in Alzheimer's disease. Brain Res 2000;887:80–89.
99. Burger D, Dayer JM. Cytokines, acute-phase proteins, and hormones: IL-1 and TNF-alpha production in contact-mediated activation of monocytes by T lymphocytes. Ann N Y Acad Sci 2002;966:464–473.
100. Weinhold B, Bader A, Poli V, Ruther U. Interleukin-6 is necessary, but not sufficient, for induction of the human C-reactive protein gene in vivo. Biochem J. 1997;325(Pt 3):617–621.
101. Gabay C, Kushner I. Acute-phase proteins and other systemic responses to inflammation. N Engl J Med 1999;340:448–454.
102. Bruun JM, Nielsen CB, Pedersen SB, Flyvbjerg A, Richelsen B. Estrogen reduces pro-inflammatory cytokines in rodent adipose tissue: studies in vivo and in vitro. Horm Metab Res 2003;35:142–146.
103. Prestwood KM, Kenny AM, Kleppinger A, Kulldorff M. Ultralow-dose micronized 17beta-estradiol and bone density and bone metabolism in older women: a randomized controlled trial. JAMA 2003;290:1042–1048.
104. Lobo RA, Bush T, Carr BR, Pickar JH. Effects of lower doses of conjugated equine estrogens and medroxyprogesterone acetate on plasma lipids and lipoproteins, coagulation factors, and carbohydrate metabolism. Fertil Steril 2001;76:13–24.
105. Prestwood KM, Kenny AM, Unson C, Kulldorff M. The effect of low dose micronized 17ss-estradiol on bone turnover, sex hormone levels, and side effects in older women: a randomized, double blind, placebo-controlled study. J Clin Endocrinol Metab 2000;85:4462–4469.

106. Yasui T, Uemura H, Tezuka M, et al. Biological effects of hormone replacement therapy in relation to serum estradiol levels. Horm Res. 2001;56:38–44.
107. Seshadri S, Beiser A, Selhub J, et al. Plasma homocysteine as a risk factor for dementia and Alzheimer's disease. N Engl J Med 2002;346:476–483.
108. Prins ND, Den Heijer T, Hofman A, et al. Homocysteine and cognitive function in the elderly: the Rotterdam Scan Study. Neurology 2002;59:1375–1380.
109. Whitmer RA, Haan MN, Miller JW, Yaffe K. Hormone replacement therapy and cognitive performance: the role of homocysteine. J Gerontol A Biol Sci Med Sci 2003;58:324–330.
110. Lorenzo J. Interactions between immune and bone cells: new insights with many remaining questions. J Clin Invest 2000;106:749–752.
111. Lorenzo JA, Naprta A, Rao Y, et al. Mice lacking the type I interleukin-1 receptor do not lose bone mass after ovariectomy. Endocrinology 1998;139:3022–3025.
112. Baugh JA, Bucala R. Macrophage migration inhibitory factor. Crit Care Med 2002;30:S27–S35.
113. Ashcroft GS, Mills SJ, Lei K, et al. Estrogen modulates cutaneous wound healing by downregulating macrophage migration inhibitory factor. J Clin Invest 2003;111:1309–1318.
114. Grady D. Postmenopausal hormones—therapy for symptoms only. N Engl J Med 2003;348:1839–1854.

8

Effects of Hypertension in Young Adult and Middle-Aged Rhesus Monkeys

Mark B. Moss and Elizabeth M. Jonak

1. INTRODUCTION

It is now clear that hypertension is among the leading risk factors for the development of stroke, cerebrovascular disease (CVD), and related disorders. Elevated blood pressure is the most common risk factor for brain hemorrhage *(1)* and virtually doubles one's risk of cardiovascular disease *(2)*. More recently, hypertension has also been implicated in the development of mild cognitive impairment (MCI) and even as a contributory factor to Alzheimer's disease (AD). Hypertension is a common condition and affects more than one-quarter of the adult population of the United States alone *(3,4)*. The effects of extremely high levels of hypertension are also well known and include a fourfold greater risk for CVD than normotensive individuals and may have marked effects on several body organs *(5,6)*. However, for the most part, hypertension is an asymptomatic disorder with a substantial number of individuals going undiagnosed or unaware of their condition. Because the incidence of hypertension increases significantly with age, together with the coming "graying of America," concern over hypertension as a major health issue will become paramount and research in the area must keep pace.

2. ANIMAL MODELS

Indeed, research initiatives toward understanding the etiology, treatment, and prevention of hypertension have moved forward on several fronts. Research approaches from the perspective of biochemistry, genetics, structural imaging, functional imaging, and physiology have been aggressively pursued in both human subjects and animal models alike. Animal studies in particular have contributed significantly to our understanding of the underlying mechanisms and pathological changes associated with hypertension and CVD. In addition to obvious reasons, animal models offer major advantages over human research for several factors. Key among these factors is the degree to which one has control over extraneous variables, such as health history, individual differences, genetic variability, the use of medications, diet, variations in exercise, and time of onset hypertension. The development of the genetic models of hypertension, such as the spontaneously hypertensive rat (SHR) and transgenic and knockout mouse models, have provided major research tools in the investigation of hypertension. Despite the availability of such extensive research tools and animal models, one area of investigation that has not received a great deal of attention is the effect of hypertension in aging. Given the strong relationship of increased incidence of hypertension with age, such a model has clear relevance and would be worthy to develop. This chapter describes the development of a multidisciplinary primate model of hypertensive CVD that has focuses on both young and middle-aged adult

From: *Current Clinical Neurology*
Vascular Dementia: Cerebrovascular Mechanisms and Clinical Management
Edited by: R. H. Paul, R. Cohen, B. R. Ott, and S. Salloway © Humana Press Inc., Totowa, NJ

monkeys, with particular emphasis on cognitive function, an important emerging outcome consequence of hypertension.

3. THE MODEL

In addition to the advantages of an animal model cited in Subheading 2., another is the ability to obtain behavioral, physiological, and morphological data from the same individual in a relatively limited time frame. Collection of the data at a narrow time point allows for greater confidence and more reliable relationships among the variables obtained. One of the variables for which timely collection is important is in cognition. What biological changes have occurred in the presence of alteration in cognition?

Although this approach typically provides reliable and precise data, its relevance to the human condition is a function of the adequacy with which the experimental animal exhibits the human traits under study. Generally, the use of animal models is indicated when the experimental methods are inconvenient or impossible to apply to human subjects (e.g., specialized preparation and treatment of tissue). Our general goal was to determine whether the rhesus monkey is a suitable animal model of human hypertensive CVD and vascular dementia (VaD). Much has been learned about various aspects of these disorders through series of clinically relevant human and animal model investigations. However, relatively few investigations have used the monkey as a model of hypertensive CVD, particularly one in which cognitive function is carefully profiled. Thus, one major objective of this model was to establish the role of hypertension in cognitive impairment and decline and the relationship of this decline to specific brain alterations. A second and related goal was to determine the mechanisms that underlie the development of neuropathology as a consequence of hypertension.

4. USE OF THE NONHUMAN PRIMATE

Nonhuman primates, particularly old-world monkeys, have served as an ideal animal model for human conditions ranging from normal aging to Parkinson's disease to immunodeficiency disease. One major advantage of using the monkey is the ability of this species to perform many of the behavioral and cognitive tasks used in studies with human subjects. Few counterparts of these tests can be used in the rodent or rabbit. The use of this species was also based on the long history of the demonstrated use of monkeys as a model for conditions affecting humans in the various fields of medical science. There exists an extensive body of knowledge about the normal and abnormal biology of this species, which is important from the standpoint of establishing correlations with observed CVD changes. Finally, whereas human life and health histories are often incomplete or nonexistent, extensive medical and social histories are available on the monkeys used for the authors' model.

Because the authors' model includes the effect of age, as well as elevated blood pressure, as the major independent variables, the issue of age-equivalency and lifespan of the rhesus monkey is key. The typical adult life span of the rhesus ranges up to 30 yr or more, and it has been estimated that the lifespan ratio of human to monkey is approximately 3:1. Therefore, the monkeys that are described below that were part of the 12-mo experimental protocol might be considered in human terms as being hypertensive for approximately 3 yr.

5. EFFECTS OF HYPERTENSION ON COGNITION

The study of the effects of hypertension on intellectual function in humans was initiated more than 50 yr ago. During this time, evidence accumulated to show that hypertension produces impairment in cognition but to a greater extent in some domains than in others. The earlier studies were conducted when antihypertensive medications were not available and variables such as age and education were typically not considered *(7–9)*. The degree of impairment described in many of these studies was likely related to subjects often having severe, uncontrolled hypertension with frank neurologic signs. Therefore, it was not surprising that many investigators concluded that hypertension not only produced marked impairments in intellectual function but also produced marked grossly visible damage to the brain.

More recent studies that have controlled for many of these factors have still shown that patients are impaired on numerous cognitive tasks, including those of general intelligence *(10,11)* and memory function *(12)*, but without evidence of frank damage to the brain. A well-controlled study by Schmidt et al. *(13)* assessed a group of individuals with hypertension and compared performance to normotensive control subjects. The researchers found that the hypertensive group was more impaired on tasks of verbal memory and total learning, but no difference in performance was observed on tasks of visual memory, attention, vigilance, and reaction time. Systolic blood pressure is a sensitive measure of cognitive status as indicated by negative correlations with Wechsler Adult Intelligence Scale (WAIS) performance in a group of male subjects with hypertension *(14)*. Deficits have also been found when hypertensive subjects were compared to normotensive subjects in WAIS performance subtest scores *(15)* and in verbal scores when studied longitudinally for 5- to 6-yr intervals *(16)*. Findings also show that with longer exposure, blood pressure measures accurately predict cognitive decline *(17)*.

In a study conducted in Sweden on 1736 community-based human subjects, both systolic and diastolic blood pressures were significantly related to baseline performance on the Mini-Mental State Examination (MMSE), and baseline systolic pressure was significantly related to follow-up performance *(18)*. Of direct relevance to the present animal model, untreated hypertension in humans has recently been found to be inversely related to both a composite index of cognitive performance and individual scores on tests of attention and memory in the Framingham Heart Study *(19–21)*. In a longitudinal study of 3735 Japanese-American men living in Hawaii, systolic blood pressure proved to be a significant predictor of reduced cognitive function 16 yr later *(22)*.

Attentional measures, such as symbol/digit substitution, continuous attention, reaction time, paired word association, and inspection time threshold, are all significantly impaired in a group of individuals with untreated mild to moderate hypertension when compared to the performance of age-matched controls *(23)*. Similarly, regression analyses revealed that part of the impairment attributed to age in a study of visual selective attention resulted from blood pressure level in a study of subjects with unmedicated mild hypertension ranging from 18 to 78 yr of age *(24)*.

Taken together, the weight of evidence strongly suggested that hypertension produces impairment in the domains of attention, memory, and executive function (abstraction and set shifting) but, to a lesser extent, in those of visuospatial skills, psychomotor speed, and verbal skills. Accordingly, the authors decided to assess the effects on cognition, particularly with regard to attention, memory, and executive function, in their primate model of hypertensive CVD.

6. INTERACTION OF HYPERTENSION AND AGE

Because the prevalence and incidence of hypertension increases with age, many studies have focused on the contribution of hypertension to age-related cognitive change *(25–27)*. However, the effects of hypertension on cognition may not be uniform across the age range. In fact, and perhaps somewhat surprisingly, the effects of high blood pressure on cognition may be greater in younger than older subjects *(28)*, and this effect is independent of demographic, psychosocial, and education-related factors *(29)*. Hypertension was negatively associated with WAIS verbal scores in younger (21 to 39 yr) but not older (45 to 65 yr) subjects, whereas its effect on performance scores was greater for younger than older subjects *(30)*. Similarly, hypertension in middle-aged adults was associated with a disproportionate decline in performance on tests of psychomotor speed and an increase in error rate on a test of visual selective attention *(24)*. In the present model, the authors have assessed the separated and combined effects of hypertension and age.

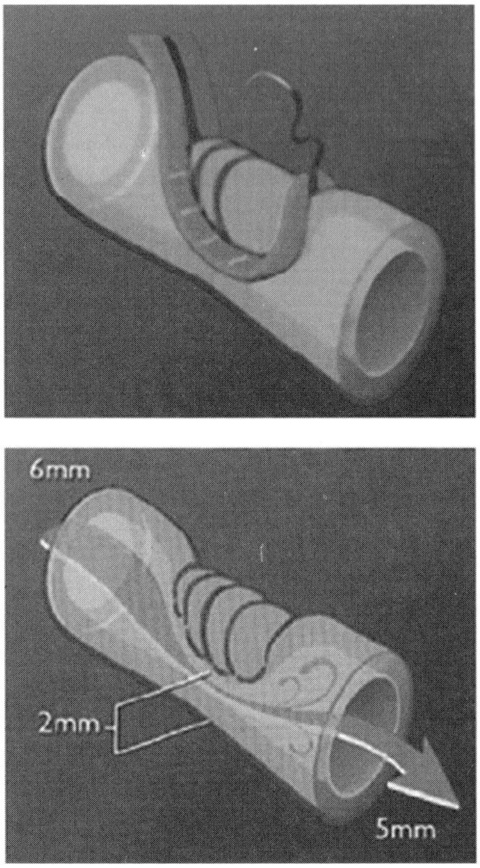

Fig. 1. Illustration depicting two stages of the partial clamping of the thoracic aorta using a vascular clamp **(A)** followed by suturing of the segment **(B)**.

7. PRODUCTION OF HYPERTENSION

The basis of this model is the production of hypertension in the monkey that is achieved by surgical coarctation of the thoracic aorta *(31)*. Before surgery, monkeys are pretrained to perform in a Wisconsin General Test Apparatus (WGTA) and an automated-touch screen apparatus. They are then assigned to one of the experimental groups or the control group in a predetermined fashion based on entry into the study. All monkeys are housed in an American Association for Acceditation of Laboratory Animal Care (AAALAC)-approved facility. At surgery, animals are initially sedated with Ketalar (ketamine hydrochloride), blood pressure is measured using an ArterioSonde, and an electrocardiogram (ECG) is recorded. The animals are anesthetized using sodium pentobarbital and are then intubated orotracheally and connected to a respirator. The monkey is placed in a lateral position with its left side up. A left anterolateral thoracotomy is performed along the fifth intercostal space. The lung is retracted medially, exposing the thoracic aorta at the posterior mediastinum. A segment of the thoracic aorta just below the level of the hilum of the left lung is mobilized and dissected without injuring the mediastinal and intercostal branches. The external diameter of the same segment is measured with a caliper. A 1-cm segment is then narrowed to luminal diameter of 2.0 to 2.5 mm using surgical calipers and a Castaneda partial occlusion vascular clamp (Pilling Instruments, Fort Washington, PA) (*see* Fig. 1).

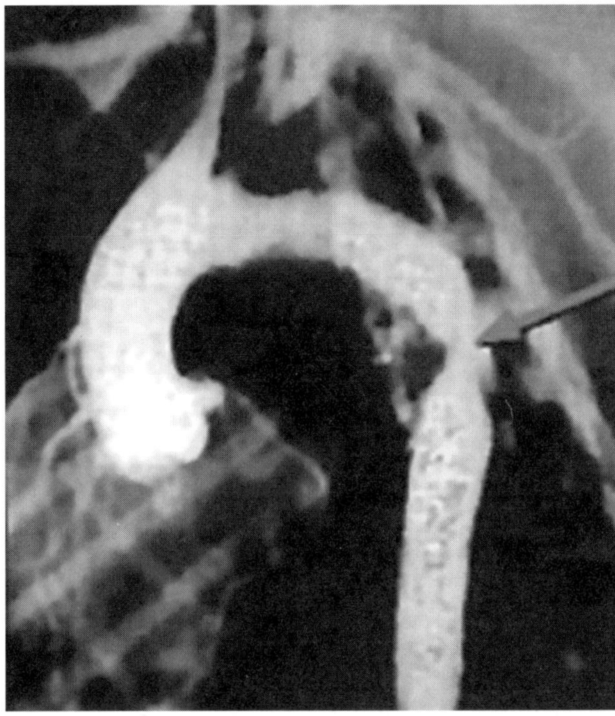

Fig. 2. Arteriogram showing the coarctation of the thoracic aorta (arrow) in the monkey.

A supporting band of umbilical tape is then drawn around the coarcted segment and sutured without further constriction of the vessel. The coarctation of the aorta results in a decrease in luminal area of approximately 75–80% (*see* Fig. 2), as indicated by autopsy findings. During the immediate 3-wk postoperative period, the monkeys are given angiotensin I converting enzyme inhibitors, diuretics, and digoxin to prevent heart failure.

During the baseline period and at 2- to 3-mo intervals throughout the experimental period, measurements are made of body weight and blood pressure.

The blood pressure in the brachial artery is monitored indirectly by the ultrasonic cuff method weekly in the postoperative period and then at 2-mo intervals with the use of the ArterioSonde *(32)*. Direct measurements of the intraarterial pressure in the brachial and femoral arteries also are performed on the day of the surgical coarctation and at 3, 6, and 12 mo after the surgery. After exposing and cannulating the brachial and femoral arteries, the arterial pressure in these arteries is simultaneously measured with strain gauge transducers attached to a Beckman dynograph recorder. Direct measurements of brachial arterial pressure were higher than the indirect measurements *(33)* (*see* Fig. 3).

8. EFFECTS OF HYPERTENSION ON COGNITION IN THE YOUNG ADULT

As part of the authors' program, the effects of hypertension on cognitive function were studied in a group of young adult rhesus monkeys ranging in age from 5 to 9 yr. Monkeys were assessed in the domains of attention, rule learning, and conceptual set-shifting using an automated task of attention, the Delayed nonmatching to sample task, and the nonhuman primate analog to the Wisconsin Card Sort Task (WCST), called the Conceptual Set Shifting Task. Their performance was compared to a group of operated controls that underwent every stage of the surgical procedures up to, but not including, the actual narrowing of the aorta.

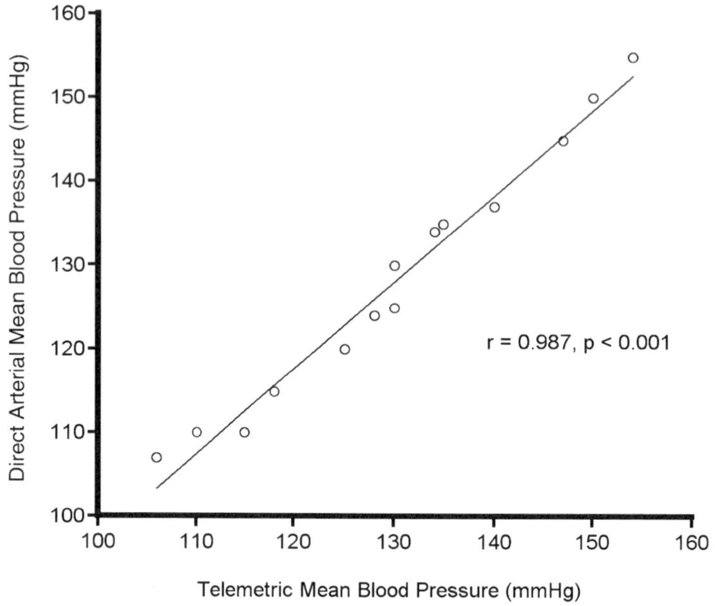

Fig. 3. The intraarterial, Doppler, and Dinamap methods of measuring systolic blood pressure; all produce values that are highly significantly correlated with one another. However, as seen on the graph, the difference between intraarterial and the Dinamap pressures is not constant because as the pressure rises, the difference between the methods increases.

8.1. Attention

Tests of attention were performed in a computer-controlled darkened testing chamber that contained a reward dispensing cup, a set of speakers, and a 19-in color computer monitor covered with a resistive touch screen. For the test of simple attention, the monkeys were required to touch the same target stimulus on the touch screen that they had seen during the pretraining phase. Mixed intertrial intervals of 5, 10, 20, 40, and 60 s were used in a pseudorandom fashion to prohibit the monkey from anticipating the appearance of the stimulus. For consistency with the pretraining phase, the target stimulus appears pseudorandomly in 1 of 12 spatial locations on the screen. When the stimulus was touched, the latency to touch was recorded, the touch screen became black, food reward was delivered, and the next intertrial interval began. If the monkey did not touch the stimulus on the screen within 60 s, a nonresponse was recorded, no reward was delivered, the touch screen became black, and the next intertrial interval began. Testing continued in this fashion for 50 trials per day for 2 consecutive days. The authors found that hypertensive monkeys evidenced a longer latency to respond than normotensive monkeys *(34)*. This finding is consistent with earlier studies in humans that even simple attention may be impaired by hypertension. When cued attention was assessed, a procedure in which the monkey is provided a cue before the onset of the stimulus to direct attention, monkeys with hypertension were still impaired relative to normotensive animals. Moreover, the authors found a significant correlation between systolic and diastolic blood pressures and the latency to respond measures ($p < 0.01$). Of note, there was no difference between both groups in the number of missed trials suggesting that motivational state did not play a factor in the findings.

Thus, in the authors' studies of attention, monkeys with hypertension were impaired on a task that required orienting to and then responding by touching a randomly presented visual stimulus. Unlike normotensive animals, hypertensive monkeys did not benefit from the presentation of a cue that preceded the target stimulus. The effect was not related to motivational state, because there was no difference in the number of missed trials. Rather, the findings suggest a reduction in the speed of processing in the stimulus–response chain.

8.2. Memory

As mentioned in the Introduction to this chapter, the weight of evidence strongly suggests that in humans, memory function is vulnerable to the effects of hypertension. The authors assessed the effect of hypertension using two tasks of memory function *(35)*, the delayed nonmatching to sample task (DNMS) and the delayed recognition span task (DRST), the latter of which has been used extensively with human subjects *(36)*.

The same animals that performed the attention tasks participated in the memory studies. Monkeys were trained initially in a WGTA and were then administered the basic condition of the DNMS and DRST tests described below. The DNMS task assesses the subject's ability to identify a novel from a familiar stimulus over varying delay intervals. Various forms of this task have been used to assess memory function in monkeys after either transection of the fornix *(37–39)* or limited removal of selected temporal lobe structures (e.g., hippocampus or amygdala) *(38–41)*. In addition, this task has been used to evaluate and quantify some aspects of recognition memory in patients with AD and normal age-matched controls *(42)*. Preoperatively, animals were administered the basic task in which the trial begins with a sample object presented over the central baited food well. The animal is permitted to displace the object and obtain the reward. Ten seconds later, the recognition trial is begun, with the sample object presented over an unbaited lateral well and a new, unfamiliar object presented over a baited lateral well. To now obtain the reward, the animal must recognize the original sample object and choose the unfamiliar, novel object. Twenty seconds later, a different sample object is presented over the baited central well, followed 10 s later by another recognition trial. The position of the two objects varied, on successive recognition trials, from left to right lateral wells in a predetermined order, and a noncorrection procedure is used. Thirty trials a day were given until the animals reached a learning criterion of 90 correct responses in 90 consecutive trials or a maximum of 1000 trials. Objects were drawn from a pool of 1500 "junk" objects, and in each daily session, 60 of the objects were used. The 1500 objects are randomly recombined to produce new sets of pairs so that the pairings presented were new and unique on each trial.

Six months postoperatively, all monkeys were readministered the DNMS basic task. After this, they were trained in an automated test apparatus described below and were administered the delayed recognition span test. The delayed recognition span task is a short-term memory test, which was designed to investigate recognition memory in monkeys after bilateral removal of the hippocampus *(43)*. It requires the subject to identify, trial-by-trial, a new stimulus among an increasing array of serially presented, familiar stimuli. The task is administered using two different classes of stimulus material, spatial location or pattern shape. This will allow the researchers to characterize any recognition memory deficits, which may occur as a general impairment, or one, which is material specific. Testing on the DRST occurred in a computer-controlled testing chamber that contains a reward dispensing cup, a set of speakers, and a 19-in color computer monitor covered with a resistive touch screen.

For the spatial condition of the DRST, the computer touch screen is programmed to display 12 nonoverlapping positions, arranged in a 3 × 4 matrix. Yellow circles are used as stimuli with the background color of the screen being black. On the first trial of the first chain of trials, a circle appeared in 1 of the 12 positions that is rewarded. The animal is allowed to touch the circle and obtain the reward. The screen is blanked and reactivated 10 s later with a second positively rewarded circle (identical to the first) on the screen with the first circle reappearing in its original location. The animal is required to touch the new circle to obtain the reward. Similarly, each successive correct response is followed by the addition of a new circle until the animal makes an error. Ten such chains of trials are presented each day, 5 d per wk, for a total of 5 wk.

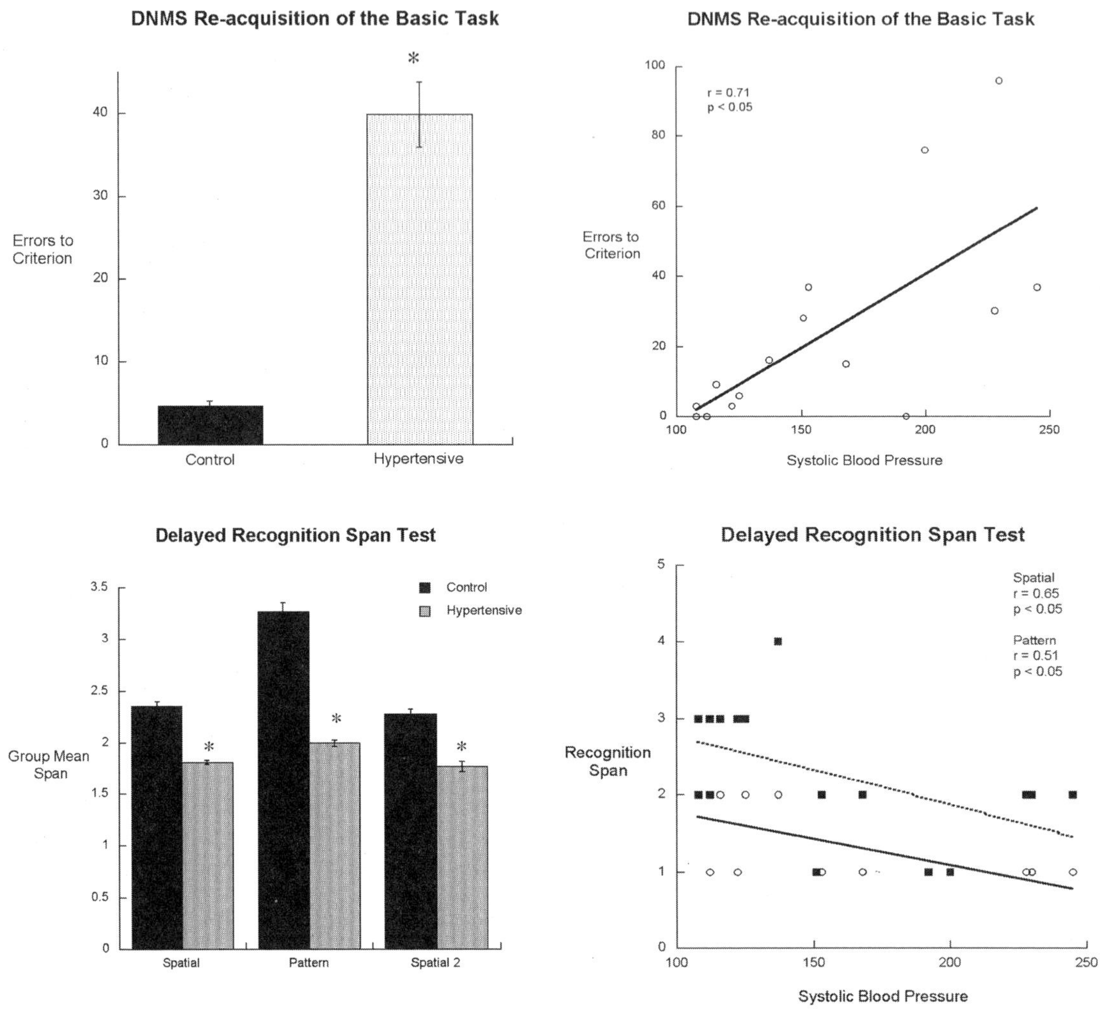

Fig. 4. Scores on the delayed nonmatching to sample and delayed recognition span test. The level of impairment on this index was significantly and linearly related to the level of both systolic and diastolic blood pressure in the monkeys in this study.

The pattern form of the DRST is administered in much the same way as the spatial form. However, for this condition of the task, on each trial the spatial location of the previously correct stimulus is changed in a predetermined random fashion so that the animal is able to identify the new stimulus based only on visual, rather than spatial, cues. The stimuli for the pattern condition were drawn from a pool of 600 "clip-art" images. The images were drawn from the pool in a predetermined fashion to ensure unique combinations on each trial.

The first findings on memory assessment revealed a significant difference among the groups on the DNMS measures at 6 mo postoperatively. Monkeys with hypertension relearned the DNMS task less efficiently than operated controls (*see* Fig. 4). On both the spatial and pattern conditions of the DRST, the performance of the hypertensive monkeys was significantly impaired with respect to the performance of the control monkeys suggesting that, in addition to attentional function, hypertension diminishes the memory "load" capacity by 6 mo (*see* Fig. 4).

Of note, again the extent of impairment on these tasks was directly related to the degree of elevation of the blood pressure (*see* Fig. 4).

8.3. Executive Function

It is now becoming clear that one of the most sensitive domains of cognitive function affected in aging and age-related disease is executive functions *(35)*. Although much is known about how memory is affected by various disease processes, little is know about the changes in executive system functions. Executive system functions encompass many cognitive skills necessary to perform high levels of cognitive abilities and include skills such as cognitive flexibility, cognitive tracking, divided attention, ability to establish and maintain set, monitoring and modification of response pattern, and abstraction. Several tests of executive system have been developed, and, in studies of humans with hypertension, performance on these tests generally has been impaired *(11,44)*.

One well-established human test of executive system function is the WCST *(45,46)*. It was developed to assess cognitive flexibility, cognitive tracking, the ability to identify abstract categories, and maintain and shift cognitive set according to changing contingencies *(47–49)*. The task requires the patient to sort a series of cards based on three stimulus dimensions: color, form, and number using feedback information from the administrator. The WCST has been used to assess deficits that are associated with a variety of disease processes and injuries. Studies with the WCST have demonstrated impaired performance by individuals owing to frontal lobe dysfunction marked by characteristic disturbances include perseverative responses, an inability to shift set once established, and an inability to use information from the environment to modify response *(50,51)*. Milner *(51)* reported that the ability to shift from one mode of solution to another on the WCST is more impaired by frontal than posterior cerebral lesions.

As part of an ongoing study of the effects of hypertension in the rhesus monkey, the authors used the principles of the WCST to develop a test of executive system functions for use with nonhuman primates *(52,53)*. This test, the Conceptual Set Shifting Task (CSST), requires the monkey to establish a cognitive set based on a reward contingency, maintain that set for a period of time, and then shift the set as the reward contingency changes. In this study, the CSST was used to assess executive system functioning and frontal lobe integrity of monkeys with sustained hypertension to further our understanding of the relationship between hypertension and cognition.

For this study, the authors used 10 of the monkeys, five of which were hypertensive and five of which were control animals. All monkeys were tested in the same automated general testing apparatus in which they had performed the attention and delayed recognition span tasks, for 80 trials/d, 5 d/wk.

The initial stage of the task began a simple three-choice discrimination. The monkey was presented with a pink square, an orange cross, and a brown 12-point star. The three appeared in pseudorandom order in nine different spatial locations on the screen. The pink square was the positive stimuli for all trials, and the monkey was rewarded with a food treat when it chose this stimuli. To reach learning criterion, the monkey had to choose the pink square for 10 consecutive trials.

The testing day after completing the discrimination task, the monkey began the CSST. On each trial of the CSST, three stimuli appeared in a pseudorandom pattern on the computer screen (*see* Fig. 5). The stimuli differed in color (red, green, or blue) and shape (triangle, star, and circle). All possible combinations of stimuli appeared on the screen for a 4-d cycle, and if more than 4 d were needed to reach criterion, the 4-d cycle was repeated until criterion was reached.

Testing consisted of an acquisition category (red) and then three concept shift categories (triangle, blue, and star). During acquisition, the monkey was required to choose the red stimulus, regardless of its shape, to obtain a food reward. Once the monkey chose this stimulus on 10 consecutive trials, the program switched the rewarded contingency during the same testing session, without alerting the monkey. The monkey now had to choose the stimulus shaped like a triangle regardless of its color to obtain a food reward. Again, when the monkey reached a criterion of 10 consecutive responses, the computer switched the rewarded contingency within the same testing session, without alerting the

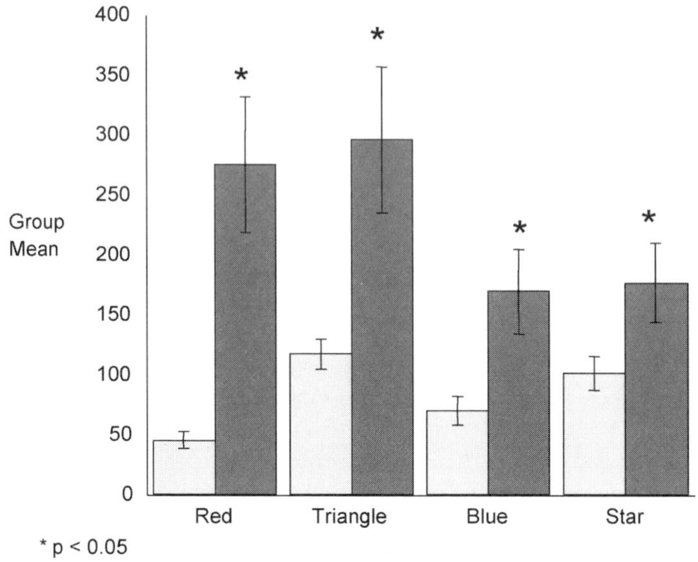

Fig. 5. Initial abstraction and subsequent set-shifting scores on the Conceptual Set-Shifting Task.

monkey. The blue stimulus then had to be chosen, regardless of its shape, to obtain a food reward. Finally, the last category, star, was rewarded, when criterion was reached on the blue category.

It was somewhat surprising that monkeys were able to perform and master this difficult "higher order" task but served to reinforce the use of the nonhuman primate as a well-suited animal model. More to the authors' surprise, they found that hypertensive monkeys were impaired at abstracting the initial concept of color and were subsequently impaired on the shifts to shape, then to color, and again when shifted back to the concept of shape (*see* Fig. 5) *(52)*.

Of particular note, and completely consistent with data from human studies of executive dysfunction in patients with frontal lobe compromise, as a group, hypertensive demonstrated a greater tendency to perseverative in its response pattern when shifting categories than normotensive monkeys. In contrast, it was clear that basic discrimination and learning skills remained intact in the hypertensive monkeys because they were as efficient as normotensive monkeys in learning the simple three-choice discrimination task.

9. EFFECTS OF HYPERTENSION IN MIDDLE-AGED NONHUMAN PRIMATES

The effects of hypertension in middle age in the nonhuman primate are perhaps even more relevant to the human condition than our studies in young hypertensive animals, because it is well known that aging is a significant risk factor for hypertension. The authors have assessed a group of five middle-aged hypertensive monkeys (ages 14–18) on the DNMS task and compared their performance to nine normotensive monkeys of the same age range. Middle-aged hypertensive monkeys, as did young hypertensive monkeys, evidenced difficulty in the acquisition of the DNMS task *(54)*. They required, on average, 250 trials and 125 errors to acquire the task. On a 2- or 10-min delay condition of the DNMS task, the middle-aged monkeys with hypertension were again significantly worse that middle aged normotensive monkeys (*see* Fig. 6).

One way to compare the degree of impairment on the DNMS task as a consequence of age and/or hypertension is to calculate the "effect" size. Figure 7 shows the effect size of age and blood pressure status for trials and errors on the task.

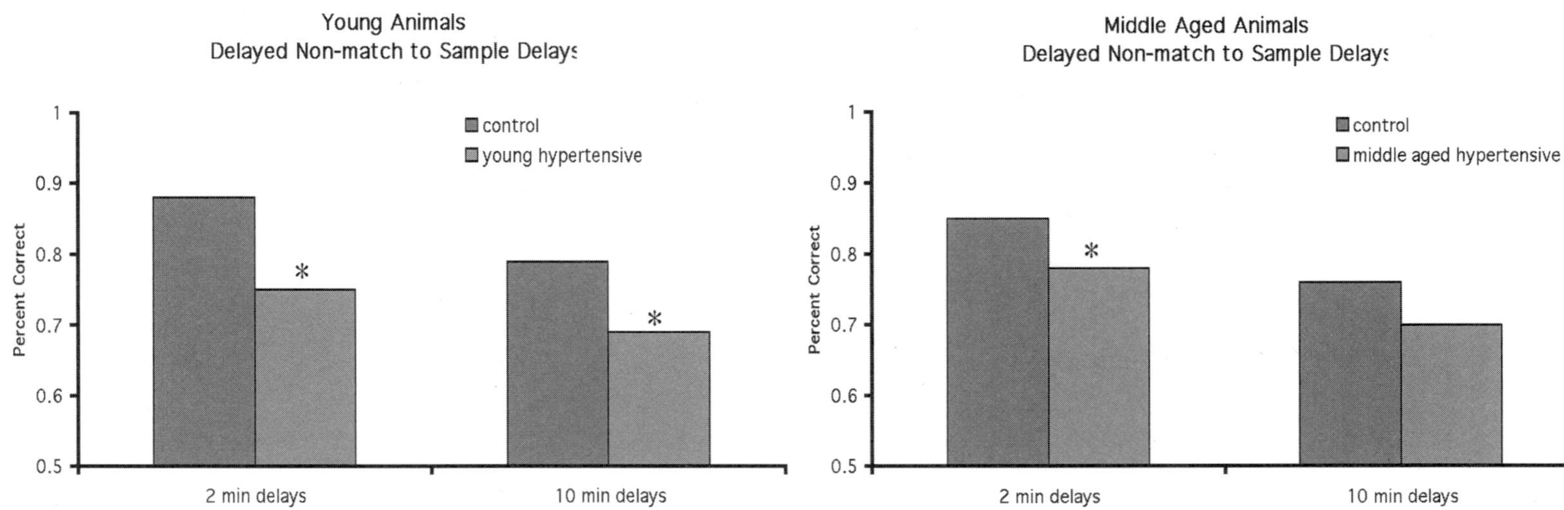

Fig. 6. Performance on two delay conditions of delayed nonmatching to sample task by normotensive and hypertensive middle-aged monkeys.

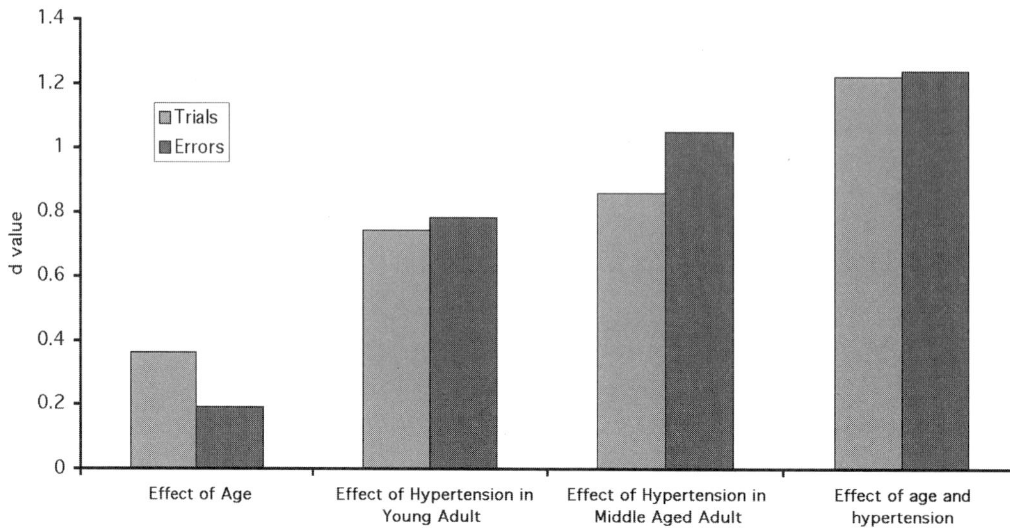

Fig. 7. Effect sizes in *d*-scores for trials and errors on delayed nonmatching to sample task acquisition: effect size for age, hypertension in young adults, hypertension in middle-aged adults, and the combination of the effect of middle age and hypertension.

As can be seen in the first set of bars, the effect of age alone had only a moderate *d* value of 0.2. That is, middle age *per se* did not markedly lessen efficiency in learning delayed nonmatching to sample. Of note, the effect of hypertension on learning DNMS in middle age (third set of bars, *d* value for errors = 1.1) relative to remaining normotensive was greater than that for hypertension in young adulthood (second set of bars, *d* value for errors = 0.8). Perhaps the finding of greatest effect was the effect of the combination of middle age and hypertension on learning relative to young adult normotensive adults (last set of bars, *d* value >1.2). Together, these initial findings suggest that the effects of middle age and hypertension are, at a minimum, additive and may, in fact, be synergistic. Additional behavioral test findings, as well as neuropathological assessment, will help determine the extent of the singular and combined effects of age and hypertension on cognition and brain integrity.

10. NEUROPATHOLOGICAL CONSEQUENCES OF HYPERTENSION

The neurobiological basis of the cognitive deficits associated with hypertension remains unclear. The authors have begun to explore the possible neuroanatomical bases for the impairment noted in attention. Yet, examinations of the brains of these animals using magnetic resonance imaging (MRI) even at 1 yr after surgery showed no evidence of stroke or infarct. Investigators *(55)* have suggested that hypertension produces subclinical pathological changes in the brain before the appearance of acute events, such as strokes. These findings are in line with those from the human literature demonstrating that hypertension produces subclinical pathological changes in the brain *(27)*.

The most conspicuous finding in the authors' model using standard Nissl and myelin stains was minute areas of infarction in both gray and white matter *(56)*. The microinfarcts were irregularly shaped and of relatively uniform size, with an average maximum diameter of slightly less than 0.5 mm. In the grey matter, these lesions were characterized by a total loss of neurons and, in the white matter, by marked loss of myelinated fibers. The microinfarcts appeared with greater frequency in the white matter of the forebrain, particularly in the capsular system and the hemispheric white matter of the corona radiata and centrum semiovale. The area with the next highest density was in the cerebral cortex, with the remainder scattered throughout the forebrain, brain stem, and cerebellum.

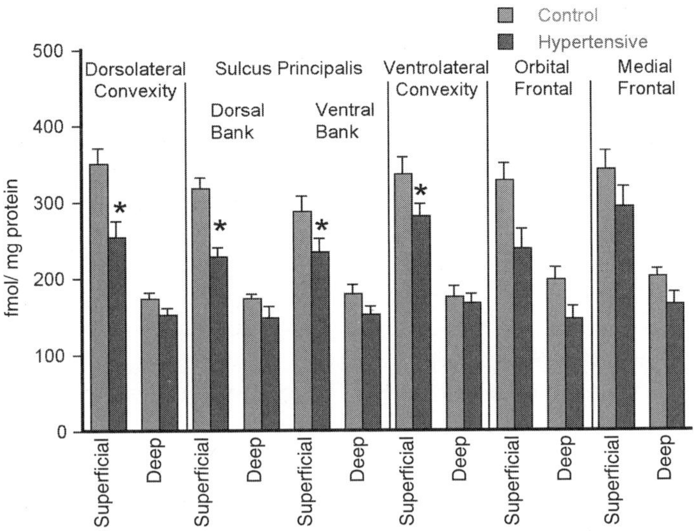

Fig. 8. Selected regions of norepinephrine and dopamine binding within the prefrontal cortex of the rhesus monkey.

The relationship of the microinfarcts observed in this primate model to the classically described focal lesions of chronic hypertension in the human brain is uncertain. The lesions are smaller than lacunar infarcts, which according to Fisher *(57)* measure 0.5 to 15 mm in diameter. They also differ from lacunar infarction because they are not associated with obvious segmental degenerative changes in penetrating arteries or vascular occlusions, conspicuous changes in the brains with lacunar infarction *(57,58)*. In contrast, the size of the microinfarcts is similar to that reported in hypertensive encephalopathy. However, the appearance of the lesions, the associated vascular changes, and the distribution pattern of the lesions are different. In human hypertensive encephalopathy, the microinfarcts observed in these hypertensive monkeys resemble those reported by Garcia et al. *(59)*. These authors studied five hypertensive monkeys with coarctations of the aorta of 2 mo to 2 yr duration. They noted grossly visible "spongy" lesions and selected these for detailed electron microscopic study. These measured 0.5 mm in diameter, were present in all five monkeys in a random pattern, and were most abundant 2 yr post coarctation. In these areas, the capillaries were dilated with flattened endothelium, interrupted endothelial linings, increased thickness and deformity of the basement membrane, and deposition of collagen and osmophilic material.

11. NEUROTRANSMITTER ALTERATIONS

As part of their investigations to assess the neurobiological basis of the cognitive decline observed as a consequence of hypertension, particularly regarding prefrontal cortical functions, the authors assessed the effect on selected neurotransmitters in the prefrontal cortex of a group of young adult hypertensive monkeys. They assessed the singular effects of chronic hypertension on dopamine and norepinephrine receptor binding in the prefrontal cortex (PFC) *(60)*. Using autoradiographic ligand-binding techniques, receptor-binding densities were quantified for one dopamine and two norepinephrine receptor subtypes (DA1, NE α 1, and NE α 2) and the norepinephrine and dopamine uptake transporters (DAU and NEU) in specific regions of the prefrontal cortex. Their findings indicate a striking decrease in DA1 (*see* Fig. 8) and NE α 1 receptor binding in the superficial layers of cortex in ventrolateral and dorsolateral convexities and ventral and dorsal banks of sulcus principalis and a marked increase in DAU receptor binding throughout all layers of the cortex of hypertensive animals.

In contrast, there was no change in NE α 2 and NEU receptor binding. The observed changes in noradrenergic receptor-binding densities in prefrontal cortices is in accord with evidence suggesting that the prefrontal cortex may be the locus for impairment of executive function in hypertension *(60)*.

12. CONCLUSION

The authors believe that the nonhuman primate monkey is a suitable model to assess the effects of hypertension on cognition and brain integrity. Their study findings demonstrate the feasibility of inducing and maintaining moderate levels of chronic hypertension in monkeys with very low mortality and little to no health complications. They also believe they have demonstrated that monkeys with hypertension evidence impairments in domains of cognitive function that parallel those seen in humans and, in several instances, using nearly identical behavioral tasks. Accordingly, the continued use of the nonhuman primate model, as well as those of rodents, should provide further insight the physiologic, neurobiologic, and genetic bases of the development, course, and effects of hypertension and hypertensive-related CVD in humans.

ACKNOWLEDGMENTS

The work described in this chapter represents the efforts of several individuals. The surgical procedures were developed and carried out by Dr. William Hollander and Dr. Somnath Prusty. The behavioral studies were conducted with significant contributions from Drs. Douglas Rosene, Ron Killiany, and Tara Moore. The authors' graduate student John Pugh, research technicians, Reese Edwards, and Jason Coole also made invaluable contributions. The studies described were funded by NIH grant R37-AG17609.

REFERENCES

1. Wolf P. Cerebrovascular risk. In: Izzo J and Black H, eds. Essentials of Hypertension. 2003, pp. 239–243.
2. Kannel WB, Wilson PWF. Cardiovascular risk factors and Hypertension. In: Izzo J and Black H, eds. Essentials of Hypertension. 2003, pp. 239–243.
3. Forette F, Boller F. Hypertension and the risk of dementia in the elderly. Am J Med 1991;90:14S–19S.
4. Kaplan NM. Hypertension: Prevalence, risks, and effect of therapy. Ann Int Med 1983;98:705–708.
5. Sandok BA, Whisnant JP. Hypertension and the brain: Clinical aspects. In: Genest J, Kuchel O, Hamet P, Cantin M, eds., Hypertension. New York, NY: McGraw-Hill, 1983, pp. 777–791.
6. Leoncini G, Viazzi F, Parodi D, et al. Mild renal dysfunction and subclinical cardiovascular damage in primary hypertension. Hypertension 2003;42:14.
7. Simonson E, Enzer N. State of motor centers in circulatory insufficiency. Arch Intern Med. 1941;68:498–512.
8. Enzer N, Simonson E, Blanksein SS. Fatigue of patients with circulatory insufficiency, investigated by means of fusion frequency of flicker. Ann Intern Med 1942;16:702–707.
9. Apter NS, Halstead WC, Heimburger RF. Impaired cerebral functions in essential hypertension. Am J Psychiatry 1951;107:808–813.
10. Wilkie F, Eisdorfer C. Intelligence and blood pressure in the aged. Science 1971;172:959–962.
11. Boller F, Vrtunski PB, Mack JL, Kim Y. Neuropsychological correlates of hypertension. Arch Neurol 1977;34:701–705.
12. Franceschi M, Tancredi O, Smirne S, Mercinelli A, Canal N. Cognitive processes in hypertension. Hypertension 1982;4:226–229.
13. Schmidt R, Fazekas F, Offenbacher H, et al. Magnetic resonance imaging white matter lesions and cognitive impairment in hypertensive individuals. Arch Neurol 1991;48:417–420.
14. Vanderploeg RD, Goldman H, Kleinman KM. Relationship between systolic and diastolic blood pressure and cognitive functioning in hypertensive subjects: an extension of previous findings. Arch Clin Neuropsy 1987;2:101–109.
15. Mazzucchi A, Mutti A, Poletti A, Ravanetti C, Novarini A, Parma M. Neuropsychological deficits in arterial hypertension. Acta Neurol Scand 1986;73:619–627.
16. Schultz NR, Elias MR, Robbins MA, et al. A longitudinal study of the performance of hypertensive and normotensive subjects on the Wechsler Adult Intelligence Scale. Psych Aging 1989;4:496–499.
17. Sands LP, Meredith W. Blood pressure and intellectual functioning in late midlife. J Gerontol 1992;47:81–84.
18. Guo Z, Fratiglioni L, Winblad B, Viitanen M. Blood pressure and performance on the Mini-Mental State Examination in the very old. Cross-sectional and longitudinal data from the Kungsholmen Project. Am J Epidemiol 1997;145:106–1113.

19. Elias MF, Wolf PA, D'Agostino RB, Cobb J, White LR. Untreated blood pressure level is inversely related to cognitive functioning: The Framingham Study. Am J Epidemiol 1993;138:353–364.
20. Elias MF, D'Agostino RB, Elias PK, Wolf PA. Neuropsychological test performance, cognitive functioning, blood pressure and age: The Framingham Heart Study. Exp Aging Res 1995a;21:369–391.
21. Elias MF, D'Agostino RB, Elias PK, Wolf PA. Blood pressure, hypertension and age as risk factors for poor cognitive performance. Exp Aging Res 1995b;21:393–417.
22. Launer LJ, Masaki K, Petrovitch H, Foley D, Havlik RJ. The association between midlife blood pressure levels and later life cognitive function. JAMA 1995;274:1846–1851.
23. Kalra L, Jackson LH, Swift CG. Psychomotor performance in elderly hypertensive patients. J Hum Hypertens 1993;7: 279–284.
24. Madden DJ, Blumenthal JA. Interaction of hypertension and age in visual selective attention performance. Health Psychol 1998;17:76–83.
25. Wallace RB, Lemke JH, Morris MC, Goodenberger M, Kohout F, Hinrichs JV. Relationship of free-recall memory to hypertension in the elderly: The Iowa 65+ rural health study. J Chronic Dis 1985;38:475–481.
26. Farmer ME, Kittner SJ, Abbott RD, Wolz MM, Wolf PA, White LR. Longitudinally measured blood pressure, anti-hypertensive medication use, and cognitive performance: The Framingham Heart Study. J Clin Epidemiol 1990;43:475–480.
27. Waldstein SR, Ryan CM, Manuck SB, Parkinson DK, Bromet EJ. Learning and memory function in man with untreated blood pressure elevation. J Consult Clin Psychol 1991;59:513–517.
28. Elias MF, Robbins MA, Schultz N, Pierce TW. Is blood pressure an important variable in research on aging and neuropsychological test performance? J Gerontol Psychol Sci 1990;45:128–135.
29. Waldstein SR, Jennings JR, Ryan CM, et al. Hypertension and neuropsychological performance in men: Interactive effects of age. Health Psychol 1996;15:102–109.
30. Schultz NR, Dineen JT, Elias MF, et al. WAIS performance for different age groups of hypertensive and control subjects during the administration of a diuretic. J Gerontol 1979;31:246–253.
31. Prusty S, Killiany RJ, Rosene DL, Hollander WH, Moss MB. Surgical production of hypertension in the non-human primate by aortic coarctation: a primate model of hypertensive cerebrovascular disease. Neurosci Meth 2003; in press.
32. Hollander W, Prusty S, Kirkpatrick B, Paddock J, Nagrai S. Role of hypertension in ischemic heart disease and cerebral vascular disease in the cynomolgus monkey with coarctation of the aorta. Circ Res 1977;40(Suppl I):I70–I83.
33. Hollander W, Prusty S, Killiany RJ, Moss, MB. Comparison of direct and indirect methods, including telemetry for measurement of blood pressure, in the hypertensive monkey. Neurosci Meth. 2003; in press.
34. Killiany RJ, TL Moore, Prusty S, Rosene DL, Moss MB. Impairment of attention in a primate model of hypertensive cerebrovascular disease. Cogn Brain Sci 2003; in press.
35. Moss MB, Killiany RJ, Prusty S, Jonak EM, Moore TL, Rosene DL. Impairment in visual recognition memory in a primate model of hypertensive cerebrovascular disease. Behav Neurosci 2003; in press.
36. Albert MS, Moss MB. Neuropsychological profiles of normal aging. In: Peters A and Morrison J, eds. Cerebral Cortex, Neurodegenerative and Age-Related Changes in Structure and Function of Cerebral Cortex. New York, NY: Plenum Press, 1998.
37. Gaffan D. Recognition impaired and association intact in the memory of monkeys after transection of the fornix. J Comp Physio Psych 1974;86:1100–1109.
38. Mahut M, Zola-Morgan S, Moss MB. Hippocampal resections impair associative learning and recognition memory in the monkey. J Neurosci 1982;2:1214–1229.
39. Saunders RC, Murray EA, Mishkin M. Further evidence that amygdala and hippocampus contribute equally to recognition memory. Neuropsychologia 1984;22:785–796.
40. Mishkin M. Memory in monkeys severely impaired by combined but not separate removal of amygdala and hippocampus. Nature 1978;273:297–298.
41. Murray EA. Medial temporal lobe structures contributing to recognition memory: the amygdaloid complex versus the rhinal cortex. In: Aggleton JP, ed. The Amygdala: Neurobiological Aspects of Emotion, Memory and Mental Dysfunction. New York, NY: Wiley-Liss, 1992, pp. 453–470.
42. Albert M, Moss MB. The assessment of memory disorders in patients with Alzheimer's disease. In: Squire L and Butters N, eds. Neuropsychology of Memory. New York, NY: Guilford Press, 1984.
43. Rehbein L. Long-term effects of early hippocampectomy in the monkey [dissertation]. Northeastern University, 1985.
44. Blumenthal JA, Madden DJ, Pierce TW, et al. Hypertension affects neurobehavioral functioning. Psychosomat Med 1993;55:44–50.
45. Berg EA. A simple objective test for measuring flexibility in thinking. J Gen Psychol 1948;39:15–22.
46. Grant DA, Berg EA. A behavioral analysis of degree of reinforcement and ease of shifting to new responses in a Weigl-type card sorting problem. J Exper Psychol 1948;34,404–411.
47. Nagahama Y, Fukuyama H, Yamauchi H, et al. Cerebral activation during performance of a card sorting task. Brain 1996;119:1667–1675.
48. Damasio AR, Anderson SW. The Frontal Lobes. In: Heilman K and Valenstein E, eds. Clinical Neuropsychology. Oxford, UK: Oxford University Press, 1993, pp.

49. Fristoe NM, Salthouse TA, Woodward JL. Examination of age-related deficits on the Wisconsin Card Sorting Task. Neuropsychology 1997;11:428–436.
50. Fuster JM. Network memory. Trends Neurosci 1997;20:451–459.
51. Milner B. Some effects of frontal lobectomy in man. In: Warren JM, Akert K, eds. The Frontal Granular Cortex and Behavior. New York, NY: McGraw-Hill, 1964, pp. 313–334.
52. Moore T, Killiany RJ, Rosene DL, Moss MB. A primate model of hypertensive cerebrovascular disease: impairment in conceptual set shifting. Behav Neurosci 2002;116:387–396.
53. Moore T, Killiany RJ, Herndon JG, Rosene DL, Moss MB. A non-human primate test of abstraction and set shifting: an automated adaptation of the Wisconsin Card Sorting Test, the Conceptual Set Shifting Task (CSST). 2003. In press.
54. Jonak EM, Moore TL, Rosene DL, Prusty S, Killiany RJ, Moss MB. Synergistic effects of aging and hypertension learning delayed non-match to sample in a monkey model of hypertensive cerebrovascular disease. Soc Neurosci Abstr 2003.
55. Shapiro AP, Miller RE, King HE, Ginchereau EH, Fitzgibbon K. Behavioral consequences of mild hypertension. Hypertension 1982;4:355–360.
56. Kemper TL, Moss MB, Hollander W, Prusty S. Microinfarction as a result of hypertension in a primate model of cerebrovascular disease. Acta Neuropathol 1999;98:295–303.
57. Fisher CM. The arterial lesion underlying lacunes. Acta Neuropathol 1969;12:1–15.
58. De Reuck J, vander Eecken H. The arterial angioarchitecture in lacunar state. Acta Neurol (Belg) 1976;76:142–149.
59. Garcia JH, Ben-David E, Conger KA, Geer JC, Hollander W. Arterial hypertension injuries brain capillaries. Definition of the lesions. Possible pathogenesis. Stroke 1981;12:410–413.
60. Moore TL, Killiany RJ, Rosene DL, Prusty S, Hollander W, Moss MB. Hypertension induced changes in monoamine receptors in the prefrontal cortex of rhesus monkeys. Neuroscience 2003;120:177–189.

III The Impact of Vascular Dementia on Cognitive, Psychiatric, and Daily Living

9

The Cognitive Profile of Vascular Dementia

Angela L. Jefferson, Adam M. Brickman, Mark S. Aloia, and Robert H. Paul

1. INTRODUCTION

Vascular dementia (VaD) refers to cognitive impairment secondary to compromise of cerebral perfusion. Although some reports document dementia with Lewy bodies (DLB) as the second most prevalent neurodegenerative cause after Alzheimer's disease (AD) *(1)*, others suggest that VaD is the second leading cause of dementia in North America *(2)*. VaD has been estimated to account for 15–25% of cognitive impairment among the elderly *(3)*. Interestingly, the extant literature has not emphasized descriptions of the cognitive profile of VaD in the same way it has for AD.

There has been longstanding theoretical and empirical interest in the link between cognition and cerebrovascular disease (CVD). However, the historic focus of such investigations emphasized cognitive syndromes associated with large-vessel territory ischemic and hemorrhagic strokes. With the advent and evolving sophistication of neuroimaging techniques (e.g., magnetic resonance imaging [MRI]), focus has begun to include small-vessel disease, because such techniques' increasing sensitivity permit both qualitative and quantitative measurement of small-vessel changes. This development has led to studies linking neuroimaging markers of small-vessel disease (e.g., disease of the white matter) and cognitive performance. For instance, Libon and others *(4)* used a 40-point leukoaraiosis scale (put forth by Junque et al. *[5]*) to quantify white matter alterations seen on MRI and link these values to neuropsychological test performances among patients with AD and ischemic vascular dementia (IVD). More recently, others have established a relationship between white matter disease and functional impairment among patients with VaD *(6)*.

Unfortunately, VaD reflects a heterogeneous condition that is defined by disparate diagnostic schemes *(7,8)* (*see* Table 1 and Chapter 2 for more information). This in some way parallels the heterogeneity seen in the frontotemporal dementia (FTD) literature *(9,10)*, because there are multiple FTD subtypes (e.g., progressive nonfluent aphasia and semantic dementia) that are frequently amalgamated when summarizing patients' cognitive profiles. The diagnostic criteria heterogeneity reflects a major limitation of VaD studies because there is poor consensus regarding causal factors, disease course, and, more importantly, for the purposes of this chapter, the neuropsychological profile of VaD.

With this scientific complexity in mind, this chapter aims to summarize the extant literature on the cognitive correlates of VaD. This chapter does not address large-vessel stroke syndromes (e.g., neglect or Balint's syndrome), because these are well described elsewhere *(11)*. Rather, the present synthesis focuses on the effect of diffuse small-vessel disease on cognitive functioning. A better understanding of the cognitive decline associated with small-vessel disease is warranted, because

From: *Current Clinical Neurology*
Vascular Dementia: Cerebrovascular Mechanisms and Clinical Management
Edited by: R. H. Paul, R. Cohen, B. R. Ott, and S. Salloway © Humana Press Inc., Totowa, NJ

Table 1
Various Diagnostic Schemes for Vascular Dementia

Diagnostic scheme (abbreviation)	Reference
1. Hachinski Ischemic Score (HIS)	Hachinski et al., 1975 *(59)*
2. Rosen Ischemic Score (RIS)	Rosen et al., 1980 *(60)*
3. Loeb Ischemic Score (LIS)	Loeb et al., 1980 *(61)*
4. International Classification of Diseases-10 (ICD-10)	World Health Organization, 1992 *(62)*
5. The State of California Alzheimer's Disease Diagnostic and Treatment Centers (ADDTC)	Chui et al., 1992 *(63)*
6. Neuroepidemiology Branch of the National Institute of Neurological Disorders Association Internationale pour la Recherche et l'Enseignement en Neurosciences (NINDS-AIREN)	Roman et al., 1993 *(30)*
7. Diagnostic and Statistical Manual-IV (DSM-IV)	American Psychological Association, 1994 *(29)*
8. Modified NINDS-AIREN–Research Criteria (NINDS-AIREN Modified)	Erkinjuntti et al., 2000 *(46)*

it may be the most common presentation of CVD *(12)*. In fact, Chui and Gontheir *(13)* purport that subcortical ischemic disease is the most common form of VaD.

This chapter first summarizes the literature pertaining to various cognitive domains, including language, visuospatial functions, and psychomotor abilities. Particular importance is placed on the executive functioning and learning and memory summaries, because these two domains reflect those most relevant to the differential diagnosis between VaD and other common dementias. The core clinical picture of VaD is summarized, followed by a discussion of a common thread theory characterizing the cognitive profile associated with VaD. The literature's primary limitations are addressed, and future directions aimed at resolving these limitations are also discussed.

2. COGNITIVE PRESENTATION OF VAD

2.1. *Language*

Language functions are cognitively mediated abilities that facilitate communication, including the most basic processing components, such as comprehension and repetition, as well as more complex skills, such as lexical retrieval necessary for confrontation naming. There is a paucity of research among the VaD literature thoroughly examining impairments in these aspects of language. Among those studies that do exist, few incorporate repetition tasks, so it is unclear if such impairment occurs. In contrast, there is more evidence for impairments in complex auditory comprehension. For example, Vuorinen et al. *(14)* found that patients with VaD performed significantly worse on a comprehension task compared to control subjects. Similarly, a more recent study by Traykov and colleagues *(15)* found that patients with VaD were impaired on an auditory comprehension task (i.e., Token Test) compared to controls.

By far, most studies including some type of language assessment emphasize naming ability deficits. One recent study conducted by Paul et al. *(16)* compared patients with mild and severe VaD on the Boston Naming Test (BNT) and found both groups were impaired relative to normative data. Furthermore, the severely impaired VaD group performed significantly worse than the mildly impaired group, suggesting worsening in naming deficits with disease progression. Similar findings have been reported when comparing patient performances to control samples *(14,17)*. In contrast, Traykov and colleagues *(15)* found no significant differences between a sample of patients with VaD and controls on a short form of the BNT, but this finding may have been secondary to a restriction of range in the abbreviated measure used.

Although the consensus from most studies is that a naming deficit is characteristic among patients with VaD, the exact nature of the deficit is less clear. It has been hypothesized by Vuorinen and colleagues *(14)* that language dissolution in VaD is secondary to a progressive breakdown in semantic processing, which may reflect a more diffuse process. Theoretically, if such naming impairments are secondary to diffuse subcortical white matter alterations as compared to strategically located lacunes, then disruption of subcortical white matter may affect information-processing networks. Furthermore, this disruption would impair naming abilities with progressive impairment over the disease course, which is supported by data from Paul and colleagues *(16)*. Nevertheless, the exact mechanism for such impairments remains unclear.

2.2. *Visuospatial Functions*

Visuospatial abilities encompass numerous cognitive components that provide information at a perceptual level that guide us in acting on our environment. This includes basic perceptual information (e.g., shape discrimination), as well as more complex visual processing components, including object recognition, facial recognition, and spatial localization. Visuoconstruction may also be conceptualized as an integrative, complex, higher level visuospatial ability that necessitates motor and planning abilities. These latter components are the focus of this discussion.

A limited amount of evidence exists regarding visuospatial impairments in VaD. Paul and colleagues *(18)* examined VaD patient performance on the Hooper Visual Organization Test (HVOT) to differentiate whether impairments in confrontation naming contributed to poor performance on this measure. Results revealed that patients with VaD were impaired on the object recognition test in comparison to normative data and HVOT performance was associated with visuoconstruction impairments (i.e., Block Design) rather than poor naming abilities (i.e., BNT). Although these results suggest that patients with VaD are impaired on visuospatial integration independent of naming deficits, it remains possible that executive difficulties contributed to poor performance on this test. Previous research has illustrated the heterogeneity of visuospatial tasks and the executive demands of tasks such as the HVOT *(19)*. It is possible that task performance impairments noted in this sample are secondary to greater executive dysfunction rather than a true deficit in object recognition capabilities. Additional studies are needed to examine this issue in detail.

The more consistent finding within the VaD literature is that of visuoconstruction deficits. Libon et al. *(20)* reported that patients with IVD performed in the impaired range relative to normal controls when asked to draw a clock to both command and copy. A qualitative analysis of these visuoconstruction deficits suggests that executive dysfunction may compromise performance, because impairments on executive control tasks were associated with clock drawing errors. Similarly, Freeman and others *(21)* found that the IVD patients' drawings of a modified Rey-Osterrieth Complex Figure were significantly impaired with notable fragmentation, perseverations, and omissions. Such visuoconstruction impairments worsen across the course of VaD, as Paul and colleagues *(16)* found a severely impaired sample of patients with VaD performed significantly worse than a mildly impaired sample on the same visuoconstruction task (i.e., Rey-Osterrieth Complex Figure).

These complex integrative visuoconstruction deficits may not be indicative of damage to those structures mediating visuospatial components, such as spatial localization or object recognition. Rather, small-vessel disease contributing to white matter disruption may affect the neural networks facilitating cognitive abilities necessary to complete visuoconstructional tasks (e.g., planning and organization). Consistent with this hypothesis, performance on working memory tasks correlates with visuoconstruction measures in patients with VaD, suggesting that monitoring performance and sustaining mental set are related to visuoconstruction abilities *(21)*. However, a primary, underlying visuoperceptual impairment among these patients cannot be ruled out, because comprehensive studies aimed at exploring the presence of such deficits have not yet been conducted.

2.3. *Psychomotor Functions*

Psychomotor functioning is a complex cognitive domain that can be loosely defined as a speeded motor response that may or may not involve some cognitive load (e.g., Trail Making Test Part A or Finger Tapping Test, respectively). Although this is somewhat of an arbitrary dichotomization, neuropsychological assessment of psychomotor functioning often involves tests of manual dexterity (i.e., "motor-based") and/or information processing speed and visuomotor tracking (i.e., "cognitive-based"). Psychomotor dysfunction can be indicative of damage to numerous brain regions, although the most commonly implicated regions include the motor strip of the cortex, subcortical white matter, basal ganglia, and cerebellum. Because the microvasculature supply source for the basal ganglia, cerebellum, and subcortical white matter becomes vulnerable with age, it is plausible that psychomotor functioning may be implicated in conditions involving microvascular disease.

Studies of psychomotor dysfunction on neuropsychological testing among VaD samples are lacking, particularly research examining performance on "motor-based" psychomotor tasks of manual dexterity and speeded motor functions. There is little doubt that VaD may result in significant disruption of subcortical motor systems, as evidenced by reports of vascular Parkinsonism *(22)*. However, few studies have empirically examined the impact of motor skills on psychomotor function in VaD. That which does exist has focused on between-group differences with AD samples with mixed results. For instance, Almkvist et al. *(23)* reported a significant difference between AD and VaD patients on a measure of fine motor speed, whereas Lamar and others *(24)* found no such between-group difference. Comparison data between normal controls and VaD patients on neuropsychological tasks assessing manual dexterity and fine motor speed are rare.

In contrast, the preponderance of literature related to this topic has emphasized those "cognitive-based" psychomotor measures with an information processing speed component (e.g., Trail Making Test, Part A and Digit Symbol). For instance, Almkvist and colleagues *(23)* found that patients with VaD performed significantly worse than patients with AD on a psychomotor speed task (i.e., Digit Symbol). This finding has been extended by more recent work in the authors' laboratory *(16)* and by others *(15)*. Specifically, patients with VaD also perform worse than control subjects on multiple measures of psychomotor speed (i.e., Digit Symbol and Trail Making Test, Part A). Furthermore, such impairments worsen during the course of the disease, as patients with severe VaD perform worse on these tasks than patients who are mildly impaired *(16)*.

Data support subcortical white matter involvement in psychomotor speed. One group of researchers found a specific relationship between subcortical hyperintensities and fine motor speed *(25)*. Furthermore, data from the authors' laboratory also support involvement of the white matter in relation to performance on tasks of psychomotor speed with an information processing component *(26,27)*. However, it is important to note that not all studies have reported significant relationships between psychomotor speed and severity of subcortical hyperintensities (for review *see* ref. *28*). Thus, future studies elucidating the underlying mechanism of psychomotor dysfunction are warranted.

In summary, recent studies by some groups have identified the cognitive-based component of psychomotor speed as a necessary element in the study of cognitive functioning in microvascular disease. However, studies are lacking with respect to the motor-based component of psychomotor speed pertaining to changes in manual dexterity and fine motor speed. Overall, there is sufficient evidence and interest to study this association more carefully with respect to both components. Such efforts may be difficult, because differentiating between the cognitive and motor aspects of psychomotor functioning is complex. Future studies are needed to elucidate the psychomotor dysfunction in patients with VaD, as well as the potential factors that might mediate such impairment.

2.4. *Learning and Memory*

Because dementia primarily involves degradation of declarative memory functioning, this discussion focuses on the ability to learn, encode, and retrieve novel material. Common or accepted diagnostic criteria for VaD *(1,2)* involve deficits in memory that reflect a substantial decline from pre-morbid levels. This essential diagnostic feature highlights the influence of AD conceptualization on VaD criteria development. Although memory deficits may not be the most prominent aspect of VaD, such impairment is generally present, though not always in the earliest stage of the disease. However, the quality of VaD memory impairment is generally one of a retrieval deficit rather than an encoding or storage deficit with relative preservation of recognition memory. Research has suggested that patients with IVD display a pattern of performance in which they have difficulty with free recall trials on declarative memory tasks *(31)*. However, when provided with a forced-choice recognition trial, these patients typically demonstrate relative preservation of encoding abilities as compared to other dementia groups (e.g., patients with AD *[31]*). Additional findings have shown that patients with subcortical IVD can be distinguished from patients with AD based on recognition memory performance *(32)*. Thus, patients with VaD do, in fact, have memory impairment, yet the pattern of such impairment suggests less difficulty formulating and storing new memories with more difficulty retrieving such memories.

This differential pattern of memory impairment may be attributed to the underlying neuropathology of VaD that disrupts subcortical structures. Such disruption affects the long white matter tracts connecting prefrontal and subcortical structures, and functional neuroimaging studies support this finding, as memory failure in vascular patients is secondary to the integrity of the prefrontal cortex *(33)*. By contrast, the entorhinal cortex and hippocampus are less affected by subcortical VaD than by other forms of dementia *(34)*; thus, there is less specific damage in the hippocampal formation where encoding is believed to occur among these patients. It appears that the neuropathology associated with VaD affects retrieval capabilities, but it does not necessarily affect those cortical substrates mediating and facilitating encoding and storage skills. This conceptualization is consistent with recognition memory performance data *(32)*, which are thought to be indicative of hippocampal integrity *(35)*.

In contrast, it is important to note that the profile of memory impairment described does not apply universally to all patients with VaD. Members of the authors' group reported impaired recognition memory performance in patients with VaD when compared to clinical norms *(16)*. However, numerous factors could explain these findings, including the heterogeneous study sample, the possibility that additional neurodegenerative processes influenced the memory performance of a subset of patients or the possibility that some patients suffered hippocampal infarctions. In support of the latter, neuropathologic studies have reported that hippocampal infarctions are common in patients with VaD, especially in the more advanced stages of the illness (*see* Chapter 3). Thus, although recognition memory function may be relatively preserved in VaD, it is possible that the profile of memory dysfunction evolves over the course of disease progression from a retrieval deficit into a more globally affected encoding problem. Additional studies following patients longitudinally are needed to elucidate such progressive changes in memory abilities.

2.5. *Executive Functioning*

Executive functioning broadly refers to the ability to conceptualize all facets of an activity and translate that conceptualization into appropriate and effective behavior *(36)*. The construct of executive functioning is multidimensional, containing several cognitive abilities, such as the capacity to program, concept formation, reasoning, cognitive flexibility, abstraction, and the ability to shift mental set. Several lines of research have suggested that executive functioning deficits are much more characteristic of VaD than primary memory impairment implied by some diagnostic criteria *(29)*. Because deficits in executive functioning are thought to be relatively more impaired *(37)*, are often present prior to the onset of frank dementia *(38)*, and correlate highly with underlying vascular pathology *(38)*, they represent the most salient and distinguishing neuropsychological feature of the disorder *(39)*.

Reported executive functioning deficits in VaD are general and not limited to specific cognitive components contained in the overall construct *(40,41)*. For example, patients with multiple subcortical lacunar infarcts have selective impairment on tests of executive functioning across several areas, including verbal fluency, semantic clustering (i.e., organization), shifting of mental set, and response inhibition *(42)*. A recent review by Looi and Sachdev *(43)* concluded that compared to patients with AD, individuals with VaD are similarly impaired on tests of language, construction, memory registration, conceptual formation, and tracking; relatively less impaired on tests of verbal long-term storage; and more impaired on measures of executive function. The review suggests that executive dysfunction is a "hallmark" of VaD, but it should be noted that this is in the context of relatively spared memory performance and relatively impaired performance across other cognitive domains. Indeed, a recent study *(32)* confirmed that recognition memory and a measure of verbal fluency best distinguish patients with VaD from patients with AD, with the patient groups displaying a double-dissociation pattern.

Consistent with the conclusion of the review noted, results of recent studies suggest that executive deficits are prominent, though not isolated, cognitive symptoms of VaD *(40)*. For example, on a comprehensive neuropsychological battery tapping several cognitive areas, Padovani and colleagues *(40)* demonstrated that individuals with VaD were impaired compared to matched controls in all domains measured. Only after close examination of the data, are somewhat larger effects in areas of executive functioning (i.e., Wisconsin Card Sorting perseverative errors) compared to other domains apparent.

Many studies that have examined executive functioning in VaD have done so in comparison to patients with AD (*see* ref. *43*) and have demonstrated that patients with VaD perform worse on indices of executive functioning in the context of better performance on tests of other cognitive domains (*see* refs. *15,37,39,40,43,44*). Although comparison studies to AD are important in establishing group differences, they have limited clinical utility because individual patient test performance during diagnostic assessment is typically compared to normative data sets and not to other clinical populations. Furthermore, AD comparison studies have contributed to the somewhat misleading notion that executive functioning is the *only* area of deficit in VaD. In fact, in addition to greater executive functioning deficits, some investigations have demonstrated equal or worse impairment across all other domains studied *(16,45)*.

In summary, executive functioning deficits may be the most prominent feature of the neuropsychological profile of VaD but should be considered in the context of deficits in several other domains. Executive functioning deficits may be a manifestation of the underlying neuropathology of VaD, as discussed in greater detail in Section 2.6.

2.6. Summary of Core Picture

The precise cognitive profile of VaD is not well understood, perhaps because of the inclusion of heterogeneous VaD subtypes and the skewed adherence to an Alzheimer's-type cognitive model seen in the various diagnostic schemes. The most commonly used diagnostic criteria (i.e., National Institute of Neurological Disorders and Stroke-Association Internationale pour la Recherche et l'Enseignement en Neurosciences [NINDS-AIREN] *[230]* and *Diagnostic and Statistical Manual of Mental Disorders*, 4th edition [DSM-IV] *[129]*) require memory impairment and deficits in at least one additional cognitive domain.

A review of the literature on neuropsychological functioning in VaD makes clear that several, if not all, cognitive domains are affected when compared to normative data or normal control samples. To illustrate this point, Figure 1 depicts neurocognitive performances of patients with mild and severe VaD. As the figure shows, the samples performed in the impaired range across all domains. Thus, the question arises whether there is a unique profile or cognitive aspect of VaD. Obviously, the nature and location of vascular neuropathology can impact cognitive functioning in the case of

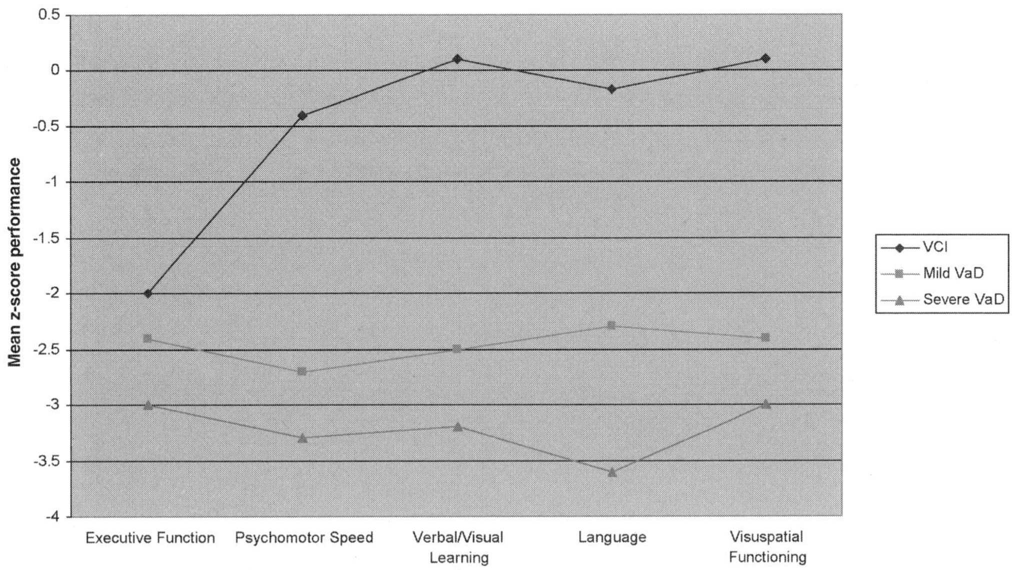

Fig. 1. Neurocognitive performances of patients with mild and severe vascular dementia (VaD) in relation to hypothetical performances of patients with vascular cognitive impairment (VCI). Data pertaining to the VCI group reflects hypothetical data, as presently there is a lack of evidence in the current literature. Data pertaining to the patients with mild and severe VaD taken from Paul et al. *(16)*. See original reference for more information regarding normative data used in patient performance conversions to z-scores as well as cognitive tasks formulating composite measures.

classic stroke syndromes. However, regarding small-vessel disease, it has been argued that impairment in executive functioning and relative preservation of recognition memory are necessary cognitive criteria for VaD *(46)*. The authors agree with this conceptualization and argue that executive deficits may represent a common symptom of most cases of VaD across the spectrum of disease severity. We believe that executive deficits are a hallmark symptom of VaD, which appear regardless of the presence or absence of cognitive dysfunction in other domains. An analogy can be drawn to the conceptualization of AD, as memory-encoding difficulties have been referred to as the *sine qua non* of AD *(47)*. Although memory difficulties are not the only clinical manifestation of AD, it is widely believed that for most, but certainly not all, cases of AD, memory dysfunction is an early and prominent symptom that is expressed throughout the course of the disease. With time, additional cognitive symptoms become apparent (e.g., deficits in language, praxis, construction, and executive function); however, memory disturbance is a cardinal feature of the disease. Similarly, the authors believe that executive deficits represent a common manifestation of VaD.

Evidence supporting this "common thread" theory of executive dysfunction may be found in studies of both preclinical and overtly demented patient samples. In almost all studies conducted among VaD cohorts, results suggest significantly impaired executive dysfunction regardless of disease severity (e.g., refs. *15,37,38,40,44*). More recent evidence *(48)* suggests that disproportionately greater executive dysfunction, as compared to other cognitive domain impairment, exist in predementia patients with CVD (i.e., the so-called syndrome of "mild cognitive impairment of the vascular type"), including work conducted by members of the authors' group *(49,50)*. Figure 1 contains a hypothetical profile of patients with vascular cognitive impairment (VCI), with disproportionately greater executive dysfunction with relative sparing of other cognitive functions. Clearly, this proposed profile should be tested in greater detail in relation to performances of patients with frank VaD.

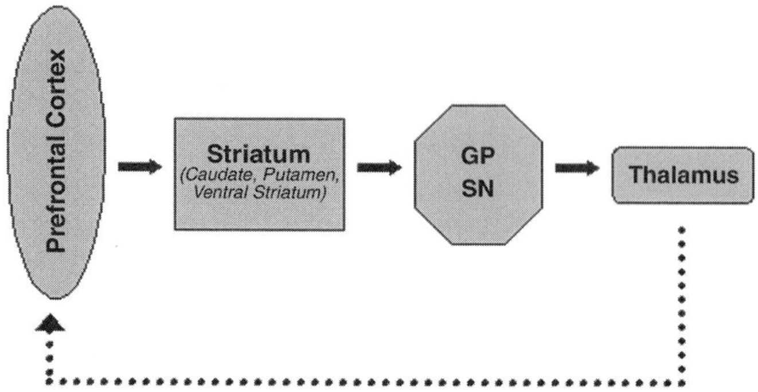

Fig. 2. Directory pathway of the prototypical frontal-subcortical (FSC) circuit (Adapted from Alexander, DeLong, & Strick *[51]*). GP, global pallidus; SN, substantia nigra.

The neuroanatomic underpinnings of executive dysfunction in VaD have traditionally been attributed to disruption of the frontal subcortical circuits initially outlined by Alexander and colleagues *(51–53)*, who described a series of parallel but functionally segregated circuits that link subcortical structures to the frontal lobes (*see* Fig. 2). More recently, these circuits were reviewed by Cummings *(54)*, who used clinical syndromes to illustrate how frontal lobe deficits can be recapitulated via damage to subcortical structures within the circuit.

The model contains six circuits, including two motor (i.e., the motor and oculomotor circuits) and four cognitive circuits (i.e., the dorsolateral prefrontal, anterior cingulate, and two orbitofrontal circuits recently described *[55]*). As Fig. 2 illustrates, the basic structure for each circuit is the same, as it originates in the frontal lobes, projects to striatum, and then projects to the globus pallidus and substantia nigra. From this point, projections are sent to specific thalamic nuclei with links from the thalamus back to the frontal lobe, thus illustrating the reciprocal and closed loop nature of the circuitry. Of note, all six circuits are parallel and contiguous, sharing common structures (illustrated by the prototypic model in Fig. 2), yet they are functionally segregated.

Perhaps the most relevant circuit to VaD is that involving the dorsolateral prefrontal cortex, as the dysexecutive syndrome that emerges from damage to this pathway is the most common clinical presentation in VaD. Indeed, there is some evidence that white matter disease in subcortical structures involved in this pathway (i.e., thalamus and basal ganglia) is associated with executive dysfunction in patients with VaD (e.g., *26*). Thus, it seems plausible that the executive dysfunction noted in both the preclinical phase and the early stage of VaD may be secondary to disruption of this circuitry. Citing functional and structural neuroimaging studies that have implicated significant frontal and striatal abnormalities underlying executive functioning deficits in VaD, Looi and Sachdev *(39)* have proposed that these frontal-subcortical circuitry abnormalities and associated cognitive deficits should be considered the most salient disturbance in VaD.

As we noted throughout this chapter, executive deficits are not the only symptom of VaD, because most studies have reported that patients with VaD exhibit relatively global cognitive deficits. Our model is based on the concept that executive deficits represent a primary feature of VaD that exists either alone or, more commonly, in the presence of cognitive deficits in additional domains of function. An analogy can be drawn with AD, where memory consolidation deficits are a common core aspect of the disease, which eventually exists in the context of other cognitive deficits. Deficits in additional cognitive areas likely represent heterogeneous locations of CVD (e.g., hippocampal lesions) and general atrophy or perhaps represent the early influence of additional comorbid neuropathologies. Because pure VaD is relatively uncommon at autopsy, the possibility is raised that AD or other neurodegenerative syndromes develop during the course of VaD, a process that would eventually influence the clinical manifestation of symptoms.

It is also worth noting the possibility that some impaired neuropsychological skills are deleteriously affected by executive deficits. For instance, visuoconstruction deficits noted in patients with VaD have been qualitatively described to include fragmentation, perseveration, and omissions *(21)*. Additional research has noted free-recall impairments with relative preservation of recognition memory performance among patients with VaD *(31)*. In both instances, these impairments were interpreted as secondary to an underlying executive deficit. This type of secondary impairment is consistent with the theoretical framework proposed by Royall and colleagues *(56,57)*, as they suggest that the cybernetic (i.e., "pilot") aspects of executive control function (ECF) interact with non-ECF cognitive domains (e.g., memory). This interaction may lead to secondary impairments in other cognitive domains that are attributable to underlying executive dysfunction.

However, although the ECF conceptualization may be a plausible explanation, investigators have yet to test whether executive functioning measures can statistically account for the visuoconstruction (e.g., ref. *21*) or free-recall impairments (e.g., ref. *31*) noted above *better* than purer measures of visuospatial functioning or memory, respectively. The extent to which executive dysfunction accounts for secondary deficits in other cognitive domains may vary as a function of disease severity, though this also has not yet been thoroughly examined. Thus, it is difficult to know at this point whether the cognitive profile of VaD can be interpreted via this ECF conceptualization.

In summary, we believe that the most accurate way to characterize the cognitive profile of VaD is that of executive dysfunction as a "common thread" symptom, regardless of disease stage. This theory does not preclude the possibility of primary deficits in other cognitive domains. Rather, theoretically, owing to the heterogeneity of the underlying pathology of VaD, brain regions involved in other domains can be affected, especially as the disease progresses. For example, although white matter disease may contribute to memory retrieval deficits in the early phase of the disease, vascular pathology in hippocampal regions may produce primary memory deficits not accounted by executive dysfunction later in the course. Furthermore, it is highly likely that these executive deficits contribute to cognitive performance in other domains, although this is unlikely to explain the global nature of cognitive impairment in this disease.

3. LIMITATIONS OF RESEARCH AND RECOMMENDED FUTURE DIRECTIONS

The preceding portion of this chapter focused on reviewing the cognitive profile of VaD. However, there are numerous limitations within the extant literature that necessitate identification and discussion. The remaining portion of this chapter identifies these limitations, focusing specifically on those that affect our understanding of the cognitive profile of VaD. Future directions for research are discussed within this context.

3.1. *Current Diagnostic Criteria*

Perhaps the primary limitation within the VaD literature is that numerous diagnostic schemes exist for VaD (*see* Table 1 and Chapter 4). These schemes are heterogeneous, because they emphasize different cognitive profiles and/or symptoms of CVD. Such heterogeneity makes it difficult to synthesize findings across study samples that are based on disparate diagnostic schemes. Furthermore, among the more popular schemes (e.g., DSM-IV *[129]* and NINDS-AIREN *[230]*) there is an emphasis on memory impairment. This necessary feature raises the possibility that some sample participants have neuropathology of mixed dementia (i.e., VaD and AD) rather than pure VaD. Another related issue is the potential for researchers to include cognitive profiles into the diagnostic process and subsequently compare patients with VaD to other patient samples or healthy controls. The tautological thinking in this approach is obvious and represents a major dilemma because including this information skews the resulting cognitive outcomes, and excluding this information raises questions regarding whether the diagnostic process was accurate.

Future research should be aimed at refining the diagnostic criteria and formulating a more unified system for research. Erkinjuntti et al. *(46)* recently proposed modified criteria to the NINDS-AIREN criteria for VaD by emphasizing a unique profile between neuropsychological functioning and neuroimaging. This modification emphasizes homogeneous subtypes of VaD and reflects a first step to resolving this problem. Future studies should examine the progression of VaD across its various stages (i.e., prodromal stage, vascular cognitive impairment no dementia, VaD, and, ultimately, death) to identify the most relevant variables for diagnostic purposes.

3.2. *Traditional VaD and AD Comparisons*

Another major concern within the literature is that the majority of research examining the cognitive profile of VaD is based on comparisons between dementia groups. That is, patients with VaD are compared to patients with AD across neuropsychological measures. This emphasizes differential performance between dementia populations over specific detection of VaD, and it does not necessarily yield a meaningful cognitive profile. In fact, the emphasis on differential performance has led to the current acceptance that executive dysfunction and preservation of recognition memory are the only areas of affliction in VaD. In reality, when compared to normal control participants, patients with VaD show impairment in almost all domains assessed yielding a much more global impairment picture (*see* ref. *16*). As Fig. 1 illustrates, patients with VaD are often significantly impaired on all cognitive domains assessed. This pattern of global impairment is maintained for both mildly and severely impaired patient subgroups. Thus, although comparison studies are important, the findings make the application of clinical assessment findings less straightforward than implied.

Additionally, even though some studies report statistically significant differences between groups, such differences are misleading, because they may not be of sufficient magnitude to be clinically relevant. For example, Lafosse and colleagues *(58)* report a statistically significant difference (i.e., $p = 0.038$) between AD and IVD patients on a free-recall trial of a serial list learning task. The *actual* difference between the two groups is less than one and a half words (i.e., AD = 1.7, IVD = 3.1 words). The clinical application of such research is limited, because it does not help a clinician make a differential diagnosis between the two dementia types. Future studies should follow patients longitudinally and use normal control comparison groups, as well as examine the clinical significance of statistical findings. Understanding how patients with VaD differ from normal controls throughout the disease course is important, because this approach parallels the clinical neuropsychological evaluation. Specifically, patients seen in a clinical setting are assessed across numerous measures, and their performances are compared to an age- and education-matched cohort to yield a profile that is interpreted based on what is known about different neurodegenerative syndromes.

Research efforts should further focus on the qualitative differences among VaD patient performances as compared to the traditional emphasis on quantitative differences. This approach is particularly important, because two patients with different types of dementia can fail the same cognitive task for different reasons. For instance, one patient may be unable to perform an object recognition task because of an anomia, whereas a second patient may have difficulty because of the executive demands of the task. Differentiating mechanisms behind impaired performances may yield important information for diagnostic purposes.

REFERENCES

1. McKeith IG, Galasko D, Kosaka E, Perry EK, Dickson DW, Hansen LA, Salmon DP et al. for the Consortium on Dementia with Lewy Bodies. Consensus guidelines for the clinical and pathologic diagnosis of dementia with Lewy Bodies (DLB): Report of the consortium on DLB international workshop. Neurol 1996;47:1113–1124.
2. Prencipe M, Ferretti, Casini AR, Santini M, Giubilei F, Culasso F. Stroke, disability, and dementia: Results of a population survey. Stroke 1997;28:531–536.
3. Roman GC. The epidemiology of vascular dementia. In: Hartmann A, Kuschinsky W, Hoyer S, eds. Cerebral ischemia and dementia. Berlin, Germany: Springer-Verlag, 1991; pp. 9–15.

4. Libon DJ, Bogdanoff B, Leopold N, Hurka R, Bonavita J, Skalina S, Swenson R, Gitlin HL, Ball SK. Neuropsychological profiles associated with subcortical white matter alterations and Parkinson's disease: Implications for the diagnosis of dementia. Arch Clin Neuropsychol 2001;16:19–32.
5. Junque C, Pujol J, Vendrell P, Bruna O, Jodar M, Ribas JC, Vinas J, Capevila A, Marti-Vilalta J L. Leuokaraiosis on magnetic resonance imaging and speed of mental processing. Arch Neurol 1990;47:151–156.
6. Boyle PA, Paul RH, Moser D, Zawacki T, Gordon N, Cohen RA. Cognitive and neurologic predictors of functional impairment in vascular dementia. Amer J Geriatr Psychiat 2003;11:103–106.
7. Bowler JV Hachinski V. Criteria for Vascular dementia: Replacing dogma with data. Neurol 2000;57:170–171.
8. Cosentino SA, Jefferson AL, Carey ME, Price CC, Davis KL, Swenson R, Libon DJ. An analysis of different diagnostic criteria for vascular dementia. The Clin Neuropsychol 2004; in press.
9. Glosser G, Gallo JL, Clark CM, Grossman M. Memory encoding and retrieval in frontotemporal dementia and Alzheimer's disease. Neuropsychol 2002;16:190–196.
10. Neary D, Snowden JS, Gustafson L, Passant U, Stuss D, Black S, Freedman M, Kertesz A, Robert PH, Albert M, Boone K, Miller BL, Cummings J, Benson DF. Frontotemporal lobar degeneration: A consensus on clinical diagnostic criteria. Neurol 1998;51:1546–1554.
11. Bogousslavsky J, Caplan LR. Stroke Syndromes, 2nd Ed. New York, NY:Cambridge University Press, 2001.
12. Jellinger KA. Vascular-ischemic dementia: an update. J Neural Transm Suppl 2002;62:1–23.
13. Chui H, Gontheir R. Natural history of vascular dementia. Alz Dis Assoc Disord 1999;13:S124–S130.
14. Vuorinen E, Laine M, Rinne J. Common pattern of language impairment in vascular dementia and in Alzheimer disease. Alz Dis Assoc Disord 2000;14:81–86.
15. Traykov L, Baudic S, Thibaudet MC, Rigaud A-S, Smagghe A, Boller F. Neuropsychological deficit in early subcortical vascular dementia: Comparison to Alzheimer's disease. Dementia Geriat Cog Disord 2002;14:26–32.
16. Paul RH, Moser D, Cohen R, Browndyke J, Zawacki T, Gordon N. Dementia severity and pattern of cognitive performance in vascular dementia. Applied Neuropsychol 2001;8:211–217.
17. Lukatela K, Cohen RA, Kessler H, Jenkins MA, Moser DJ, Stone WF, Gordon N, Kaplan RF. Dementia Rating Scale performance: A comparison of Vascular and Alzheimer's dementia. J Clin Exper Neuropsychol 2000;22:445–454.
18. Paul RH, Cohen RA, Moser D, Ott B, Zawacki T, Gordon N. Performance on the Hooper Visual Organizational Test in patients diagnosed with subcortical vascular dementia: Relation to naming performance. Neuropsychiatry, Neuropsychology, Behav Neurol 2001;14:93–97.
19. Libon DJ, Glosser G, Malamut BL, Kaplan E, Goldberg E, Swenson R, Sands LP. Age, executive functions, and visuospatial functioning in healthy older adults. Neuropsychol 1994;8:38–43.
20. Libon DJ, Malamut BL, Swenson R, Sands LP, Cloud BS. Further analyses of clock drawings among demented and nondemented older subjects. Arch Clin Neuropsychol 1996;11:193–205.
21. Freeman RQ, Giovannetti T, Lamar M, Cloud BS, Stern RA, Kaplan E, Libon DJ. Visuoconstruction problems in dementia: Contribution of executive systems functions. Neuropsychol 2000;14:415–426.
22. Yamanouchi H, Nagura H. Neurological signs and frontal white matter lesions in vascular parkinsonism. A clinicopathologic study. Stroke 1997;28:965–969.
23. Almkvist O, Backman L, Basun H, Wahlund LO. Patterns of neuropsychological performance in Alzheimer's disease and vascular dementia. Cortex 1993;29:661–673.
24. Lamar M, Carew TG, Resh R, Goldberg E, Podell K, Cloud BS, Kennedy C, Kaplan E, Libon DJ. Perseverative behavior in Alzheimer's disease and subcortical ischemic vascular dementia. Neuropsychol 1997;11:523–534.
25. Ylikoski R, Ylikoski A, Erkinjuntti T, Sulkava R, Raininko R, Tilvis R. White matter changes in healthy elderly persons correlate with attention and speed of mental processing. Arch Neurol 1993;50:818–824.
26. Moser DJ, Cohen RA, Paul RH, Paulsen JS, Ott BR, Gordon NM, Bell S, Stone WM. Executive function and magnetic resonance imaging subcortical hyperintensities in vascular dementia. Neuropsychiatry, Neuropsychol, Behav Neurol 2001;14:89–92.
27. Cohen RA, Paul RH, Ott BR, Moser DJ, Zawacki TM, Stone W, Gordon N. The relationship of subcortical MRI hyperintensities and brain volume to cognitive function in vascular dementia. J Internat Neuropsychol Soc 2002;8:743–752.
28. Campbell JJ, Coffey CE. Neuropsychiatric significance of subcortical hyperintensity. J Neuropsychiatry Clin Neurosci 2001;13:261–288.
29. American Psychiatric Association. Diagnostic & Statistical Manual-IV (DSM-IV). Washington, DC: American Psychiatric Association, 1994.
30. Roman GC, Tatemichi TK, Erkinjuntti T, Cummings JL, Masdeu JC, Garcia JH, Amaducci L, Orgogozo J-M, Brun A, Hofman A, Moody DM, O'Brien MD, et al. Vascular dementia: Diagnostic criteria for research studies. Report of the NINDS-AIREN International Workshop. Neurology 1993;43:250–260.
31. Libon DJ, Mattson RE, Glosser G, Kaplan E, Malamut BL, Sands LP, Swenson R, Cloud BS. A nine-word dementia version of the California Verbal Learning Test. Clin Neuropsychol 1996;10:237–244.
32. Tierney MC, Black SE, Szalai JP, Snow G, Fisher RH, Nadon G, Chui HC. Recognition memory and verbal fluency differentiate probable Alzheimer's disease from subcortical ischemic vascular dementia. Arch Neurol 2001;58:1654–1659.

33. Reed BR, Eberling JL, Mungas D, Weiner MW, Jagust WJ.Memory failure has different mechanisms in subcortical stroke and Alzheimer's disease. Ann Neurol 2000;48:275–284.
34. Du AT, Schuff N, Laakso MP, Zhu XP, Jagust WJ, Yaffe K, Kramer JH, Miller BL, Reed BR, Norman D, Chui HC, Weiner MW. Effects of subcortical ischemic vascular dementia and AD on entorhinal cortex and hippocampus. Neurol 2002;58:1635–1641.
35. Milner B, Corkin S, Teurber H-L. Further analysis of the hippocampal amnesic syndrome: 14-year follow-up study of H.M. Neuropsychologia 1968;6:215–234.
36. Lezak MD. Neuropsychological Assessment, 3rd Ed. New York, NY: Oxford University Press, 1995.
37. Kertesz A, Clydesdale S. Neuropsychological deficits in vascular dementia vs Alzheimer's disease. Frontal lobe deficits prominent in vascular dementia. Arch Neurol 1994;51:1226–1231.
38. Kramer JH, Reed BR, Mungas D, Weiner MW, Chui HC. Executive dysfunction in subcortical ischaemic vascular disease. J Neurol, Neurosurg, Psychiat 2001;72:217–220.
39. Looi JCL, Sachdev PS. Vascular dementia as a frontal subcortical system dysfunction. Psychological Medicine, 2000; 30:997–1003.
40. Padovani A, DiPiero V, Bragoni M, Iacoboni M, Gualdi GF, Lenzi GL. Patterns of neuropsychological impairment in mild dementia: A comparison between Alzheimer's disease and multi-infarct dementia. Acta Neurol Scand 1995;92: 433–442.
41. Yuspeh RL, Vanderploeg RD, Crowell TA, Mullan M. Differences in executive functioning between Alzheimer's disease and subcortical ischemic vascular dementia. J Clin Experimen Neuropsych 2002;24:745–754.
42. Wolfe N, Linn R, Babikian VL, Knoefel JE, Albert ML. Frontal systems impairment following multiple lacunar infarcts. Arch Neurol 1990;47:129–132.
43. Looi JCL, Sachdev PS. Differentiation of vascular dementia from AD on neuropsychological tests. Neurol 1999;53: 670–678.
44. Tei H, Miyazaki A, Iwata M, Osawa M, Nagata Y, Maruyama S. Early stage Alzheimer's disease and multiple subcortical infarction with mild cognitive impairment: Neuropsychological comparison using an easily applicable test battery. Dementia Geriat Cogn Disord 1997;8:355–358.
45. Cannata AP, Alberoni M, Franceschi M, Mariani C. Frontal impairment in subcortical ischemic Vascular dementia in comparison to Alzheimer's disease. Dementia Geriat Cogn Disord 2001;13:101–111.
46. Erkinjuntti T, Inzitari D, Pantoni L, Wallin A, Scheltens P, Rockwood K, Roman GC, Chui H, Desmond DW. Research criteria for subcortical vascular dementia in clinical trials. J Neurotransm 2000;59:23–30.
47. Kertesz A, Mohs RC. Cognition. In Gauthier S, ed. Clinical Diagnosis and Management of Alzheimer's Disease. London, UK: Martin Dunitz, 1999.
48. Frisoni GB, Galluzzi S, Bresciani L, Zanetti O, Geroldi C. Mild cognitive impairment with subcortical features: Clinical characteristics and outcome. J Neurol 2002;249:1423–1432.
49. Garrett KD, Browndyke JN, Whelihan W, Paul RH, DiCarlo M, Moser DJ. The neuropsychological profile of vascular cognitive impairment - no dementia: Comparisons to patients at risk for cerebrovascular disease and vascular dementia. Arch Clin Neuropsych 2004; in press.
50. Paul RP, Cohen RA, Gunstad J, Browndyke J, Jefferson AL, Brickman A. Does brain size matter? Neuroimaging markers of cognitive decline in patients with vascular cognitive impairment - no dementia. Poster presentation. Gothenburg, Sweden: The 1st Congress of the International Society for Vascular Behavioral & Cognitive Disorders (VAS-COG), August 2003.
51. Alexander GE, DeLong MR, Strick PL. Parallel organization of functionally segregated circuits linking basal ganglia and cortex. Ann Rev Neurosci 1986;9:357–381.
52. Alexander GE, Crutcher MD. Functional architecture of basal ganglia circuits: neural substrates of parallel processing. Trends Neurosci 1990;13:266–271.
53. Alexander GE, Crutcher MD, DeLong MR. Basal ganglia thalamocortical circuits: parallel substrates for motor, oculomotor, 'prefrontal' and 'limbic' functions Prog Brain Res 1990;85:119–146.
54. Cummings J. Frontal-subcortical circuits and human behavior. Arch Neurol 1993;50:873–880.
55. Middleton FA, Strick PL. A revised neuroanatomy of frontal-subcortical circuits. In: Lichter DG, Cummings JL, eds., Frontal-subcortical circuits in psychiatric and neurological disorders. New York, NY: The Guilford Press, 2001; pp. 44–58.
56. Royall DR, Lauterbach EC, Cummings JL, Reeve A, Rummans TA, Kaufer DI, Lafrance Jr. WC, Coffey CE. Executive control function: A review of its promise and challenges for clinical research. J Neuropsych Clin Neurosci 2002; 14:377–405.
57. Roman GC, Royall DR. Executive control function: A rational basis for the diagnosis of vascular dementia. Alz Dis Assoc Disord 1999;13:S69–S80.
58. Lafosse JM, Reed BR, Mungas D, Sterling SB, Wahbeh H, Jagust WJ. Fluency and memory differences between Ischemic Vascular Dementia and Alzheimer's disease. Neuropsychol 1997;11:514–522.
59. Hachinski V, Illif LK, Zilkha E, Du Boulay G, McAllister V, Marshall J, Ross Russell RW, Symon L. Cerebral blood flow in dementia. Arch Neurol 1975;32:632–637.

60. Rosen WG, Terry R, Fuld PA, Katzman R, Peck A. Pathological verification of ischemic score in the differentiation of dementias. Ann Neurol 1980;7:486–488.
61. Loeb C. Clinical diagnosis of multi-infarct dementia. In: Amaducci L, ed., Aging of the Brain & Dementia, Vol. 13. New York, NY: Raven Press, 1980; pp. 251–260.
62. World Health Organization. International Statistical Classification of Diseases and Related Health Problems, 10th Ed. Los Angeles, CA: Practice Management Information Corporation, 1992.
63. Chui HC, Victoroff JI, Margolin D, Jagust W, Shankle R, Katzman R. Criteria for the diagnosis of ischemic vascular dementia proposed by the State of California Alzheimer's Disease Diagnostic and Treatment Centers. Neurol 1992;42: 473–480.

10

Progression of Cognitive Impairments Associated With Cerebrovascular Disease

Sally Stephens, Raj Kalaria, Rose Anne Kenny, and Clive Ballard

1. INTRODUCTION

Vascular dementia (VaD) is the second most frequent form of dementia, accounting for 10 to 20% of cases, and vascular factors contribute to the development of dementia in many patients with Alzheimer's disease (AD). For example, a recent review of consortium data concluded that all patients with AD experienced degeneration of the microvasculature and more than 30% of patients with AD exhibited additional cerebrovascular pathology. Therefore, it is evident that cerebrovascular disease (CVD) is a major substrate of cognitive impairment in the majority of people with dementia.

2. PATHOGENESIS OF DEMENTIA RELATED TO CEREBROVASCULAR DISEASE

VaD can be defined as a clinical syndrome of acquired clinical impairment resulting from brain injury owing to cerebrovascular disorder *(1)*; therefore, it is a heterogeneous disorder or group of disorders. The profile of cognitive deficits in patients with VaD have often been described as patchy, and the pathophysiology incorporates interactions between many vascular processes, different types of CVD, vascular risk factors (hypertension and apolipoprotein E [apo E]), and changes in the brain (white matter lesions [WMLs] and atrophy). This lack of clarity has made it difficult to clarify the relationship between CVD and specific aspects of cognition. The following is a description of the types of lesions that may result in the symptoms of VaD based on the National Institute of Neurological Disorders and Stroke-Association Internationale pour la Recherche et l'Enseignement en Neurosciences (NINDS-AIREN) criteria *(2)*. They can be grouped into multiinfarct dementia (MID), strategic single infarct dementia, white matter disease, hypoperfusion, and hemorrhagic dementia.

1. MID involves multiple large complete infarcts usually from large-vessel occlusions involving cortical and subcortical areas resulting in a clinical syndrome of dementia.
2. Strategic single infarct dementia results from small localized ischemic damage occurring in cortical and subcortical areas of the brain that results in specific clinical syndromes. For example, infarcts to the angular gyrus result in the onset of fluent aphasia, alexia with agraphia, memory disturbance, spatial disorientation, and constructional disturbances.
3. Small-vessel disease or microvascular disease results from lesions that occur in either cortical or subcortical areas of the brain and often involve white matter. The lesions result in an occlusion of a single arteriolar or arterial lumen that leads to complete lacunar infarct. Critical stenosis of multiple small vessels can also occur, resulting in hypoperfusion and complete infarctss.
4. White matter disease or leukoaraiosis is frequently noted on structural brain imaging. The frequency of white matter disease rises steadily with age. It is associated with hypertension, cigarette smoking, low plasma vitamin E, lacunar infarcts, low education, and hypoxic-ischemic disorders.

From: *Current Clinical Neurology*
Vascular Dementia: Cerebrovascular Mechanisms and Clinical Management
Edited by: R. H. Paul, R. Cohen, B. R. Ott, and S. Salloway © Humana Press Inc., Totowa, NJ

Table 1
Proportions of Patients With VaD With Specific Types of Cerebrovascular Pathology

Pathological feature	Vascular dementia (%)
Cerebral amyloid angiopathy	30
Microvascular degeneration [a]	10
All infarctions	100
Microinfarcts	60
Intracerebral hemorrhages	10
White matter lesions [b]	70
Cardiovascular disease (aortic)	60

[a] Focal or diffuse small-vessel disease involving blood vessels with smooth muscle may be present in most cases of VaD.

[b] Diffuse periventricular white matter lesions may be present in almost all cases of AD.

Data from refs. *4, 14–16*.

5. Hypoperfusion results from a global brain ischemia secondary to cardiac arrest or profound hypertension or from restricted ischemia that has occurred in the border zones between two main arterial territories. Hemorrhagic dementia occurs because of chronic subdural hematoma, sequelae of subarachnoid hemorrhage, and a cerebral hematoma and is often associated with amyloid angiopathy.

The pathogenesis of VaD is complex and incompletely understood, and, in addition to the vascular lesions described in the NINCDS AIRENS criteria, it is likely that concurrent atrophy may also be associated with dementia, especially in older stroke patients *(3)*. How the pattern of progression relates to the underlying neuropathological substrates, both cerebrovascular and neurodegenerative, is a fundamental question. What is known about the various potential substrates of progressive decline is reviewed below.

2.1. White Matter Lesions

Ischemic WMLs associated with lipohyalinosis and narrowing of the lumen of the small perforating arteries, as well as arterioles that nourish the deep white matter, have been amply described in AD *(4–10)*. Neuropathological correlative studies comparing magnetic resonance imaging findings with postmortem neuropathological examination have determined that the hyperintense deep WMLs, identified on magnetic resonance imaging (MRI) in more than 80% of patients with VaD *(11)*, consist mainly of demyelination, reactive gliosis, and arteriosclerosis *(12)*. It is apparent that these lesions are only progressive in a modest proportion of patients *(13)*, but it is unclear what factors and/or lesion characteristics determine their propensity to progress. The overall frequency of these lesions in patients with VaD is summarized in Table 1.

Neuroimaging and neuropathological studies of cross-sectional design, comparing patients with and without dementia in the context of CVD, suggest that diffuse white matter changes and microvascular disease are the main predictors of dementia *(17,18)*, even in the absence of significant plaque or tangle pathology *(18)*. In community populations of older people, an association between executive dysfunction and the severity of white matter hyperintensities (WMH) has been reported *(19,20)*. Within the context of CVD, the overall severity of MRI WMH is related to the speed of cognitive processing in patients with subcortical ischemic VaD *(21)* and with executive performance, but not global cognition, in people with more heterogenous VaD *(22)*. A study focusing on stroke patients, including those with and without dementia, identified an association between the severity of periventricular WMH and executive dysfunction, although no association was seen between executive performance and the severity of WMH in the watershed areas *(23)*. In a cohort of stroke patients without dementia, the severity of WMH in key fronto-striatal circuits was also associated with a similar pattern of cognitive deficits, including impairments of attention, cognitive processing speed, and working memory *(24)*. Hence, white matter ischemic lesions are a substrate of dementia and specific cognitive impairments in patients with CVD.

2.2. *Large and Multiple Infarcts and Microinfarcts*

In relation to CVD, several neuropathological studies have clearly indicated that 50 mL of infarcted brain tissue is a sufficient substrate for dementia *(25)*, although infarcts in strategically important sites can also lead to dementia syndromes *(2,26,27)*. In addition, infarcts in key areas may lead to specific cognitive deficits. For example, subcortical lacunae are associated with executive dysfunction *(23)*. However, it is also apparent that the size and distribution of cortical or subcortical infarcts are not the main substrates of dementia in many people with CVD *(17)*. The role of large and multiple areas of infarction as a cause of cognitive dysfunction is, therefore, unclear within the context of CVD, although some of the apparent disparities may be explained by age differences in the various studies. For example, many of the studies indicating that infarction is not a key substrate of dementia in the context of CVD *(17)* or emphasizing the potential importance of atrophy *(3,28)*, have studied patient cohorts with an older mean age. Therefore, the authors would hypothesize that infarction is the key association of dementia in younger patients with CVD but may be less important in older patients.

2.3. *Cerebral Amyloid Angiopathy and Related Hemorrhages*

Cerebral amyloid angiopathy (CAA) involves the leptomeninges, small pial vessels, and intracortical arterioles, as well as brain capillaries *(29)*. The lesions are characterized by sporadic focal deposits in surface vessels to complete infiltration of numerous meningeal and intracortical vessels throughout all cortical lobes *(30)*. The characteristic cerebral distribution of CAA also implicates that the process may be largely limited to brain vessels associated with a tight or continuous endothelium and when exposed to molecular triggers that may include soluble Aβ itself that may even originate in perivascular plaques. Weller et al. *(31)* have suggested that the characteristic vascular deposition of amyloid is related to the lack of clearance of Aβ via the interstitial drainage pathways.

CAA compromise vascular function promotes chronic hypoperfusion *(32)* and leads to lobar or intracerebral hemorrhages *(16,33)*. Although numerous authors have speculated about the relative importance of CAA in patients with AD, the potential importance of these lesions as a substrate of cognitive decline in patients with cognitive deficits related to CVD is unclear and likely to be most important in patients with a presentation of mixed AD/VaD.

2.4. *Microvascular Pathophysiology and Degeneration*

Profound changes in the cerebral microvessels are evident in a minority of patients with VaD. Several elegant studies using morphological and biochemical methods have demonstrated abnormalities in various cellular elements of cerebral microvessels or capillaries, including degeneration of vascular smooth muscle cells (SMCs) *(34,35)*, focal constrictions and SMC irregularities *(36)*, degeneration and focal necrotic changes of the endothelium *(30,37)*, vascular basement membrane alterations accompanied by accumulation of collagen *(38,39)*, loss of perivascular nerve plexus *(40)*, decreased mitochondrial content and increased pinocytotic vesicles *(41)*, and loss of tight junctions *(42)*. Both the length and the number of degenerated microvessel profiles were significantly correlated with neocortical Aβ deposits, but there was no apparent relationship between the degenerated microvessels and neurofibrillary tangles or existing pyramidal neurones. The relationship with the severity of Aβ deposition and the higher frequency of microvasculature degeneration in VaD indicates that this is related to concurrent AD. The potential effect on cognitive function has not been determined.

2.5. Section Summary

Because of the multiple possible substrates of cognitive impairment, the authors hypothesize that the progression of cognitive impairment would relate to the differential progression of these lesions. There may be important age-related differences in the relative importance of different types of vascular lesion and related neurodegenerative change. The likely contribution of AD pathology is also complex and probably includes an effect on key vascular processes, such as CAA and microvascular pathology, as well as atrophy intrinsic to the neurodegenerative process. Given the complexities, longitudinal clinicopathological studies are needed to clarify these issues.

3. PROFILE OF COGNITIVE IMPAIRMENT IN PATIENTS WITH CEREBROVASCULAR DISEASE

The profile of cognitive impairments in people with dementia related to CVD may give important information regarding aspects of cognition that are most likely to be impaired in these individuals and may be the cognitive domains at greatest risk of further deterioration. The cognitive deficits that are characteristic of AD include progressive loss of short-term and long-term memory, language, and orientation. Constructional praxis, visual perception, attention, and executive function are relatively unimpaired until the latter stages of AD *(43,44)*. In comparison, patients with VaD are likely to have a relative preservation of long-term memory, especially in the early stages of the dementia *(45)* and greater deficits in frontal executive functioning (planning, organization, abstraction, category fluency initiation, reasoning, mental flexibility, sequencing, fine motor performance, and the allocation of attentional resources) than patients with AD *(46–50)*.

4. PROGRESSION OF COGNITIVE DEFICITS IN ESTABLISHED DEMENTIA ASSOCIATED WITH CEREBROVASCULAR DISEASE

It is often suggested that the rate of cognitive and behavioral progression of VaD differs according to etiology, type of brain lesion, lesion site, and clinical syndrome. For example, dementia related to large or strategic areas of cortical infarction is usually characterized by an abrupt onset of cognitive impairment and behavioral change, whereas in MID, there is a more stepwise progression with cognitive impairments and aphasia. Subcortical VaD is seldom stepwise in progression and has an insidious onset in more than half the patients, with a course that is usually slowly progressive. However, many people experience an overlap of different types of cerebrovascular pathology.

Overall, the rate of decline is similar in both VaD and AD. The clinical view of a stepwise progression of VaD has not been demonstrated or validated in studies. For example, in a study by Ballard et al. *(51)* 193 patients—101 with AD, 64 with dementia with Lewy bodies (DLB), and 38 with VaD— completed annual Mini-Mental State Examination (MMSE) schedules, with 154 of these also completing the Cambridge Examination for Mental Disorders in the Elderly (CAMCOG). During 1 yr, the magnitude of cognitive decline (MMSE, 4–5 points and CAMCOG, 12–14 points) was similar in each of the dementias. In a study reported by Bowler et al. *(45)*, the evolution of AD and VaD and mixed dementia (AD with infarcts) were compared using the extended scale for dementia (ESD). A total of 120 patients with definite or probable AD, 12 patients with definite or probable VaD, and 36 patients with definite or probable mixed dementia were grouped as having an early, moderate, or advanced stage of disease according to the ESD. AD, VaD, and mixed dementia evolved similarly as assessed using cognitive domains obtained by subdivision of the ESD in a patient population derived from a memory clinic and by analyzing VaD as a single entity. Although suggesting similar overall rates of progression, more frequent assessments would be necessary to determine whether the progression was insidious or stepwise.

In contrast, in a longitudinal epidemiologic study of black Americans with AD, VaD, or stroke without dementia, Nyenhius et al. *(52)*, reported that the people with AD experienced the expected progression of cognitive impairment but it wasn't until the fourth year of follow-up that the VaD group showed significant cognitive deterioration.

In clinical trials, patients with VaD receiving placebo treatment deteriorate less rapidly than would be expected in patients with AD, with many not experiencing significant decline during 6–12 mo. For example, Erkinjuntti et al. *(53)* evaluated the efficacy of galatamine in probable VaD and AD with CVD. Placebo-treated patients with AD and CVD experienced the expected cognitive decline, but the subgroup with probable VaD showed no cognitive deterioration. They suggested that the cognitive stability of the probable VaD patients would be as expected, because patients must have stable CVD to meet inclusion criteria for the study. Patients with unstable cardiovascular or cerebrovascular disease who may have more rapid progression were excluded. In a much earlier study *(54)*, 70 patients with MID were randomized into an aspirin-treated group and an untreated control group for an exploratory investigation to determine any effects of 325 mg aspirin daily on cognitive performance. The control group did not receive placebo, but evaluations were conducted blindly. The index group ($n = 37$, mean age 67.1 yr) received 325 mg of aspirin by mouth once daily, while the control group ($n = 33$, mean age 67.6 yr) was followed and treated similarly, except that they received no aspirin. Patients were evaluated at 1-yr intervals. Significant improvements were demonstrated for cognitive performance scores ($p < 0.0001$) among aspirin-treated patients, compared to untreated controls at each of three annual follow-up evaluations, with many of the aspirin-treated patients experiencing no significant cognitive decline. Aspirin is allowed as a concurrent medication in clinical trials of other agents, such as cholinesterase inhibitors, and is another potential reason for the apparently good outcome of placebo-treated patients.

The evidence from different sources is highly discrepant. Most of the studies indicating a similar rate of decline in patients with VaD and AD have been based on psychiatric cohorts, and it is possible that differences in outcome regarding progression may be a consequence of sample bias because such patients may be more likely to have a mixture of cerebrovascular and neurodegenerative pathologies and less likely to have clear-cut strokes. However, it is equally plausible that the clinical trials have included a biased group of good prognosis patients. Hence, there are numerous important issues to clarify regarding the progression of cognitive deficits in patients with dementia and CVD.

There is little work focusing on the progression of impairments of specific aspects of cognitive function in patients with dementia with CVD. Bowler et al. *(45)* reported relative preservation of memory in the early stages of the dementia; however, with increasing severity of dementia, memory impairment in VaD accelerated and became similar in magnitude to that seen in patients with AD. The relative pattern of progression of executive and attentional impairments in AD and VaD requires clarification.

In Bowler et al.'s *(45)* study, the differences between AD and mixed AD/VaD were greater than those between mixed dementia and VaD, suggesting an important role for the ischemic component of mixed dementia. In a separate study, Nyenhius et al. *(52)* reported that the profile of cognitive deficits in patients with progressive cognitive decline in the context of CVD was suggestive of mixed dementia (AD and VaD) rather that AD or VaD alone, with relatively greater memory impairment rather than spatial or language deficits. This acceleration of memory deficits is consistent with the Bowler study. Therefore, concurrent neurodegeneration may play an important role in the progression of cognitive deficits in patients with CVD.

5. VASCULAR COGNITIVE IMPAIRMENT

The early detection of preclinical dementia has become an important focus of clinical research to enable the early identification, investigation, and, potentially, treatment of at-risk individuals. Hachinski and Bowler *(55)* first described the concept of vascular cognitive impairment (VCI) as an umbrella term encompassing all levels of cognitive decline related to CVD, from the earliest steps to severe dementia. Rockwood et al. *(56)* divided VCI into four groups: VCI that does not meet the criteria for dementia (i.e., aphasia after left middle cerebral artery infarction); VCI, no dementia

(CIND); VCI that met the criteria for dementia (i.e., dementia in the setting of multiple cortical and subcortical strokes; VaD), and VCI presenting with other dementing illnesses (i.e., VCI plus AD, mixed AD/VaD). Since then, the concept has been divided again into a collection of syndromes. These include vascular CIND, cortical VaD (equivalent to MID), subcortical VaD, hyperfusion or cardiogenic dementia, hemorrhagic dementia, hereditary VaD, and mixed dementia (AD with evidence of CVD) *(57)*. However, much of the more recent literature refers to VCI as a predementia syndrome in the context of CVD. This is useful in focusing on a group of patients, probably at high risk of developing dementia *(57)*, for whom there are no established diagnostic criteria.

The closest to a diagnostic approach has been adopted with the concept of vascular CIND, which uses a combination of clinical and global cognitive criteria to identify cognitive impairment in the absence of dementia and then assigns cases as vascular CIND on the basis of likely etiology. Graham et al. *(58)* diagnosed CIND in patients from the Canadian Study of Health and Aging (CSHA) study based on the exclusion of dementia and the presence of various categories of impairment identified in a clinical examination and in a battery of neuropsychological tests. CIND cases came from those who were below the modified MMSE cut-off point but did not have dementia. Di Carlo et al. *(59)* used the concept CIND in a longitudinal study for an Italian population. Their criteria for CIND required the exclusion of dementia, a CAMCOG total score lower than 80, and a clinical judgment based on direct examination, evaluation of neuropsychological tests, informant interview, Hamilton Depression Scale, and assessment of functional activities according to the Pfeffer Questionnaire.

Although these criteria have good face validity, their value in predicting dementia has not been fully established. The CSHA published findings of their cohort *(60)* that were divided into those with no cognitive impairment (NCI) and those with CIND. At follow-up 5 yr later, persons with CIND were more likely than those with NCI to receive a diagnosis of dementia (47 vs 15%). The Kungsholmen study *(61)* reported on a group of subjects 75 and older with CIND. They showed that 35% of subjects with mild CIND (1 SD below age and education norms in the MMSE) progressed to dementia between baseline and follow-up. However, 25% of the subjects also improved within this time. These variations in progression rates occur throughout all the previously published data on progression to dementia in early cognitive impairment *(62–64)* and probably result from the definition of the criteria and the length of follow-up that each study uses. The basis of all these reports has been a mixed cohort of subjects with early cognitive deficits; there has been no specific focus on VCI.

One study that has investigated subjects with vascular CIND is a follow-up study from the CSHA, in which 44% of people meeting criteria for vascular CIND developed dementia during the 5 yr of follow-up *(65)*. Although this highlights the high risk of dementia in patients with vascular CIND and is hence a landmark study, there are numerous important questions that remain unanswered. For example, as the comparative frequency of incident dementia was not examined in a group of patients with CVD but no evidence of cognitive dysfunction, it has not been clearly established that a diagnosis of vascular CIND identified a group at greater risk of subsequent cognitive decline than other individuals with CVD. In addition, although it is extremely important that memory dysfunction was significantly associated with the 5-yr incidence of dementia, the predictors of dementia during a shorter time course may have been different and the comparative value of vascular CIND and other criteria for VCI was not examined. These issues need further clarification in subsequent studies.

Regarding the pattern of cognitive decline in this group, the researchers found that incident dementia cases performed significantly worse at baseline on test of memory (i.e., free and cued recall BCRT) and category fluency (animal naming) than those who did not develop dementia. These deficits tie in with those often associated with AD; therefore, it is not surprising that almost half of those who progressed to dementia were diagnosed with AD or mixed AD/VaD at follow-up.

A large proportion of studies have included a range of participants with CVD, which will have hence included patients with a spectrum of different types of cerebrovascular lesion with or without concurrent neurodegeneration. One approach to clarifying the nature of impairments specifically related to CVD is to focus specifically on stroke patients. Twenty five percent of stroke survivors

Table 2
Profile of Cognitive Impairments

	Stroke survivors $n = 150$	Elderly controls $n = 30$	AD $n = 57$	Evaluation stroke vs controls	Evaluation stroke vs AD
CAMCOG total	83.2 ± 8.8	96.1 ± 7.4	64.8 ± 15.3	$T = 7.5$ $p < 0.0001$	$T = 8.5$ $p < 0.0001$
Memory	20.8 ± 3.1	23.4 ± 3.1	10.2 ± 5.7	$T = 3.9$ $p < 0.0001$	$T = 13.2$ $p < 0.0001$
SRT	619.1 ± 415.6	400.1 ± 103.1	634.4 ± 338.0	$T = 5.6$ $p < 0.0001$	$T = 0.25$ $p = 0.80$
CRT	756.4 ± 279.9	569.9 ± 82.0	814.4 ± 415.6	$T = 6.8$ $p < 0.0001$	$T = 1.2$ $p = 0.26$
Vig Acc	92.4 ± 15.5	98.9 ± 2.5	84.4 ± 5.6	$T = 3.5$ $p = 0.001$	$T = 2.5$ $p = 0.01$
Spatial working memory	2388.1 ± 1507.5	1480.1 ± 531.7	3194.0 ± 2379.4	$T = 4.7$ $p < 0.0001$	$T = 3.7$ $p < 0.0001$

Abbr: AD, Alzheimer's disease; CAMCOG, Cambridge Examination for Mental Disorders in the Elderly; CRT, choice reaction time; SRT, simple reaction time.

develop dementia within 12 mo of having a stroke *(66–70)*, with even higher incidence rates in older stroke survivors *(1,71)*. However, few studies have examined the detailed profile of cognitive impairment in these patients. Rao et al. *(72)* examined the profile of cognitive deficits in a small group of 25 stroke survivors, identifying greater impairment than controls across the majority of cognitive domains examined, including attention, planning, and memory. Their results are difficult to interpret because it was unclear how many of the patients had dementia. In a much larger study where stroke patients with dementia were excluded, attention, memory, orientation, and verbal fluency were all significantly more impaired in stroke patients than in the control group *(1)*. More recently, Leeds et al. *(73)* confirmed the presence of a dysexecutive syndrome after stroke. A preliminary report from a larger ongoing study conducted by the authors' group in Newcastle, UK, described in detail the profile of cognitive impairments specifically in older stroke survivors (>75 yr of age) without dementia *(74)*. The study sample consisted of 259 subjects (150 elderly stroke survivors, 57 AD, and 30 elderly controls). Neuropsychological evaluations were undertaken using the CAMCOG and the Cognitive Drug Research computerized system. The CAMCOG is a 107-item standardized paper-and-pencil test, which is well tolerated and sensitive for the identification of dementia in stroke patients. The schedule includes a detailed evaluation of memory on three subscales (new learning, remote memory, and visual memory). The COGDRAS-D is a computerized assessment battery that has been widely used for the evaluation of attention/processing speed and executive function in patients with dementia and elderly controls. Specific tasks include simple reaction time (SRT), choice reaction time (CRT), a numerical working memory task, and a visuospatial working memory task.

In comparison with age-matched controls, global cognitive deficits are evident, although the most striking decrements are in cognitive processing speed, apparent on both attention and working memory tasks (the latter involving a strong component of executive functioning). In addition, digit vigilance accuracy, an attentional task independent of processing speed, was also significantly more impaired in stroke patients. There were significant but less pronounced deficits of memory. The profile of cognitive impairments is summarized in Table 2. To put this in context, the severity of deficits in cognitive processing speed and the magnitude of impairment in vigilance accuracy was similar in older stroke patients without dementia and patients with AD, although the stroke patients had much less pronounced impairment of memory.

Table 3
Early Cognitive Impairments in Stroke Patients

n = 150	Threshold (1 SD) from elderly control group (n = 30)	Meeting specific sets of criteria for early cognitive deficits (%)	
Memory	CAMCOG memory <20	MCI 26	(17)
Global cognition	CAMCOG total <89	CIND 48	(32)
Choice reaction time	>570 ms	AACD 110	(73)
Spatial working memory (accuracy)	<61%	AACD 31	(21)
Spatial working memory (reaction time)	>2781.1 ms	AACD 21	(14)
Digit vigilance accuracy	<96.4	AACD 67	(45)

Abbr: AACD, Aging associated cognitive decline; CAMCOG, Cambridge Examination for Mental Disorders in the Elderly; CIND, vascular dementia, no dementia; MCI, mild cognitive impairment.

5.1. Criteria for Early Cognitive Impairment in Stroke Patients

There are several studies that have now attempted to examine the frequency of VCI, mainly using the concept of vascular CIND, with prevalence rates varying from 15 to 20% in clinical settings *(75,76)*. As part of an ongoing study in Newcastle, criteria for AACD, MCI, and CIND were applied to the same sample of older stroke patients without dementia to examine potential differences in the number of patients identified as having VCI. To do this, age-related cut-offs on the appropriate cognitive tasks were obtained from an age-matched control group. For each computerized task, performance 1 SD below the performance level of the control group was taken to indicate the presence of AACD from that cognitive domain. Patients were defined as having MCI if they performed 1.5 SD below the level of the control group on the total CAMCOG memory score. Patients were defined as having CIND if they scored lower than 80 on the total CAMCOG score and met the clinical criteria *(59)*. The relative prevalence of mildbut potentially significant VCI varied enormously depending on the criteria and concept used as well as which cognitive domain was assessed. Criteria based on abnormalities of processing speed identify a much larger proportion of patients than criteria focusing on memory. This is important in highlighting the different profile of early cognitive impairments in stroke patients compared to those typically reported in the context of AD. The breakdown is shown in more detail in Table 3.

Studies focusing on patients with VaD or who have experienced strokes indicate that attention, processing speed, and executive function are the most frequently and most severely impaired aspects of cognition. In addition, criteria using these aspects of cognition identify higher frequencies of VCI. However, given the disparity in frequencies between different criteria, they cannot all be identifying meaningful patient groups, and because impairments are most prevalent in a particular cognitive domain, this does not necessarily indicate that this is also the best early markers of subsequent cognitive decline. It is also possible that memory deficits, although less severe, may be an important predictor of subsequent dementia, as indicated from the CSHA for patients with vascular CIND related to a broader spectrum of underlying vascular lesions *(65)*.

In an initial report from the authors' group in Newcastle of 115 older stroke patients (>75) without dementia 3 mo poststroke followed-up for 12 mo *(77)*, 10% experienced a significant deterioration in cognitive performance. Unfortunately, none of the widely used criteria for early cognitive impairment, including MCI, CIND, or AACD, predicted people at higher risk of progressive cognitive decline. In addition, based on a detailed neuropsychological evaluation, only greater impairment of expressive language performance was significantly associated with a higher risk of progressive cognitive decline. The report from the CSHA focusing on a broader group of patients with VCI also indicated that baseline performance on attentional and executive tasks did not predict subsequent dementia. Also consistent with the current report, expressive language function was associated with the development of dementia, particularly impairments of category fluency. Baseline memory performance was associated with decline in the Canadian study but not the current report; this may be explained by the different time frame of follow-up and memory impairments may be a better predictor of more delayed onset of dementia. Therefore, the authors hypothesize that memory impairments may be a marker of concurrent atrophy that may predict more delayed dementia, whereas vascular events and small-vessel disease may be more important in people developing progression of cognitive deficits over a shorter time frame. It is imperative to try and improve the early identification of people at risk of delayed dementia. Study of putative risk factors, MRI characteristics (such as atrophy or extensive white matter hyperintensities), and relevant genetic polymorphisms may give important additional information.

Perhaps more important than the people who experienced significant cognitive decline was the larger proportion (50%) of people experiencing some improvement in cognition, with 16% experiencing significant (>2 points on the MMSE) delayed improvements. Although there are reports of longer term improvements in functional abilities, it has generally been assumed that there is little improvement in cognition beyond 3 mo poststroke. The current study supports the conclusions of previous preliminary observations and studies of younger stroke patients *(78)* that delayed improvement is possible and indicates that it is even more frequent in older stroke patients. The findings are also consistent with the improvements seen in a proportion of people with more general early cognitive impairment *(61)*. However, there are key implications for understanding the profile of change in patients with VCI as progression of early cognitive deficits is far from inevitable. Longer duration follow-up studies are needed to determine the pattern of change.

6. SUBSTRATES OF COGNITIVE IMPAIRMENT IN VCI

Several preliminary studies have been completed in patients with VCI. Bowler et al. *(79)* reported an association between VCI and atrophy, but no correlation was seen with deep WMH. However, a trend toward an association was seen between VCI and periventricular hyperintensities, which probably reflects ventricular enlargement as the two are strongly associated. Conversely, Garde et al. *(80)* reported an association between early VCI and deep WMH in the Rotterdam study. In Newcastle, the authors have reported preliminary findings from a study examining the relationship between atrophy and WMH on MRI and the profile of cognitive deficits amongst older stroke patients without dementia *(24)*. Significant associations were evident between cognitive impairments and both the severity of WMLs and atrophy in key fronto-striatal areas. Processing speed, attentional measures, and executive function were associated with hyperintensities in the internal capsule, caudate, and thalamus. Lesions in these areas are likely to disrupt topographical fronto-striato-thalamo-frontal circuits of which two, those involving the dorsolateral prefrontal cortex and anterior cingulate cortex, have particularly been implicated in executive function and attentional tasks *(81–82)*.

These data from several largely preliminary studies appear at first sight to be highly contradictory, with different studies indicating that different processes may be more important in the development of VCI or dementia. However, these discrepancies seem inevitable when considering the different patterns of vascular and neurodegenerative pathologies, that can lead to cognitive impairment in an individual patient with CVD. The complexities lie in the different types of pathology that occur in patients with cognitive impairments. Therefore, it is important to understand how different pathologies are linked to vascular risk factors and to determine whether dementia is caused by one type of pathology or a combination of these processes. In doing so, a potential opportunity for primary and secondary prevention is provided.

7. CONCLUSIONS

The study of CVD and the cognitive impairment that can follow is of high priority. Elderly stroke survivors especially are at a particularly increased risk of developing dementia and would benefit greatly from targeted interventions for secondary prevention. However, although secondary prevention studies are important, validated evidence-based criteria defining individuals at high risk of dementia are a necessary prerequisite. As yet, there are no reliable criteria for detecting those who fall into this group. The prevalence of early cognitive impairment varies enormously depending on the criteria used. There is still a large amount of longitudinal data to collect to identify the precursors of dementia be it cognitive deficits, neuropathological substrates, or a combination of both.

REFERENCES

1. Tatemichi TK, Desmond D, Stern Y, et al. Cognitive impairment after stroke: frequency, pattern and relationship to functional abilities J Neurol Neurosurg Psychiatry 1994;57:202–207.
2. Roman GC, Tatemichi T, Erkinjuntti T, Cummings JL, Masden JC, Garcia JH. Vascular dementia: diagnostic criteria for research studies. Report of the NINDS AIRENS International Workshop. Neurology 1993;43:250–260.
3. Cordoliani-Mackowiak MA, Henon H, Pruvo JP, Pasquier F, Leys D. Poststroke dementia: influence of hippocampal atrophy. Arch Neurol. 2003;60:583–590.
4. Brun A, Englund E. A white matter disorder in dementia of the Alzheimer type: a pathoanatomical study. Ann Neurol 1986;19:253–262.
5. Blennow K, Wallin A, Uhlemann C, Gottfries C. White-matter lesions on CT in Alzheimer patients: relation to clinical symptomatology and vascular factors. Acta Neurol Scand 1991;83:187–193.
6. Diaz FJ, Merskey H, Hachinski VC, et al. Improved recognition of leukoaraiosis and cognitive impairment in Alzheimer's disease. Arch Neurol 1991;48:1022–1025.
7. Englund E. Neuropathology of white matter changes in Alzheimer's disease and vascular dementia. Dement Geriatr Cogn Disord 1998;9(Suppl 1):6–12.
8. Leys D, Pruvo JP, Parent M, et al. Could Wallerian degeneration contribute to "leuko-araiosis" in subjects free of any vascular disorder? J Neurol Neurosurg Psychiatr 1991;54:46–50.
9. Scheltens P, Barkhof F, Valk J, et al. White matter lesions on Magnetic Resonance Imaging in clinically diagnosed Alzheimer's disease. Evidence for a heterogeneity. Brain 1992;115:735–748.
10. Skoog I. Risk factors for vascular dementia. A review. Dementia 1994;5:137–144.
11. Barber R, Scheltens P, Gholkar A, et al. White matter lesions on magnetic resonance imaging in dementia with Lewy bodies, Alzheimer's disease, vascular dementia, and normal aging. J Neurol Neurosurg Psychiatry 1999;67:66–72.
12. Van Gijn G. Leukoariosis and vascular dementia. Neurology 1998;51(Suppl 3):S3–S8.
13. Schmidt R, Schmidt H, Kapeller P, et al. The natural course of MRI white matter hyperintensities. J Neurolog Sci. 2002;203–204:253–257.
14. Kalaria RN. Cerebral vessels in ageing and Alzheimer's disease. Pharm Therap 1996;72:193–214.
15. Kalaria RN. Apolipoprotein E, arteriosclerosis and Alzheimer's disease. Lancet 1997;349:1174–1175.
16. Premkumar DRD, Cohen DL, Hedera P, Friedland RP, Kalaria RN. Apolipoprotein E e4 alleles in cerebral amyloid angiopathy and cerebrovascular pathology in Alzheimer's disease. Am J Pathol 1996;148:2083–2095.
17. Esiri MM, Wilcock GK, Morris JH. Neuropathological assessment of the lesions of significance in vascular dementia. J Neurol Neurosurg Psychiatry 1997;63:749–753.
18. Ballard C, McKeith I, O'Brien J, et al. Neuropathological substrates of dementia and depression in vascular dementia, with a particular focus on cases with small infarct volumes. Dementia 2000;11:59–65.
19. DeCarli C, Murphy DG, Tranh M, et al. The effect of white matter hyperintensity volume on brain structure, cognitive performance, and cerebral metabolism of glucose in 51 healthy adults. Neurology 1995;45:2077–2084.
20. O'Brien JT, Wiseman R, Burton EJ, et al. Cognitive associations of subcortical white matter lesions in older people. Ann NY Acad Sci 2002;977:436–444.
21. Mungas D, Jagust WJ, Reed BR, et al. MRI predictors of cognition in subcortical ischemic vascular disease and Alzheimer's disease. Neurology 2001;57:2229–2235.
22. Cohen RA, Paul RH, Ott BR, et al. The relationship of subcortical MRI hyperintensities and brain volume to cognitive function in vascular dementia. J Int Neuropsychol Soc 2002;8:743–752.
23. Vataja R, Pohjasvaara T, Mantyla R, et al. MRI correlates of executive dysfunction in patients with ischemic stroke. J Neurol Neurosurg Psychiatry, in press.
24. Burton EJ, Ballard C, Stephens S, et al. Hyperintensities and fronto-subcortical atrophy on MRI are substrates of mild cognitive deficits after stroke dementia and geriatric cognitive disorders. 2003;16:113–118.
25. Tomlinson BE, Blessed G, Roth M. Observations on the brains of demented old people. J Neurolog Sci 1970;11:205–242.
26. Tatemichi TK, Desmond DW, Prohovnik I, et al. Confusion and memory loss from capsular genu infarction: a thalamocortical disconnection syndrome? Neurology 1992;42:1966–1979.
27. Erkinjuntti T, Haltia M, Palo J, Sulkava R, Paetau A. Accuracy of the clinical diagnosis of vascular dementia: a prospective clinical and post-mortem neuropathological study. J Neurol Neurosurg Psychiatry 1988;51:1037–1044.

28. Henon H, Durieu I, Guerouaou D, Lebert F, Pasquier F, Leys D. Poststroke dementia: incidence and relationship to prestroke cognitive decline. Neurology 2001;57:1216–1222.
29. Cohen D L, Hedera P, Premkumar DRD, Friedland RP, Kalaria RN. Amyloid-β angiopathies masquerading as Alzheimer's disease. Ann N Y Acad Sci 1997;826:390–395.
30. Kalaria RN, Hedera P. Differential degeneration of the endothelium and basement membrane of capillaries in Alzheimer's disease. Neuroreport 1995;6:477–480.
31. Weller RO, Massey A, Newman TA, Hutchings M, Kuo YM, Roher AE. Cerebral amyloid angiopathy: amyloid beta accumulates in putative interstitial fluid drainage pathways in Alzheimer's disease. Am J Pathol 1998;153:725–733.
32. De Jong GI, De Vos RAI, Jansen Steur ENH, Luiten PGM. Cerebrovascular hypoperfusion: a risk factor for Alzheimer's disease? Ann N Y Acad Sci 1997;826:56–74.
33. Olichney JM, Hansen LA, Hofstetter CR, Grundman M, Katzman R, Thal LJ. Cerebral infarction in Alzheimer's disease is associated with severe amyloid angiopathy and hypertension. Arch Neurol 1995;52:702–708.
34. Kawai M, Kalaria RN, Cras P, et al. Degeneration of amyloid precursor protein-containing smooth muscle cells in cerebral amyloid angiopathy. Brain Res 1993;623:142–146.
35. Perry G, Smith MA, McCann CE, Siedlak SL, Jones PK, Friedland RP. Cerebrovascular muscle atrophy is a feature of Alzheimer's disease. Brain Res 1998;791:63–66.
36. Kimura T, Hashimura T, Miyakawa T. Observations of microvessels in the brain with Alzheimer's disease by scanning electron microscopy. Jpn J Psychiatry Neurol 1991;45:671–676.
37. Kalaria RN, Hedera P. Beta-amyloid vasoactivity in Alzheimer's disease [letter]. Lancet 1996; 347:1492–1493.
38. Kalaria RN, Pax AB. Increased collagen content of cerebral microvessels in Alzheimer's disease. Brain Res 1995;705:349–352.
39. Perlmutter LS, Chui HC. Microangiopathy, the vascular basement membrane and Alzheimer's disease: a review. Brain Res Bull 1990;24:677–686.
40. Scheibel AB, Duong T, Tomiyasu U. Denervation microangiopathy in senile dementia, Alzheimer type. Alz Dis Assoc Dis 1987;1:19–37.
41. Claudio L. Utrastructural features of the blood-brain barrier in biopsy tissue from Alzheimer's disease patients. Acta Neuropathol 1996;91:6–14.
42. Stewart PA, Hayakawa K, Akers MA, Vinters HV. A morphometric study of the blood brain barrier in Alzheimer's disease. Lab Invest 1992;67:34–742.
43. Huff FJ, Belle SH, Nebes RD, Holland AL, Boller F. Cognitive deficits and clinical diagnosis of Alzheimer's disease. Neurology 1987;37:1119–1124.
44. Becker JT, Boller F, Lopez Saxton J, Mcgonigle KL. The natural history of Alzheimer's disease: description of study cohort and accuracy of diagnosis. Arch Neurol 1994;51:585–594.
45. Bowler JV, Eliasziw M, Steenhuis R, et al. Comparative evolution of Alzheimer's disease, vascular dementia, and mixed dementia . Arch Neurol 1997;54:697–703.
46. Almkvist O, Backman L, Basun H, Wahlund L.O. Patterns of neuropsychological performance in Alzheimer's disease and vascular dementia. Cortex 1993;29:661–673.
47. Mendez MF, Ashla-Mendez M. Differences between multi-infarct dementia and Alzheimer's disease on unstructured neuropsychological tasks. J Clin Exper Neuropsychol; 13:923–932.
48. Villardita C, Grioli S, Lomeo C, Cattaneo C Parini J. Clinical studies with oxiracetam in patients with dementia of Alzheimer type and multi-infarct dementia of mild to moderate degree. Neuropsychobiology 1992;25:24–28.
49. Padovani A, Di Piero V, Bragoni. M, Iacoboni M, Gualdi GF. Lenzi GL. Patterns of neuropsychological impairment in mild dementia: a comparison between Alzheimer's disease and multi-infarct dementia. Acta Neurologica Scandinavica 1995;92:433–442.
50. Lafosse JM, Reed BR, Mungas D, Sterling SB, Wahbeh H, Jagust WJ. Fluency and memory differences between ischemic vascular dementia and Alzheimer's disease. Neuropsychology 1997;11:514–522.
51. Ballard C, O'Brien J, Morris CM, et al. The progression of cognitive impairment in dementia with Lewy bodies, vascular dementia and Alzheimer's disease. Int J Geriatr Psychiatry 2001:5:499–503.
52. Nyenhius DL, Gorlick PB. Vascular dementia: a contemporary review of epidemiology, diagnosis, prevention, and treatment. J Am Geriatr Soc 1998;46:1437–1448.
53. Erkinjuntti T, Kurz A, Gauthier S, Bullock R, Lilienfeld S, Damaraju CV. Efficacy of galatamine in probable vascular dementia and Alzheimer's disease combined with cerebrovascular disease: a randomized trial. Lancet. 2002;359:1283–1290.
54. Meyer JS, Rogers RL, McClintic K, Mortel KF, Lotfi J. Randomized clinical trial of daily aspirin therapy in multi-infarct dementia. A pilot study. J Am Geriatr Soc 1989;37:549–555.
55. Hachinski VC, Bowler J. Vascular dementia. Neurology 1993;43:2159–2160.
56. Rockwood K, Bowler J, Erkinjuntti T, Hachinski V, Wallin A. Subtypes of vascular dementia. Alz Dis Assoc Disord 1999;13(Suppl 3):S59–S65.
57. Rockwood K. Vascular cognitive impairment and vascular dementia. J Neurolog Sci 2002;203-204:23–27.
58. Graham JE, Rockwood K, Beattie L, et al. Prevalence and severity of cognitive impairment with and without dementia in an elderly population. Lancet 1997;349:1793–1796.

59. Di Carlo A, Baldersreschi M, Amaducci L, et al. Cognitive impairment without dementia in older people: prevalence, vascular risk factors, impact on disability. The Italian Logitudinal Study on Aging. J Am Geriatr Soc 2000;48:775–782.
60. Tuokko H, Frerichs R, Graham J, et al. Five year follow-up of cognitive impairment with no dementia. Arch Neurol 2003;60:577–582.
61. Palmer K, Wang H, Backman L, Winblad B, Fratiglioni L. Differential evolution of cognitive impairment in nondemented older persons: Results from the Kungsholmen project. Am J Psychiatry 2002;159:436–442.
62. Johansson B, Zarit SH. Early cognitive markers of the incidence of dementia and mortality: a longitudinal study of the oldest old. Int J Geriatr Psychiatry 1997;12:53–59.
63. Peterson RC, Smith GE, Waring SC, Ivnik RJ, Tangalos EG, Kokmen E. Mild cognitive impairment: clinical characterization and outcome. Arch Neurol 1999;56:303–308.
64. Ritchie K, Ledesert B, Touchon J. Subclinical cognitive impairment: epidemiology and clinical characteristics. Comp Psychiatry 2000;41:61–65.
65. Ingles JL, Wentzel C, Fisk, JD, Rockwood K. Neuropsychological predictors of incident dementia in patients with vascular cognitive impairment, without dementia. Stroke 2002;8:1999–2002.
66. Sacco RL, Shi T, Zemenillo MC, et al. Predictors of onset and occurrence of dementia after hospitalized cerebral infarctions in an urban community: The Northern Manhattan Stroke Study. Neurology 1994;44:626–634.
67. Barba R, Martinez-Espinosa S, Rodriguez-Garcia E, Pondal M, Vivancos J, Del Ser T. Post-stroke dementia. Clinical features and risk factors. Stroke 2000;31:1494–1501.
68. Desmond DW, Moroney JT, Paik MC, et al. Frequency and clinical determinants of dementia after ischemic stroke. Neurology 2000;54:1124–1131.
69. Kokmen E, Whisnant JP, O'Fallon WF, et al. Dementia after ischemic stroke: a population based study in Rochester, Minnesota (1960–1984). Neurology 1996;46:154–159.
70. Tatemichi TK, Desmond DW, Paik M, et al. Clinical determinants of dementia related to stroke. Ann Neurol 1993;33:568–575.
71. Pohjasvaara T, Erkinjuntti T, Vataja R, Kaste M. Clinical determinants of post-stroke dementia in the Helsinki Stroke Aging Memory study (SAM) cohort. Stroke 1997;28:785–792.
72. Rao R, Jackson S, Howard R. Neuropsychological impairment in stroke, carotid stenosis, and peripheral vascular disease, a comparison with healthy community residents. Stroke 1999;30:2167–2173.
73. Leeds L, Meara RJ, Woods R, Hobson JP. A comparison of the new executive functioning domains of the CAMCOG-R with existing tests of executive function in elderly stroke survivors. Age Ageing 2001;30:251–251.
74. Ballard C, Stephens S, McLaren A, et al. Neuropsychological deficits in older stroke patients. Ann NY Acad Sci 2002;977:179–182.
75. Rockwood K, Wentzel C, Hachinski V, Hogan DB, MacKnight C, McDowell I. Prevalence and outcomes of vascular cognitive impairment. Vascular Cognitive Impairment Investigators of the Canadian Study of Health and Aging. Neurology 2000; 2:447–451.
76. Szatmari S, Fekete I, Csiba L, Kollar J, Sikula J. Bereczki D. Screening of vascular cognitive impairment on a Hungarian cohort. Psychiatry Clin Neurosci 1999;53:39–43.
77. Ballard C, Rowan E, Stephens S, Wesnes K, Kalaria R, Kenny R. A prospective follow up study between 3 and 15 months post stroke: Improvements and decline in cognitive function amongst dementia free stroke survivors over the age of 75. Stroke, in press.
78. Desmond DW, Moroney JT, Sano M, Stern Y. Recovery of cognitive function after stroke. Stroke 1996;27:179–183.
79. Bowler JV. Vascular cognitive impairment. Intl Psychogeriatrics, in press.
80. Garde E, Mortensen EL, Krabbe K, Rostrup E, Larsson HB. Relation between age related decline in intelligence and cerebral white matter hyperintensities in healthy octogenarians: a longitudinal study. Lancet 2000;356:628–634.
81. Alexander GE, DeLong MR, Strick PL. Parallel organization of functional segregated circuits linking basal ganglia and cortex [review] [128 refs]. Annu Rev Neurosci 1986;9:357–381.
82. Dubois B, Pillon B. Cognitive deficits in Parkinson's disease. J Neurol 1997;244:2–8.

11

Neuropsychiatric Correlates of Vascular Injury

Vascular Dementia and Related Neurobehavioral Syndromes

Anand Kumar, Helen Lavretsky, and Ebrahim Haroon

1. INTRODUCTION

Vascular dementia (VaD) is the second most common type of dementia following Alzheimer's disease (AD) and accounts for 10 to 20% of dementia cases *(1,2)*. VaD is commonly associated with behavioral disturbances that impair overall functioning and often require active intervention *(3)*. However, unlike AD, where there is an extensive literature describing the phenomenology and management of behavioral and psychological symptoms, the neuropsychiatric features of VaD have received less clinical and scientific attention.

Despite the paucity of studies on the neuropsychiatric correlates of VaD, certain consistent behavioral patterns have been identified in patients with VaD. These observations permit us to compare behavioral profiles in patients with VaD to patients diagnosed with degenerative disorders and other clinical brain disorders of presumed vascular etiology. The primary focus of this chapter is the behavioral manifestations of patients diagnosed clinically with VaD. However, to fully appreciate the behavioral/neuropsychiatric manifestations of vascular injury to the brain, it is necessary to go beyond traditional nosological categories and also examine the behavioral correlates of stroke and subclinical cerebrovascular disease (CVD). The second segment of this chapter comprises a description of the behavioral correlates of vascular injury to the brain in patients with stroke and subclinical ischemic vascular disease. The authors conclude by discussing some of the newer neuroimaging approaches and their role in elucidating mechanisms and pathways that may be relevant to the study of vascular disease and its effect on behavioral disorders.

The study of behavioral changes in VaD has been impeded, in part, by variability in the clinical criteria used to diagnose VaD *(1)*. The *International Classification of Diseases* (ICD-10), and the *Diagnostic and Statistical Manual of Mental Disorders*, 4th ed. (DSM-IV) for psychiatric disorders, although broad based, comprise the primary diagnostic/classificatory stems for the diagnosis of behavioral disorders. ICD-10 specifically suggests that personality is relatively well preserved in VaD but allows for personality changes that may occur with features of "apathy, disinhibition, or accentuation of previous traits, such as egocentricity, paranoid attitudes, or irritability." The ischemia score that is frequently used to identify VaD includes several behavioral items. The DSM-IV *(4)* criteria are even more sketchy and recognize only three possible comorbid behavioral disturbances in patients diagnosed with VaD: delirium, delusions, and depressed mood. The National Institute of Neurological Disorders and Stroke-Association Internationale pour la Recherche et l'Enseignement en Neurosciences (NINDS-AIREN) criteria for VaD and the criteria from the State of California Alzheimer Disease Diagnostic and Treatment Centers (SCADDTC) operationalize clinical criteria

From: *Current Clinical Neurology*
Vascular Dementia: Cerebrovascular Mechanisms and Clinical Management
Edited by: R. H. Paul, R. Cohen, B. R. Ott, and S. Salloway © Humana Press Inc., Totowa, NJ

Table 1
Primary Behavioral Abnormalities That Characterize VaD and Related Clinical Brain Disorders

Symptoms	Vascular dementia	Alzheimer dementia	Poststroke depression	Vascular depression
Memory	+++	++++	+++	++
Executive function	++++	++++	+++	+++
Delusions	++++	++++	++	++
Visual hallucinations	++++	++++		
Auditory hallucinations	+++	+++		
Delusional misidentification	++++	+++		
Anxiety	++++	+++	++++	
Apathy/abulia		++++	++++	+
Wandering behavior	++++	+++	++	
Depression	++++	+++	++++	++++
Irritability	+++	+++	++++	
Aggression	++++	++	++++	
Mania	++	++	+++	
Obsessive-compulsive symptoms	+++	+++		
Eating disorder	++	++	+++	
Pathological emotionalism	++++	+++		

for the diagnosis of VaD *(5,6)*. The NINDS-AIREN criteria attach significance to emotional incontinence, mood, and personality changes *(6)*. The California criteria list illusions, delusions, hallucinations, and psychosis as "features that do not constitute strong evidence either for or against the diagnosis of probable ischemic vascular dementia (IVD) and do not mention mood disturbances."

Research into behavioral disturbances in VaD has been further complicated by traditional approaches to the study of behavioral and psychological correlates of dementia, which separate different types of behaviors but combine dementing illnesses of different etiology. An additional complication is that numerous patients have overlapping clinical features of AD and VaD, or frontal-temporal dementia (FTD), which can only be confirmed by autopsy. Relatively few studies have examined the broad spectrum of behavioral symptoms between major dementias, such as AD and VaD, or FTD *(7)*. The predominant emphasis has been on traditional domains of neuropsychiatric impairment, such as depression, psychosis, and anxiety, and in comparing the prevalence of these behaviors in patients with VaD and AD.

Although there is some overlap in the behavioral features in patients diagnosed with VaD and those with AD, the prevalence of individual behavioral features and the overall behavioral profile vary across diagnostic categories (*see* Table 1). Ballard and colleagues *(8)* noted greater rates of depression and anxiety but no difference in psychotic symptoms among patients diagnosed with VaD compared to those with AD. Aharon-Peretz et al. *(9)* found a similar spectrum of behavioral disturbances in patients with VaD and white matter and lacunar infarctions compared to patients with AD who were matched by age and dementia severity. A recent report *(10)* identified the relationship between a subcortical brain syndrome expressed in psychomotor retardation and depression in patients with three dementia types: AD, VaD, and FTD. Bathgate et al. *(7)* observed a greater prevalence of many behavioral disturbances, including sleep and appetite disturbance, among the patients with FTD compared to the AD group, with patients with VaD having intermediate rates of behavioral disturbances. The primary behavioral abnormalities that characterize VaD and related clinical brain disorders follow.

1.1. Depression

Many, although not all, studies demonstrate a higher prevalence of mood disorders in patients diagnosed with VaD when compared with patients with AD *(8,11,12)*. The prevalence of depression ranges from 20 to 50% in patients with VaD and between 3 and 30% in patients diagnosed with AD in most reports *(11)*. Most studies were cross-sectional and used samples in ambulatory programs and inpatient settings. In a population-based study of the prevalence of dementia using widely accepted clinical criteria, Newman et al. found that patients with VaD had a significantly higher prevalence of major depression when compared with the AD group *(12)*. In one study, extrapyramidal features and a positive grasp reflex correlated significantly with depression, whereas pyramidal signs showed no relationship to mood in the VaD group *(13)*. Also in that study, patients with VaD had more neurovegetative signs when compared with patients with AD. The correlation between the positive grasp reflex and mood in the VaD group was interpreted as evidence supporting a role for disruption of afferent frontal circuits in depression *(8,12)*. In addition, in patients with VaD, extrapyramidal features correlated strongly with both behavioral and physical features of depression *(13)*. In patients with VaD, depression has been reported to be less common in mildly impaired patients as opposed to patients with AD, where mood disorders are more commonly present in patients with early dementia *(3,8,12)*. Also, patients with VaD and depression performed poorly on tests of attention and concentration when compared with patients with VaD without depression *(3,6,8,12)*. This raises the possibility that depression additionally compromises cognition in patients with VaD. Patients with VaD are also reported to show decreased affect/slowing and psychomotor retardation when compared with patients with AD *(14)*. The differences in psychomotor slowing between the groups were also reported to be independent of the severity of white matter disease.

Studies of behavior and mood in patients with both VaD and AD have several methodological limitations *(3,7,8,12)*. These include small sample sizes, different approaches to diagnosing depression and dementia, the cross-sectional nature of the assessments, and the variability in the time interval in assessments after the acute vascular event. Despite these methodological pitfalls, the emerging consensus is that mood disorders are more frequent in dementia secondary to vascular injury than in patients clinically diagnosed with AD. The consistently higher prevalence of depression in patients with VaD has resulted in some classificatory systems using depression as an important clinical feature that helps in distinguishing VaD from AD. Both major depressive disorder and less severe forms of clinical depression occur in patients with VaD and AD. These findings have implications for the pathophysiology of mood disorders and the management of these disorders in clinical settings. There are little data pertaining specifically to manic and hypomanic features in VaD, although some studies indicate prevalence rates of 1–2% comparable to those observed in AD *(3,15–17)*.

1.2. Psychosis

Most studies of psychosis in VaD describe the prevalence and symptoms/signs of psychosis and compare them to comparable phenomena in patients with AD. Psychotic symptoms that have been described in VaD include delusions (8–50%), visual hallucinations (14–60%), and delusional misidentifications (19–30%) *(3,8,18)*. The most commonly studied psychotic features are delusions, which have a mean prevalence of 33% *(3)*. The most commonly occurring delusions are paranoid delusions and delusions of pathological jealousy that are associated with right hemispheric lesions. Delusions, delusional misidentification, and visual hallucinations were present to a comparable degree in both AD and VaD groups. Delusions in patients with dementia have been interpreted as an adaptive response resulting from progressive cognitive deterioration often reflecting the patient's inability to cope with reality. Both visual and auditory hallucinations have been described in patients with VaD and AD. On occasion, they are difficult to clearly distinguish from delusions and confabulations.

In AD, psychosis has been linked to greater severity of cognitive impairment with the prevalence in excess of 60% in some samples, although the evidence for that is less consistent in VaD *(8,18,19)*.

Factors predisposing to psychosis in patients with focal strokes include cerebral atrophy and development of seizures *(20)*, as well as personal and family history of psychosis preceding stroke.

Most common stroke lesions associated with psychotic symptoms occur in temporoparietal and temporoparietal-occipital regions, deep gray matter, or frontal white matter ischemic lesions *(20)*. White matter lesions (WMLs) are the most frequently identified cerebral abnormality in patients with late-onset psychosis that may serve as a prodrome for dementia *(21,22)*.

1.3. *Anxiety*

Anxiety symptoms were also more common in patients with VaD when compared with patients diagnosed with AD. In one study, 70% of patients diagnosed with VaD had two or more anxiety symptoms, a finding that is consistent with the high frequency of anxiety in stroke patients *(8)*. The frequency of anxiety symptoms in patients with AD in this study was approximately 38% and was consistent with previous reports. Anxiety symptoms were more common in patients with VaD with Mini-Mental State Examination (MMSE) scores of less than 10 *(8)*. This is in contrast to the AD group, where anxiety was more frequently observed in patients with MMSE scores greater than 22. A higher percentage of VaD patients was also diagnosed with generalized disorder when compared with the AD group (53 vs 27%) *(8)*. Although most patients with two or more anxiety symptoms were not concurrently depressed, a subgroup of patients with anxiety also met criteria for Major Depressive Disorder (MDD). The effect of vascular lesions on pathways and neurotransmitter systems has been suggested as a possible mechanism by which vascular injury contributes to both mood and anxiety in these patients. Sultzer and colleagues *(23)* reported that cortical metabolic dysfunction identified by positron emission tomography (PET) was related to ischemic subcortical lesions identified on magnetic resonance imaging (MRI). Anxiety, depression, and overall severity of neurobehavioral symptoms were correlated with the extent of white matter ischemia in subjects with VaD.

1.4. *Agitation and Aggression*

In addition to the classical domains of mood and psychosis, other behavioral features are also frequently observed in patients with both AD and VaD. These include wandering behaviors, such as pacing, aimless wandering, and following the caregiver *(15)*. Additional behavioral features observed in patients diagnosed with dementia include different forms of aggression, such as physical and verbal aggression. A recent population study identifies irritability in 18% of patients with VaD compared to 20% in those with AD *(24,25)*. These behaviors increase the morbidity associated with these disorders and complicate long-term clinical management. They are often the precipitating cause of placement in nursing homes and other long-term care settings.

1.5. *Obsessive-Compulsive Disorder*

Obsessive-compulsive disorder (OCD) or symptoms may develop in VaD after basal ganglia strokes and striatal lesions with predominance of combined bilateral or unilateral lesions of caudate and putamen nuclei *(26)*. VaD of Binswanger's type is reportedly associated with greater obsessive and compulsive behaviors compared to AD. The subjects with dementia with obsessive-compulsive symptoms typically have no awareness of their behaviors, unlike patients with idiopathic OCD *(27)*. Other behavioral abnormalities, such as anorexia, bulimia, binge eating, or compulsive craving for food or alcohol, may also occur with VaD after stroke. Only anecdotal reports of such cases exist in the stroke literature *(28)*.

2. SUBCORTICAL VASCULAR DISEASE AND BEHAVIOR

Clinically and pathophysiologically, there are different types of strokes, depending on the location and the nature of the underlying vascular insult. The term VaD is overly broad and includes patients with heterogeneous cerebrovascular compromise. The most widely studied form is cortical stroke involving the gray matter. Other common forms of stroke are typically subcortical and include lacunar strokes and white matter ischemia. The most common type of vascular disease (stroke type) associated with VaD is the lacunar stroke *(29)*. Most lacunes affect the subcortical nuclei, the caudate nucleus, globus pallidus, and the thalamus. Lacunes also occur in connecting fibers of frontal subcortical circuits and produce a clinical syndrome similar to that seen in other subcortical diseases. Aharon-Peretz et al. *(29)* reported that the rate of cognitive and behavioral decline observed in the majority (i.e., 83%) of patients with VaD was determined by the severity of cognitive and behavioral impairment at baseline and by the occurrence of new strokes. Clinically, the dementia associated with subcortical lacunar infarction is characterized by slowing of information processing, memory deficit, impaired executive functions, and gait dysfunction *(30)*. These are frequently accompanied by personality and mood alterations. In lacunar infarcts, behavioral changes may be more prominent than intellectual deficits, suggesting that behavioral differences are important in VaD. Comparison of patients with infarcts with patients without infarcts suggests that symptoms of depression, apathy, and perseveration are associated with lacunar infarcts.

3. BINSWANGER'S DISEASE

Binswanger's disease may be considered a relatively distinct vascular/behavioral syndrome with certain unique clinical, pathophysiological, and neuroimaging characteristics *(31,32)*. The typical clinical picture is that of a patient in the sixth or seventh decade, more often a male, with long-standing and poorly controlled hypertension and diabetes. Memory loss and dementia are often, though not invariably, part of the clinical picture. Aphasia and amnestic intervals are observed, together with focal motor signs, dysarthria, gait disturbances, ataxia, incontinence, and Parkinsonism. Behavioral changes may be seen early in the clinical picture even before the motor and cognitive features become clinically apparent. Depression and mood disturbances are common in Binswanger's disease. Manic features may be seen early on, though abulia often develops later in the illness. The overall picture is slowly progressive, and a history of stroke is common through the course of the illness. Extensive WMLs on MRI is common, and the disease is conceptualized as a subcortical ischemic encephalopathy predominantly of the white matter. Diagnosis requires a combination of clinical and neuroimaging evidence and should not be made exclusively on the basis of neuroimaging evidence of white matter ischemia. Pathologically confirmed cases of Binswanger's disease are few *(30,33)*.

Other types of vascular lesions contributing to significant cognitive and behavioral impairment include a combination of clinical cortical and "strategic" subcortical infarcts (e.g., thalamus and anterior limb of genu of the internal capsule), as well as subclinical or "silent" strokes in the deep white matter that may be progressive or nonprogressive *(34)*. It is also possible that chronic exposure to risk factors for CVD, such as elevated plasma lipids or diabetes mellitus, can be associated with microcirculatory disturbances, microangiopathy, and lacunar infarction and lead to cognitive and behavioral signs and symptoms *(34)*.

4. VASCULAR BEHAVIORAL SYNDROMES

In the clinical arena, it is common practice to classify disorders based on the most striking clinical manifestations. For example, when memory and related cognitive features dominate the clinical picture in patients with stroke and vascular disease, it is customary to categorize these patients as having a "VaD." This occurs even though depression and other behavioral features may comprise an important part of the symptom complex requiring pharmacological and psychosocial intervention. Similarly, when a mood disturbance is the most clinically apparent feature after vascular insult, the term "poststroke depression" is commonly used to characterize the syndrome, even though cognitive impairment may coexist and complicate management and functional recovery. The clinical/behavioral manifestations of vascular injury depend largely on the location of the vascular injury and its effect on neuronal circuits and connectivity. Ischemic compromise to the brain over time frequently involves multiple regions, and, consequently, the clinical features are diverse and vary over time.

This clinical heterogeneity leads to classificatory difficulties, which, in turn, lead to nosological ambiguity. In keeping with this approach, VaD and poststroke depression may be best conceptualized as neurobehavioral syndromes resulting from ischemic injury to brain regions and circuits. Both the focal and the remote effect of lesions (diaschisis) on the brain may contribute to the clinically diverse picture. Therefore, the authors discuss the behavioral manifestations of vascular injury to the brain outside the context of what is commonly considered "VaD." Cognitive impairment, especially impairment in executive functions and aspects of memory, is commonly observed in these states though patients may not meet criteria for clinical dementia.

5. STROKE AND BEHAVIOR

There are numerous related neuropsychiatric syndromes and symptoms occurring after stroke. A comprehensive assessment is usually needed to distinguish among related disorders. The most commonly described behavioral symptoms described in association with CVD are depression, apathy, anxiety, and emotional lability *(35–37)*. Aggression and agitation, psychosis, and disturbances of sleep, appetite, and sexual functioning have also been described in this patient group. The best studied syndrome in the context CVD is depression. Depression has been identified as a risk factor for VaD, along with more common vascular risk factors in the recent report from the Canadian Study of Health and Aging (CSHA) *(38)*.

5.1. Poststroke Depression

Depression after vascular injury to the cerebral hemispheres is now a well-recognized clinical entity. Poststroke depression (PSD) may present as minor or major depression and occur within 12–24 mo after the cerebrovascular accident *(39)*. Depression occurs in 20–50% in the first year poststroke *(40,41)*. Poststroke depression is a heterogeneous phenomenon, which can occur in patients of different ages, but mainly in middle-aged and older adults. According to recent studies of the subtypes of poststroke depression *(42,43)*, the prevalence of major depression ranges from 0 to 25%; minor depression occurs in 10–30% of patients after stroke *(44)*. However, after a comprehensive review of the literature, Primeau *(45)* concluded that depression may be as common in patients with stroke as in the elderly with other physical illnesses.

5.1.1. Phenomenology and Course

Despite its high prevalence, depression after a stroke remains a controversial issue because of an unresolved debate about causality of depression. It involves complex relationship between focal neurological deficits, cognitive impairment, disability, and comorbid psychiatric and physical conditions *(46)*. Phenomenology of poststroke major depression is similar to that of "functional" major depression *(44)*. Numerous studies have assessed the duration of poststroke depression *(47,48)*. The majority of patients with major depression experience remission within the first year. However, in a minority of patients, depression becomes chronic and persists for more than 3 yr after the stroke *(49)*. On the other hand, minor depression was more variable, with both short- and long-term depression occurring in these patients *(44)*. In a 12-mo prospective study, depression was diagnosed in 53% of patients at 3 mo poststroke and was associated with impairment in memory, nonverbal problem solving, and attention and psychomotor speed. The presence of dysphasia also increased the risk of major depression *(46)*. A few studies examined the effect of PSD on outcome after stroke. Most frequently, such studies demonstrate greater functional impairment in depressed patients compared with their nondepressed counterparts *(50)*. Although early reports demonstrated a link between the proximity of the lesion to the left frontal pole and depression, this finding has been inconsistently observed in subsequent studies. In addition, at least two systematic reviews *(51,52)* have not provided any evidence to support the role of any specific lesion locations in the development of PSD.

5.1.2. Cognitive Changes in PSD

Although mood changes and their effect on recovery and disability in PSD have received attention, cognitive changes have also been identified in patients diagnosed with PSD *(53–58)*. Some investigators have found clearcut associations between depression and cognitive changes ascertained using standard neuropsychological tests at both 3- and 12-mo intervals after stroke *(59)*. Patients with PSD performed poorly on tests of nonverbal problem solving, attention, memory, and psychomotor speed after controlling for the effect of dysphasia *(58)*. The cognitive changes persisted in PSD patients 12 mo after the stroke, although the relationship between mood and cognition was stronger in the immediate poststroke period *(59)*. In another study, patients with executive function impairment poststroke scored higher on the Beck depression scale but not on other clinical instruments *(57)*. Other investigators have also reported significant correlations between mood and cognitive changes early on in the poststroke period *(60)*. However, in this study, improvement in mood was not associated with a corresponding improvement in cognition, thereby indicating that both processes might occur concurrently, albeit independently, after acute vascular injury *(60)*. Cognitive and mood changes are important components of the behavioral spectrum that follows vascular injury to the brain and probably reflect injury to overlapping circuits in the brain *(61)*.

Hypomania may arise after stroke and represent a secondary mood disorder or may be a continuation of long-standing bipolar disorder, which has become unstable with the onset of organic brain disease. The phenomenology of this state is similar to that observed in primary hypomania, and mood-congruent delusions and hallucinations may occur. Manic-like symptoms are associated more frequently with right-sided lesions *(62,63)* and right thalamic lesions *(64,65)*.

5.2. Apathy

Apathy is defined as diminished motivation not attributable to decreased levels of consciousness, cognitive impairment, or emotional distress *(66)*. Apathy occurs in up to 20% of patients after stroke *(35,67)*, and its presence depends, to some degree, on lesion location *(67–73)*. Apathy may or may not coexist with depression. Differentiating the syndromes of apathy and depression is sometimes difficult because of overlapping or coexisting clinical features. Abulia is a more profound state of psychomotor retardation characterized by flat affect, reduced motor responses, fixed gaze, blank face, perseverations, and lack of awareness of condition *(74)*. Abulia can result from strokes disrupting fronto-subcortical pathways, such as anterior cingulate and capsular lesions *(35)*.

5.3. Agitation and Aggression

Outbursts of apparent anger and periods of agitation and aggression are common in stroke *(64)*. A range of negative emotions, such as irritability, hostility, bitterness, frustration, and rage, may be present in stroke victims. The presence of dementia and aphasia, as well as disinhibition, after frontal lobe injury may facilitate agitated behaviors. Aggression after stroke, although often observed clinically after frontal lobe infarcts, has not been systematically studied. Several areas of the brain have been proposed as the ones facilitating aggression after injury and include the amygdala, hypothalamus, cingulum, temporal, and frontal lobes *(64)*.

5.4. Anxiety

Anxiety and nervousness are most frequently experienced during the first year after stroke *(64)*. Several studies suggested a significant relationship between generalized anxiety disorder and CVD *(75–77)*. Generalized anxiety disorder (GAD) after stroke is a common and long-lasting affliction that interferes substantially with social life and functional recovery. In a population-based cohort of 80 patients with acute stroke, the prevalence of the GAD was about 28%, and this number did not change during 3 yr of follow-up *(78)*. Comorbidity with major depression was high and worsened the prognosis of depression. Anxiety disorder without depression may be associated with right posterior lesions in stroke patients *(79)*, and, in general, anxiety is more common with cortical rather than subcortical lesions *(62)*. Emotional lability after stroke has numerous names (e.g., pathological laughing and crying or "emotional incontinence") which may be upsetting for patients and their families. Although emotional lability is a cause of such signs as crying and looking sad, it may not necessarily reflect clinical depression. Many patients find their condition embarrassing and attribute it to their inability to control emotions but not to sadness.

Changes in appetite, sexual dysfunction, and sleep disturbances have all been reported in poststroke patients. Lesions in specific limbic and brain stem regions have been implicated in their pathophysiology. Collectively, these behavioral abnormalities substantially increase the morbidity associated with stroke and often require active clinical management.

6. GENETIC FACTORS

Another less common cause of familial stroke and VaD is cerebral autosomal dominant arteriopathy with subcortical infarcts and leukoencephalopathy (CADASIL). Associated histopathology is fairly consistent typically demonstrating granular thickening of cerebral arterioles. Stroke, depression, and seizures are frequently part of the clinical picture in CADASIL. CADASIL has been localized to chromosome 19, and the notch 3 gene has been implicated in its etiology *(80)*.

7. VASCULAR DEPRESSION

Although the most readily recognized form of vascular depression is PSD, there is increasing awareness that "subclinical" CVD—cerebrovascular risk factors in the absence of overt stroke—might contribute to mood disorders, especially in the elderly. Even though VaD typically follows one or more clinically obvious brain infarctions, there is growing consensus that vascular factors contribute to depression and cognitive impairment in a subgroup of patients with late-life major depression. This thesis is supported by the following observations: data from computed tomography (CT) and MRI neuroimaging studies, which identify hyperintensities in such patients; the association of hyperintensities with age and cerebrovascular risk factors; and the pathophysiological evidence indicating that hyperintensities are associated with widespread diminution in cerebral perfusion *(81)*. The neuropathological correlates of hyperintensities are diverse and represent ischemic changes together with demyelination, edema, and gliosis *(81–83)*. However, the putative link between hyperintensities and vascular disease forms the basis of the vascular theory of depression. Patients with clinically defined vascular depression experience greater cognitive dysfunction, disability, and retardation but less agitation and guilt feelings than patients with nonvascular depression. Krishnan et al. *(84)* examined the specific clinical and demographic characteristics of elderly patients with vascular depression as defined by the presence of vascular lesions in MRI. Elderly patients with MRI-defined vascular depression were older and had a later age of onset, more apathy, and a lower incidence of family history of depression than elderly patients with nonvascular depression *(84)*. In a study of patients with the DSM-III-R criteria for depression, "silent cerebral infarctions" were reported in 65% of patients *(85)*. Future studies should examine the validity of this proposed depressive subtype and its relationship to other depressive subtypes.

In comparison to normal control subjects and other neuropsychiatric groups, high rates of abnormality have been consistently observed in MRI evaluations of elderly patients with major depressive disorder *(83,85,86)*. These abnormalities appear as areas of increased signal intensity bright regions in balanced (mixed T1- and T2-weighted), T2-weighted, and fluid-attenuated inversion recovery (FLAIR) images *(81)*. High-intensity lesions occur in the periventricular and deep white matter regions and in subcortical and brain stem areas. Collectively, these three types of abnormalities have been referred to as leukoaraiosis or encephalomalacia. The rate of these findings is higher in geriatric depression compared with normal controls *(82,86)* or patients diagnosed with AD *(87)* and may be comparable to that in MID *(88)*. However, cerebrovascular abnormalities are not restricted to old age or unipolar depression. MRI hyperintensities are commonly reported in middle-aged unipolar and young bipolar patients relative to controls or in bipolar patients with familial bipolar disorder *(89,90)*. MRI hyperintensities found in late onset unipolar depression and bipolar disorder have been attributed to CVD on the basis that these abnormalities are commonly associated with vascular risk factors *(4,39,40,42,43,46,47,49,64,66–72,75–79,82–87,89–112)*. More recent observations *(82,83)* suggest that in the elderly, smaller brain volumes and hyperintensities may provide complimentary, albeit autonomous pathways to late-life MDD. Vascular and nonvascular medical comorbidity contribute to high-intensity lesions, which, in turn, lead to MDD. Smaller frontal brain volumes represent a complementary path.

8. EXECUTIVE DYSFUNCTION

Although frontal system pathology is common in AD, FTD, VaD, and many other degenerative dementias *(113)*, VaD disproportionately affects frontal systems *(57,114,115)*. Subcortical lesions indirectly affect frontal cortical metabolism, particularly if they include lacunar infarctions of the basal ganglia and thalamus or anterior periventricular hyperintensities. A depression-executive dysfunction syndrome in late-life has been proposed *(116)*. Impairment of executive functions in patients with late-life depression may identify a subgroup of patients who present with increased disability, poor treatment response, relapse, and recurrence. Vascular compromise to specific prefrontal circuits may provide the neurobiological basis for both mood and cognitive changes in these patient groups. Increased high-intensity lesions in the prefrontal regions are associated with impaired executive functions in patients with late-life depression and may be a reliable in vivo marker of ischemic compromise in a subgroup of patients *(117)*.

9. SUMMARY

Vascular injury to the brain results in a broad spectrum of behavioral changes of which disturbances of cognition, mood, psychosis and anxiety are perhaps the best characterized and understood. The nature and location of the vascular injury and predisposing risk factors most likely determine the clinical picture and overall outcome. These behaviors often lead to increased suffering and caregiver burden and precipitate nursing home placements. A better understanding of these behaviors, their pathophysiology, and approaches to their management is likely to improve the quality of life of patients and their families and reduce the care cost for the society.

Modern magnetic resonance-based approaches, such as diffusion tensor imaging, magnetization transfer, and two-dimensional spectroscopy have the potential to elucidate physiological changes in focal brain regions and discrete white matter tracts. Together with valid neuropsychological and other behavioral measures, they can be exploited to help develop a more sophisticated understanding of the relationship between brain biology and behavioral changes in the context of vascular compromise. The study of specific, well-characterized clinical samples including patients with transient ischemic attacks who are at high risk for developing stroke and patients with subcortical stroke has the potential to further clarify the biological basis of behavioral changes in patients with VaD and related neurobehavioral syndromes.

ACKNOWLEDGMENT

This work was supported in part by the MH55115, MH 61567 and KO2-MH02043 (AK); K23-MH01948 (HL).

REFERENCES

1. Bowler JV, Hachinski V. Vascular dementia. In: Feinberg TE, Farah MJ, eds. Behavioral Neurology and Neuropsychology. New York, NY: McGraw-Hill, 1997, pp. 589–603.
2. Rocca WA, Hofman A, Brayne C, et al. The prevalence of vascular dementia in Europe: facts and fragments from 1980-1990 studies. EURODEM-Prevalence Research Group. Ann Neurol 1991;30:817–824.

3. Ballard C, O'Brien JT. Behavioural and psychological symptoms. In: Erkinjuntti T, Gauthier S, eds. Vascular Cognitive Impairment. London,UK: Martin Dunitz Ltd, 2002, pp. 237–252.
4. American Psychiatric Association. Diagnostic and Statistical Manual of Mental Disorders: DSM-IV. Washington, DC: American Psychiatric Association, 1994.
5. Chui HC, Victoroff JI, Margolin D, Jagust W, Shankle R, Katzman R. Criteria for the diagnosis of ischemic vascular dementia proposed by the State of California Alzheimer's Disease Diagnostic and Treatment Centers. Neurology 1992;42(3 Pt 1):473–480.
6. Roman GC, Tatemichi TK, Erkinjuntti T, JL, et al. Vascular dementia: diagnostic criteria for research studies. Report of the NINDS-AIREN International Workshop. Neurology 1993;43:250–260.
7. Bathgate D, Snowden JS, Varma A, Blackshaw A, Neary D. Behaviour in frontotemporal dementia, Alzheimer's disease and vascular dementia. Acta Neurol Scand 2001;103:367–378.
8. Ballard C, Neill D, O'Brien J, McKeith IG, Ince P, Perry R. Anxiety, depression and psychosis in vascular dementia: prevalence and associations. J Affect Disord 2000;59:97–106.
9. Aharon-Peretz J, Kliot D, Tomer R. Behavioral differences between white matter lacunar dementia and Alzheimer's disease: a comparison on the neuropsychiatric inventory. Dement Geriatr Cogn Disord 2000;11:294–298.
10. Lind K, Edman A, Karlsson I, Sjogren M, Wallin A. Relationship between depressive symptomatology and the subcortical brain syndrome in dementia. Int J Geriatr Psychiatry 2002;17:774–778.
11. Hebert R, Lindsay J, Verreault R, Rockwood K, Hill G, Dubois MF. Vascular dementia : incidence and risk factors in the Canadian study of health and aging. Stroke 2000;31:1487–1493.
12. Newman SC. The prevalence of depression in Alzheimer's disease and vascular dementia in a population sample. J Affect Disord 1999;52:169–176.
13. Simpson S, Allen H, Tomenson B, Burns A. Neurological correlates of depressive symptoms in Alzheimer's disease and vascular dementia. J Affect Disord 1999;53:129–136.
14. Hargrave R, Geck LC, Reed B, Mungas D. Affective behavioural disturbances in Alzheimer's disease and ischaemic vascular disease. J Neurol Neurosurg Psychiatry 2000;68:41–46.
15. Hope T, Keene J, Fairburn C, McShane R, Jacoby R. Behaviour changes in dementia 2: Are there behavioral syndromes? Int J Geriatr Psychiatry 1997;12:1074–1078.
16. Hope T, Keene J, Gedling K, Cooper S, Fairburn C, Jacoby R. Behaviour changes in dementia. 1: Point of entry data of a prospective study. Int J Geriatr Psychiatry 1997;12:1062–1073.
17. Lyketsos CG, Lopez O, Jones B, Fitzpatrick AL, Breitner J, DeKosky S. Prevalence of neuropsychiatric symptoms in dementia and mild cognitive impairment: results from the cardiovascular health study. JAMA 2002;288:1475–1483.
18. Burns A, Jacoby R, Levy R. Psychiatric phenomena in Alzheimer's disease. I: Disorders of thought content. Br J Psychiatry 1990;157:72–74.
19. Jeste DV, Wragg RE, Salmon DP, Harris MJ, Thal LJ. Cognitive deficits of patients with Alzheimer's disease with and without delusions. Am J Psychiatry 1992;149:184–189.
20. Edwards-Lee T, Cummings JL. Focal lesions and psychosis. In: Bogousslavsky J, Cummings JL, eds. Behavior and Mood Disorders in Focal Brain Lesions. Cambridge, MA: Cambridge University Press, 2000, pp. 419–436.
21. Lesser IM, Hill-Gutierrez E, Miller BL, Boone KB. Late-onset depression with white matter lesions. Psychosomatics 1993;34:364–367.
22. Miller BL, Lesser IM, Boone K, et al. Brain white-matter lesions and psychosis. Br J Psychiatry 1989;155:73–78.
23. Sultzer DL, Mahler ME, Cummings JL, Van Gorp WG, Hinkin CH, Brown C. Cortical abnormalities associated with subcortical lesions in vascular dementia. Clinical and position emission tomographic findings. Arch Neurol 1995; 52:773–780.
24. Lyketsos CG, Steinberg M, Tschanz JT, Norton MC, Steffens DC, Breitner JC. Mental and behavioral disturbances in dementia: findings from the Cache County Study on Memory in Aging. Am J Psychiatry 2000;157:708–714.
25. Paradiso S, Robinson RG, Arndt S. Self-reported aggressive behavior in patients with stroke. J Nerv Ment Dis 1996; 184:746–753.
26. Etcharry-Bouyx F, Dubas F. Obsessive-compulsive disorders in association with focal brain lesions. In: Bogousslavsky J, Cummings JL, eds. Behavior and Mood Disorders in Focal Brain Lesions. Cambridge, MA: Cambridge University Press, 2000, pp. 304–326.
27. Lawrence RM. Is the finding of obsessional behavior relevant to the differential diagnosis of Vascular Dementia of the Binswanger Type? Behav Neurol 2000;12:149–154.
28. Ghika J. Mood and behavior in disorders of the basal ganglia. In: Bogousslavsky J, Cummings JL, eds. Behavior and mood disorders in focal brain lesions. Cambridge, MA: Cambridge University Press, 2000, pp. 122–201.
29. Aharon-Peretz J, Daskovski E, Mashiach T, Tomer R. Natural history of dementia associated with lacunar infarctions. J Neurol Sci 2002;203-204:53–55.
30. Cummings JL. Vascular subcortical dementias: clinical aspects. Dementia 1994;5:177–180.
31. Babikian V, Ropper AH. Binswanger's disease: a review. Stroke 1987;18:2–12.
32. Caplan LR, Schoene WC. Clinical features of subcortical arteriosclerotic encephalopathy (Binswanger disease). Neurology 1978;28:1206–1215.

33. Mahler ME, Cummings JL. Behavioral neurology of multi-infarct dementia. Alzheimer Dis Assoc Disord 1991;5:122–130.
34. Tatemichi TK, Desmond DW, Prohovnik I. Strategic infarcts in vascular dementia. A clinical and brain imaging experience. Arzneimittelforschung 1995;45:371–385.
35. Starkstein SE, Fedoroff JP, Price TR, Leiguarda R, Robinson RG. Apathy following cerebrovascular lesions. Stroke 1993;24:1625–1630.
36. Starkstein SE. Relationship between anxiety disorders and depressive disorders in patients with cerebrovascular injury. Arch Gen Psychiatry 1990;47:246–251.
37. Starkstein SE, Fedoroff JP, Price TR, Leiguarda R, Robinson RG. Catastrophic reaction after cerebrovascular lesions: frequency, correlates, and validation of a scale. J Neuropsychiatry Clin Neurosci 1993;5:189–194.
38. The Canadian Study of Health and Aging Working Group. The Canadian study of health and aging: study methods and prevalence of dementia. Can Med Assoc J 1994;150:899–913.
39. Kumar A, Cummings J. Depression in neurodegenerative disorders and related conditions in Alzheimer's disease and related conditions. In: Gothier S, Cummings J, eds. Alzheimer's Disease and Related Disorders. London, UK: Martin Dunitz, 2001, pp. 123–141.
40. House A, Dennis M, Mogridge L, Warlow C, Hawton K, Jones L. Mood disorders in the year after first stroke. Br J Psychiatry 1991;158:83–92.
41. Robinson RG, Bolduc PL, Price TR. Two-year longitudinal study of poststroke mood disorders: diagnosis and outcome at one and two years. Stroke 1987;18:837–843.
42. Chemerinski E, Robinson RG. The neuropsychiatry of stroke. Psychosomatics 2000;41:5–14.
43. Eastwood MR, Rifat SL, Nobbs H, Ruderman J. Mood disorder following cerebrovascular accident. Br J Psychiatry 1989;154:195–200.
44. Robinson RG. Neuropsychiatric consequences of stroke. Annu Rev Med 1997;48:217–229.
45. Primeau F. Post-stroke depression: a critical review of the literature. Can J Psychiatry 1988;33:757–765.
46. Kauhanen M, Korpelainen JT, Hiltunen P, et al. Poststroke depression correlates with cognitive impairment and neurological deficits. Stroke 1999;30:1875–1880.
47. Lipsey JR, Spencer WC, Rabins PV, Robinson RG. Phenomenological comparison of poststroke depression and functional depression. Am J Psychiatry 1986;143:527–529.
48. Morris PL, Robinson RG, Raphael B. Prevalence and course of depressive disorders in hospitalized stroke patients. Int J Psychiatry Med 1990;20:349–364.
49. Astrom M, Adolfsson R, Asplund K. Major depression in stroke patients. A 3-year longitudinal study. Stroke 1993;24: 976–982.
50. Parikh RM, Robinson RG, Lipsey JR, Starkstein SE, Fedoroff JP, Price TR. The impact of poststroke depression on recovery in activities of daily living over a 2-year follow-up. Arch Neurol 1990;47:785–789.
51. Morris PL, Robinson RG. Personality neuroticism and depression after stroke. Int J Psychiatry Med 1995;25:93–102.
52. Robinson RG, Starr LB, Kubos KL, Price TR. A two-year longitudinal study of post-stroke mood disorders: findings during the initial evaluation. Stroke 1983;14:736–741.
53. Censori B, Manara O, Agostinis C, et al. Dementia after first stroke. Stroke 1996;27:1205–1210.
54. Ebrahim S, Nouri F, Barer D. Cognitive impairment after stroke. Age Ageing 1985;14:345–348.
55. Kase CS, Wolf PA, Kelly-Hayes M, Kannel WB, Beiser A, D'Agostino RB. Intellectual decline after stroke: the Framingham Study. Stroke 1998;29:805–812.
56. Pohjasvaara T, Erkinjuntti T, Vataja R, Kaste M. Dementia three months after stroke. Baseline frequency and effect of different definitions of dementia in the Helsinki Stroke Aging Memory Study (SAM) cohort. Stroke 1997;28:785–792.
57. Pohjasvaara T, Leskela M, Vataja R, et al. Post-stroke depression, executive dysfunction and functional outcome. Eur J Neurol 2002;9:269–275.
58. Rasquin SM, Verhey FR, Lousberg R, Winkens I, Lodder J. Vascular cognitive disorders: memory, mental speed and cognitive flexibility after stroke. J Neurol Sci 2002;203–204:115–119.
59. Downhill JE, Jr., Robinson RG. Longitudinal assessment of depression and cognitive impairment following stroke. J Nerv Ment Dis 1994;182:425–431.
60. Andersen G, Vestergaard K, Riis JO, Ingeman-Nielsen M. Dementia of depression or depression of dementia in stroke? Acta Psychiatr Scand 1996;4:272–278.
61. Tekin S, Cummings JL. Frontal-subcortical neuronal circuits and clinical neuropsychiatry: an update. J Psychosom Res 2002;53:647–654.
62. Starkstein SE, Mayberg HS, Berthier ML, et al. Mania after brain injury: neuroradiological and metabolic findings. Ann Neurol 1990;27:652–659.
63. Starkstein SE, Bryer JB, Berthier ML, Cohen B, Price TR, Robinson RG. Depression after stroke: the importance of cerebral hemisphere asymmetries. J Neuropsychiatry Clin Neurosci 1991;3:276–285.
64. Birkett DP. The Psychiatry of Stroke. American Psychiatric, Inc., Washington, DC, 1996.
65. Cummings JL, Mendez MF. Secondary mania with focal cerebrovascular lesions. Am J Psychiatry 1984;141:1084–1087.
66. Levy ML, Cummings JL, Fairbanks LA, et al. Apathy is not depression. J Neuropsychiatry Clin Neurosci 1998;10: 314–319.

67. Finset A, Andersson S. Coping strategies in patients with acquired brain injury: relationships between coping, apathy, depression and lesion location. Brain Inj 2000;14:887–905.
68. Cummings JL. Frontal-subcortical circuits and human behavior. Arch Neurol 1993;50:873–880.
69. Duffy JD, Kant R. Apathy secondary to neurologic disease. Psychiatr Ann 1997;27:39–43.
70. Marin RS. Apathy and related disorders of diminished motivation. American Psychiatric Press Review of Psychiatry 1996;15:205–242.
71. Marin RS. Differential diagnosis of apathy and related disorders of diminished motivation. Psychiatr Ann 1997;27:30–33.
72. Marin RS. Differential diagnosis and classification of apathy. Am J Psychiatry 1990;147:22–30.
73. Okada K, Kobayashi S, Yamagata S, Takahashi K, Yamaguchi S. Poststroke apathy and regional cerebral blood flow. Stroke 1997;28:2437–2441.
74. Fisher CM. Honored guest presentation: abulia minor vs. agitated behavior. Clin Neurosurg 1983;31:9–31.
75. Coyle PK, Sterman AB. Focal neurologic symptoms in panic attacks. Am J Psychiatry 1986;143:648–649.
76. Mathew RJ, Wilson WH, Nicassio PM. Cerebral ischemic symptoms in anxiety disorders. Am J Psychiatry 1987; 144:265.
77. Schultz SK, Castillo CS, Kosier JT, Robinson RG. Generalized anxiety and depression. Assessment over 2 years after stroke. Am J Geriatr Psychiatry 1997;5:229–237.
78. Astrom M. Generalized anxiety disorder in stroke patients. A 3-year longitudinal study. Stroke 1996;27:270–275.
79. Castillo CS, Starkstein SE, Fedoroff JP, Price TR, Robinson RG. Generalized anxiety disorder after stroke. J Nerv Ment Dis 1993;181:100–106.
80. Adair JC. Is it Alzheimer's? Hosp Pract (Off Ed) 1998;33:35–36, 51.
81. Sackeim HA. Brain structure and function in late-life depression. In: Morihisa JM, ed. Washington, DC: Advance in Brain Imaging. American Psychiatric Publishing, Inc., 2001, pp. 83 –122.
82. Kumar A, Bilker W, Jin Z, Udupa J. Atrophy and high intensity lesions: complementary neurobiological mechanisms in late-life major depression. Neuropsychopharmacology 2000;22:264–274.
83. Kumar A, Mintz J, Bilker W, Gottlieb G. Autonomous neurobiological pathways to late-life major depressive disorder: clinical and pathophysiological implications. Neuropsychopharmacology 2002;26:229–236.
84. Krishnan KR, Hays JC, Blazer DG. MRI-defined vascular depression. Am J Psychiatry 1997;154:497–501.
85. Fujikawa T, Yokota N, Muraoka M, Yamawaki S. Response of patients with major depression and silent cerebral infarction to antidepressant drug therapy, with emphasis on central nervous system adverse reactions. Stroke 1996;27:2040–2042.
86. Coffey CE, Wilkinson WE, Weiner RD, et al. Quantitative cerebral anatomy in depression. A controlled magnetic resonance imaging study. Arch Gen Psychiatry 1993;50:7–16.
87. Erkinjuntti T, Gao F, Lee DH, Eliasziw M, Merskey H, Hachinski VC. Lack of difference in brain hyperintensities between patients with early Alzheimer's disease and control subjects. Arch Neurol 1994;51:260–268.
88. Zubenko GS, Sullivan P, Nelson JP, Belle SH, Huff FJ, Wolf GL. Brain imaging abnormalities in mental disorders of late life. Arch Neurol 1990;47:1107–1111.
89. Dupont RM, Jernigan TL, Butters N, et al. Subcortical abnormalities detected in bipolar affective disorder using magnetic resonance imaging. Clinical and neuropsychological significance. Arch Gen Psychiatry 1990;47:55–59.
90. Figiel GS, Krishnan KR, Rao VP, et al. Subcortical hyperintensities on brain magnetic resonance imaging: a comparison of normal and bipolar subjects. J Neuropsychiatry Clin Neurosci 1991;3:18–22.
91. Adler R, MacRitchie K, Engel GL. Psychologic processes and ischemic stroke (occlusive cerebrovascular disease). I. Observations on 32 men with 35 strokes. Psychosom Med 1971;33:1–29.
92. Akiskal HS, Bolis CL, Cazzullo C, et al. Dysthymia in neurological disorders. Mol Psychiatry 1996;1:478–491.
93. Alexander GE, DeLong MR, Strick PL. Parallel organization of functionally segregated circuits linking basal ganglia and cortex. Annu Rev Neurosci 1986;9:357–381.
94. Alexopoulos GS, Meyers BS, Young RC, Campbell S, Silbersweig D, Charlson M. 'Vascular depression' hypothesis. Arch Gen Psychiatry 1997;54:915–922.
95. Beaulieu M, Coyle JT. Postnatal development of aminergic projections to frontal cortex: effects of cortical lesions. J Neurosci Res 1983;10:351–361.
96. Bolla-Wilson K, Robinson RG, Starkstein SE, Boston J, Price TR. Lateralization of dementia of depression in stroke patients. Am J Psychiatry 1989;146:627–634.
97. Bush BA. Major life events as risk factors for post-stroke depression. Brain Inj 1999;13:131–137.
98. Carney RM, Rich MW, Tevelde A, Saini J, Clark K, Jaffe AS. Major depressive disorder in coronary artery disease. Am J Cardiol 1987;60:1273–1275.
99. Coffey CE, Figiel GS, Djang WT, Saunders WB, Weiner RD. White matter hyperintensity on magnetic resonance imaging: clinical and neuroanatomic correlates in the depressed elderly. J Neuropsychiatry Clin Neurosci 1989;1:135–144.
100. Everson SA, Goldberg DE, Kaplan GA, Julkunen J, Salonen JT. Anger expression and incident hypertension. Psychosom Med 1998;60:730–735.
101. Fedoroff JP, Starkstein SE, Parikh RM, Price TR, Robinson RG. Are depressive symptoms nonspecific in patients with acute stroke? Am J Psychiatry 1991;148:1172–1176.

102. Gass CS, Lawhorn L. Psychological adjustment following stroke: An MMPI study. Psychological Assessment 1991;3:628–633.
103. Goldstein K. The organism. A holistic approach to biology derived from pathological data in man. New York, NY: American Book, 1939.
104. Gross CR, Shinar D, Mohr JP, et al. Interobserver agreement in the diagnosis of stroke type. Arch Neurol 1986;43:893–898.
105. Hamilton M. A rating scale for depression. J Neurol Neurosurg Psychiatry 1960;23:56–61.
106. Herrmann M, Bartels C, Schumacher M, Wallesch CW. Poststroke depression. Is there a pathoanatomic correlate for depression in the postacute stage of stroke? Stroke 1995;26:850–856.
107. Kempster PA, Gerraty RP, Gates PC. Asymptomatic cerebral infarction in patients with chronic atrial fibrillation. Stroke 1988;19:955–957.
108. Krishnan KR, Ellinwood EH, Jr., Goli V. Structural brain changes revealed by MRI. Am J Psychiatry 1988;145:1316.
109. Lavretsky H, Kumar A. Clinically significant non-major depression: old concepts, new insights. Am J Geriatr Psychiatry 2002;10:239–255.
110. Marin RS, Fogel BS, Hawkins J, Duffy J, Krupp B. Apathy: a treatable syndrome. J Neuropsychiatry Clin Neurosci 1995;7:23–30.
111. Matsumoto Y, Uyama O, Shimizu S, et al. Do anger and aggression affect carotid atherosclerosis? Stroke 1993;24:983–986.
112. Mayberg HS, Parikh RM, Morris PL, Robinson RG. Spontaneous remission of post-stroke depression and temporal changes in cortical S2-serotonin receptors. J Neuropsychiatry Clin Neurosci 1991;3:80–83.
113. Royall DR, Lauterbach EC, Cummings JL, et al. Executive control function: a review of its promise and challenges for clinical research. A report from the Committee on Research of the American Neuropsychiatric Association. J Neuropsychiatry Clin Neurosci 2002;14:377–405.
114. Ishii N, Nishihara Y, Imamura T. Why do frontal lobe symptoms predominate in vascular dementia with lacunes? Neurology 1986;36:340–345.
115. Wolfe N, Linn R, Babikian VL, Knoefel JE, Albert ML. Frontal systems impairment following multiple lacunar infarcts. Arch Neurol 1990;47:129–132.
116. Alexopoulos GS, Kiosses DN, Klimstra S, Kalayam B, Bruce ML. Clinical presentation of the "depression-executive dysfunction syndrome" of late life. Am J Geriatr Psychiatry 2002;10:98–106.
117. Salloway S, Malloy P, Kohn R, et al. MRI and neuropsychological differences in early- and late-life-onset geriatric depression. Neurology 1996;46:1567–1574.

12

Functional Impairment in Vascular Dementia

Patricia A. Boyle and Deborah Cahn-Weiner

1. INTRODUCTION

Vascular dementia (VaD) is associated with cognitive, physical, and functional impairments and is a major source of disability among the elderly *(1,2)*. Much of the disability reported among patients with VaD is attributable to declines in activities of daily living (ADLs). ADLs are composed of instrumental and basic self-care abilities (IADLs and BADLs, respectively); IADLs include complex behaviors, such as cooking, housekeeping, and medication management, and BADLs include more basic tasks, such as grooming and feeding *(3)*. ADL impairments result in a diminished quality of life for patients and their caregivers *(4)* and an increased use of healthcare services *(5)*. ADL dysfunction also often precipitates nursing home placement *(5,6)*.

The assessment of ADLs represents an important component of the evaluation of patients with VaD, and an understanding of the determinants of ADL dysfunction can facilitate improved patient care. This chapter reviews ADL assessment methods, the course of ADL declines, and the determinants of ADL impairment among patients with VaD. The potential use of neuropsychological tests of executive function as a marker for ADL impairment is discussed, and recommendations for clinical practice and future research are provided.

2. WHY IS IT IMPORTANT TO FORMALLY ASSESS ADLs IN PATIENTS WITH VaD?

The assessment of ADLs constitutes an important component of the diagnosis, tracking, and management of patients with VaD. The *Diagnostic and Statistical Manual of Mental Disorders*, 4th ed., text revision (DSM-IV-TR) *(7)* and National Institute of Neurological Disorders and Stroke-Association Internationale pour la Recherche et l'Enseignement en Neurosciences (NINDS-AIREN) *(8)* criteria for VaD require the presence of cognitive deficits sufficient to cause significant declines in social or occupational functioning and clarify that ADL impairments must be the result of cognitive deficits, not the physical impairments resulting from stroke. Although ADLs can be assessed informally (via unstructured interviews between healthcare providers and patients' families), formal ADL evaluations typically provide more detailed and reliable information and help to clarify the severity of the dementia and the extent to which ADL impairments are the result of cognitive vs physical limitations. Therefore, formal ADL evaluations are strongly recommended.

In addition to the diagnostic use of formal ADL assessments, such evaluations provide reliable baseline estimates of functional status. Using these estimates, clinicians and researchers can identify areas in which assistance is needed, implement targeted treatment and management strategies, and track a patient's stability or decline over time. ADL impairments often lead to nursing home placement among individuals with dementia, and an awareness of a patient's specific deficits can facilitate

From: *Current Clinical Neurology*
Vascular Dementia: Cerebrovascular Mechanisms and Clinical Management
Edited by: R. H. Paul, R. Cohen, B. R. Ott, and S. Salloway © Humana Press Inc., Totowa, NJ

the implementation of appropriate compensatory strategies to prolong in-home living. Moreover, functional status is increasingly recognized as an important outcome in pharmacologic and other intervention studies *(9)*, and ADL assessments can help to determine treatment effectiveness.

3. ADL ASSESSMENT TECHNIQUES

There exists no single measure specifically designed for the assessment of ADLs in patients with VaD; however, there are several widely available, reliable ADL assessment instruments for use with patients with dementia. Examples include the Lawton & Brody ADL Scale (LB ADL) *(10)*, the Progressive Deterioration Scale (PDS) *(11)*, the Disability Assessment for Dementia (DAD) *(12)*, and the Alzheimer Disease Cooperative Study ADL Scale (ADCS/ADL) *(13)*. These scales differ regarding their focus on IADLs vs BADLs, respectively, but are similar in that most are completed by an informant (e.g., a caregiver or relative who spends a considerable amount of time with the patient in the home environment and who can report on the individual's functional abilities) rather than the patient himself or herself. Informant-based measures are strongly recommended because of the unreliability of dementia patients' self-reports; however, it is noteworthy that potential biases can affect informant ratings. For example, informants may underexaggerate or overexaggerate ADL deficits, depending on the informant's own mental health and/or their knowledge of the patient's functional status, which often is determined by the amount of contact the caregiver has with the patient. Furthermore, gender-based or cultural biases may affect assessment results (e.g., a man may be rated as "dependent" in housekeeping because he never participated in that activity). Some of the more recently developed scales (e.g., the ADCS-ADL Scale) make provisions for areas in which an informant cannot provide an accurate rating because of participant's limited undertaking or involvement in a specific task.

Most widely used ADL scales include items designed to assess IADLs and BADLs specifically, in addition to providing a measure of overall ADL performance. Therefore, informants are asked to provide ratings of the dementia patient's ability to perform individual IADL and BADL skills (e.g., bathing, grooming, and medication management). Ratings typically indicate independence, partial dependence, or dependence on a given skill. Total IADL, BADL, and ADL scores then are derived by summing performances across relevant items, and total ADL scores reflect an individual's overall level of functional capability.

Individual ADL assessment instruments are weighted differentially toward IADLs or BADLs, and the selection of an ADL assessment instrument typically depends on the severity of the dementia population being evaluated. IADLs decline earlier in the course of dementia than do BADLs, and scales that emphasize IADLs are most useful for outpatients with mild-moderate dementia. In contrast, scales that emphasize BADLs are most useful for inpatients or those with severe dementia. When assessing patients with VaD, the use of instruments that assess nonmotor-based skills rather than motor-based abilities (e.g., walking and transferring) is recommended, given the physical limitations commonly associated with stroke. Table 1 provides information on some commonly used ADL scales and offers recommendations regarding the population for which individual instruments are most appropriate.

4. COURSE OF ADL DECLINE AMONG PATIENTS WITH VaD

Although ADL declines have been extensively studied in individuals with Alzheimer's disease (AD), relatively few studies have examined the course of ADL declines among patients with VaD. The paucity of research investigating the ADLs in VaD may, in part, reflect the demands and challenges associated with studying a disorder with multiple subtypes (e.g., VaD resulting from strokes vs small-vessel disease). VaD subpopulations can be difficult to characterize, and the subtypes of VaD likely are associated with different trajectories of decline. For example, individuals with VaD owing to large-vessel strokes would be expected to follow a stepwise course of deterioration in func-

Table 1

Four Commonly Used Activities of Daily Living Assessment Scales

Scale name	Recommended population
Progressive Deterioration Scale (PDS)	Mild stage
Alzheimer Disease Cooperative Study ADL Scale (ADCS/ADL)	Mild stage
Lawton & Brody ADL Scale (LB ADL)	Mild and moderate stages
Disability Assessment for Dementia (DAD)	Moderate stage

tioning, whereas individuals with VaD owing to small-vessel disease would be expected to show a more gradual, progressive decline. Therefore, understanding the course of ADL declines in VaD requires a careful evaluation of the subpopulation of VaD patients being studied.

Placebo-controlled, randomized clinical trials investigating the efficacy of pharmacologic agents for treating the cognitive symptoms of dementia provide some data regarding the course of ADL declines in VaD. Such trials typically include mild to moderately impaired patients with VaD resulting from multiple strokes, and rates of functional decline often are compared to those of AD patients. In one study, Erkinjuunti et al. *(14)* evaluated ADL declines among placebo-treated, mild-moderately impaired VaD patients (Mini-Mental State Examination [MMSE] scores 10–25) enrolled in a 6-mo clinical trial. Functional abilities were assessed using the DAD, and individuals in the placebo group declined very slowly, showing an overall ADL decline of 4.5% during 6 mo. In two comparable studies of patients with AD, untreated patients with AD showed a decline of 5.1–5.8% on the DAD during 6 mo and 11.6–13.1% during 1 yr. The slower ADL decline among patients with VaD as compared to patients with AD has been corroborated in additional studies *(15,16)*, and it is generally accepted that the rate of functional decline is slower among patients with VaD than among patients with AD.

More recently, investigators have begun to evaluate ADLs in patients with VaD resulting from small-vessel disease and/or chronic ischemia, and initial studies have focused on the course of IADL declines in mild-moderately impaired patients. As is the case with VaD owing to stroke, VaD owing to small-vessel disease is associated with a progressive decline in ADLs that is slower than or approximately equivalent to that reported among individuals with AD. The authors recently examined the course of IADL declines during a 1-yr period in a sample of 30 patients with VaD of moderate severity. IADLs were measured using the LB ADL scale, and results indicated a 15% decline in IADLs during 1 yr *(17)*. Although this study used a different ADL measure than the ones used in the studies described, it is important to acknowledge that a 15% decline translates to the complete loss of a single IADL skill or the partial loss of two IADLs. The loss of even one IADL skill has significant functional implications; for example, the loss of the ability to maintain one's medications or to cook for oneself results in an increased need for care and may even precipitate nursing home placement.

Taken together, the available studies suggest that there is a progressive deterioration of ADLs in patients with VaD, as in AD. Although the rate of ADL decline is slower among patients with VaD than among AD patients, the nature of ADL declines is similar. IADLs decline earlier than do BADLs in both groups, and, ultimately, all patients with dementia are at-risk for functional disability.

5. DETERMINANTS OF FUNCTIONAL IMPAIRMENT IN VaD

Patients with VaD exhibit diverse cognitive, physical, and behavioral symptoms, and there are multiple possible contributors to ADL dysfunction in VaD. Several studies have reported significant associations between global cognitive impairment (commonly measured by the MMSE) and ADL dysfunction in VaD *(18,19)*; however, given that diagnostic criteria for VaD specify the presence of *cognitive* deficits sufficient to cause functional impairment *(7,8)*, surprisingly few studies have examined associations between *specific* cognitive deficits and ADLs in patients with VaD. An understanding of the neuropsychological determinants of functional impairment is essential for the early identification of patients at high-risk for ADL dysfunction and for the implementation of targeted interventions to reduce disability in patients with VaD.

One recent study sought to examine predictive associations between specific cognitive domains and IADLs in patients with AD and VaD resulting from small-vessel disease *(20)*. These authors examined the contributions of attention, memory, verbal fluency, and visuospatial abilities to IADLs across diagnoses. Although AD and VaD patients display different cognitive profiles, memory was the only cognitive function associated with functional impairment across diagnoses. More specifically, regression analyses revealed that memory impairment accounted for approximately 34% of IADL impairment among the patients with VaD. These findings provide initial support for the role of memory impairment as a determinant of functional status in VaD. However, this study failed to use adequate measures of executive functions, making it difficult to determine the relative contribution of executive functions vs memory to ADL performance in these two groups.

The authors also have begun to investigate the use of neuropsychological tests for predicting IADLs and BADLs, respectively, among patients with VaD resulting from small-vessel disease. Their findings suggest a complex relationship between cognitive and other functions and ADL performance, such that IADLs and BADLs are subserved by different abilities. This is not surprising, because the performance of IADLs requires significantly more cognitive capacity than the performance of BADLs, which are more routine or overlearned. A discussion of the factors associated with IADL vs BADL impairment and the implications of this research follows.

6. PREDICTING IADLS

Executive dysfunction is arguably the most salient neuropsychological feature of VaD *(21–24)*, and executive dysfunction has emerged as a reliable determinant of IADL impairment in healthy *(25,26)* and demented elderly *(27–29)*. Executive functions include complex thinking abilities, mental flexibility/set shifting, and behavioral initiation and persistence *(30)*, and it follows logically that these abilities are required for independent living. The authors have demonstrated unique and significant associations between executive dysfunction and IADL impairment in two recent cross-sectional studies of patients with VaD. Furthermore, preliminary evidence suggests that baseline evaluations of executive dysfunction also may serve as an indicator of *future* functional declines in patients with VaD.

In an initial study, the authors examined cross-sectional associations between cognitive functions and IADLs in a sample of 32 patients with VaD *(31)*. ADLs were measured using the LB ADL scale, and the authors predicted that executive dysfunction, but not other cognitive functions, would be significantly associated with IADL impairment. As predicted, executive dysfunction correlated highly with IADL performance and was the only cognitive domain that correlated significantly with IADLs. Attention, memory, and visuospatial skills did not correlate significantly with IADLs in this population. Moreover, performance on one single, commonly used measure of executive functioning explained 40% of the variance in IADLs, even after accounting for dementia severity. These findings provided initial evidence of a strong and unique relationship between executive dysfunction and IADL impairments in patients with VaD.

In a follow-up study, the authors *(32)* examined cross-sectional associations between executive dysfunction, subcortical neuropathology, and IADLs in an independent sample of 29 patients with VaD. The authors hypothesized that executive dysfunction and MRI-defined subcortical neuropathology would correlate significantly with IADL dysfunction but that other cognitive functions would not. Multiple regression analyses revealed that these two factors accounted for a total of 42% of the variance in IADLs; more specifically, executive dysfunction accounted for 28% of the variance in IADLs, and subcortical neuropathology explained an additional 14% of the variance. Again, other cognitive functions (e.g., memory, attention, and visuospatial skills) did not correlate significantly with IADLs.

Based on these findings that indicate a powerful association between executive dysfunction and IADL impairment, the authors recently sought to examine whether early executive dysfunction serves as predictor of *future* IADL declines *(17)*. Cognitive and functional abilities were assessed at baseline and at a 1-yr follow-up in a sample of 29 patients with VaD resulting from small-vessel disease. The authors hypothesized that: (1) baseline performance on executive tests would significantly predict IADL impairment at 1 yr and (2) baseline estimates of subcortical neuropathology would add to this prediction. Results indicated that baseline performance on all executive tests correlated significantly with IADLs at 1 yr, whereas performance on tests examining *other* cognitive functions did not. Moreover, regression analysis revealed that baseline performance on executive tasks explained 52% of the variance in IADLs at the 1-yr follow-up. However, contrary to their expectation, subcortical neuropathology did not explain unique variance in IADLs after accounting for executive dysfunction. Therefore, these findings suggest a unique and powerful predictive relationship between baseline executive dysfunction and IADL *declines* in patients with VaD.

7. PREDICTING BADLS

Although executive dysfunction is a useful indicator of IADL dysfunction in VaD, other factors are associated with BADL impairment. In the study described in Section 6. *(31)*, the authors also investigated the contributions made by cognitive vs motor impairments in the prediction of BADLs. Because (1) performance of BADLs is less cognitively demanding than performance of IADLs and (2) motor dysfunction can lead to impairments in basic self-care abilities even in cognitively intact individuals, the authors hypothesized that motor dysfunction would emerge as a significant predictor of BADLs. As predicted, stepwise regression analyses revealed that motor performance alone accounted for a significant proportion of the variance in BADLs. In contrast to the findings reported for IADLs, cognitive functions (e.g., attention, memory, executive functions, and visuospatial skills) were not significantly associated with BADL performance in the authors' sample. Similar findings were reported by Bennet et al. *(33)* and suggest a dissociation between the cognitive deficits that subserve IADL impairments and the motor functions that subserve BADL impairments in VaD.

8. SUMMARY

Executive dysfunction is arguably the most salient neuropsychological deficit seen among patients with VaD *(21–24)*, and increasing evidence suggests that there is a strong and unique predictive association between executive dysfunction and IADL impairment in VaD. Individuals with more severe executive impairment are likely to show greater functional declines (regardless of dementia severity or other cognitive deficits) and, more importantly, individuals who show significant executive impairment at baseline evaluations are likely to show more severe functional impairment after 1 yr. Therefore, prominent early executive dysfunction may serve as a marker for future functional declines.

It is important to acknowledge that executive functions are multifaceted and involve planning, motivation, goal-directedness, mental flexibility, and resistance to interference. Impairment in a single or multiple aspects of executive functions may be sufficient to produce IADL impairment, and further research is needed to determine the level of executive dysfunction sufficient to produce IADL impairment and to determine the extent to which specific components of executive dysfunction are predictive of functional declines. It is likely that impaired initiation/motivation and mental flexibility in particular may impede performance of the complex behavioral repertoires necessary for activities such as medication management and bill paying; therefore, individuals with executive cognitive impairment may be unable to perform IADLs because of their inability to manage the competing demands associated with real-world tasks. The authors are conducting studies to determine the relative contribution of specific components of executive functions to IADL impairment in VaD.

In addition to demonstrating the importance of executive cognitive abilities in determining IADLs, the available studies also provide evidence of a dissociation between the functions that subserve IADLs and BADLs, respectively. Whereas executive dysfunction and possibly memory are important determinants of IADL impairment, motor and other physical functions are associated with BADL impairment. Thus, there exists a complex relationship between cognitive, motor, and functional deficits in VaD.

Given the consistency among studies indicating the presence of significant executive dysfunction among patients with VaD and the increasing evidence of its functional significance, thorough evaluations of executive abilities are recommended for all patients with VaD. Such evaluations may aid in the identification of individuals at highest risk for disability and provide important information regarding treatment planning and long-term care options. Healthcare providers should closely monitor those individuals with marked executive dysfunction early in the course of the illness, because these individuals may be at increased risk for progressive IADL declines.

9. RECOMMENDATIONS FOR FUTURE RESEARCH

The studies reviewed herein provide evidence of the potential use of neuropsychological tests of executive dysfunction for predicting functional declines in VaD; however, additional research is greatly needed to clarify the nature and course of ADL dysfunction in VaD subpopulations and to examine the extent to which pharmacological and nonpharmacological interventions may slow the course of ADL declines. Prospective studies that evaluate well-characterized subpopulations of VaD patients over several years; assess a wider array of cognitive, motor, and behavioral features; and use comprehensive ADL evaluations are encouraged and will provide more comprehensive information for use in clinical practice. Importantly, the factors associated with functional impairment in VaD may change with the course of the disease, and future investigations should seek to clarify the predictors of ADL impairment among patients with VaD of varying degrees of severity.

Determination of the *specific* cognitive predictors of functional disability in subpopulations of patients with VaD has been understudied and represents an important research goal. The early identification of those patients at high risk for functional disability may facilitate the use of targeted compensatory interventions aimed to maintain in-home living. For example, although such interventions have not yet been tested, interventions aimed to compensate for executive cognitive impairments may help to maintain in-home living. Therefore, the ability to identify and treat patients with VaD at increased risk for functional disability may have significant emotional, financial, and public health implications. Understanding the specific predictors of ADL dysfunction ultimately may improve treatment options for patients with VaD and reduce the disability associated with VaD.

REFERENCES

1. Aguero-Torres HL, Fratiglioni L, Winblad B. Natural history of Alzheimer's disease and other dementias: review of the literature in the light of the findings from the Kungsholmen Project. Intl J Geriatric Psychiatry 1998;13:755–66.
2. Cummings JL. Vascular subcortical dementias: clinical aspects. Dementia 1994;5:177–180.
3. Lawton MP, Brody EM. Assessment of older people: self-maintaining and instrumental activities of daily living. Gerontologist 1969;9:179–86.
4. Severson MA, Smith GE, Tangalos EG, et al. Patterns and predictors of institutionalization in community-based dementia patients. J Amer Geriatrics Soc 1994;42:181–185.
5. Hope T, Keene J, Gedling K, Fairburn CG, Jacoby R. Predictors of institutionalization for people with dementia living at home with a carer. Intl J Geriatric Psychiatry 1998;13:682 –690.
6. Vetter PH, Krauss S, Steiner O, et al. Vascular dementia versus dementia of Alzheimer's type: do they have differential effects on caregivers' burden? J Gerontol Behav Psychol Sci Soc 1999;54:S93–S98.
7. American Psychiatric Association. Diagnostic criteria from the DSM-IV-TR. Washington, DC: American Psychiatric Association, 2000, pp. 90–91.
8. Roman GC, Tatemichi TK, Erkinjutti T, et al. Vascular dementia: diagnostic criteria for research studies. Report of the NINDS-AIREN International Workshop. Neurology 1993;43:250–260.

9. Gauthier S, Rockwood K, Gelinas I, et al. Outcome measures for the study of activities of daily living in vascular dementia. Alzheimer Dis Assoc Disord 1999;13(Suppl 3),143–147.
10. Lawton MP, Brody EM. Assessment of older people; self-maintaining and instrumental activities of daily living. Gerontologist 1969;9(3):179–186.
11. DeJong R, Osterland O, Roy G. Measurement of quality of life changes in patients with Alzheimer's disease. Clin Ther 1989;11:545–554.
12. Gelinas L, Gauthier L, McIntyre M, Gauthier S. Development of a functional measure for persons with Alzheimer's disease. Amer J Occup Ther 1999;53:471–481.
13. Galasko D, Bennet D, Sano M, et al. An inventory to assess activities of daily living for clinical trials in Alzheimer's disease. Alzheimer Dis Assoc Disord 1997;11:S33–S39.
14. Erkinjuntti T, Lilienfeld S. Galantamine shows efficacy in patients with Alzheimer's disease with cerebrovascular components or probable vascular dementia. Neurology 2001;56(Suppl 3):A340.
15. Kitter B, for the European/Canadian Propentofylline Study Group. Clinical trials of Propentofylline in vascular dementia. Alzheimer Dis Assoc Disord 1999;13(Suppl 3):S166–S171.
16. Nyenhuis DL, Gorelick PB, Freels S, Garron D. Cognitive and functional decline in African Americans with VaD, AD, and stroke without dementia. Neurology 2002;58:56–61.
17. Boyle P, Paul R, Moser D, Cohen R. Executive dysfunction predicts ADL declines in patients with vascular dementia. Clin Neuropsychol 2004: in press.
18. Mitnitski AB, Graham JE, Mogilner AJ, Rockwood K. The rate of decline in function in Alzheimer's disease and other dementias. J Gerontolog Biolog Sci Med Soc 1999;54:M65–M69.
19. Paul RH, Cohen RA, Moser D, Browndike J, Zawacki T, Gordon N. Performance on the Mattis Dementia Rating Scale in patients with vascular dementia: relationships to neuroimaging findings. J Geriatric Psychiatry Neurol 2001;14:33–36.
20. Tomaszewski Farias S, Mackin S, Mungas D, Reed B, Jagust W. Differences in degree of impaired daily functioning in different dementia types [abstract]. Arch Clin Neuropsychol 2001;17:735.
21. Almkvist O. Neuropsychological deficits in vascular dementia in relation to Alzheimer's disease: reviewing evidence for functional similarity or divergence. Dementia 1994;5(3–4):203–209.
22. Libon DL, Bogdanoff B, Swenson R, et al. Neuropsychological profiles associated with subcortical white matter alterations and Parkinson's disease: Implications for the diagnosis of dementia. Arch Clin Neuropsychol 2001;16:19–32.
23. Roman GC, Royall DR. Executive control function: a rational basis for the diagnosis of vascular dementia. Alzheimer Dis Assoc Disord 1999;13(S3):69–80.
24. Royall DR, Roman DC. Differentiation of vascular dementia from Alzheimer's disease on neuropsychological tests. Neurology 2000;55:604–606.
25. Bell-McGinty S, Podell K, Franzen M, Baird A, Williams M. Standard measures of executive function in predicting IADLs in older adults. Intl J Geriatric Psychiatry 2002;17(9):828–834.
26. Grigsby J, Kaye K, Baxter J, Shetterly S, Hamman R. Executive cognitive abilities and functional status among community-dwelling older persons in the San Luis Valley Health and Aging Study. J Amer Geriatric Soc, 1998;46: 590–596.
27. Boyle P, Malloy P, Salloway S, Cahn-Weiner D, Cohen R, Cummings JL. Executive dysfunction and apathy predict functional impairment in Alzheimer disease. Amer J Geriatric Psychiatry 2003;11:214–221.
28. Chen ST, Sultzer DL, Hinkin C, Mahler M, Cummings JE. Executive dysfunction in Alzheimer's disease: association with neuropsychiatric symptoms and functional impairment. J Neuropsychiatry Clin Neurosci 1998;10:426–432.
29. Norton LE, Malloy PF, Salloway S. The impact of behavioral symptoms on activities of daily living in patients with dementia. Amer J Geriatric Psychiatry 2001;9:41–48.
30. Lezak MD. Neuropsychological Assessment. New York, NY: Oxford University Press, Inc., 1995.
31. Boyle P, Cohen R, Paul R, Moser D, Gordon N. Cognitive and motor impairments predict functional declines in vascular dementia. International J Geriatric Psychiatry, 2002;17:164–169.
32. Boyle P, Paul R, Moser D, Zawacki T, Gordon N, Cohen R. Cognitive and neurologic predictors of functional impairment in vascular dementia. Amer J Geriatric Psychiatry 2003;11:103–106.
33. Bennett HP, Corbett AJ, Gaden S, Grayson DA, Kril JJ, Broe GA. Subcortical vascular disease and functional decline: a 6- year predictor study. J Amer Geriatric Soc, 2002;50:1969–1977

IV Neuroimaging of Vascular Dementia

13

Functional Brain Imaging of Cerebrovascular Disease

Ronald Cohen, Lawrence Sweet, David F. Tate, and Marc Fisher

1. INTRODUCTION

One of the greatest challenges facing clinicians involved in the management of patients with cerebrovascular disease (CVD) is the detection and measurement of cerebral ischemia and associated metabolic changes that lead to infarctions in the brain *(1–4)*. Before the development of computed tomography (CT) methods, the diagnosis of stroke was largely dependent on the analysis of clinical signs and symptoms *(5)*. Although clinical findings may suggest an evolving stroke in a small proportion of patients, in most cases, cognitive and behavioral impairments are observed in the aftermath of a stroke that has caused a brain lesion resulting from infarction *(1–9)*. The use of standard CT and magnetic resonance imaging (MRI) as routine clinical procedures greatly facilitated the detection of brain abnormalities associated with stroke *(10–23)*, although these structural brain imaging methods have had only limited value in routine clinical management. Standard CT and MRI methods are excellent for detecting cerebral infarctions *(15,19,23)*, but physiologically abnormal tissue that is not completely necrotic often goes undetected *(24–26)*. The development of ultrafast and serial structural imaging methods has improved the early diagnosis of stroke *(18,19,25–28)*, but these methods still have limitations *(29,30)*.

These clinical challenges are amplified among patients with chronic CVD, particularly those with vascular dementia (VaD) *(31–34)*. Although the occurrence of a single large-vessel stroke is usually obvious to the patient or his or her family or doctors, smaller strokes frequently go undetected *(35,36)*. This is particularly true for small-vessel disease that affects the brain's white matter and subcortical systems. In such cases, detection of an evolving infarction is usually not possible. The clinical challenge is to determine whether the patient is having multiple small strokes with an accumulation of cerebral infarctions over time and to correlate observed functional decline with increases in lesion volume on brain imaging. Ultimately, it is extremely difficult for clinicians to draw firm conclusions from such analysis.

Dramatic strides have been made during the past decade in the development of functional neuroimaging techniques *(37–50)*. The term *functional brain imaging* often has been used to refer to techniques such as functional magnetic resonance imaging (fMRI) and positron emission tomography (PET) that enable the visualization and quantification of physiological brain processes associated with cognitive and behavioral functioning *(37–39)*. In this chapter, the term "functional brain imaging" is used more broadly to refer to all methods sensitive to the physiological mechanisms underlying brain function. Although traditional brain imaging methods are directed at neuroanatomic structure, many of the newer methods provide a window into neural mechanisms, ranging from metabolic characteristics to hemodynamic function to higher level cognitive processes. These techniques

From: *Current Clinical Neurology*
Vascular Dementia: Cerebrovascular Mechanisms and Clinical Management
Edited by: R. H. Paul, R. Cohen, B. R. Ott, and S. Salloway © Humana Press Inc., Totowa, NJ

Table 1
Functional Imaging Methods and Their Research and Clinical Value in Studying Vascular Dementia

Imaging method	Potential research and clinical values
Diffusion-weighted imaging (DWI)	• Quantifying penumbra volumes • Measuring evolution of infarction • Characterize physiology of ischemia
Diffusion tensor imaging	• Characterizing brain tissue integrity • Examining white matter and subcortical connectivity • Provides directional information for functional white matter pathways • Uses physiology to characterize structural connectivity
Perfusion-weighted imaging	• Quantified measure of blood flow and volume across brain regions • Provides sensitive early measure of potential lesion • Can be combined with DWI to correlate infarction development with diminished tissue perfusion • Physiological measure of ischemia
Magnetic resonance spectroscopy	• Characterize metabolic abnormalities secondary to cerebral ischemia • Biochemical indices
Functional magnetic resonance imaging	• Characterize functional neuroanatomic correlates of cognitive and behavioral sequela of stroke and vascular dementia • Used to measure cognition
Single photon emission tomography	• Provides relative cerebral blood flow measure • Can be used with subtraction methods to characterize functional neuroanatomic relationships • Used to measure both physiology and cognition • Can be used to study neurotransmitters and receptor systems
Positron emission tomography	• Provides absolute cerebral blood flow measure • Can be used with subtraction methods to characterize functional neuroanatomic relationships • Used to measure both physiology and cognition • Methodologically more demanding and expensive • Can be used to study neurotransmitors and receptor systems

include numerous methods that involve MRI, including diffusion-weighted imaging (DWI), perfusion-weighted imaging (PWI), diffusion tensor imaging (DTI), and fMRI imaging. Magnetic resonance spectroscopy (MRS) methods have also been developed that enable the measurement of metabolic abnormalities occurring in brain tissue as a result of neuropathological processes. Before the development of MRI methods, radiological techniques were developed, including PET and single photon emission computed tomography (SPECT). These methods rely on the detection of radioactive agents given to the patient before imaging is conducted. These MRI and radiological methods provide different types of information about brain functions and vascular dynamics that may help to better understand factors associated with the development of VaD. Each of these methods also has limitations and drawbacks that may affect their clinical use.

Table 1 summarizes the types of information that can be most directly derived from each method. Some of these methods are reviewed in greater detail in this chapter. However, first it is worth considering the general rationale and constraints that have bearing on clinical use of functional imaging methods for chronic CVD and VaD.

1.1. Rationale

Standard CT and MRI methods provide excellent spatial resolution for detecting neuroanatomic abnormalities in the brain, but they do not provide temporal resolution and are not useful for measuring brain processes and mechanisms. Functional brain imaging techniques provide both spatial and temporal resolution *(47)* and different sensitivities to brain processes and physiological processes. Furthermore, certain techniques can be used to measure biochemical abnormalities associated with brain metabolic changes and, therefore, can provide a window into the pathophysiology of brain diseases.

Functional neuroimaging methods provide several potential types of information that may be of great value for the analysis and clinical management of patients with VaD: (1) methods for directly relating cognitive and behavioral data to regional brain activity associated with cerebrovascular abnormalities, (2) methods for measuring and correlating cognitive and behavioral outcome after treatment with specific changes in brain activity, (3) methods for measuring and quantifying alterations in brain tissues that affect blood diffusion associated with cerebral ischemia, (4) methods for measuring and quantifying cerebral blood flow (CBF) in specific brain regions, (5) methods for examining the relationship between brain regions and pathways and the effects of tissue damage on functional connectivity, and (6) methods for measuring alterations in metabolic activity associated with vascular damage. Each of these methods has tremendous potential clinical use that is now only beginning to be explored.

1.2. Methodological Constraints

Functional brain imaging methods have great clinical potential, but they also have certain drawbacks that may affect their eventual utility. Some of these are general limitations common to all methods. First, it is important to note that all of these methods require sophisticated equipment, making routine clinical assessment more difficult to accomplish *(48)*. Most of these methods are not currently available as routine clinical tests, nor are most reimbursed by insurance companies. The technical demands of functional brain imaging require considerable expertise and infrastructure *(49)*. To translate these methods for clinical use, a team of specialists is needed, including the involvement of physicists, cognitive scientists, and physiologists, along with MR technicians. Typically, this is not possible except at large teaching hospitals.

Another limitation arises from the variability that exists across scanners and even across imaging sessions when the same scanner is used. This variability is less of problem for structural brain imaging, because typically multiple redundant sweeps across the brain occur and subtle variances across acquisitions are corrected for by averaging. Functional brain imaging uses the variation in blood oxygen level dependent (BOLD) signal over time, because consistent temporal variations can be correlated with task conditions to extract unique activation associated with specific task associated processes. However, the fact that there is less data redundancy when constructing functional images also amplifies the chance of error associated with any variations across time and between scanners.

Variability across scanners can result in distortions of signal intensity and localization *(48,49)*. This represents an obvious problem if clinical judgments are based on signal intensity or the relationship of different areas of regional activation. That different companies make scanners contributes to part of this problem. Although the general characteristics of scanners made by different companies may be similar, signal intensity parameter differences could greatly affect interpretation of findings. Even though efforts are underway to develop standards across scanners, this is issue is not fully resolved and currently affects clinical application.

Numerous methodological issues influence the standardization of functional imaging data and the ability to generalize findings across studies *(50–52)*. One standardization issue relates to the lack of adequate normative data for most brain neuroimaging methods. For example, fMRI studies have employed paradigms derived from a range of different cognitive tasks but most have employed relatively small sample sizes of normal control subjects *(50)*. Most of these studies were not conducted with goal of developing normative data for how people's brains respond during particular paradigms. With only limited efforts to date to establish normative databases with reliability and validity data for people across different age groups, it is difficult to interpret findings from a single patient *(51)*. Statistically, significant group differences in brain activity may reflect relatively subtle effects that are not readily apparent in the results from a single patient. Accordingly, before most techniques can become clinically useful, there is much standardization that needs to be accomplished for each of the functional brain imaging methods.

Methods that require the use of radiation (SPECT and PET) also have limitations related to health and safety. Although single assessments are generally not a problem with SPECT or PET, repeated measurements is more of a problem because it involves repeated exposure to radiation. Furthermore, these methods do not provide great spatial or temporal resolution. Even though SPECT and PET methods are discussed briefly, most of the focus of this chapter is on MR-based methods. The authors will not review studies of MRS, because it is beyond the scope of this chapter. However, MRS is another important MR-based method that enables analysis of the metabolic and biochemical characteristics of brain tissue. With MRS, it is possible to examine cellular changes associated with ischemia and other pathophysiological factors *(46)*. It can also be used to examine neurotransmitter characteristics in particular brain tissues, providing similar information to what is available from radiological approaches.

In the remainder of this chapter, the authors: (1) summarize the assumptions and basic methods underlying each of these brain imaging approaches, (2) describe methodological constraints that affect their clinical application, (3) review efforts to date to apply these methods to the study of CVD (particularly VaD), and (4) discuss how these methods could be applied in the future for the study and clinical assessment of VaD. Because relatively few studies have applied these methods directly to VaD, the authors focus much of their review on brain neuroimaging studies of healthy people who are both young and elderly and brain disorders that affect VaD (e.g., Alzheimer's disease [AD] and stroke). The authors then present existing data from studies of VaD and chronic CVD.

2. DIFFUSION-WEIGHTED IMAGING

DWI represents an important extension of standard MR methods. DWI provides a unique and powerful method for imaging subtle differences in water content and diffusion across different tissue types. Because DWI is particularly sensitive to the structural changes related to ischemic events *(53,54)*, it is particularly interesting to cerebrovascular researchers. Currently, two primary methods exist, DWI and DTI, which is an adaptation of DWI that enables measurement of directional diffusion across the brain. The basic principles of DWI and DTI methods, findings from studies using these methods with clinical populations, and their potential use for the clinical management of VaD are briefly reviewed.

2.1. Methodological Considerations

Diffusion-weighted MRI is complicated, and only the basic principles of this imaging technique are discussed in this chapter. For a more detailed description of diffusion-weighted physics, the reader is referred to additional outside sources *(55–57)*. Diffusion imaging relies on the basic principal of random molecular diffusion. Diffusion refers to the physical phenomena of "random" or isotropic movement of molecules through a medium. In biological tissues, this movement is not entirely random or uniform but dependent on physiological and physical characteristics of the particular tissue type. By measuring rates of diffusion, it is possible to contrast the physiological characteristics of brain tissue at different points in time. In DWI, diffusion coefficients are derived that reflect the degree of motion of water molecules within a region of interest. In living tissue, the "isotropic" motion is restricted by the presence of various structural components of tissue (i.e., cellular membranes, organelles, and macromolecules), as well as the size, shape, orientation, and spacing between these cellular microstructures. This restriction in molecular motion—called anisotropic motion—can be imaged and used to infer basic information regarding the histological integrity and connectivity of the cells within living tissue. For example, because of the shape and size of neuronal cell bodies, gray matter structures do not restrict the randomness of molecular movement like highly oriented and myelinated white matter fiber tracts. Thus, diffusion within gray matter structures is generally higher than that observed in white matter.

Furthermore, subtle cellular changes resulting from alterations in ionic content, inflammation, and other pathophysiological processes can be detected by DWI because of its sensitivity to intracellular fluid dynamics and its effect on the cell's structural characteristics *(53,58,59)*. Accordingly, temporal information derived from DWI can provide a useful window into how brain tissue changes with time. Tissue that is completely healthy with normal physiological function will have different diffusion characteristics than dysfunctional tissue in which abnormal ionic channel function and biochemical disturbances are occurring. This effect is evident when one examines the results of studies that have examined the evolution of stroke in laboratory animals *(60–63)*. As the stroke evolves, there are points in time when an infarction is not yet evident on structural imaging involving standard T1 or T2 MRI but where clear changes are apparent on DWI. These changes lend potential insights into the effects of cerebral ischemia on the development of penumbra, which is tissue that is physiologically dysfunctional but still living.

2.2. DTI Method

Diffusion within brain tissues measured by DWI yields a numerical value called the apparent diffusion coefficient (ADC), which indicates the degree to which water moves freely throughout the tissue within the region of interest. ADC values are readily determined using standard DWI methods. However, these methods do not provide information about the diffusion along directional pathways, because ADC is generally measured within a single plane.

During the past several years, DWI techniques have been extended to enable the measurement of diffusion along multiple planes, yielding information regarding diffusion directionality. These methods, referred to as DTI, are based on there being a restriction of diffusion parallel to the spatial orientation of brain tissue that is organized in directional pathways (directional anisotropy). This results because the diffusion of water is faster parallel to the direction of the white matter tract than perpendicular. Because white matter fibers are highly organized, the direction and magnitude of restricted diffusion along white matter tissue can be imaged to provide additional information regarding the integrity and connectivity of white matter pathways within the brain. By contrasting differences in diffusion across spatial orientations, it is possible to characterize the direction of diffusion and visualize these pathways. There is now considerable empirical evidence supporting the ability of DTI to delineate white matter pathways and enabling investigators the means of examining structural abnormalities along these pathways (*see* Fig. 1).

Furthermore, DTI provides an index of the directional coherence of the particular pathways being imaged called fractional anisotropy (FA). FA is a numerical representation of the degree of anisotropy or directional diffusion within the white matter fibers. This measure of directional coherence provides information about how highly organized the pathway is and its integrity. DTI data can also be analyzed to determine the correlation of spatial orientation between different regions of brain tissue. This value, called the lattice anisotropy (LA) coefficient, provides another way of examining the connectivity of brain tissue and the integrity of the white matter pathways and interconnected brain systems.

2.3. Clinical Evidence From Diffusion Imaging

Given the type of information that can be derived from DWI, clinical researchers have directed considerable attention to using DWI to gain insights into the characteristics of diseased and injured brain tissue (central nervous system [CNS]). Some of these efforts have direct relevance to VaD, including studies of acute stroke; leukoaraiosis, cases of cerebral autosomal dominant arteriopathy with subcortical infarcts and leukoencephalopathy (CADASIL), and studies of normal aging and dementia.

2.4. Cerebrovascular Disorders

During the past decade, DWI has been studied as a potential neurodiagnostic tool for measuring the evolution of cerebral infarction. The guiding principle is that during the early stages of stroke, patients often present with subtle clinical deficits and normal findings on CT scan, making it difficult for the clinicians to determine whether the patients are actually experiencing a stroke. DWI provides a mechanism by which clinicians can detect stroke early in its course and measure tissue changes associated with ischemia.

Laboratory studies in which arterial occlusion was induced in cats demonstrated that ischemic brain tissue begins to show changes in DWI indices that are readily apparent within minutes of the occlusion. The changes in diffusion characteristics within the affected tissue result in bright hyperintense regions on imaging that are easily distinguished from unaffected tissue *(61,62)*. These DWI signal changes occur despite the lack of significant abnormalities indicative of stroke on CT. Thus, one of the primary clinical uses of DWI is to investigate the impact and extent of ischemic events in patients who are presenting with acute stroke and/or acute transient ischemic attacks (TIAs).

Interestingly, studies of stroke demonstrate a temporal evolution of diffusion characteristics within the ischemic region *(63–68)*. These changes are similar in both animal models of stroke and human studies in clinical samples, which show initial reduction of ADC during the acute phase of the stroke. The decrease in ADC is followed by a normalization and gradual increase in ADC during chronic stages of stroke.

More specifically, DWI studies have shown a reduction in ADC (60–70% reduction) within the hyperintense regions during the early stages of a stroke *(65)*. These changes in the diffusion characteristics are believed to be related to the failure of ionic pumping and the resultant cytotoxic edema. This energy-dependent pump is susceptible to the acute loss of energy when the blood flow is reduced during ischemic events. Once the pump fails, the cell begins to swell as osmotically obligated extracellular water flows into the cell. This movement of water decreases the extracellular space and is correlated with reductions of the ADC value. Over time, cell lyses and macrophage activity increase in the affected areas, leading to vasogenic edema. This physiological change leads to a renormalization of ADC values, followed by a gradual increase in ADC in older infarct areas *(65,66)*. This is opposite to what is observed in acute phases of stroke and likely reflects the increased diffusion of water molecules in the extracellular space.

Studies also demonstrate temporal changes in the diffusion anisotropy (directional diffusion) over time, which, once again, are similar in both animal models and human clinical studies *(67–69)*. In the acute phases of the stroke, anisotropy is generally increased. This is believed to be related to the decrease in space between the myelin bundles and the increased membrane tortuosity, resulting in additional restriction of water movement, except in the plane parallel to the axon bundles. As the cells begin to lose their structural integrity, anisotropy is significantly reduced in the affected regions when compared to normal tissue within the same subject. In fact, Werring et al. demonstrated that anisotropy remains reduced in the infarct 2 to 6 mo after the stroke *(70)*.

Thus, the observed changes in diffusion are useful in understanding the distinct time course or evolution of ischemic related injuries. It also demonstrates the unique ability of diffusion-weighted techniques in understanding the various underlying pathological changes in the connectivity and integrity of tissue at the cellular level, despite the current resolution limitations of structural MRI techniques.

The major limitation of the method is clinical feasibility, because it requires that patients be scanned early in the course of acute stroke (i.e., within the first few hours) and that they remain still for the duration of the scan because DWI is more susceptible to the effects of motion than other

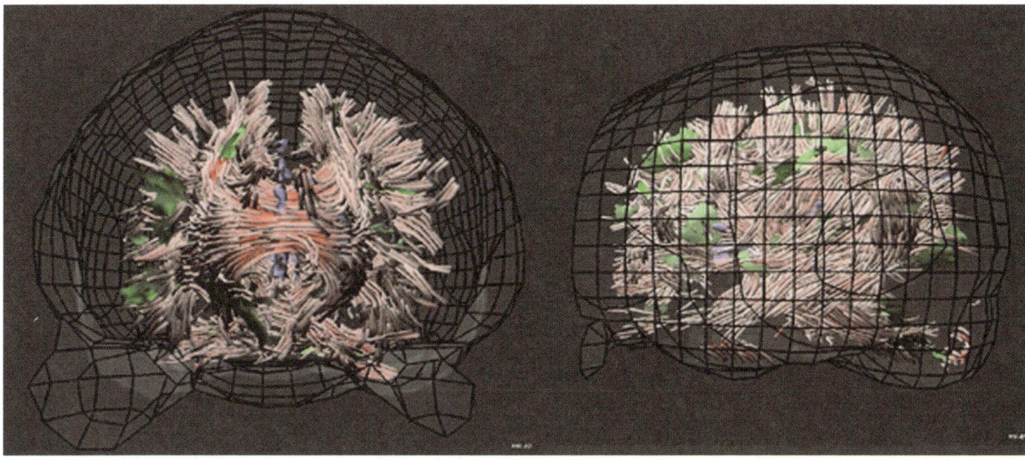

Fig. 1. These are three-dimensional images of diffusion tensor maps. Tractography is s a common way of visualizing the complicated directional diffusion data collected during the imaging session. This method allows the investigator or clinician to view all of the major white matter pathways throughout the brain and make inferences about the functional connectivity and integrity of these connections. *Note:* Coronal view on the left and Sagital view on the right. (Images courtesy of David Laidlaw, PhD, Brown University Computer Science Department.)

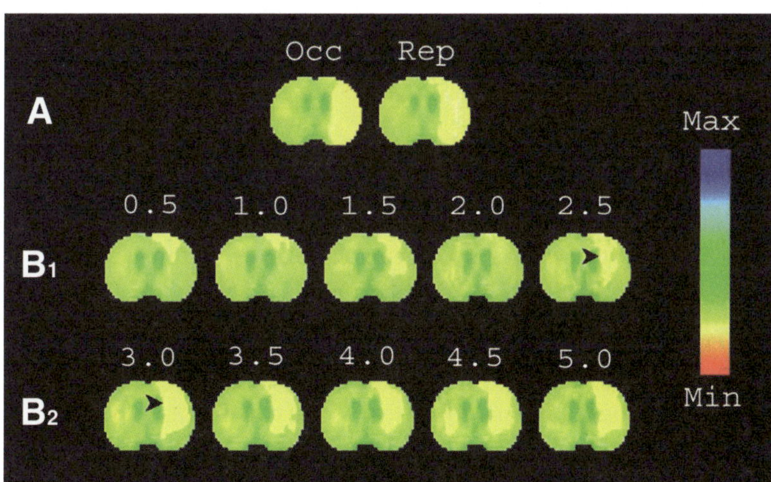

Fig. 2. Diffusion-weighted images (DWI) of the brain following occlusion of the middle cerebral artery in rats. The two pictures in line A depict both a complete infarction (Occ) when no reperfusion has occurred and a brain immediately following occlusion. The pictures in B_1 and B_2 show the brain at 30 min intervals. As cortical ischemia persists over this time period, infarction volume increases as shown by an increase in yellow areas on the brain image. The black arrows show the time point at 3 h when the infarction has fully developed and there is a reduced chance of tissue recovery with reperfusion.

imaging techniques. Furthermore, the clinicians have been slow to adopt this diagnostic method, although increasingly it is being included in clinical trials of new therapies to treat stroke. Therefore, it is likely to become a more routine part of clinical assessment during the next several years. Though the primary focus of DWI in CVD has been measuring the evolution of infarction acutely after large-vessel occlusion, the principles underlying its use in assessing cerebral ischemia before complete infarction could be applied to patients with more chronic diffuse cerebral ischemic disease, which presumably is the substrate of most cases of VaD (*see* Fig. 2).

2.5. Small-Vessel Ischemic Disease

The occurrence of diffuse changes in periventricular and subcortical white matter observed on both CT and MRI have been identified as a significant finding in VaD *(71,72)*. These findings are believed to reflect the accumulation of infarctions of small vessels that are abundant in subcortical areas. Unlike large-vessel infarctions, which are easier to link to specific clinical cerebrovascular events, these subcortical and periventricular white matter findings have a more gradual development course. Accordingly, DWI could provide unique insights into the evolution of infarctions in patients who show such changes, because it should provide evidence of brain tissue dysfunction associated with chronic ischemic disease. Yet, to date there are relatively few DWI studies of patients with small-vessel ischemic disease, although recent research has been directed at using DTI to characterize subcortical white matter injury.

In one study, Jones et al. used DTI methods to compare measures of mean diffusivity and anisotropy in a group of nine patients with small-vessel ischemic disease, defined by the appearance of periventricular white matter changes on conventional MRI *(73)*. All of the patients had a clinical history of lacunar stroke and/or a subcortical dementia believed to be of vascular origin. Their findings showed an elevation in mean diffusivity (restricted movement) and reduced anisotropy (restricted directional movement) in patients with leukoaraiosis compared to controls. For example, in the right subcortical white matter, the mean diffusivity was significantly elevated in patients with leukoaraiosis when compared to controls, whereas fractional anisotropy was significantly reduced. Jones et al. attributed these findings to the proliferation of glial tissue and increases in extracellular space, which are commonly observed in the histopathological studies of leukoaraiosis *(73,74)*.

2.6. Cerebral Autosomal Dominant Arteriopathy With Subcortical Infarcts and Leukoencephalopathy (CADASIL)

This genetically determined (autosomal dominant) small-artery disease linked to mutations on chromosome 19 causes a progressive degeneration of white matter pathways, severe motor disability, pseudobulbar palsy, and dementia *(75)*. A hallmark of CADASIL is the presence of white matter hyperintensities (WMHs) on T2-weighted MRI. Yet, the extent of MRI hyperintensities varies across CADASIL patients, and severity of dementia is not consistently related to the extent of white matter abnormalities on T2-weighted MRI, because patients with dementia can have similar lesions as asymptomatic CADASIL patients. Because of its sensitivity to subtle dysfunction in white matter, DTI offers a means of better characterizing changes associated with cognitive decline.

Chabriat et al. used DTI to characterize white matter connectivity in CADASIL *(76)*. Sixteen symptomatic CADASIL patients and 10 age-matched controls were studied, with mean diffusivity and diffusion anisotropy measured within and outside hyperintense areas identified on T2-weighted MRIs. There was a 60% increase in mean diffusivity with similar reduction in diffusion anisotropy in hyperintense regions. Normal-appearing white matter (using T2-weighted images) also had increased mean diffusivity compared to controls, indicating more subtle changes not observed in T2 imaging. Changes in diffusivity and anisotropy were associated with cognitive functioning measured by the Mini-Mental State Examination (MMSE) and disability on a physical handicap scale (Rankin). In contrast, standard T2 MRIs have shown little or no relationship with these measures in CADASIL *(77)*.

DTI diffusivity and anisotropy findings were attributed to changes in extracellular space in these patients with CADSIL. This expansion in extracellular space is believed to be caused by the loss of white matter structural components, such as astrocytes, axons, and myelin, which is characteristic of patients with CADSIL *(78)*. These nonspecific changes in white matter have been observed in clinicopathological postmortem studies, which have documented significant increases in extracellular space. This is similar to the findings in patients with leukoaraiosis mentioned in Section 2.5. Thus, diffusion imaging techniques are a useful technique in monitoring disease progression among patients with CADASIL.

2.7. DWI in Aging and Dementia

Studies of normal neuronal development and aging using diffusion imaging created a great deal of excitement during the early stages of DTI development. DTI clearly demonstrated pronounced age-related region-specific increases in diffusion anisotropy during childhood and early adolescence *(79,80)*. Although not directly compared, the DTI findings are related to the regional specific increases in white matter volume (owing to myelination) observed in developmental studies of normal aging children and adolescents.

In aging studies, diffusion imaging studies have shown significant declines in white matter organization and order as participants age *(81–84)*. These declines in anisotropy (FA) most likely result from the microstructural changes found in normal aging; namely loss of myelin and axonal fibers. These changes lead to increases in extracellular space, which, in turn, alter the diffusion imaging results. Furthermore, these changes in anisotropy appear even in the absences of abnormal morphological findings on conventional T1-, T2-, or proton density-weighted MR images.

DWI and DTI have also proved useful in studying the effects of abnormal aging, as in the case of Alzheimer's disease (AD). The medial temporal lobes and associated limbic and paralimbic structures (e.g., hippocampus and entorhinal cortex) are affected early in AD, producing prominent impairments in the encoding and storage of new memory *(85,86)*. MRI studies of AD readily show the loss of hippocampal volume, and there are even some morphological changes in large white matter fiber tracts, such as the corpus callosum. The changes in white matter are believed to be secondary to neuronal cell death in the affected gray matter nuclei in the brain.

There have been several studies of AD using DWI. In a study looking at the effect of diagnostic classification of AD on diffusion characteristics, Hanyo et al. demonstrated a stepwise decrease in regional anisotropy that was related to the classification of participants as having "possible" and "probable" AD *(87)*. They demonstrated reductions in anisotropy in the white matter tracts of the temporal stem in the "possible" AD group that was significantly lower than that of age-matched controls. Additional reductions in anisotropy were demonstrated in temporal stem among "probable" AD when compared to the "possible" AD participants. These significant findings were found, despite normal diffusivity within the hippocampus. Reductions in the temporal stem anisotropy despite normal diffusivity within the hippocampus was believed to be related to the accumulation of cell inclusion material known to be caused by AD (plaques and neurofibrillary tangles), which would restrict the directional diffusivity of water along the axonal pathways obstructed by such cellular debris.

Recently, Kantarci et al. studied regional diffusivity of water in a group of normally aging individuals and compared them to the findings in patients with mild cognitive impairment (MCI) and AD *(88)*. Measures of ADC and anisotropy (anisotropy index) were compared for several regions of interest, including the gray matter thalami and hippocampal structures and the frontal, temporal, parietal, occipital, and posterior cingulate white matter. A single significant difference in ADC values was noted in the hippocampus when comparing the MCI group and controls. This difference in hippocampal ADC for patients with MCI was similar to that of patients with AD. Additional significant differences in the temporal stem, occipital, parietal, posterior cingulate, and hippocampus were noted when comparing AD patients and controls. Mean ADC was nearly always higher in patients with MCI than in controls and lower than patients with AD for each of the regions of interest, although these differences were not significant. These trends toward difference are believed to be related to the many patients presenting with isolated memory impairment who will convert to AD in their lifetime. Therefore, MCI is often viewed as being on the continuum between normal aging and AD. Additionally, there is neuropathological evidence of neurofibrillary conditions in postmortem studies of patients with isolated memory problems, such as patients with MCI.

Hanyu et al. compared the diffusion imaging characteristics in the cerebral white matter of patients with AD with periventricular hyperintensities, a group of patients with VaD of the Binswanger type, and age-matched controls *(89)*. Patients with AD and Binswanger's disease had similar nonsignificantly different ADC values in the anterior and posterior white matter that were significantly higher than controls. Ratios designed to look at the directional diffusion characteristics were also significantly higher in the dementia groups when compared to controls. However, the patients with AD had higher ratios in the posterior white matter, and patients with Binswanger's disease had higher ratios in the anterior white matter.

These several studies taken together indicate the sensitivity of diffusion imaging to the pathophysiological changes that occur in several disease states related to VaD. During the next several years, it is expected that more studies in VaD will be conducted using diffusion imaging because measure of diffusivity and anisotropy have the potential to distinguish between subtle types of microstructural damage in types of dementia. Additionally, regional analyses of white matter involvement are likely to demonstrate differences between dementia types, which could lead to more specific classification of dementia, as well as impact treatment.

3. PERFUSION-WEIGHTED IMAGING

PWI uses fast gradient-echo or spin-echo pulse sequences to observe the movement of a paramagnetic contrast agent through capillaries over time. Usually a bolus of an exogenous nonionizing contrast agent, such as gadolinium, is administered intravenously. This leads to magnetic field inhomogeneities and, therefore, greater T2 signal attenuation in brain regions with greater blood perfusion. Noninvasive methods have also been developed that magnetically label blood to be used as an endogenous contrast agent. This is done by manipulating proton spins before the blood reaches the region of interest (ROI) *(90–92)*. These methods are typically named arterial spin labeling (ASL). Several perfusion characteristics can be derived from contrast PWI or ASL. These include cerebral blood volume (CBV), the ratio of blood volume to tissue volume; CBF, the volume of blood delivered to the tissue volume per minute; and mean transit time (MTT), the average time it takes the contrast to pass through the tissue.

PWI applied to neurological disorders is a growing field of research with a growing list of clinical applications. For example, PWI is useful in predicting neurological outcome in head injury *(93)*, cardiac surgery *(94,95)*, and epilepsy *(96)*. However, studies of stroke have been the most common experimental and clinical application, and several studies of patients with brain tumors and internal carotid artery occlusion have also been reported. The following sections describe the use of PWI in selected patient populations most relevant to CVD.

3.1. *Leukoaraiosis*

Of special relevance to VaD is a PWI study of eight patients with ischemic leukoaraiosis. Patients exhibited less CBF in white matter ROIs and greater CBV in gray matter ROIs compared to healthy control participants. MTTs were longer among the patients in superior white matter. The authors concluded that white matter hypoperfusion might underlie leukoaraiosis *(97)*.

3.2. *Alzheimer's Dementia*

Studies have demonstrated the diagnostic use of PWI and ASL among patients with AD. One group compared 19 patients with AD to 18 age-matched healthy control participants. They demonstrated less bilateral temporoparietal PWI-CBV among the patients and diagnosed with a sensitivity of 88–95% and specificity of 96% *(98–100)*. Alsop and colleagues *(101)* demonstrated less ASL-measured CBF in temporal, parietal, and frontal cortices among 18 patients with AD compared to 11 age-matched control subjects. These investigations concluded that PWI is a good alternative to SPECT and PET in this population. It is noteworthy that these patients with AD exhibited cortical hypoperfusion, whereas patients with leukoaraiosis *(97)* exhibited white matter hypoperfusion.

3.3. Stroke

Cerebral ischemia has been the most frequently studied neuropathy using PWI. These studies have shown that PWI is useful in the diagnosis of stroke, identification of ischemic tissue, prediction of infarct volume, and the evaluation of treatment outcome *(102–110)*. Specifically, increased CBF, increased CBV, and decreased MTT suggest that tissue is involved in acute ischemia *(106,111)*, whereas CBF and CBV predict final infarct volume *(104–106,111)*. In individual unilateral stroke patients, PWI values from the affected hemisphere are often compared to these measures from the unaffected hemisphere to identify and determine the volume of ischemic tissue. When the PWI-identified abnormal tissue volume exceeds the volume identified by DWI, the excess tissue is in danger of permanent infarct *(110–117)*. Thus, PWI can be used in addition to DWI to identify ischemic tissue in danger of infarct, and when combined both methods are more sensitive and specific than either alone. However, PWI has unique value in identifying TIAs and subarachnoid hemorrhage *(118)*. In summary, the use of PWI in identifying ischemic tissue is evident in its growing use in clinical settings. It appears to have the potential to better identify ischemic events not identified by DWI images and may, therefore, be of special value in the study and clinical treatment of VaD.

3.4. Other Cerebrovascular Applications

Abnormal PWI findings have been associated with chronic occlusive carotid artery disease in a series of studies *(119–122)*. In these studies, perfusion response rate (time to peak response) was a more reliable marker of carotid disease severity than CBV. Therefore, PWI can be used as a reliable indicator of chronic occlusive carotid artery disease. Another study of giant aneurisms of the intracranial internal carotid artery found that less CBF and more variable blood volume were strong predictors of recovery on functional measures after bypass surgery *(123)*. Such studies show how PWI can be applied beyond acute stroke to the study of chronic CVD.

Because of its sensitivity to subtle vascular abnormalities and changes in perfusion, PWI has been demonstrated to aid in the identification and diagnostic classifications of tumors and in evaluating treatment outcome. Lower CBF and CBV have been observed in areas of edema surrounding meningioma *(124)*, and greater CBV has been used to differentiate brain tumors from pyogenic cerebral abscess *(125)* and AIDS-related toxoplasmosis *(126)*. Sugahara and colleagues *(127)* found greater CBV in recurring neoplasm than nonneoplastic enhancing tissue after resection. Different PWI characteristics may be useful in distinguish between types of tumors *(128,129)*. Two studies have also reported volume to be a useful measure in determining the grade of gliomas *(129,130)*. These advances represent an improvement over traditional contrast MRI resulting from identification, classification, and differentiation of tumors compared to traditional methods (e.g., PET and SPECT). PWI is advantageous because of its lower cost, safety, and imaging resolution.

3.5. Advantages and Future Directions

Compared to PET, SPECT, and structural MRI, PWI has been demonstrated to be as sensitive and specific to several neurological disorders (e.g., AD and stroke). In some instances, PWI better detects and differentiates pathology (e.g., tumor or transient ischemia). Improved spatial resolution is an important feature that may prove advantageous in future studies of VaD. Other clear advantages of ASL-based PWI over traditional methods include availability, cost, no radiation, and noninvasiveness.

Although few clinical studies using ASL have been published *(96,131–132)*, they represent a promising future direction. This method can even be used as an alternative to BOLD fMRI *(133)*.

Despite the additional advantages of noninvasiveness and the ability to image areas of high BOLD susceptibility artifact, ASL techniques are less frequently used in part because of the lack of availability of pulse sequences and lower signal-to-noise ratios. Other disadvantages of this method for PWI are lower signal-to-noise ratios, only partial brain coverage, low signal change, and vascular artifacts, the need for complicated methods to control for arterial artifact *(134–136)*. Variable delays in arterial dispersion of labeled bolus in patients may also be confound for certain PWI methods *(137)*.

4. FUNCTIONAL MAGNETIC RESONANCE IMAGING

MRI methods have been developed during the past 13 yr that enable cognitive neuroscientists to measure brain activation associated with various cognitive and behavioral tasks. These methods, commonly referred to as fMRI, capitalize on the subtle variations in vascular hemodynamics that occur in the brain during the course of a single imaging session. With traditional MRI aimed at high-resolution depiction of brain anatomy and structural abnormalities, these physiological variations are a source of error, which are averaged out by collecting redundant scans with as much control of head position as possible. However, variations in MR signal that occur on a moment-to-moment basis contain much useful information about metabolic differences across brain areas. When MRI acquisition is coupled with precise experimental tasks that enable this variation to be fractionated by different cognitive conditions, it is possible to obtain data that reflect physiological brain changes associated with specific cognitive processes (*see* Fig. 3).

The most common fMRI technique involves the measurement of BOLD that occur as people perform cognitive tasks. BOLD takes advantage of the magnetic properties of hemoglobin for use as an endogenous contrast agent. The principle behind BOLD is that deoxyhemoglobin is paramagnetic, whereas oxyhemoglobin is not. It has been observed that neural activity leads to the delivery of an excess of oxyhemoglobin. A smaller deoxyhemoglobin to oxyhemoglobin ratio in the capillary beds surrounding active neurons yields a more homogenous magnetic field and a greater MR signal. Although increased neural activity results in vasodilation and greater delivery of oxygen-rich blood, the intervening mechanisms have not been well established. For example, CBF and volume also affect BOLD signal *(138)*.

Since the first reports of noncontrast echoplanar BOLD *(139)* and the application to human experiments 2 yr later *(140–142)*, BOLD fMRI has rapidly diversified in terms of cognitive domains and populations studied. The earliest studies examined primary visual and motor cortices among healthy participants; however, the technique was soon applied to investigations of higher order cognitive functions of every cognitive domain (e.g., memory, language, attention, and emotional functioning). fMRI investigators have increasingly directed their attention to participants of all ages and several psychiatric and neurologic populations. Healthy cognitive functioning *(143–159)*, as well as developmental disorders, such as epilepsy *(160–164)*, dyslexia *(165–172)*, and attention-deficit/hyperactivity disorder (ADHD) *(173–175)* have been studied among children. Psychiatric disorders studied include substance abuse (cocaine *[176–180]*, nicotine *[181–184]*, and alcohol *[185–190]*), anxiety disorders (phobias *[191–193]* and obsessive-compulsive disorder *[194,195]*), schizophrenia *(196–203)*, and personality disorders (antisocial *[204]*). Neurological populations studied include patients with multiple sclerosis *(205–208)*, Parkinson's disease *(209–214)*, and AD *(215–219)*. VaD studies have yet to appear; however, other chronic cerebrovascular disorders have been studied. These include acute stroke and stroke recovery *(220–225)*, arteriovenous malformation *(226,227)*, migraine headaches *(228,229)*, and CADASIL *(230)*.

fMRI data acquisition sessions involve stimulus presentation and usually some type of behavioral response. BOLD signal is sampled in repeated acquisitions of a brain volume during a carefully designed stimulus presentation protocol. Brain volumes may include the whole brain or selected slices in any plane. For example, one whole-brain volume might be acquired every 3 s. These resulting raw data undergo several preprocessing steps to yield a time-dependent signal course for each pixel of each slice (i.e., each voxel). Repetitions are assigned to appropriate experi-

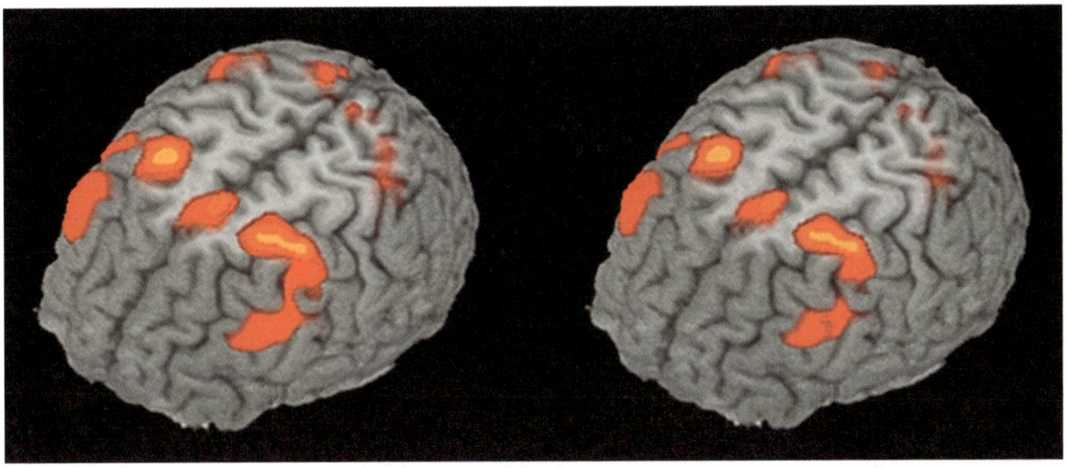

Fig. 3. These three-dimensional brain maps illustrate the active regions of the brain across 17 healthy control subjects performing a working memory task commonly used in fMRI studies. Active regions are shown in red and represent regional changes in blood flow compared to each subject's individual resting brain state.

mental conditions, which may be contrasted within an individual, summarized for group comparisons, or both.

The raw BOLD signal obtained from each voxel of an individual is typically converted to a standardized metric according to some theoretical model to allow comparison across subjects or time. For example, a simple method is subtracting an individual's mean baseline signal from mean signal during the experimental condition. These mean difference scores may be compared to a hypothetical mean of zero (i.e., the null hypothesis) using a one-sample student's *t*-test for each voxel. Other methods, such as cross-correlation and multiple regression, can be used to determine how closely each voxel's time course is related to the time course of the stimulation. Thus, individual data sets are assigned a value per voxel that corresponds to the voxel's intensity change between conditions (e.g., difference scores or *t* values) or relatedness to the stimulus presentation (e.g., *r* values).

The term "activation" is usually used to denote voxels in which intensity of the MR signal or the relatedness of the MR signal to the task presentation exceeds a significance threshold that is usually corrected for multiple comparisons. Volumes of activation may be quantified by counting the number of voxels exceeding the threshold. Grouped statistical comparisons are performed once the individual dependent variable is calculated and the ROI is specified. Associated behavioral data, if recorded, are used to validate that participants adequately performed the task and to test performance related experimental hypotheses.

The early BOLD fMRI experiments used subtraction and cross-correlation analyses of block designs to demonstrate task associated BOLD response in primary motor or visual processing areas. For example, Bandettini and colleagues *(231)* identified brain voxels most related to the time course of a self-paced finger-tapping task. fMRI studies of higher order cognitive processes, such as language *(232)* and executive functions *(233)*, began to appear soon after using similar cross-correlation methods. Early studies typically did not examine the whole brain and tended to include small sample sizes. However, these methods were soon applied to experiments employing whole-brain imaging and larger sample sizes. For example Rao and colleagues *(234)* reported a whole-brain network of cortical and subcortical brain structures that exhibited activity associated with a conceptual reasoning paradigm among eleven healthy adults. Another major advance in fMRI was the development of linear multiple regression methods to identify activity associated with rapid presentation of stimulus trials *(235–238)*. This advance grew out of the findings that BOLD responses could be detected after brief stimuli (<1 s) and that responses to such stimuli were additive and approximately linear *(237–240)*. These were significant advances because event-related designs could be developed that did not require long interstimulus intervals to allow the hemodynamic response to return to baseline *(237)*. Event-related designs also provided more flexibility than the blocked design, which had been the predominant neuroimaging paradigm during decades of PET research. Other advantages of event-related design include observation of the evolution of activity over short periods of time (e.g., 10 s) *(240)* and the ability to retrospectively bin stimulus events into different conditions based on performance *(241)*.

Although these studies contribute to the understanding of healthy brain function, they have also laid a methodological and theoretical foundation with which we may contrast patient populations. The methods and findings of fMRI studies of stroke, AD, and healthy geriatric populations are particularly relevant in guiding future studies of patients with chronic CVD, such as VaD.

4.1. Comparison Groups

Several fMRI studies of older adults have appeared since the mid 1990s *(242–264)* that may be useful to help us differentiate expected from unexpected hemodynamic changed among older adults. This is crucial because uncontrolled studies of VaD may identify fMRI changes among their older participants that are related to aging rather than VaD *per se*. On the other hand, VaD may end up presenting an extreme example of normal aging that is qualitatively similar but quantitatively extreme. Most fMRI studies of older adults have focused on cognitive domains in which patients with VaD typically demonstrate impairment, memory encoding, working memory, and motor functions. However, a few have examined emotional perception, sensory perception (vision *[255]* and olfaction *[254]*), and executive functions (dual task *[258]* and Stroop interference *[260]*).

Among the studies of memory encoding, the most common findings are less prefrontal activity in expected areas *(243,244)* but more bilateral activity, particularly if older participants performed equally to younger participants *(244–247)*. In contrast, greater prefrontal activation has been reported among older adults who performed well during verbal working memory tasks *(248,249)*. A robust finding across motor studies is that older adults demonstrate decreased BOLD activity within primary motor and somatosensory areas *(250,251)*. There is some evidence that greater supplementary motor association areas recruitment occurs compared to younger controls *(252)*. Studies of basic perception, such as vision and olfaction have also reported less activity compared to younger control participants *(253–255)*, whereas more complex perception facial emotion has been associated with less activity in expected regions *(256,257)*.

Some higher order cognitive functions other than memory have been studied among older adults. Dual task performance has yielded similar patterns of activity between younger and older groups; however, each task alone continued to elicit dorsolateral prefrontal cortex activation among the older group but not the younger group *(258)*. Attentional interference tasks have shown a pattern of increased and more bilateral prefrontal and parietal activation pattern among equal performers *(259)* and produced less frontal and parietal activity among older participants with lower scores *(260)*.

Taken together, the major findings of fMRI studies of older adults suggest that BOLD signal declines with age-related declines in cognitive performance and perception. Furthermore, a compensatory bilateral frontal activation pattern emerges, particularly when participants are matched to younger controls for performance. These trends in fMRI studies of older adults point to the importance of understanding normal changes in aging brain function that may be mistaken as a result of a dementia. The cognitive domains studied among older adults (executive, memory, and motor functioning) provide an excellent foundation of what to expect in studies of VaD, because they are areas of deficit in this population. Because hemodynamic properties normally change with advancing age, it is possible that these finding among healthy older adults will be evident among patients with VaD but with greater effects. Unfortunately, to date, fMRI aging research has tended to map and compare activation patterns, but few have examined why lower BOLD signal is evident among older adults. Visual and motor studies have revealed longer hemodynamic lags, later peak intensity, more intersubject variability, and lower signal-to-noise ratios *(253,261,262)*. Lower BOLD signal has also been confirmed with near-infrared spectroscopy (NIRS) *(263,264)*, suggesting that it is not a fMRI methodological artifact. Attenuated hypercapnic BOLD signal response among older participants compared you younger participants during a finger-tapping task suggests that older cerebral vessels may not normally dilate *(250)*. These age effects on BOLD signal are not be surprising, given other vascular changes occur in older adults, such as slower capillary refill times and an increased incidence of CVD.

4.2. Dementia

Although fMRI studies of VaD have not yet appeared, memory, language, and visuospatial abilities have been examined among patients with AD. These patients tend to present a picture of shifting activity, typically less activity in expected regions and greater activity in other regions suggestive of compensatory neural mechanisms. Several fMRI memory studies among patients with mild AD reported less BOLD signal, or the lack of expected activation, in the temporal lobe compared to healthy control participants who performed better *(215–217)*. For example, one study demonstrated less hippocampal activity and less behavioral accuracy among patients with mild AD compared to younger healthy control participants while encoding face-name associations (Spurling). Meanwhile, greater recruitment of visual association and parietal cortices was evident in this and another study of patients with AD *(215,217)*. Compensatory recruitment has also been suggested in fMRI studies of other cognitive domains. Language tasks, such as lexical fluency among elderly at high genetic risk for AD and verbal categorization among patients with mild AD, also suggest compensatory recruitment in parietal and frontal regions, respectively. A study of line orientation among patients with mild AD revealed lower parietal and greater occipitotemporal activity compared to control participants *(218)*, suggesting compensation of the impaired dorsal visuospatial stream by the ventral visual object identification stream *(214)*. It is important to note that atrophy significantly contributed to their findings. Atrophy was directly studied in another study of verbal categorization, where it was positively correlated with inferior frontal activity but unrelated to temporal activity *(219)*. These studies suggest compensatory mechanisms shift activation patterns even before the onset of AD and point to the importance of accounting for brain atrophy in fMRI studies of AD.

4.3. Stroke

The majority of fMRI studies of stroke populations focus on recovery of language and motor functions subsequent to large vessel infarcts or lacunes. The few studies of stroke patients who have aphasia have demonstrated that their language dysfunction is associated with greater contralateral and perilesional activation than expected from healthy control groups. Furthermore, greater bilateral activity and greater perilesional activity were associated with better language recovery *(220,221)*.

The most consistent finding from investigations of recovery of motor functions (typically hemiparetic patients) are increased ipsilateral primary somatosensory area activity compared to healthy control participants *(222–225)*. An interesting finding is that this ipsilateral recruitment effect has been enhanced by a single dose of Fluoxetine *(224)*. These findings also suggest that greater bilateral activity may be transient if the infarct has not caused significant damage to the primary motor areas (i.e., becomes lateralized again once patients recover function) *(225)*.

One group studied motor function among patients with CADASIL without hemiparesis or other focal motor symptoms *(230)*. They found decreased laterality in primary motor area compared to control participants and an inverse relationship between white matter injury and laterality. Therefore, ipsilateral recruitment of motor areas may not be limited to patients exhibiting hemiparesis.

In summary, older participants and these neurologic patients tend to exhibit shifting BOLD signal activity during cognitive performance, including motor skills and sensory perception. A pattern has emerged across these groups, where less activation is evident in expected regions, whereas overall activity becomes more bilateral, particularly when groups are matched for performance. Intrahemispheric and more frequently interhemispheric compensation models have been proposed in all of these populations.

4.4. Future Directions

fMRI of patients with chronic CVD remains a topic of little research but great potential. It is likely that similar deviations in brain function will be discovered in patients with VaD as they have among other patient populations. However, verification of the validity of BOLD studies among this population is particularly important, given the compromise of cerebrovasculature and our incomplete understanding of the mechanisms underlying BOLD response. This may involve replication of studies of healthy controls, research aimed at a better understanding the effects of healthy aging on BOLD signal, and clarification of the meaning of relatively greater or less signal among patients in general (e.g., successful compensation or inefficient activity). An exciting possibility is group contrasts of dementia subtypes (e.g., VaD vs AD) that may provide a better understand of different functional pathologies and clearer diagnoses. fMRI of neurologic patients also provides an excellent method to evaluate neuropsychological models' brain dysfunction and the efficacy of medications.

Technical advances, such as application of nonechoplanar sequences to reduce susceptibility artifacts, higher field strength magnets, and more powerful (and more uniform) preprocessing and statistical analysis techniques, may produce significant advances in our understanding of chronic CVD. With the emerging finding of BOLD signal decline among older healthy adults resulting from hemodynamic factors, it is crucial to understand how much of the BOLD signal decline is related to these factors in patients with disorders directly affecting hemodynamics. Understanding these intervening hemodynamic mechanisms is crucial to interpreting BOLD data from patients with compromised cerebrovascular systems because the data may not be interpreted as usual.

4.5. Advantages

fMRI has several advantages over older functional neuroimaging techniques that include better feasibility, better resolution, more design flexibility, and availability. fMRI, as typically performed, already has the advantage of investigating concurrent relationships among BOLD response, cognitive performance, and structural pathology. Furthermore, additional MR-related data may be collected in the same fMRI session (e.g., fluid attenuated inversion recovery [FLAIR], PWI, DWI, and DTI) with little additional inconvenience to the patient (i.e., more time). BOLD fMRI is also noninvasive, repeatable, and less expensive than PET, allowing more design flexibility, including longitudinal studies. Typical fMRI spatial resolution is 3–5 mm^3, with a whole-brain temporal resolution of approximately 3–4 s but can exceed 1 mm^3 or well below 1 s. A good balance of spatial and temporal resolution is chosen based on the study questions, with an inherent trade-off between these two types of parameters. Thus, smaller regions and more transient cognitive processes can be observed using fMRI compared to other functional neuroimaging techniques. However, fMRI designs have been evolving with even greater flexibility, particularly with the introduction of event-related designs since the late 1990s *(235–238)*. Finally, fMRI has the advantage of the proliferation of MRI systems in most large medical settings. Standard clinical MRI scanners may be easily upgraded to run fMRI sequences with minimal additional costs.

4.6. Disadvantages

There are several special considerations in fMRI experiments, including patients with VaD. Subject screening and selection must be more carefully considered than with younger and healthy adults. For example, regardless of whether they are patients, older adults tend to have more medical issues leading to MR contraindications. Contraindications preclude scanning of individuals with ferrous implants; however, even nonferrous implants may heat up or produce image artifacts. Safety is also a special consideration with patients who may not be able to follow instructions or may forget that they still have a set of keys in their pocket. Eyesight, movement, comfort level, and body morphometry (size and shape) tend to be greater issues in older adults and patients.

When studying any clinical population, or healthy people for that matter, investigators must consider the effects of loud scanner noise, the potential danger of a magnetic environment, motion artifacts, claustrophobia, and susceptibility artifacts. Scanner noise and movement artifact make verbal responding unfeasible and often lead to more sophisticated responding and stimulus presentation paradigms. These paradigms may be more confusing to patients with cognitive problems than standard neuropsychological testing. Other stimulus presentation issues include the need for MR-compatible equipment (safe and functional) and the ability to present stimuli to participants who are lying in a narrow MRI bore. Averaging and temporal smoothing of BOLD signal is necessary to gain reliable data because observed signal changes are typically less than 10%, even during the more robust response to motor and visual stimulation paradigms. Generalizability of findings may be a problem because acquisition, preprocessing, statistical analysis, thresholding of significant effects, and technology differ from site to site. Finally, fMRI research with patient population is expensive. It depends on specialized equipment and highly trained personnel from several different disciplines, such as clinicians, radiologists, biomedical engineers, physicists, statisticians, neuroscientists, computer programmers, and information technologists.

5. RADIOLOGICAL METHODS

Radiological methods, such as SPECT and PET provided the primary means of functional brain imaging before the recent development of MR-based techniques. Both PET and SPECT involve the introduction of a radioactive tracer into the blood and subsequent imaging of radioactivity emitted from the brain. The premise underlying such imaging is that the quantity of radioactivity that is emitted after a period of time is dependent on the perfusion and metabolic rates of different tissue within the brain. These methods can be used to assess CBF, which is of obvious interest for patients with CVD. Reviews have been written during the past several years that provide more detailed discussion of evidence regarding the use of SPECT and PET for the assessment of dementia and cerebrovascular disorders *(38)*.

5.1. Rationale for Radiological Measures

The primary advantage of radiological over MRI-based functional imaging methods stems from the fact that radiological methods provide a more direct measure of the metabolic response of the brain tissue being imaged, as well as a measure of CBF. Both SPECT and PET work because brain tissue metabolizes blood at different rates based on the physiological characteristics of the tissue and the functions it is performing. Radioactivity introduced into the blood is used to measure these metabolic differences. With MRI-based methods, inferences about metabolism must be made based on the information known about the hemodynamic characteristics of blood under different conditions.

Radiological methods have some other methodological advantages over MRI-based methods. They are less vulnerable to artifact associated with spaces in the brain, such as sinuses. Consequently, activation in orbital frontal regions can be imaged more easily with PET than with most MRI methods.

Of all the currently available functional imaging methods, SPECT has been most widely used in clinical practice. There are numerous reasons for this, including that it is reimbursed by many insurance companies and the technology is less expensive to implement than is PET. The majority of clinical studies involving SPECT have involved baseline analyses of patients during rest, although it also been used to a more limited extent in cognitive paradigms in which brain activation during task performance is compared to a control condition of resting.

PET has been largely used as a research tool. It was the first method to show reliable task-dependent differences in regional brain activation associated with cognition *(265,267)*. It is quite useful for imaging brain activity associated with cognitive and behavioral processes. It is also useful for studying specific neurotransmitter systems that have been tagged with specific ligands. Although in theory MR-based methods can be developed to be used for this purpose, currently, PET provides an easier means of studying neurotransmitter systems.

5.2. Methodological Limitations

Numerous methodological differences exist between MRI and radiological techniques. The most obvious difference is that radiological techniques require the introduction of radioactivity into the body of the patient, whereas MRI does not. Although the quantity of radioactivity used in any single imaging session is not great enough to pose a health risk, the cumulative effect of multiple scanning sessions is of concern. Consequently, it is difficult to use either of these methods for clinical applications in which repeated measurement is required. This poses a significant limitation for use in VaD when the goal is measuring brain changes over time.

Another limitation is that SPECT and PET usually do not provide the spatial or temporal resolution that can be achieved with MRI. To characterize the neuroanatomy underlying observed activation findings, it is necessary to coregister the radiological data with structural data obtained from MRI or some other imaging method. This requires an additional methodological step and introduces error associated with matching to different types of data. Even with coregistration, radiological methods have limited spatial resolution, so that it is not possible to image small brain regions. This is particularly true for standard SPECT methods. Data from SPECT usually need to analyzed relative to a reference brain area, such as the cerebellum. PET does not require this and provides a better absolute measure of metabolic activity.

The temporal resolution of SPECT and PET is also limited compared to MRI-based techniques. SPECT has the poorest temporal resolution and has a relatively long time period to construct a single functional image, usually approximately 20–30 min. This usually means that only one task or behavior can be performed during the period before scanning, and the image reflects the average activity during this period. This disadvantage may actually be beneficial in certain cases, because it is possible to have the patient engage in a task outside of the scanner during the time after injection. This makes it easier to do certain types of ecologically relevant tasks with SPECT.

PET has higher temporal resolution, so it is possible to image the brain during different conditions within a single scanning session. However, the time required to capture activation is still much greater than 1 s, so that it is not possible to image the components of cognitive or physiological processes that are occurring during brief time periods. Consequently, PET does not lend itself to event-related paradigms in which processing during individual trials is examined. Furthermore, PET has been used in only a limited fashion in clinical practice, largely because of the high cost associated with procedure and methodological difficulties associated with its routine use.

Although SPECT and PET have value because of this methodological difference, in practice, MRI-based methods can provide similar information, at less cost and risk. Nonetheless, radiological methods represent another potentially important approach to functional brain assessment and should be considered when studying VaD.

5.3. Clinical Evidence for Use in VaD

Both SPECT and PET have been studied extensively among patients with dementia, most notably AD, although there are emerging data on VaD. There is also a large body of research on how patients respond on SPECT and PET after a stroke. For the most part, data from PET parallels findings from MRI studies discussed earlier.

5.4. SPECT Studies of Dementia and Stroke

Of all functional methods described in this chapter, SPECT has been most widely used in the clinical assessment of patients with dementia, particularly AD. Reduced bilateral parietal lobe-resting activation has been reported to be a strong correlate of AD in numerous studies *(268–269)*. Clinicians often incorporate such SPECT findings to help with differential diagnosis of AD from other types of dementia, although, unfortunately, there are many clinical exceptions to this general finding.

With respect to stroke, there are numerous studies showing that SPECT activation decreases in regions of the brain with infarcts *(267,270–272)*. This is not surprising, because brain tissue that is necrotic should show an absence of blood flow and metabolism. Strategic infarcts involving critical subcortical structures, such as the thalamus, cause not only reduced activation in the affected area but also hypoperfusion of adjacent cortical areas *(273)*. The primary problem with SPECT is that because it lacks spatial and temporal resolution, it is difficulty to derive precise measurements that would enable determination of dysfunctional brain tissue (penumbra) before complete infarction. Consequently, the data obtained from SPECT among patients with stroke largely mirrors structural MRI data.

During the past several years, several investigations of SPECT in VaD have been conducted. These studies have yielded mixed results regarding the presumed cerebrovascular etiology of VaD. The authors studied SPECT in a group of patients with VaD assessed as part of a treatment outcome study and observed global decrements in cortical activation that were related to dementia severity *(274)*. Decreased SPECT activation was correlated with whole-brain volume but not the extent of subcortical hyperintensities on MRI. Regional differences in brain activation were not found, nor was dementia related to activation decrements in specific brain regions, such as the frontal lobes. These findings suggested an indirect relationship between subcortical pathology associated with small-vessel white matter disease and dementia in these patients. A complex relationship between cerebrovascular etiology and brain atrophy exists in VaD. The lack of a clear relationship between CBF on SPECT and hyperintensities of the subcortical white matter has been described by other investigators as well.

SPECT studies conducted in Japan have yielded results with greater specificity of SPECT abnormality in VaD. For example, Yoshikawa et al. compared patients with VaD secondary to small-vessel ischemic disease and healthy controls on SPECT using a CBF method involving three-dimensional fractal analysis *(275)*. Patients with VaD had two abnormal patterns, with globally reduced blood flow in the whole brain and reductions in blood flow in the frontal lobes. Some patients exhibited both patterns, whereas other exhibited one or the other.

5.5. PET Studies

Before the development of fMRI, PET provided the best means of measuring brain activation associated with cognitive and behavioral processes. The cognitive neuroscience literature is replete with studies in which PET was used to analyze the brain regions involved in specific cognitive processes in healthy adults. For example, in an early study, PET was used to demonstrate that different brain regions activated during the language processing in relationship to the requirement for phonological, orthographic, or semantic operations. PET has also been used to characterize the functional neuroanatomy of learning and memory, attention, and most other domains of cognition.

More recently, PET has been used to study cognition in clinical disorders, including AD and stroke. These studies typically show diminished activation of strategic brain regions that are essential for a cognitive operation, or conversely increased activation of collateral brain regions, presumably in compensation for diminished processing capacity of the brain structures normally involved in the operation. The literature in this regard mirrors that discussed earlier regarding fMRI and is not reviewed in detail. PET does provide a useful means of studying the cognitive dysfunction associated with dementia.

PET has also been used in a manner similar to SPECT to characterize cerebral hypoperfusion among patients with stroke and dementia. The rationale underlying these efforts is that to understand the underlying mechanisms it is necessary to assess the relationship between CBF, metabolism, related biochemical processes, and the location and time course of brain tissue damage. Accordingly, PET has been used to examine how infarction affects the metabolic characteristics of brain tissue in patients with VaD. For example, De Reuck et al. *(272)* compared stroke patients with and without VaD on PET using Cobalt-55 imaging, which enables characterization of new vs. old infarctions. Both stroke patients with and without VaD showed an interesting pattern of decreased uptake of Colbalt-55 that was reduced in deep gray matter nuclei and white matter but was the same in cortical areas compared to the cerebellum. Those patients with VaD showed greater Colbalt-55 uptake, which was interpreted as indicating that stroke patients with progressive cognitive decline have PET findings that reflect ischemic effects on white matter.

Other investigators have used PET to differentiate VaD from AD. Nagata et al. *(276)* found that the metabolic rate of oxygen was abnormal in the parietal temporal lobe of patients with AD. In contrast, vascular reactivity measured by PET was abnormal in the patients with VaD but not the patients with AD. This study illustrates how PET and other functional imaging methods can be used in the differential diagnosis of dementia.

6. CONCLUSIONS

Numerous functional brain imaging methods have been discussed in this chapter that have potential value for the study and clinical management of VaD. Relatively few of these methods have been adopted for routine clinical use, although it is likely that they will play a greater role in the future. Currently, only SPECT is widely used in clinical studies of dementia. DWI is beginning to be used in clinical stroke studies and will likely be used to an even greater extent as new drugs are tested and efforts are made to study the evolution of infarction. Other MR-based methods, such as DTI and fMRI, hold particular promise for future efforts to evaluate patients with VaD. However, further research is needed to develop standardized methods for clinical use, to gain a full understanding of how patients with VaD respond on these tasks, and to establish normative data on which clinical decision making can be based.

REFERENCES

1. Reivich M, Waltz AG Circulatory and metabolic factors in cerebrovascular disease. In: Cerebrovascular Survey Report. Bethesda, MD: NINCDS Monographs, 1980, pp. 55–134.
2. Caplan LR. Stroke: A clinical approach. 2nd Ed. Boston, MA: Butterworths, 1993.
3. Zorowitz R, Walker J. Predicting length of stay, functional outcome, and aftercare in the rehabilitation of stroke patients. The dominant role of higher-order cognition. Stroke 1994;24:1794–1800.
4. Wunderlich MT, Ebert AD, Kratz T, Goertler M, Jost S, Herrmann M. Early neurobehavioral outcome after stroke is related to release of neurobiochemical markers of brain damage. Stroke 1999;30:1190–1195.
5. Adams RD, Victor M, Roper AH. Principles of neurology. 7th Ed. New York, NY: McGraw Hill, 2001.
6. Tatemichi TK, Desmond DW, Stern Y, et al. Cognitive impairments after stroke: frequency, patterns, and relationship to functional abilities. J Neurol Neurosurg Psychiat 1994;57:202–207.
7. Corbett A, Bennett H, Kos S. Cortical dysfunction following subcortical infarction. Arch Neurol 1994;51:999–1007.
8. Burton E, Ballard C, Stephens S, et al. Hyperintensities and fronto-subcortical atrophy on MRI are substrates of mild cognitive deficits after stroke. Dementia Geriatric Cogn Disord. 2003;16:113–118.

9. Bracco L, Campani D, Baratti E, et al. Relation between MRI features and dementia in cerebrovascular disease patients with leukoaraisosis: a longitudinal study. J Neurol Sci 1993;120:131–136.
10. Masdeu JC, Azar-Kia B, Rubino FA. Evaluation of recent cerebral infarction by computerized tomography. Arch Neurol 1977;34:417–421.
11. Kinkel WR. Classification of stroke by neuroimaging technique. Stroke 1990;21(Suppl):II7–II8.
12. Marks MP, Holmgren EB, Fox AJ, Patel S, von Kummer R, Froehlich J. Evaluation of early computed tomographic findings in acute ischemic stroke. Clinical trial. Multicenter study. Randomized controlled trial. Stroke 1999;30:389–392.
13. Tei H, Uchiyama S, Koshimizu K, Kobayashi M, Ohara K. Correlation between symptomatic, radiological and etiological diagnosis in acute ischemic stroke. Acta Neurol Scand. 1999;99:192–195.
14. Kinkel PR, Kinkel WR, Jacobs L. Nuclear magnetic resonance imaging in patients with stroke. Semin Neurol. 1986; 6:43–52.
15. Mirsen TR, Lee DH, Wong CJ, et al. Clinical correlates of white-matter changes on magnetic resonance imaging scans of the brain. Arch Neurol 1991;48:1015–1021.
16. Kertesz A, Black SE, Nicholson L, Carr T. The sensitivity and specificity of MRI in stroke. Neurology 1987;37: 1580–1585.
17. Brown JJ, Hesselink JR, Rothrock JF. MR and CT of lacunar infarcts. AJR Amer J Roentgenol 1988;151:367–372.
18. Schellinger PD, Jansen O, Fiebach JB, Hacke W, Sartor K. A standardized MRI stroke protocol: comparison with CT in hyperacute intracerebral hemorrhage [comment]. Stroke 1999;30:765–768.
19. Helgason CM, Chomka E, Louie E. The potential role for ultrafast cardiac computed tomography in patients with stroke. Stroke 1989;20:465–472.
20. Toni D, Fiorelli M, De Michele M, et al. Clinical and prognostic correlates of stroke subtype misdiagnosis within 12 hours from onset [erratum appears in Stroke 1996;27:152]. Stroke 1995;26:1837–1840.
21. Hommel M, Besson G, Le Bas JF, et al. Prospective study of lacunar infarction using magnetic resonance imaging. Stroke 1990;21:546–554.
22. Leary MC, Saver JL. Annual incidence of first silent stroke in the United States: a preliminary estimate. Cerebrovasc Dis 2003;16:280–285:2003.
23. Barest GD, Sorensen AG, Gonzalez RG. Magnetic resonance imaging of cerebral infarction. Top Magnet Resonance Imag 1998;9:199–207.
24. Longstreth WT Jr., Manolio TA, Arnold A, et al. Clinical correlates of white matter findings on cranial magnetic resonance imaging of 3301 elderly people. The Cardiovascular Health Study [comment]. Stroke 1996;27: 1274–1282.
25. Longstreth WT Jr, Dulberg C, Manolio TA, et al. Incidence, manifestations, and predictors of brain infarcts defined by serial cranial magnetic resonance imaging in the elderly: the Cardiovascular Health Study [comment]. Stroke 2002;33: 2376–2382.
26. Donnan GA, Davis SM. Neuroimaging, the ischaemic penumbra, and selection of patients for acute stroke therapy. Lancet Neurol 2002;1:417–425.
27. Neumann-Haefelin T, Kastrup A, de Crespigny A, et al. Serial MRI after transient focal cerebral ischemia in rats: dynamics of tissue injury, blood-brain barrier damage, and edema formation. Stroke 2000;31:1965–72; discussion 1972–1973.
28. Grotta JC, Chiu D, Lu M, et al. Agreement and variability in the interpretation of early CT changes in stroke patients qualifying for intravenous rtPA therapy [comment]. Stroke 1999;30:1528–1533.
29. Bhadelia RA, Anderson M, Polak JF, et al. Prevalence and associations of MRI-demonstrated brain infarcts in elderly subjects with a history of transient ischemic attack. The Cardiovascular Health Study. Stroke 1999;30:383–388.
30. Lang EW, Daffertshofer M, Daffertshofer A, et al. Variability of vascular territory in stroke. Pitfalls and failure of stroke pattern interpretation. Stroke 1995;26:942–945.
31. Roman CG, Tatemichi T, Erkinjunntti T, et al. Vascular dementia: diagnostic criteria for research studies. Neurology 1993;43:250–260.
32. Kertez A, Polk M, Carr T. Cognition and white matter changes on magnetic imaging in dementia. Arch Neurol 1990; 47:387–391.
33. Miyashita K, Naritomi H, Sawada T, et al. Identification of recent lacunar lesions in cases of multiple small infarctions by magnetic resonance imaging. Stroke 1988;19:834–839.
34. Wolfe N, Babikian VL, Linn RT, et al. Are multiple cerebral infarcts synergistic? Arch Neurol 1994;51:211–215.
35. Price TR, Manolio TA, Kronmal RA, et al. Silent brain infarction on magnetic resonance imaging and neurological abnormalities in community-dwelling older adults. The Cardiovascular Health Study. CHS Collaborative Research Group. Stroke 1997;28:1158–1164.
36. Kwa VI, Franke CL, Verbeeten B Jr, Stam J. Silent intracerebral microhemorrhages in patients with ischemic stroke. Amsterdam Vascular Medicine Group [comment]. Ann Neurol 1998;44:372–377.
37. Jezzard P, Mathews PM, Smith SM. Functional MRI: an introduction to methods. Oxford, UK: Oxford University Press, 2001.

38. Van Heertum RL, Tikofsky RS. Positron emission tomography and single-photon emission computed tomography brain imaging in the evaluation of dementia. Sem in Nuclear Med. 2003;33:77–85.
39. Fisher M, Albers GW. Applications of diffusion-perfusion magnetic resonance imaging in acute ischemic stroke. Neurology 1999;52:1750–1756.
40. Warach S, Chien D, Li W, Ronthal M, Edelman RR. Fast magnetic resonance diffusion-weighted imaging of acute human stroke. Neurology 1992;42:1717–1723.
41. Schramm P, Schellinger PD, Fiebach JB, et al.Comparison of CT and CT angiography source images with diffusion-weighted imaging in patients with acute stroke within 6 hours after onset. Stroke 2002;33:2426–2432.
42. Wardlaw JM, Keir SL, Bastin ME, Armitage PA, Rana AK. Is diffusion imaging appearance an independent predictor of outcome after ischemic stroke? Neurology 2002;59:1381–1387.
43. Arenillas JF, Rovira A, Molina CA, et al. Prediction of early neurological deterioration using diffusion- and perfusion-weighted imaging in hyperacute middle cerebral artery ischemic stroke. Stroke 2002;33:2197–2203.
44. Jaillard A, Hommel M, Baird AE, et al. Significance of early CT signs in acute stroke. A CT scan-diffusion MRI study. Cerebrovasc Dis 2002;13:47–56.
45. Fiebach JB, Schellinger PD, Jansen O, et al. CT and diffusion-weighted MR imaging in randomized order: diffusion-weighted imaging results in higher accuracy and lower interrater variability in the diagnosis of hyperacute ischemic stroke. Stroke 2002;33:2206–2210.
46. Gadian DG, Allen K, van Bruggen N, et al. Applications of NMR spectroscopy to the study of experimental stroke in vivo. Stroke 1993;24:I57–I59; discussion I66-8.
47. Menon RS, Goodyear BG. Spatial and temporal resolution in fMRI. In: Jezzard P, Mathews PM, Smith SM, eds. Functional MRI: An introduction to methods. Oxford, UK: Oxford University Press, 2001.
48. Glover GH. Hardware for functional MRI. In: Jezzard P, Mathews PM, Smith SM, eds. Functional MRI: An introduction to methods. Oxford, UK: Oxford University Press, 2001.
49. Savoy R. The scanner as a psychophysiology laboratory. In: Jezzard P, Mathews PM, Smith SM., eds. Functional MRI: An introduction to methods. Oxford, UK: Oxford University Press, 2001.
50. Worsley KJ. Statistical analysis of activation images. In: Jezzard P, Mathews PM, Smith SM, eds. Functional MRI: An introduction to methods. Oxford, UK: Oxford University Press, 2001.
51. Brammer MJ. Head motion and its correction. In: Jezzard P, Mathews PM, Smith SM, eds. Functional MRI: An introduction to methods. Oxford, UK: Oxford University Press, 2001.
52. Jenkinson M. Registration, atlases and cortical flattening. In: Jezzard P, Mathews PM, Smith SM, eds. Functional MRI: An introduction to methods. Oxford, UK: Oxford University Press, 2001.
53. Sotak CH. The role of diffusion tensor imaging in the evaluation of ischemic brain injury—a review. NMR Biomed 2002;15:561–569.
54. Allder SJ, Moody AR, Martel AL, et al. Differences in the diagnostic accuracy of acute stroke clinical subtypes defined by multimodal magnetic resonance imaging. J Neurol Neurosurg Psychiatry 2003;74:886–888.
55. Beaulieu C. The basis of anisotropic water diffusion in the nervous system—a technical review. NMR Biomed 2002;15:435–455.
56. Le Bihan D, van Zijl P. From the diffusion coefficient to the diffusion tensor. NMR Biomed 2002;15:431–434.
57. Bammer R. Basic principles of diffusion-weighted imaging. Euro J Neuroradiol 2003;45:169–184.
58. Sullivan EV, Pfefferbaum A. Diffusion tensor imaging in normal aging and neuropsychiatric disorders. Euro J Radiol, 2003;45:244–255.
59. Moseley M. Diffusion tensor imaging and aging—a review. NMR Biomed 2002;15:553–5560.
60. Moseley ME, Cohen YC, Kucharczyk J, et al. Diffusion-weighted MR imaging of anisotropic water diffusion in cat central nervous system. Radiology 1990;176:439–445.
61. Moseley ME, Kucharczyk J, Asgari HS, Norman D. Anisotropy in diffusion-weighted MRI. Magnet Resonance Med 1991;19:321–326.
62. Mintorvitch J, Moseley ME, Chileuitt L, et al. Comparison of diffusion- and T2-weighted MRI for the early detection of cerebral ischemia and reperfusion in rats. Magnet Resonance Med 1991;18:39–50.
63. Fuhai L, Siva MD, Kai-Feng L, et al. Secondary decline in apparent diffusion coefficient and neurological outcomes after a short period of focal brain ischemia in rats. Ann Neurol 2000;48:236–244.
64. Zelaya F, Flood N, Chalk JB, et al. An evaluation of the time dependence of the anisotropy of the water diffusion tensor in acute human stroke. Magnet Resonance Imag 1999;17:331–348.
65. Carano RAD, Li F, Irie K, et al. Multispectral analysis of the temporal evolution of cerebral ischemia in the rat brain. J Magnet Resonance Imag 2000;12:842–858.
66. Helpern JA, Dereski MO, Knight RA, et al. Histopathological correlations of nuclear magnetic resonance imaging parameters in experimental cerebral ischemia. Magnet Resonance Imag 1993;11:241–246.
67. Knight RA, Dereski MO, Helpern JA, Ordidge RJ, Chopp M. MRI assessment of evolving focal cerebral ischemia: comparison with histopathology in rats. Stroke 1994;25:1252–1262.
68. Zelaya F, Flood N, Chalk JB, et al. An evaluation of the time dependence of the anisotropy of the water diffusion tensor in acute human stroke. Magnet Resonance Imag 1999;17:331–348.

69. Yang Q, Tress BM, Barber PA, et al. Serial study of apparent diffusion coefficient and anisotropy in patients with acute stroke. Stroke 1999;20:2382–2390.
70. Werring DJ, Toosy AT, Clark CA, et al. Diffusion tensor imaging can detect and quantify corticospinal tract degeneration after stroke. J Neurol Neurosurg Psychiatry 2000;69:269–272.
71. Bigler ED, Kerr B, Tate DF, et al. Role of white matter lesions, cerebral atrophy, and APOE on cognition in older persons with and without dementia: the Cache County, Utah, study of memory and aging. Neuropsychology 2003;17: 339–352.
72. Cohen RA, Paul RH, Ott BR, et al. The relationship of subcortical MRI hperintensities and brain volume to cognitive function in vascular dementia. J Intl Neuropsychol Soc 2002;8:743–752.
73. Jones DK, Lythgoe D, Horsfield MA, et al. Characterization of white matter damage in ischemic leukoaraiosis with diffusion tensor MRI. Stroke 1999;30:393–397.
74. Pantoni L, Garcia JH. Pathogenesis of leukoaraiosis: a review. Stroke 1997;28:652–659.
75. Dichgans M, Mayer M, Uttner I, et al. The phenotypic spectrum of CADASIL: clinical findings in 102 cases. Ann Neurol 1998;44:731–739.
76. Chabriat H, Pappata S, Poupon C, et al. Clinical severity in CADASIL related to ultrastructural damage in white matter: in vivo study with diffusion tensor MRI. Stroke 1999;30:2637–2643.
77. Chabriat H, Levy C, Taillia H, et al. Patterns of MRI lesions in CADASIL. Neurology 1998;51:452–457.
78. Baudrimont M, Dubas F, Joutel A, Tournier-Lasserve E, Bausser M. Autosomal dominant leukoencephalopathy and subcortical ischemic strokes: a clinicopathological study. Stroke 1993;24:122–125.
79. Neil JJ, Shiran SI, McKinstry RC, et al. Normal brain in human newborns: apparent diffusion coefficient and diffusion anisotropy measured by using diffusion tensor MR imaging. Radiology 1998;209:57–66.
80. Paus T, Collins DL, Evans AC, et al. Maturation of white matter in the human brain: a review of magnetic resonance studies. Brain Res Bull 2001;54:255–266.
81. Pfefferbaum A, Sullivan EV, Hedehus M, et al. Age-related decline in brain white matter anisotropy measured with spatially corrected echo-planar diffusion tensor imaging. Magnet Resonance Med 2000;44:259–268.
82. Sullivan EV, Adalsteinsson E, Hedehus M, et al. Equivalent disruption of regional white mater microstructure in aging healthy men and women. Neuroreport 2001;12:99–104.
83. Chun T, Filippi CG, Zimmerman RD, Ulug AM. Diffusion changes in the aging human brain. Amer J Neuroradiol 2000;21:1078–1083.
84. Nusbaum AO, Tang CY, Buchsbaum MS, Wei TC, Atlas SW. Regional and global changes in cerebral perfusion with normal aging. Amer J Neuroradiol 2001;22:136–142.
85. Brun A. Regional rather than global pathology decides symptoms in senile dementia of Alzheimer's disease. Neurobiol Aging 1994;15:367–368.
86. Braak H, Braak E. Morphological criteria for the recognition of Alzheimer's disease and the distribution pattern of cortical changes related to this disorder. Neurobiol Aging 1994;15:355–356.
87. Hanyu H, Sakurai H, Iwamoto T, et al. Diffusion-weighted MR imaging of the hippocampus and temporal white matter in Alzheimer's disease. J Neurol Sci 1998;156:195–200.
88. Kantarci K, Jack CR, Jr., Xu YC, et al. Mild cognitive impairment and Alzheimer's disease: regional diffusivity of water. Radiology 2001;219:101–107.
89. Hanyu H, Asano T, Sakurai H, et al. Diffusion-weighted and magnetization transfer imaging of the corpus callosum in Alzheimer's disease. J Neurol Sci 1999;167:37–44.
90. Rosen BR, Turner R, Hunter GJ, Fordham JA. MR depicts perfusion of brain and heart. Diagnostic Imag 1991;13: 105–110.
91. Detre JA, Alsop DC. Perfusion magnetic resonance imaging with continuous arterial spin labeling: methods and clinical applications in the central nervous system. Euro J Radiol 1999;30:115–124.
92. Wong EC, Luh WM, Liu TT. Turbo ASL: arterial spin labeling with higher SNR and temporal resolution. Magnet Resonance Med 2000;44:511–515.
93. Garnett MR, Blamire AM, Corkill RG, et al. Abnormal cerebral blood volume in regions of contused and normal appearing brain following traumatic brain injury using perfusion magnetic resonance imaging. J Neurotrauma 2001;18: 585–593.
94. Wityk RJ, Goldsborough MA, Hillis A, et al. Diffusion- and perfusion-weighted brain magnetic resonance imaging in patients with neurologic complications after cardiac surgery. Arch Neurol 2001;58:571–576.
95. Restrepo L, Wityk RJ, Grega MA, et al. Diffusion- and perfusion-weighted magnetic resonance imaging of the brain before and after coronary artery bypass grafting surgery. Stroke. 2002;33:2909–2915.
96. Wolf RL, Alsop DC, Levy-Reis I, et al. Detection of mesial temporal lobe hypoperfusion in patients with temporal lobe epilepsy by use of arterial spin labeled perfusion MR imaging. AJR Amer J Neuroradiol. 2001;22:1334–1341.
97. Markus HS, Lythgoe DJ, Ostegaard L, O'Sullivan M, Williams SC. Reduced cerebral blood flow in white matter in ischaemic leukoaraiosis demonstrated using quantitative exogenous contrast based perfusion MRI. J Neurol Neurosurg Psychiatry 2000;69:48–53.
98. Maas LC, Harris GJ, Satlin A, et al. Regional cerebral blood volume measured by dynamic susceptibility contrast MR imaging in Alzheimer's disease: a principal components analysis. J Magnet Resonance Imag 1997;7:215–219.

99. Harris GJ, Lewis RF, Satlin A, et al. Dynamic susceptibility contrast MRI of regional cerebral blood volume in Alzheimer's disease. Amer J Psychiatry 1996;153:721–724.
100. Harris GJ, Lewis RF, Satlin A, et al. Dynamic susceptibility contrast MR imaging of regional cerebral blood volume in Alzheimer disease: a promising alternative to nuclear medicine. AJNR Am J Neuroradiol. 1998;19:1727–1732.
101. Alsop DC, Detre JA, Grossman M. Assessment of cerebral blood flow in Alzheimer's disease by spin-labeled magnetic resonance imaging. Ann Neurol 2000;47:93–100.
102. Kidwell CS, Saver JL, Mattiello J, et al. Thrombolytic reversal of acute human cerebral ischemic injury shown by diffusion/perfusion magnetic resonance imaging. Ann Neurol. 2000;47:462–469.
103. Singer OC, de Rochemont Rdu M, Foerch C, et al. Relation between relative cerebral blood flow, relative cerebral blood volume, and mean transit time in patients with acute ischemic stroke determined by perfusion-weighted MRI. J Cereb Blood Flow Metab 2003;23:605–611.
104. Zhu M, Dai J, Li S. Cerebral angiography and MR perfusion images in patients with ischemic cerebral vascular disease. Chin Med J (Engl). 2002;115:1687–1691.
105. Schaefer PW, Romero JM, Grant PE, et al. Perfusion magnetic resonance imaging of acute ischemic stroke. Semin Roentgenol 2002;37:230–236.
106. Flacke S, Urbach H, Folkers PJ, et al. Ultra-fast three-dimensional MR perfusion imaging of the entire brain in acute stroke assessment. J Magn Reson Imag 2000;11:250–259.
107. Rordorf G, Koroshetz WJ, Copen WA, et al. Regional ischemia and ischemic injury in patients with acute middle cerebral artery stroke as defined by early diffusion-weighted and perfusion-weighted MRI. Stroke 1998;29:939–943.
108. Arenillas JF, Rovira A, Molina CA, et al. Prediction of early neurological deterioration using diffusion- and perfusion-weighted imaging in hyperacute middle cerebral artery ischemic stroke. Stroke 2002;33:2197–2203.
109. Sorensen AG, Copen WA, Ostergaard L, et al. Hyperacute stroke: simultaneous measurement of relative cerebral blood volume, relative cerebral blood flow, and mean tissue transit time. Radiology 1999;210:519–527.
110. Beaulieu C, de Crespigny A, Tong DC, et al. Longitudinal magnetic resonance imaging study of perfusion and diffusion in stroke: evolution of lesion volume and correlation with clinical outcome. Ann Neurol 1999;46:568–578.
111. Parsons MW, Yang Q, Barber PA, et al. Perfusion magnetic resonance imaging maps in hyperacute stroke: relative cerebral blood flow most accurately identifies tissue destined to infarct. Stroke 2001;32:1581–1587.
112. Wu O, Koroshetz WJ, Ostergaard L, et al. Predicting tissue outcome in acute human cerebral ischemia using combined diffusion- and perfusion-weighted MR imaging. Stroke 2001;32:933–942.
113. Uno M, Harada M, Yoneda K, et al. Can diffusion- and perfusion-weighted magnetic resonance imaging evaluate the efficacy of acute thrombolysis in patients with internal carotid artery or middle cerebral artery occlusion? Neurosurgery 2002;50:28–34; discussion 34-5.
114. Baird AE, Benfield A, Schlaug G, et al. Enlargement of human cerebral ischemic lesion volumes measured by diffusion-weighted magnetic resonance imaging. Ann Neurol 1997;41:581–589.
115. Barber PA, Darby DG, Desmond PM, et al. Prediction of stroke outcome with echoplanar perfusion- and diffusion-weighted MRI. Neurology 1998;51:418–426.
116. Neumann-Haefelin T, Wittsack HJ, Wenserski F, et al. Diffusion- and perfusion-weighted MRI: the DWI/PWI mismatch region in acute stroke. Stroke 1999;30:1591–1597.
117. Karonen JO, Vanninen RL, Liu Y, et al. Combined diffusion and perfusion MRI with correlation to single-photon emission CT in acute ischemic stroke: ischemic penumbra predicts infarct growth. Stroke 1999;30:1583–1590.
118. Rordorf G, Koroshetz WJ, Copen WA, et al. Diffusion- and perfusion-weighted imaging in vasospasm after subarachnoid hemorrhage. Stroke 1999;30:599–605.
119. Kajimoto K, Moriwaki H, Yamada N, et al. Cerebral hemodynamic evaluation using perfusion-weighted magnetic resonance imaging: comparison with positron emission tomography values in chronic occlusive carotid disease. Stroke 2003;34:1662–1666.
120. van Osch MJ, Rutgers DR, Vonken EP, et al. Quantitative cerebral perfusion MRI and CO2 reactivity measurements in patients with symptomatic internal carotid artery occlusion. Neuroimage 2002;17:469–78.
121. Kim JH, Lee EJ, Lee SJ, et al. Reliability of perfusion MR imaging in symptomatic carotid occlusive disease. Cerebral blood volume, mean transit time and time-to-peak. Acta Radiol 2002;43:360–364.
122. Kikuchi K, Murase K, Miki H, et al. Measurement of cerebral hemodynamics with perfusion-weighted MR imaging: comparison with pre- and post-acetazolamide 133Xe-SPECT in occlusive carotid disease. AJNR Am J Neuroradiol 2001;22:248–254.
123. Caramia F, Santoro A, Pantano P, et al. Cerebral hemodynamics on MR perfusion images before and after bypass surgery in patients with giant intracranial aneurysms. AJNR Am J Neuroradiol. 2001;22:1704–1710.
124. Uematsu H, Maeda M, Itoh H. Peritumoral brain edema in intracranial meningiomas evaluated by dynamic perfusion-weighted MR imaging: a preliminary study. Eur Radiol 2003;13:758–762.
125. Chan JH, Tsui EY, Chau LF, et al. Discrimination of an infected brain tumor from a cerebral abscess by combined MR perfusion and diffusion imaging. Comput Med Imaging Graph 2002;26:19–23.
126. Ernst TM, Chang L, Witt MD, et al. Cerebral toxoplasmosis and lymphoma in AIDS: perfusion MR imaging experience in 13 patients. Radiology 1998;208:663–669.

127. Sugahara T, Korogi Y, Tomiguchi S, et al. Posttherapeutic intraaxial brain tumor: the value of perfusion-sensitive contrast-enhanced MR imaging for differentiating tumor recurrence from nonneoplastic contrast-enhancing tissue. AJNR Am J Neuroradiol 2000;21:901–909.
128. Hartmann M, Heiland S, Harting I, et al. Distinguishing of primary cerebral lymphoma from high-grade glioma with perfusion-weighted magnetic resonance imaging. Neurosci Lett 2003;338:119–122.
129. Cho SK, Na DG, Ryoo JW, et al. Perfusion MR imaging: clinical utility for the differential diagnosis of various brain tumors. Korean J Radiol 2002;3:171–179.
130. Yang D, Korogi Y, Sugahara T, et al. Cerebral gliomas: prospective comparison of multivoxel 2D chemical-shift imaging proton MR spectroscopy, echoplanar perfusion and diffusion-weighted MRI. Neuroradiology 2002;44:656–666.
131. Siewert B, Schlaug G, Edelman RR, Warach S. Comparison of EPISTAR and T2*-weighted gadolinium-enhanced perfusion imaging in patients with acute cerebral ischemia. Neurology 1997;48:673–679.
132. Detre JA, Alsop DC, Vives LR, et al. Noninvasive MRI evaluation of cerebral blood flow in cerebrovascular disease. Neurology 1998;50:633–641.
133. Yee SH, Liu HL, Hou J, et al. Detection of the brain response during a cognitive task using perfusion-based event-related functional MRI. Neuroreport 2000;11:2533–2536.
134. Rempp KA, Brix G, Wenz F, et al. Quantification of regional cerebral blood flow and volume with dynamic susceptibility contrast-enhanced MR imaging. Radiology 1994;193:637–641.
135. Ostergaard L, Johannsen P, Host-Poulsen P, et al. Cerebral blood flow measurements by magnetic resonance imaging bolus tracking: comparison with [(15)O]H2O positron emission tomography in humans. J Cereb Blood Flow Metab 1998;18: 935–940.
136. Schreiber WG, Guckel F, Stritzke P, et al. Cerebral blood flow and cerebrovascular reserve capacity: estimation by dynamic magnetic resonance imaging. J Cereb Blood Flow Metab 1998;18:1143–1156.
137. Ostergaard L, Chesler DA, Weisskoff RM, et al. Modeling cerebral blood flow and flow heterogeneity from magnetic resonance residue data. J Cereb Blood Flow Metab 1999;19:690–699.
138. Buxton RB, Frank LR. A model for the coupling between cerebral blood flow and oxygen metabolism during neural stimulation. J Cereb Blood Flow Metab. 1997;17:64–72.
139. Ogawa S, Lee TM, Nayak AS, et al. Oxygenation-sensitive contrast in magnetic resonance image of rodent brain at high magnetic fields. Magn Reson Med 1990;14:68–78.
140. Ogawa S, Tank DW, Menon R, et al. Intrinsic signal changes accompanying sensory stimulation: functional brain mapping with magnetic resonance imaging. Proc Natl Acad Sci USA 1992;89:5951–5955.
141. Bandettini PA, Wong EC, Hinks RS, Tikofsky RS, Hyde JS.Time course EPI of human brain function during task activation. Magn Reson Med 1992;25:390–397.
142. Kwong KK, Belliveau JW, Chesler DA, et al. Dynamic magnetic resonance imaging of human brain activity during primary sensory stimulation. Proc Natl Acad Sci USA 1992;89:5675–5679.
143. Ahmad Z, Balsamo LM, Sachs BC, Xu B, Gaillard WD. Auditory comprehension of language in young children: Neural networks identified with fMRI. Neurology 2003;60:1598–1605.
144. Gaillard WD, Sachs BC, Whitnah JR, et al. Developmental aspects of language processing: fMRI of verbal fluency in children and adults. Hum Brain Mapping 2003;18:176–185.
145. Gaillard WD, Balsamo LM, Ibrahim Z, Sachs BC, Xu B. fMRI identifies regional specialization of neural networks for reading in young children. Neurology 2003;60:94–100.
146. Peterson BS, Vohr B, Kane MJ, et al. A functional magnetic resonance imaging study of language processing and its cognitive correlates in prematurely born children. Pediatrics 2002;110:1153–1162.
147. Adleman NE, Menon V, Blasey CM, et al. A Developmental fMRI Study of the Stroop Color-Word Task. Neuroimage 2002;16:61–75.
148. Bunge SA, Dudukovic NM, Thomason ME, Vaidya CJ, Gabrieli JD. Immature frontal lobe contributions to cognitive control in children: evidence from fMRI. Neuron 2002;33:301–11.
149. Klingberg T, Forssberg H, Westerberg H. Increased brain activity in frontal and parietal cortex underlies the development of visuospatial working memory capacity during childhood. J Cogn Neurosci 2002;14:1–10.
150. Holland SK, Plante E, Weber Byars A, et al. Normal fMRI brain activation patterns in children performing a verb generation task. Neuroimage 2001;14:837–843.
151. Gaillard WD, Pugliese M, Grandin CB, et al. Cortical localization of reading in normal children: an fMRI language study. Neurology 2001;57:47–54.
152. Serafini S, Steury K, Richards T, et al. Comparison of fMRI and PEPSI during language processing in children. Magn Reson Med 2001;45:217–225.
153. Nelson CA, Monk CS, Lin J, et al. Functional neuroanatomy of spatial working memory in children. Dev Psychol 2000; 36:109–116.
154. Gaillard WD, Hertz-Pannier L, Mott SH, et al. Functional anatomy of cognitive development: fMRI of verbal fluency in children and adults. Neurology 2000;54:180–185.
155. Thomas KM, King SW, Franzen PL, et al. A developmental functional MRI study of spatial working memory. Neuroimage 1999;10:327–338.

156. Booth JR, Macwhinney B, Thulborn KR, et al. Functional organization of activation patterns in children: whole brain fMRI imaging during three different cognitive tasks. Prog Neuropsychopharmacol Biol Psychiatry. 1999;23:669–682.
157. Ulualp SO, Biswal BB, Yetkin FZ, Kidder TM. Functional magnetic resonance imaging of auditory cortex in children. Laryngoscope 1998;108:1782–1786.
158. Casey BJ, Cohen JD, Jezzard P, et al. Activation of prefrontal cortex in children during a nonspatial working memory task with functional MRI. Neuroimage 1995;2:221–229.
159. Hertz-Pannier L, Gaillard WD, Mott SH, et al. Noninvasive assessment of language dominance in children and adolescents with functional MRI: a preliminary study. Neurology 1997;48:1003–1012.
160. Boor S, Vucurevic G, Pfleiderer C, et al. EEG-related Functional MRI in Benign Childhood Epilepsy with Centrotemporal Spikes. Epilepsia 2003;44:688–692.
161. Liegeois F, Connelly A, Salmond CH, et al. A direct test for lateralization of language activation using fMRI: comparison with invasive assessments in children with epilepsy. Neuroimage 2002;17:1861–1867.
162. Holloway V, Gadian DG, Vargha-Khadem F, et al. The reorganization of sensorimotor function in children after hemispherectomy. A functional MRI and somatosensory evoked potential study. Brain 2000;123:2432–2444.
163. Graveline CJ, Mikulis DJ, Crawley AP, Hwang PA. Regionalized sensorimotor plasticity after hemispherectomy fMRI evaluation. Pediatr Neurol 1998;19:337–342.
164. Stapleton SR, Kiriakopoulos E, Mikulis D, et al. Combined utility of functional MRI, cortical mapping, and frameless stereotaxy in the resection of lesions in eloquent areas of brain in children. Pediatr Neurosurg 1997;26:68–82.
165. Aylward EH, Richards TL, Berninger VW, et al. Instructional treatment associated with changes in brain activation in children with dyslexia. Neurology 2003;61:212–219.
166. Shaywitz BA, Shaywitz SE, Pugh KR, et al. Disruption of posterior brain systems for reading in children with developmental dyslexia. Biol Psychiatry 2002;52:101–110.
167. Georgiewa P, Rzanny R, Gaser C, et al. Phonological processing in dyslexic children: a study combining functional imaging and event related potentials. Neurosci Lett 2002;318:5–8.
168. Seki A, Koeda T, Sugihara S, et al. A functional magnetic resonance imaging study during sentence reading in Japanese dyslexic children. Brain Dev 2001;23:312–316.
169. Corina DP, Richards TL, Serafini S, et al. fMRI auditory language differences between dyslexic and able reading children. Neuroreport 2001;12:1195–1201.
170. Temple E, Poldrack RA, Salidis J, et al. Disrupted neural responses to phonological and orthographic processing in dyslexic children: an fMRI study. Neuroreport 2001;12:299–307.
171. Georgiewa P, Rzanny R, Hopf JM, et al. fMRI during word processing in dyslexic and normal reading children. Neuroreport 1999;10:3459–3465.
172. Levin HS, Scheller J, Rickard T, et al. Dyscalculia and dyslexia after right hemisphere injury in infancy. Arch Neurol 1996;53:88–96.
173. Durston S, Tottenham NT, Thomas KM, et al. Differential patterns of striatal activation in young children with and without ADHD. Biol Psychiatry 2003;53:871–878.
174. Anderson CM, Polcari A, Lowen SB, Renshaw PF, Teicher MH. Effects of methylphenidate on functional magnetic resonance relaxometry of the cerebellar vermis in boys with ADHD. Am J Psychiatry 2002;159:1322–1328.
175. Bush G, Frazier JA, Rauch SL, et al. Anterior cingulate cortex dysfunction in attention-deficit/hyperactivity disorder revealed by fMRI and the Counting Stroop. Biol Psychiatry 1999;45:1542–1552.
176. Lee JH, Telang FW, Springer CS Jr, Volkow ND. Abnormal brain activation to visual stimulation in cocaine abusers. Life Sci 2003;73:1953–1961.
177. Wexler BE, Gottschalk CH, Fulbright RK, et al. Functional magnetic resonance imaging of cocaine craving. Am J Psychiatry 2001;158:86–95.
178. Li SJ, Biswal B, Li Z, et al. Cocaine administration decreases functional connectivity in human primary visual and motor cortex as detected by functional MRI. Magn Reson Med 2000;43:45–51.
179. Gollub RL, Breiter HC, Kantor H, et al. Cocaine decreases cortical cerebral blood flow but does not obscure regional activation in functional magnetic resonance imaging in human subjects. J Cereb Blood Flow Metab 1998;18:724–734.
180. Breiter HC, Gollub RL, Weisskoff RM, et al. Acute effects of cocaine on human brain activity and emotion. Neuron 1997;19:591–611.
181. Kumari V, Gray JA, Fytche DH, et al. Cognitive effects of nicotine in humans: an fMRI study. Neuroimage 2003;19: 1002–1013.
182. Due DL, Huettel SA, Hall WG, Rubin DC. Activation in mesolimbic and visuospatial neural circuits elicited by smoking cues: evidence from functional magnetic resonance imaging. Am J Psychiatry 2002;159:954–960.
183. Jacobsen LK, Gore JC, Skudlarski P, et al. Impact of intravenous nicotine on BOLD signal response to photic stimulation. Magn Reson Imaging 2002;20:141–145.
184. Bloom AS, Hoffmann RG, Fuller SA, et al. Determination of drug-induced changes in functional MRI signal using a pharmacokinetic model. Hum Brain Mapping 1999;8:235–244.
185. Parks MH, Morgan VL, Pickens DR, et al. FMRI activation associated with self-paced finger tapping in chronic alcohol-dependent patients. Alcohol Clin Exp Res 2003;27:704–711.

186. Wrase J, Grusser SM, Klein S, et al. Development of alcohol-associated cues and cue-induced brain activation in alcoholics. Eur Psychiatry 2002;17:287–291.
187. Schneider F, Habel U, Wagner M, et al. Subcortical correlates of craving in recently abstinent alcoholic patients. Am J Psychiatry 2001;158:1075–1083.
188. George MS, Anton RF, Bloomer C, et al. Activation of prefrontal cortex and anterior thalamus in alcoholic subjects on exposure to alcohol-specific cues. Arch Gen Psychiatry 2001;58:345–352.
189. Tapert SF, Brown GG, Kindermann SS, et al. fMRI measurement of brain dysfunction in alcohol-dependent young women. Alcohol Clin Exp Res 2001;25:236–245.
190. Levin JM, Ross MH, Mendelson JH, et al. Reduction in BOLD fMRI response to primary visual stimulation following alcohol ingestion. Psychiatry Res 1998;82:135–146.
191. Paquette V, Levesque J, Mensour B, et al. Change the mind and you change the brain: effects of cognitive-behavioral therapy on the neural correlates of spider phobia. Neuroimage 2003;18:401–409.
192. Schneider F, Weiss U, Kessler C, et al. Subcortical correlates of differential classical conditioning of aversive emotional reactions in social phobia. Biol Psychiatry 1999;45:863–871.
193. Birbaumer N, Grodd W, Diedrich O, et al. fMRI reveals amygdala activation to human faces in social phobics. Neuroreport 1998;9:1223–1226.
194. Adler CM, McDonough-Ryan P, Sax KW, et al. fMRI of neuronal activation with symptom provocation in unmedicated patients with obsessive compulsive disorder. J Psychiatr Res 2000;34:317–324.
195. Levine JB, Gruber SA, Baird AA, Yurgelun-Todd D. Obsessive-compulsive disorder among schizophrenic patients: an exploratory study using functional magnetic resonance imaging data. Compr Psychiatry 1998;39:308–311.
196. Schlosser R, Gesierich T, Kaufmann B, et al. Altered effective connectivity during working memory performance in schizophrenia: a study with fMRI and structural equation modeling. Neuroimage 2003;19:751–763.
197. Jessen F, Scheef L, Germeshausen L, et al. Reduced hippocampal activation during encoding and recognition of words in schizophrenia patients. Am J Psychiatry 2003;160:1305–1312.
198. Walter H, Wunderlich AP, Blankenhorn M, et al. No hypofrontality, but absence of prefrontal lateralization comparing verbal and spatial working memory in schizophrenia. Schizophr Res 2003;61:175–184.
199. Hofer A, Weiss EM, Golaszewski SM, et al. An FMRI study of episodic encoding and recognition of words in patients with schizophrenia in remission. Am J Psychiatry 2003;160:911–918.
200. Lawrie SM, Whalley HC, Job DE, Johnstone EC. Structural and functional abnormalities of the amygdala in schizophrenia. Ann N Y Acad Sci 2003;985:445–460.
201. Schroder J, Wenz F, Schad LR, Baudendistel K, Knopp MV. Sensorimotor cortex and supplementary motor area changes in schizophrenia. A study with functional magnetic resonance imaging. Br J Psychiatry 1995;167:197–201.
202. Volz HP, Gaser C, Hager F, et al. Brain activation during cognitive stimulation with the Wisconsin Card Sorting Test–a functional MRI study on healthy volunteers and schizophrenics. Psychiatry Res 1997;75:145–157.
203. Callicott JH, Ramsey NF, Tallent K, et al. Functional magnetic resonance imaging brain mapping in psychiatry: methodological issues illustrated in a study of working memory in schizophrenia. Neuropsychopharmacology 1998;18:186–196.
204. Schneider F, Habel U, Kessler C, et al. Functional imaging of conditioned aversive emotional responses in antisocial personality disorder. Neuropsychobiology 2000;42:192–201.
205. Sweet L, Rao S, Primeau P, Mayer A, Cohen R. Functional Magnetic Resonance Imaging of Working Memory among Multiple Sclerosis Patients. In press.
206. Sweet L, Rao S, Primeau P, Durgerian S, Cohen R. FMRI response to increased verbal working memory demands among patients with multiple sclerosis. In press.
207. Penner IK, Rausch M, Kappos L, Opwis K, Radu EW. Analysis of impairment related functional architecture in MS patients during performance of different attention tasks. J Neurol 2003;250:461–472.
208. Staffen W, Mair A, Zauner H, et al. Cognitive function and fMRI in patients with multiple sclerosis: evidence for compensatory cortical activation during an attention task. Brain 2002;125:1275–1282.
209. Lewis SJ, Dove A, Robbins TW, Barker RA, Owen AM. Cognitive impairments in early Parkinson's disease are accompanied by reductions in activity in frontostriatal neural circuitry. J Neurosci 2003;23:6351–6356.
210. Peters S, Suchan B, Rusin J, et al. Apomorphine reduces BOLD signal in fMRI during voluntary movement in Parkinsonian patients. Neuroreport 2003;14:809–812.
211. Grossman M, Cooke A, DeVita C, et al. Grammatical and resource components of sentence processing in Parkinson's disease: an fMRI study. Neurology 2003;60:775–781.
212. Rowe J, Stephan KE, Friston K, Frackowiak R, Lees A, Passingham R. Attention to action in Parkinson's disease: impaired effective connectivity among frontal cortical regions. Brain 2002;125:276–289.
213. Jech R, Urgosik D, Tintera J, et al. Functional magnetic resonance imaging during deep brain stimulation: a pilot study in four patients with Parkinson's disease. Mov Disord 2001;16:1126–1132.
214. Haslinger B, Erhard P, Kampfe N, et al. Event-related functional magnetic resonance imaging in Parkinson's disease before and after levodopa. Brain 2001;124:558–570.
215. Kato T, Knopman D, Liu H. Dissociation of regional activation in mild AD during visual encoding: a functional MRI study. Neurology 2001;57:812–816.

216. Small SA, Nava AS, Perera GM, Delapaz R, Stern Y. Evaluating the function of hippocampal subregions with high-resolution MRI in Alzheimer's disease and aging. Microsc Res Tech. 2000;51:101–108.
217. Sperling RA, Bates JF, Chua EF, et al. fMRI studies of associative encoding in young and elderly controls and mild Alzheimer's disease. J Neurol Neurosurg Psychiatry 2003;74:44–50.
218. Prvulovic D, Hubl D, Sack AT, et al. Functional imaging of visuospatial processing in Alzheimer's disease. Neuroimage 2002;17:1403–1414.
219. Johnson SC, Saykin AJ, Baxter LC, et al. The relationship between fMRI activation and cerebral atrophy: comparison of normal aging and Alzheimer disease. Neuroimage 2000;11:179–187.
220. Cao Y, Vikingstad EM, George KP, Johnson AF, Welch KM. Cortical language activation in stroke patients recovering from aphasia with functional MRI. Stroke 1999;30:2331–2340.
221. Zahn R, Huber W, Drews E, et al. Recovery of semantic word processing in transcortical sensory aphasia: a functional magnetic resonance imaging study. Neurocase 2002;8:376–386.
222. Johansen-Berg H, Rushworth MF, Bogdanovic MD, et al. The role of ipsilateral premotor cortex in hand movement after stroke. Proc Natl Acad Sci U S A 2002;99:14518–14523.
223. Marshall RS, Perera GM, Lazar RM, et al. Evolution of cortical activation during recovery from corticospinal tract infarction. Stroke 2000;31:656–661.
224. Pariente J, Loubinoux I, Carel C, et al. Fluoxetine modulates motor performance and cerebral activation of patients recovering from stroke. Ann Neurol 2001;50:718–729.
225. Feydy A, Carlier R, Roby-Brami A, et al. Longitudinal study of motor recovery after stroke: recruitment and focusing of brain activation. Stroke 2002;33:1610–1617.
226. Ozdoba C, Nirkko AC, Remonda L, Lovblad KO, Schroth G. Whole-brain functional magnetic resonance imaging of cerebral arteriovenous malformations involving the motor pathways. Neuroradiology 2002;44:1–10.
227. Lazar RM, Marshall RS, Pile-Spellman J, et al. Interhemispheric transfer of language in patients with left frontal cerebral arteriovenous malformation. Neuropsychologia 2000;38:1325–1332.
228. Cao Y, Aurora SK, Nagesh V, Patel SC, Welch KM. Functional MRI-BOLD of brainstem structures during visually triggered migraine. Neurology 2002;59:72–78.
229. Smith M, Cros D, Sheen V. Hyperperfusion with vasogenic leakage by fMRI in migraine with prolonged aura. Neurology 2002;58:1308–1310.
230. Reddy H, De Stefano N, Mortilla M, Federico A, Matthews PM. Functional reorganization of motor cortex increases with greater axonal injury from CADASIL. Stroke 2002;33:502–508.
231. Bandettini PA, Jesmanowicz A, Wong EC, Hyde JS. Processing strategies for time-course data sets in functional MRI of the human brain. Magn Reson Med 1993;30:161–173.
232. Binder JR, Rao SM, Hammeke TA, et al. Functional magnetic resonance imaging of human auditory cortex. Ann Neurol 1994;35:662–672.
233. D'Esposito M, Detre JA, Alsop DC, et al. The neural basis of the central executive system of working memory. Nature 1995;378:279 –281.
234. Rao SM, Bobholz JA, Hammeke TA, et al. Functional evidence for subcortical participation in conceptual reasoning skills. Neuroreport 1997;8:1987–1993.
235. Buckner RL, Bandettini PA, O'Craven KM, et al. Detection of cortical activation during averaged single trials of a cognitive task using functional magnetic resonance imaging. Proc Natl Acad Sci USA 1996;93:14,878–14,883.
236. Zahran E, Aguire G, D'Esposito M. A trial-based experimental design for fMRI. Neuroimage 1997;6:122–138.
237. Dale AM, Buckner RL. Selective averaging of rapidly presented individual trials using fMRI. Hum Brain Mapping 1997;5:329–340.
238. Josephs O, Turner R, Friston K. Event-related fMRI. Hum Brain Mapping 1997;5:243–248.
239. Boynton GM, Engel SA, Glover GH, Heeger DJ. Linear systems analysis of functional magnetic resonance imaging in human V1. J Neurosci 1996;16:4207–4221.
240. Cohen JD, Perlstein WM, Braver TS, et al. Temporal dynamics of brain activation during a working memory task. Nature 1997;386:604–607.
241. Wagner AD, Schacter DL, Rotte M, et al. Building memories: remembering and forgetting of verbal experiences as predicted by brain activity. Science 1998;281:1188–1191.
242. Rosen AC, Rao SM, Harrington DL, et al. Functional MRI correlates of cognitive-motor learning [abstract]. J Int Neuropsychol Soc 1996;2:49.
243. Stebbins GT, Carrillo MC, Dorfman J, et al. Aging effects on memory encoding in the frontal lobes. Psychol Aging 2002;17:44–55.
244. Rosen AC, Prull MW, O'Hara R, et al. Variable effects of aging on frontal lobe contributions to memory. Neuroreport 2002;13:2425–2428.
245. Morcom AM, Good CD, Frackowiak RS, Rugg MD. Age effects on the neural correlates of successful memory encoding. Brain 2003;126:213–229.
246. Cabeza R, Anderson ND, Locantore JK, McIntosh AR. Aging gracefully: compensatory brain activity in high-performing older adults. Neuroimage 2002;17:1394–1402.

247. Cabeza R. Cognitive neuroscience of aging: contributions of functional neuroimaging. Scand J Psychol 2001;42:277–286.
248. Mencl WE, Pugh KR, Shaywitz SE, et al. Network analysis of brain activations in working memory: behavior and age relationships. Microsc Res Tech 2000;51:64–74.
249. Grossman M, Cooke A, DeVita C, et al. Age-related changes in working memory during sentence comprehension: an fMRI study. Neuroimage 2002;15:302–317.
250. Riecker A, Grodd W, Klose U, et al. Relation between regional functional MRI activation and vascular reactivity to carbon dioxide during normal aging. J Cereb Blood Flow Metab 2003;23:565–573.
251. Hesselmann V, Zaro Weber O, Wedekind C, et al. Age-related signal decrease in functional magnetic resonance imaging during motor stimulation in humans. Neurosci Lett 2001;308:141–144.
252. Hutchinson S, Kobayashi M, Horkan CM, et al. Age-related differences in movement representation. Neuroimage 2002;17:1720–1728.
253. Huettel SA, Singerman JD, McCarthy G. The effects of aging upon the hemodynamic response measured by functional MRI. Neuroimage 2001;13:161–175.
254. Suzuki Y, Critchley HD, Suckling J, et al. Functional magnetic resonance imaging of odor identification: the effect of aging. J Gerontol A Biol Sci Med Sci 2001;56:M756–M760.
255. Ross MH, Yurgelun-Todd DA, Renshaw PF, et al. Age-related reduction in functional MRI response to photic stimulation. Neurology 1997;48:173–176.
256. Gunning-Dixon FM, Gur RC, Perkins AC, et al. Age-related differences in brain activation during emotional face processing. Neurobiol Aging 2003;24:285–295.
257. Lidaka T, Sadato N, Yamada H, et al. An fMRI study of the functional neuroanatomy of picture encoding in younger and older adults. Brain Res Cogn Brain Res 2001;11:1–11.
258. DiGirolamo GJ, Kramer AF, Barad V, et al. General and task-specific frontal lobe recruitment in older adults during executive processes: a fMRI investigation of task-switching. Neuroreport 2001;12:2065–2071.
259. Nielson KA, Langenecker SA, Garavan H. Differences in the functional neuroanatomy of inhibitory control across the adult life span. Psychol Aging 2002;17:56–71.
260. Milham MP, Erickson KI, Banich MT, et al. Attentional control in the aging brain: insights from an fMRI study of the stroop task. Brain Cogn 2002;49:277–296.
261. Taoka T, Iwasaki S, Uchida H, et al. Age correlation of the time lag in signal change on EPI-fMRI. J Comput Assist Tomogr 1998;22:514–517.
262. D'Esposito M, Zarahn E, Aguirre GK, Rypma B. The effect of normal aging on the coupling of neural activity to the bold hemodynamic response. Neuroimage 1999;10:6–14.
263. Mehagnoul-Schipper DJ, van der Kallen BF, Colier WN, et al. Simultaneous measurements of cerebral oxygenation changes during brain activation by near-infrared spectroscopy and functional magnetic resonance imaging in healthy young and elderly subjects. Hum Brain Mapping 2002;16:14–23.
264. Hock C, Müller-Spahn F, Schuh-Hofer S, et al. Age dependency of changes in cerebral hemoglobin oxygenation during brain activation: a near-infrared spectroscopy study. J Cereb Blood Flow Metab 1995;15:1103–1108.
265. Pardo JV, Fox PT, Raichle ME. Localization of a human system for sustained attention by positron emission tomography. Nature 1991;349:61–64.
266. Petersen SE, Fox PT, Posner MI, et al. Positron emission tomographic studies of the cortical anatomy of single word processing. Nature 1988;331:585–589.
267. Starkstein SE, Sabe L, Vazquez S, et al. Neuropsychological, psychiatric, and cerebral blood flow findings in vascular dementia and Alzheimer's disease. Stroke 1996;27:408–414.
268. Lee BC, Mintun M, Buckner RL, Morris JC. Imaging of Alzheimer's disease. J Neuroimag 2003;13:199–214.
269. Albert MS. Detection of very early Alzheimer disease through neuroimaging. Alzhemier Dis Assoc Disord. 2003;2(Suppl):S63–S65.
270. Szelies B, Mielke R, Kessler J, Heiss WD. EEG power changes are related to regional cerebral glucose metabolism in vascular dementia. Clin Neurophysiol. 1999;110:615–620
271. De Reuck J, Decoo D, Hasenbroekx MC, et al. Acetazolamide vasoreactivity in vascular dementia: a positron emission tomographic study. Euro Neurol 1999;41:31–36.
272. De Reuck J, Santens P, Strijckmans K, Lemahieu I. European Task Force on Age-Related White Matter Changes. Cobalt-55 positron emission tomography in vascular dementia: significance of white matter changes. J Neurol Sci. 2001;193:1–6.
273. Szirmai I, Vastagh I, Szombathelyi E, Kamondi A. Strategic infarcts of the thalamus in vascular dementia. J Neurol Sci 2002;203–204:91–97.
274. Cohen RA, Paul RH, Zawacki TM, et al. Single photon emission computed tomography, magnetic resonance imaging hyperintensity, and cognitive impairments in patients with vascular dementia. J Neuroimaging 2001;11:253–260.
275. Yoshikawa T, Murase K, Oku N, et al. Heterogeneity of cerebral blood flow in Alzheimer disease and vascular dementia. AJNR Am J Neuroradiol 2003;24:1341–1347.
276. Nagata K, Sato M, Satoh Y, et al.Hemodynamic aspects of Alzheimer's disease. Ann N Y Acad Sci 2002;977:391–402.

14

Contributions of Subcortical Lacunar Infarcts to Cognitive Impairment in Older Persons

Dan Mungas

1. INTRODUCTION

Alzheimer's disease (AD) and cerebrovascular disease (CVD) are generally considered the most common causes of cognitive impairment and dementia in older persons and are independent but frequently comorbid pathological processes. It is well established that AD is a major contributor to cognitive impairment and dementia, but the effects of CVD are less clear. Not only is there controversy about the magnitude of CVD effects in general, but CVD is also pathologically heterogenous and there also are important questions about how specific manifestations of CVD relate to cognition.

CVD varies according to type (e.g., ischemic vs hemorrhagic), location (cortical, subcortical, or white matter), size of affected vessels (small vs large artery involvement), and degree of vascular pathology. There is little question that large cortical infarcts, even single infarcts, can cause substantial cognitive impairment and dementia. Subcortical CVD also is interesting for several reasons. Subcortical ischemic vascular disease (SIVD), including subcortical lacunar infarcts (lacunes) and white matter hyperintensities (WMH), is relatively common in older people in general *(1–4)* and is frequently present in patients seen at dementia clinics *(1)*.

Advances in imaging technology have facilitated routine detection of relatively small lacunes and WMH in clinical settings, but scientific understanding of the significance of these changes has lagged behind. SIVD typically results from occlusions of the deep penetrating arterioles and arteries that feed the basal ganglia, thalamus, white matter, and internal capsule. Unlike large-vessel ischemia, which results in cortical strokes with acute onset and focal neurologic dysfunction, SIVD can present similarly to AD, with insidious onset and gradual progression and without obvious focal neurologic symptoms. These similarities in clinical presentation and age of onset make the differential diagnosis between AD and SIVD challenging but clinically important and point to the need for better understanding of how SIVD contributes to cognitive decline. This chapter focuses on how one component of SIVD, lacunar infarction, relates to cognition.

1.1. *Cerebral Infarcts, Cognitive Impairment, and Dementia*

Cerebral infarcts have been linked to dementia since the classic work of Tomlinson and colleagues *(5)*. More recently, Schneider et al. *(6)* found that neuropathologically identified cerebral infarcts were associated with at least a twofold increased risk for dementia. Although these studies did not separately examine effects of subcortical infarcts, there is evidence that subcortical infarcts are specifically related to dementia. Another pathological series from the Nun study *(7)* showed a link between subcortical infarcts and dementia. Subcortical infarcts were important moderators of the effect of AD pathology on cognition. Patients with a given amount of AD pathology who had

From: *Current Clinical Neurology*
Vascular Dementia: Cerebrovascular Mechanisms and Clinical Management
Edited by: R. H. Paul, R. Cohen, B. R. Ott, and S. Salloway © Humana Press Inc., Totowa, NJ

infarcts were more likely to be demented than those with equal AD changes who didn't have infarcts. Tatemichi and colleagues *(8,9)* found an increased risk for dementia in poststroke patients associated both with large cortical infarction (3.9 times increased risk) and small lacunar infarction (2.7 times). Similar results were reported from a European epidemiological study in which participants received magnetic resonance imaging (MRI) scans; silent cerebral infarcts more than doubled the risk for dementia *(4)*.

Lacunar infarction has significant effects on cognition short of dementia. For example, mild cognitive changes have been reported after single infarcts *(10)*. In this study, cognitive changes were subtle but involved multiple cognitive domains. Vermeer et al. *(4)* described more specific effects, showing that silent thalamic lacunes were related to longitudinal decline in memory performance, whereas silent nonthalamic lacunes were associated with decline in psychomotor speed. Interestingly, cognitive decline was apparent only in those who had additional lacunes after the baseline MRI. Van der Werf et al. *(11)* identified specific cognitive changes associated with specific lesions of the thalamus and dissociated these relationships from the effects of broader CVD. They found specific associations between mamillothalamic tract damage and episodic memory and between several specific thalamic nuclei and executive function.

Literature to date provides consistent evidence that cerebral infarcts are associated with cognitive impairment and dementia. There is more specific evidence linking subcortical lacunes to both dementia and decline on continuous cognitive measures, and lacune effects on cognition are present even when lacunes are clinically silent. Thalamic lacunes, in particular, have important relationships with cognition. Thus, there is considerable support for an association between lacunes and cognitive impairment.

1.2. Frontal-Subcortical Circuits and SIVD

Neural circuits connecting subcortical gray matter structures, especially the thalamus and basal ganglia, with frontal cortex and the medial temporal lobes have important significance for understanding cognitive impairment resulting from SIVD and lacunes. Discrete frontal-subcortical circuits have been linked to both cognitive and behavioral changes *(12)*. The dorsolateral prefrontal circuit is particularly important for cognition, and it has been linked to executive function, which is a frontally mediated cognitive domain. This circuit involves projections from dorsolateral prefrontal cortex to the dorsolateral head of the caudate to the globus pallidus and substantia nigra and then to the ventral anterior and dorsomedial nuclei of the thalamus and back to dorsolateral prefrontal cortex. Subcortical gray matter structures and white matter tracts in this circuit are perfused by small penetrating arterioles and are vulnerable to SIVD ischemic lesions. The interconnection of the subcortical nuclei and pathways in this circuit with dorsolateral prefrontal cortex provides a conceptual basis for expecting selective deficits of executive function associated with the two primary types of SIVD, lacunes, and WMH.

The medial temporal limbic-diencephalic memory system is a second neural network that has important significance for understanding how subcortical lacunes might affect memory and cognition. This is a complex circuit that includes the hippocampus and amygdala in the medial temporal lobe, the septal nuclei, mammillary bodies, and the anterior cingulate gyrus and orbital frontal cortex. In addition, the anterior thalamic nucleus and the medial dorsal nucleus of the thalamus are important components of this circuit. This circuit has interconnections with other frontal-subcortical circuits. Bilateral lesions affecting these thalamic nuclei have been observed to cause a dementia syndrome with dense amnesia *(13,14)*. Disruption of this system by ischemic lesions of the thalamus is another important mechanism linking SIVD and cognitive impairment.

1.3. Previous Related Studies on SIVD, AD, and Cognitive Impairment

This chapter reports results from a longitudinal, multicenter project examining the contributions of SIVD and AD to cognitive impairment and dementia. Subcortical lacunes identified using MRI are an important focus in this project and have been a primary independent variable in numerous studies. However, in addition, quantitative measures of other components of brain structure also have been examined in conjunction with lacunes, which facilitates evaluation of the relative contributions of different structural changes to cognitive decline. A consistent finding from the researchers' project is that cortical gray matter (CGM) volume and hippocampal (HC) volume are more important determinants of cognitive status than are SIVD components, lacunes, and WMH. This general pattern of results was observed when dementia was the primary outcome *(15)* and when specific neuropsychological tests of memory, language, and executive function were outcomes *(16)*. In the latter study, thalamic lacunes had the strongest relationship with cognitive measures, but these effects were weak and were not independent of WMH, CGM, and HC. In a study of baseline MRI predictors of longitudinal decline in global cognition, HC and CGM again were the primary determinants of cognitive change, but presence of lacunes moderated the effect of HC such that baseline HC predicted cognitive decline in those without lacunes but not in those with lacunes. In a study of cognitively normal participants, defined by the Clinical Dementia Rating (CDR) *(17,18)*, lacunes were associated with subtle but significant cognitive changes in visual memory and executive function *(19)*. These changes were specific, because lacunes were not related to verbal memory, language, or spatial ability. Another approach involved using positron emission tomography (PET) to examine effects of lacunes on regional brain function *(20)*. This study found that subcortical lacunes were associated with decreased global cortical glucose metabolism but also showed a stronger, more specific relationship between lacunes and frontal lobe metabolism. In a second PET study, Reed et al. *(21)* found dorsolateral frontal metabolism to be associated with cognitive decline in patients with lacunes.

In summary, the researchers' work has shown that lacunes are related to subtle cognitive impairment, especially of executive abilities, and are also associated with decreased cortical glucose metabolism, particularly in the frontal lobes. However, lacunes' effects have been weak in comparison with the effects of WMH, CGM, and HC. One explanation for this pattern of results is that lacunes might simply be an epiphenomenon of broader CVD. That is, lacunes may be a marker for broader CVD, but cognitive changes resulting from CVD may result from WMH and cortical ischemic injury that are also part of the broader CVD. The extent to which lacunes uniquely contribute to cognitive impairment is an important question for further research. Other interpretations for the relatively weak lacune effects in the researchers' studies are possible, and consequently, there is a need for research examining some of these possibilities. In particular, methodological issues regarding lacune localization and how lacunes are measured might have important implications.

1.4. Purpose of Study

The purpose of this study was to extend the researchers' work and address questions not adequately answered in previous literature. The researchers were interested in both methodological and substantive questions. They examined effects of subcortical lacunes on cognitive function and compared these effects with effects of other structural brain variables, including WMH, CGM, and HC. This study had several goals and was designed to test specific hypotheses. First, it examined the relative benefits of lacune volume vs number of lacunes in accounting for cognition and tested the hypothesis that lacune volume is more sensitive to cognitive differences. Second, it addressed the issue of strategic localization of lacunes and specifically tested the hypothesis that lacunes in specific subcortical regions are differentially associated with cognition. It also examined the relative strength of effects of volume of lacunes within specific regions vs total volume of lacunes. Third, it evaluated whether lacunes make a contribution to cognitive function independent of WMH and tested the hypothesis that lacunes have specific effects on cognition that transcend nonspecific effects of SIVD. Fourth, it examined relative effects of lacunes in comparison with other volumetric brain measures to address relative contributions of these brain components to cognition and, ultimately, to clarify the importance of lacunes as a pathological substrate for impaired cognition.

Table 1
Demographic Characteristics and Global Cognitive Status of Subject Sample

Gender	Number (%) male	98 (59.4)
	Number (%) female	67 (40.6)
Education (yr)	Mean (SD)	14.6 (3.3)
	Range	5–23
Age (yr)	Mean (SD)	75.6 (7.2)
	Range	56–90
MMSE	Mean (SD)	25.1 (5.3)
	Range	1–30

Abbr: MMSE, Mini-Mental State Exam.

2. METHOD

2.1. Participants

Participants in this study were recruited from three academic dementia centers and were evaluated as part of a multicenter collaborative study of contributions of SIVD and AD to cognitive impairment and dementia. All participants received a comprehensive clinical evaluation that included a detailed medical history, a neurological examination, appropriate laboratory tests, and neuropsychological testing with a standardized test battery. In addition, participants received an MRI scan of the brain at the baseline evaluation, and some had a subsequent, second MRI scan. Individuals with cortical infarcts at the time of the baseline scan were excluded. Participants were diagnosed at a multidisciplinary case conference using National Institute of Neurological and Communicative Diseases and Stroke/Alzheimer's Disease and Related Disorders Association (NINCDS/ADRDA) diagnostic criteria *(22)* for AD and State of California Alzheimer Disease Diagnostic and Treatment Centers (SCADDTC) criteria *(23)* for ischemic vascular dementia. A diagnosis of mixed dementia required that the patient met criteria for both AD and IVD, and in the judgment of the clinical team, both etiologies were believed to contribute relatively equally to the dementia symptoms. The institutional review boards at all participating institutions approved this study, and subjects or their legal representatives gave written informed consent for participation.

Recruitment was targeted to fill six groups defined by three levels of cognitive impairment crossed with presence vs absence of subcortical lacunes. The levels of cognitive impairment were: (1) normal—defined by a CDR *(17,18)* total score of 0.0, (2) impaired (CDR = 0.5), and (3) demented (CDR $\geq$1.0). A single neuroradiologist reviewed all MRI scans to determine the presence of lacunes.

This study was based on a sample of 165 participants that included the full range of cognitive function and had broad variability in presence of SIVD. The most recent MRI scan for participants in the overall project was identified, and individuals who had complete MRI data from this scan and also had complete neuropsychological test data from a visit within 6 mo of the index scan were selected. Demographic characteristics and global cognitive function (Mini-Mental State Examination [MMSE]) *(24)* are presented in Table 1. There were 59 cognitively normal individuals (22 with lacunes), 46 of whom were cognitively impaired (25 with lacunes), and 60 who were demented (25 with lacunes). This sample was diverse in both cognitive function and presence/degree of SIVD.

2.2. MRI Methods

Volumetric MRI variables were computerized measures of WMH, CGM, HC, and lacunes within specific structures: thalamus, putamen, caudate, globus pallidus, and white matter. All volumes were normalized to total intracranial volume. Number of lacunes in each region identified by the neuroradiologist was also recorded and included as an independent variable.

Lacunes were small (>2 mm) areas of the brain with increased signal relative to cerebrospinal fluid (CSF) on proton density MRI in subcortical gray and white matter. Lacunes were differentiated from perivascular spaces, which can be particularly prominent below the anterior commissure and putamen and at bends in the course of penetrating arterioles. Isointense lesions on pseudo-proton density MRI (as opposed to "true" proton density, which is obtained when extrapolated to TE = 0) at the level of the anterior commissure or inferior putamen were termed perivascular spaces; outside that region they were defined as cavitated lacunes if they were greater than or equal to mm at maximum width. Lesions that met either of these criteria were considered lacunes for purposes of this study.

Image acquisition and data management and transmission previously have been described *(15)*. A computerized segmentation algorithm was used to classify brain MRI pixels into CGM, subcortical gray matter, white matter, WMH, ventricular CSF, and sulcal CSF. In addition, total intracranial volume was computed by summing all pixels within the intracranial vault. Segmentation methods have been previously reported *(15)*. Intraclass correlation coefficients across independent raters ($n = 10$) were: 0.93 for percent of white matter; 0.99 for percent of white matter hyperintensity; 0.95 for CGM; 0.99 for sulcal CSF; and 0.99 for ventricular CSF.

Automated hippocampal volumetry was conducted using a commercially available high dimensional brain-mapping tool (Medtronic Surgical Navigation Technologies, Louisville, CO), which combined a coarse and then a fine transformation to match cerebral MR images with a template brain *(25)*. Global landmarks were placed at external boundaries of the target brain by manual adjustment of the angle and dimension of a three-dimensional box in orthogonal MR images. The next step was manual selection of 22 control points as local landmarks for hippocampal segmentation: one at the hippocampal head, one at the tail, and four per image (i.e., at the superior, inferior, medial, and lateral boundaries) on five equally spaced images perpendicular to the long axis of the ipsilateral hippocampus. This step was repeated for the contralateral hippocampus. Using both the global and the local landmarks, a coarse transformation was computed using landmark matching. Automated hippocampal morphometry was then performed by a fluid image matching transformation *(26)*.

2.3. *Neuropsychological Measures*

All participants received a standardized battery of neuropsychological tests in common clinical use. Several specific tests were used to derive psychometrically matched measures of global cognition, memory, and executive function that were the primary outcomes in this study. Details of scale derivation and validation have been previously reported *(27)*. Global cognition was a composite measure derived from trials 1 and 2 of the word list learning task of the Memory Assessment Scales (MAS) *(28)*, Wechsler Memory Scale-Revised *(29)* Digit span forward and backward, animal category fluency *(30,31)*, and letter fluency for the letter "A" *(32)*. Memory was derived from delayed and cued recall and selected immediate recall trials of the MAS word list-learning task. Scores were primarily determined by delayed free and cued recall and by supraspan recall from the immediate recall trials. The executive scale used letter fluency (F, A, and S) *(32)*, digit span backward, visual span backward *(29)*, and the Initiation-Perseveration subscale of the Mattis Dementia Rating Scale *(33)* as donor scales.

Scale construction of the global, memory, and executive measures was guided by methods associated with item response theory (IRT) *(34,35)*, a modern and widely used approach to large-scale psychometric test development. Scale construction methods were based on a larger sample of 400 from this project and are described in detail elsewhere *(27)*. Briefly, IRT analyses yield two important scale level functions or curves that describe the basic psychometric properties of the scale. The test information curve (TIC) represents scale reliability at each point on the ability continuum, whereas the test characteristic curve (TCC) describes the expected test score at each ability point. Ability essentially refers to capacity to successfully perform the task or tasks incorporated in the scale and can be estimated roughly by scale total score. The three composite measures had TICs showing high reliability ($r \geq .90$) from approximately 2.0 SD below the mean of the cognitively diverse overall development sample to 2.0 SD above the mean. These measures have a broad range of measurement without appreciable floor or ceiling effects for participants in this sample and have linear measurement properties across this broad ability range *(27)*. They also are near-normally distributed, which presents important advantages for statistical analyses.

The global, memory, and executive measures were transformed so that scores were referenced to the distribution of the cognitively normal without lacunes recruitment group, so that the scale of measurement corresponded to a traditional scale with a mean of 100 and standard deviation of 15. Thus, a score of 85 represents 1 SD below the mean of the normal participants without lacunes.

2.4. Data Analysis

The three matched cognitive measures, global, memory, and executive, were the primary outcomes of interest. Multistage linear regression analyses were used to evaluate the relationship of MRI variables to cognitive function. In the first stage of analysis, lacune volumes in the five specific subcortical regions were entered as independent variables predicting each of the three cognitive variables. Effects of specific lacune locations were then compared with total volume of lacunes. In the second stage of analysis, lacune number was entered as the independent variable. In the third stage, lacune volume and WMH were independent variables; in the fourth stage, CGM was added to the two variables from step three; and in the fifth stage, HC was added to the variables from the previous step. Effect size estimates were calculated in two ways. First, the R^2 value associated with using a specific independent variable as a predictor of each dependent variable was used to quantify the strength of that simple bivariate relationship. R^2 is an index of the amount of variance in the dependent variable accounted for by the independent variable, or variables in more complex models. Second, estimates of incremental effect sizes were calculated to determine strength of a given independent variable independent of the contribution of other independent variables in a model. The R^2 value was calculated for the full model, including the MRI effect of interest and an R^2 was also calculated for a model missing the effect of interest. The incremental effect size for that variable was the R^2 for the full model minus the R^2 for the model without the effect of interest.

3. RESULTS

3.1. Localization of Lacunes

Volumes of lacunes within the five subcortical regions (white matter, caudate, putamen, globus pallidus, and thalamus) were entered as joint independent variables in separate models to explain global, memory, and executive as dependent variables. Lacunes entered jointly were significantly related to global ($F[5,159] = 2.37$, $p = 0.04$) and executive ($F[5,159] = 5.26$, $p = 0.0002$) but were not related to memory ($p = 0.38$). White matter ($F[1,159] = 8.15$, $p = 0.005$) and thalamic ($F[1,159] = 7.74$, $p = 0.006$) lacune volumes were independently related to executive, but only thalamic lacune volume (F[1,159]) = 4.71, $p = 0.03$) was significantly related to Global. Table 2 shows simple bivariate R^2 explained by thalamic and white matter lacunes and total R^2 explained by all lacune locations jointly. Total lacune effects were strongest for executive, accounting for approximately 14% of the variance in this variable. White matter and thalamic lacunes each explained approximately 8% of the variance in executive. Thalamic lacunes explained approximately 4% of the variance in global, but lacune effects for global and memory were otherwise limited.

Total volume of lacunes in all regions was next included as the lone independent variable. This variable was significantly related to global (F[1,163]) = 8.53, $p < 0.004$, $R^2 = 0.050$) and executive ($F[1,163] = 20.57$, $p < 0.0001$, $R^2 = 0.112$) but not to Memory ($p > 0.14$, $R^2 = 0.013$). Variance in cognitive variables explained by total lacune volume also is shown in Table 2. Comparing the effect sizes in Table 2 shows that total lacune volume is nearly as effective in accounting for cognitive performance as is using lacune volumes within all five specific structures. Consequently, total lacune volume was used to characterize lacune effects in subsequent analyses.

Table 2
Variance in Cognition (Global, Memory, Executive) Explained by Different Combinations of Magnetic Resonance Imaging Variables

	Cognitive variable		
Effects in model	Global	Memory	Executive
Volume of thalamic lacunes	.043	.021	.076
Volume of white matter lacunes	.035	.009	.084
Volumes of lacunes in all regions [a]	.069	.033	.142
Total number of lacunes	.022	.005	.060
Total volume of lacunes (LAC)	.050	.013	.112
LAC + WMH	.164	.098	.216
LAC + WMH + CGM	.265	.254	.283
LAC + WMH + CGM + HC	.366	.504	.344

Note: Tabled values are R^2 values from regression analyses with the cognitive variables as dependent variables and the indicated magnetic resonance imaging variables as independent variables. All volumes were normalized to total intracranial volume.

[a] Thalamus, caudate, putamen, globus pallidus, and white matter.

Abbr: CGM, cortical gray matter volume; HC, hippocampal volume.

3.2. *Number of Lacunes*

Numbers of lacunes within each of the five specific regions were entered jointly as independent variables in next analysis stage. Global ($p > 0.37$, $R^2 = 0.033$) and memory ($p > 0.33$, $R^2 = 0.035$) were not significantly related to number of lacunes in the five regions. Executive was significantly associated with the five regions entered jointly (F[5,159] = 2.33, $p < 0.05$, $R^2 = 0.068$), but only thalamic lacune number approached significance as an individual effect (F[1,159] = 3.83, $p < 0.06$). Total number of lacunes in all five regions entered as a lone independent variable was significantly related to executive (F[1,163] = 10.48, $p < 0.002$, $R^2 = 0.060$), but not to global ($p < 0.06$) or memory ($p > 0.38$). Relationships of lacune volumes from prior analyses were consistently stronger than analogous relationships with lacune numbers (*see* Table 2), and, indeed, total lacune volume accounted for almost twice the variance as did total number of lacunes. These results indicate that lacune volume is consistently superior to lacune number in explaining cognitive function.

3.3. *Lacunes and White Matter Hyperintensity*

Total lacune volume and WMH were entered as joint independent variables in the next stage of analysis. The overall models for all three dependent variables were statistically significant: global (F[2,162] =15.93, $p < 0.0001$, $R^2 = 0.164$), memory (F[2,162] = 8.79, $p = 0.0002$, $R^2 = 0.098$), executive (F[2,162] = 22.29, $p < 0.0001$, $R^2 = 0.216$). Global (F[1,162] = 22.22, $p < 0.0001$) and memory (F[1,162] = 15.27, $p < 0.0001$) were significantly related to WMH but not lacune volume. Executive was independently related to both lacune volume (F[1,162] = 6.82, $p = 0.01$) and WMH (F[1,162] = 21.42, $p < 0.0001$). These results show specific lacune volume effect independent of generalized SIVD for executive but not for global or memory.

3.4. *Lacunes, White Matter Hyperintensity, Cortical Gray Matter, and Hippocampus*

CGM was added as an independent variable to the model from the previous step that included WMH and lacune volume. Global (overall $R^2 = 0.265$) was significantly related to WMH (F[1,161] = 4.88, $p < 0.3$) and CGM (F[1,161] = 22.14, $p < 0.0001$) but not lacune volume. Memory (overall $R^2 = 0.254$) was significantly related only to CGM (F[1,161] = 33.74, $p < 0.0001$). Executive (overall

Table 3
Regression Coefficients, Standard Errors, and Standardized Betas for Effect of Total Lacune Volume on Executive in Models With Different Combinations of Magnetic Resonance Imaging Variables

Effects in model	Regression coefficient	Standard error	Standardized beta
Total lacune volume	–10153.9	2238.7	–.33
LAC + WMH	–5990.7	2294.1	–.20
LAC + WMH + CGM	–5851.9	2200.2	–.19
LAC + WMH + CGM + HC	–7534.9	2156.0	–.25

Abbr: LAC, total volume of lacunes; WMH, white matter hyperintensity volume; CGM, cortical gray matter volume; HC, hippocampal volume. All volumes were normalized to total intracranial volume.

$R^2 = 0.283$) was independently related to all three MRI components: lacune volume (F[1,161] = 7.07, $p < 0.009$), WMH (F[1,161] = 5.89, $p < 0.02$), CGM (F[1,161] = 15.17, $p < 0.0001$). These results show that CGM is strongly related to all three cognitive variables and incrementally improves the prediction of these variables beyond effects of lacunes and WMH (*see* Table 2). These results continue to show specific lacune effects for executive but not global or memory.

A final model added HC to lacune volume, WMH, and CGM from the previous analysis. HC was significantly and independently related to all three dependent variables: global (F[1,160] = 25.46, $p < 0.0001$), memory (F[1,160] = 80.71, $p < 0.0001$), executive (F[1,160] = 14.84, $p = 0.0002$). Hippocampal volume explained 10.1% of the variance in global beyond that explained by lacunes, WHM, and CGM; for memory, HC incrementally explained 25.0% of the variance and, for executive, incrementally explained 6.1% of variance (*see* Table 2). Global also was independently but weakly related to lacune volume (F[1,160] = 4.27, $p < 0.05$) and WMH (F[1,160] = 6.4, $p < 0.02$). Memory was independently related only to HC. Executive also was related to lacune volume (F[1,160] = 12.21, $p = 0.0006$) and WMH (F[1,160] = 7.02, $p < 0.009$). CGM was not related to any of the three cognitive variables independent of HC. These results show that HC has important, broadly based relationships with cognition, but CGM effects were not independent of HC. Lacunes and WMH were significantly related to both global and executive, but SIVD effects were strongest for executive. There were specific lacune effects on executive.

Table 2 shows that even for executive, lacune effects were smaller than were the effects of WMH, CGM, and HC. WMH clearly added explanatory power for all three cognitive variables beyond that associated with lacunes. CGM made a clear incremental contribution to all three variables, as did HC, especially for memory, where the variance accounted for was doubled. Table 3 shows the regression coefficients and standard errors, as well as standardized betas, for the lacune effect on executive for models involving (1) lacunes alone, (2) lacunes plus WMH, (3) lacunes, WMH, and CGM, and (4) lacunes, WMH, CGM, and HC. Standardized beta is a standardized regression coefficient that provides comparable estimates of independent effect size across different variables and models. Its square can be roughly interpreted as the amount of independent variance accounted for by the effect of interest. The regression coefficient for lacunes was attenuated by approximately 50% when WMH was added to the model but was not further attenuated by the addition of CGM. The coefficient increased moderately when HC was added. Standardized betas show a similar pattern; independent variance accounted for by lacunes was more than halved when WMH was added, was not affected by CGM, and increased slightly when HC was added. These results indicate that part of the effect of lacune volume on executive is shared with WMH and may reflect nonspecific SIVD. Approximately 4–5% of the variance in executive is unique to lacunes.

3.5. Interrelationship of MRI Variables

Pearson correlation coefficients were calculated to assess intercorrelation of total volume of lacunes, WMH, CGM, and HC. Lacunes were significantly related both to WMH (Pearson r = 0.39) and CGM (r = –0.21). CGM was more strongly related to WMH (r = –0.51) and HC (0.53). HC was weakly related to WMH (r = 0.19) but not to lacunes (r = 0.07, $p > 0.35$). Becuause CGM had bivariate relationships with the other three MRI variables, a regression analysis was performed to evaluate independent relationships of the other variables with CGM. WMH and HC were both independent predictors of CGM ($p < 0.0001$), but lacune volume was not related independent of WMH and HC. WMH independently accounted for approximately 17% of CGM variance and HC for approximately 21%.

4. DISCUSSION

Subcortical lacunes showed a pattern of differential relationships to cognitive abilities. Having psychometrically matched measures of cognitive domains was an important strength of this study that facilitates identification of differential effects. Lacunes were most strongly related to executive function but were not related to memory. There was a weak relationship with the global cognitive measures, which may reflect the presence of an executive component in the global measure. Total volume of subcortical lacunes was as effective in accounting for cognition as was volume of lacunes in specific subcortical structures. Thalamic lacunes, as expected based on previous literature, were most strongly related to cognition, but unexpectedly, white matter lacunes were as strongly related to executive function as thalamic lacunes. Lacune volume consistently was more strongly associated with cognition than was lacune number.

Total lacune volume accounted for approximately 11% of the variance in executive function but less than 5% of variance in memory and the global cognition measure. The lacune effect on executive function was independent of WMH, CGM, and HC. This lacune effect was substantially attenuated by the addition of WMH but was not further diminished by adding CGM and HC as explanatory variables. These results suggest that lacunes have both nonspecific and specific effects on cognition. That is, lacunes are an indicator of more generalized CVD that is associated with cognitive changes and results in nonspecific effects that are shared with WMH, another indicator of generalized CVD. However, lacunes also had a more specific effect on executive function that was independent of WMH. Lacune effects were somewhat stronger in this study than in a previous similar study from this project *(16)*. Part of this difference may relate to selecting a subject sample defined by the most recent available scan. This may have resulted in greater variability in both cognitive function and AD and SIVD pathology owing to differential longitudinal change across participants in these variables.

WMH had a greater effect than lacunes on cognition in this study and may be a better index of the extent of generalized CVD. The specific lacune effect on executive function was modest, accounting for approximately 5% of the variance, but this was independent of all other volumetric brain components examined. Results from this study showed that thalamic and white matter lacunes were more strongly related to executive function than lacunes in other locations, which did not further contribute to executive function. It may be that there are more specific characteristics of white matter lacunes that affect cognition, and, specifically, white matter lacunes disrupting tracts of the dorsolateral prefrontal-thalamic circuit may be especially important. A limitation of this study was that specific localization of white matter lacunes was not available. Similarly, more precise delineation of lacunes in the other structures might be important, and, for example, lacunes in the dorsolateral head of the caudate might have a more evident effect. Further studies with more specific localization of lacunes might lead to a better understanding of how these lacunes affect cognition.

Results from this study support a selective effect of lacunes on executive function and a broader effect of CVD on cognition. AD is well established as a major contributor to cognitive impairment, AD and CVD frequently co-occur, and it is difficult to directly measure extent of AD pathology in living patients. Better understanding of relative contributions of AD and CVD would have important clinical implications, would help in clinical diagnosis of AD and CVD contributions to dementia. This is more than an academic issue and will be increasingly important as effective and specific treatments for AD become available.

This study used MRI variables to make inferences about AD and CVD contributions to cognition. Lacunes and WMH are direct measures of SIVD. HC is generally considered a marker for AD pathology *(36,37)* There is evidence that CGM is affected by both AD and CVD *(15,16)*. In this study and in previous work from this project, CGM was as highly correlated with WMH and with HC, and the relationship of CGM and WMH was independent of effects of HC. CVD affects on CGM could have several mechanisms, including deafferentation of cortical neurons due to SIVD changes as well as direct ischemic injury to the cortex related to generalized vascular insufficiency that also affects subcortical structures. Small-vessel disease is particularly important for subjects in this study because participants with identifiable cortical strokes were excluded from enrollment. Cortical microinfarcts have been implicated as an important pathological component of CVD *(38)*, would likely be a result of small vessel CVD, are an important pathology in the neuropathology series, and might be associated with reduced CGM in patients with SIVD.

Results from this study did not support the hypothesis that CVD effects on CGM have effects on cognition beyond the SIVD associated with lacunes and WMH. That is, although CGM greatly improved prediction of cognition beyond that associated with lacunes and WMH, CGM effects were no longer significant when HC was added as an explanatory variable. This would suggest that the increased explanation of cognition associated with adding CGM to lacunes and WMH resulted from the ability of CGM to index AD. HC is likely a more specific index of AD and in the full model accounted for the AD variance in cognition that CGM had explained in the previous model lacking AD.

The lack of a CGM effect independent of HC is somewhat inconsistent with previous cross-sectional *(16)* and longitudinal *(39)* results from this project that have shown CGM effects independent of HC. However, previous studies have shown the same general pattern in which both CGM and HC make major contributions to explaining cognition beyond the contributions of lacunes and WMH.

Based on this study and previous work, a pattern has emerged that has generated the following hypothetical explanation of the contributions of AD and CVD to cognitive impairment. The specific role of lacunes in producing cognitive impairment is to interfere with frontal lobe function that affects executive components of cognition. Broader CVD indexed by WMH and possibly CGM also has a likely effect on cognition in general, particularly executive abilities. Relative contributions of AD and CVD differ by cognitive domain. AD is a much stronger determinant of memory impairment, which is not surprising because the hippocampus, a critical anatomical substrate for memory, is severely affected by AD. Executive function is more complexly determined by AD, generalized CVD, and specific effects of lacunes, and results from this study suggest that these pathologies make relatively equal contributions to executive decline.

This formulation would suggest that the relative impairment of executive function and memory would have important implications for the diagnosis of AD vs CVD. AD would be more likely if memory is most prominently impaired, whereas CVD would be most likely with executive but not memory impairment. The neuropsychological profile would be less informative when both memory and executive function are impaired. This might result from AD as a lone pathology, but could also reflect combined effects of AD on memory and CVD on executive function. These conclusions are based on using volumetric MRI measures to make inferences about underlying AD and CVD pathologies. There is a need for validation of the hypotheses generated from these studies of the relationship of cognition to volumetric MRI using direct measures of neuropathology. Results from the neuropathology series from this project will soon be available and will facilitate direct tests of hypotheses generated from structural imaging correlations with cognition.

ACKNOWLEDGMENTS

Supported by grants AG12435 and AG10129 from the National Institute on Aging, Bethesda, MD, and by the California Department of Health Services Alzheimer's Disease Program, contracts 98-14970 and 98-14971. Michael Weiner directed the Imaging Core that produced the quantitative MRI data for this project. Helena Chui was the overall principal investigator for this project, and along with William Jagust, provided the scientific leadership that made this study possible.

REFERENCES

1. DeCarli C. The role of cerebrovascular disease in dementia. Neurology 2003;9:123–136.
2. Longstreth WT, Jr., Bernick C, Manolio TA, Bryan N, Jungreis CA, Price TR. Lacunar infarcts defined by magnetic resonance imaging of 3660 elderly people: the Cardiovascular Health Study. Arch Neurol 1998;55:1217–1225.
3. Longstreth WT, Jr., Dulberg C, Manolio TA, et al. Incidence, manifestations, and predictors of brain infarcts defined by serial cranial magnetic resonance imaging in the elderly: the Cardiovascular Health Study. Stroke 2002;33:2376–2382.
4. Vermeer SE, Prins ND, den Heijer T, Hofman A, Koudstaal PJ, Breteler MMB. Silent brain infarcts and the risk of dementia and cognitive decline. N Engl J Med 2003;348:1215–1222.
5. Tomlinson BE, Blessed G, Roth M. Observations on the brains of demented old people. J Neurolog Sci 1970;11:205–242.
6. Schneider JA, Wilson RS, Cochran EJ, et al. Relation of cerebral infarctions to dementia and cognitive function in older persons. Neurology 2003;60:1082–1088.
7. Snowdon DA, Greiner LH, Mortimer JA, et al. Brain infarction and the clinical expression of Alzheimer disease: the nun study. JAMA 1997;277:813–817.
8. Tatemichi TK, Desmond DW, Paik M, et al. Clinical determinants of dementia related to stroke. Ann Neurol 1993;33: 568–575.
9. Tatemichi TK, Desmond DW, Mayeux R, et al. Dementia after stroke: baseline frequency, risks, and clinical features in a hospitalized cohort. Neurology 1992;42:1185–1193.
10. Van Zandvoort MJ, De Haan EH, Kappelle LJ. Chronic cognitive disturbances after a single supratentorial lacunar infarct. Neuropsychiatry Neuropsychol Behav Neurol 2001;14:98–102.
11. Van der Werf YD, Scheltens P, Lindeboom J, Witter MP, Uylings HBM, Jolles J. Deficits of memory, executive functioning and attention following infarction in the thalamus; a study of 22 cases with localised lesions. Neuropsychologia 2003;41:1330–1344.
12. Cummings JL. Frontal subcortical circuits and human behavior. Arch Neurol 1993;50:873–80.
13. Stuss DT, Guberman A, Nelson R, Larochelle S. The neuropsychology of paramedian thalamic infarction. Brain Cogn 1988;8:348–378.
14. Katz DI, Alexander MP, Mandell AM. Dementia following strokes in the mesencephalon and diencephalon. Arch Neurol 1987;44:1127–1133.
15. Fein G, Di Sclafani V, Tanabe J, et al. Hippocampal and cortical atrophy predict dementia in subcortical ischemic vascular disease. Neurology 2000;55:1626–1635.
16. Mungas D, Jagust WJ, Reed BR, et al. MRI predictors of cognition in subcortical ischemic vascular disease and Alzheimer's disease. Neurology 2001;57:2229–2235.
17. Hughes CP, Berg L, Danziger WL, Coben LA, Martin RL. A new clinical scale for the staging of dementia. Br J Psychiatry 1982;140:566–572.
18. Morris JC. The Clinical Dementia Rating (CDR): current version and scoring rules. Neurology 1993;43:2412–2414.
19. Kramer JH, Reed BR, Mungas D, Weiner MW, Chui HC. Executive dysfunction in subcortical ischaemic vascular disease. J Neurol Neurosurg Psychiatry 2002;72:217–220.
20. Kwan LT, Reed BR, Eberling JL, et al. Effects of subcortical cerebral infarction on cortical glucose metabolism and cognitive function. Arch Neurol 1999;56:809–814.
21. Reed BR, Eberling JL, Mungas D, Weiner M, Jagust WJ. Frontal lobe hypometabolism predicts cognitive decline in patients with lacunar infarcts. Arch Neurol 2001;58:493–497.
22. McKhann G, Drachman D, Folstein M, Katzman R, Price D, Stadlan EM. Clinical diagnosis of Alzheimer's disease: Report of the NINCDS-ADRDA Work Group under the auspices of Department of Health and Human Services Task Force on Alzheimer's Disease. Neurology 1984;34:939–944.
23. Chui HC, Victoroff JI, Margolin D, Jagust W, Shankle R, Katzman R. Criteria for the diagnosis of ischemic vascular dementia proposed by the State of California Alzheimer's Disease Diagnostic and Treatment Centers. Neurology 1992; 42:473–480.
24. Folstein M, Folstein S, McHugh PR. Mini-mental state: a practical method for grading the cognitive state of patients for the clinician. J Psychiatric Res 1975;12:189–198.
25. Csernansky JG, Wang L, Joshi S, et al. Early DAT is distinguished from aging by high dimensional mapping of the hippocampus. Dementia of the Alzheimer type. Neurology 2000;55:1636–1643.

26. Haller JW, Christensen GE, Joshi SC, et al. Hippocampal MR imaging morphometry by means of general pattern matching. Radiology 1996;199:787–791.
27. Mungas D, Reed BR, Kramer JH. Psychometrically matched measures of global cognition, memory, and executive function for assessment of cognitive decline in older persons. Neuropsychology, in press.
28. Williams JM. Memory Assessment Scales. Odessa, FL: Psychological Assessment Resources,1991.
29. Wechsler D. Wechsler Memory Scale-Revised (WMS-R). San Antonio, TX: The Psychological Corporation, 1987.
30. Morris JC, Heyman A, Mohs RC, et al. The Consortium to Establish a Registry for Alzheimer's Disease (CERAD). Part I. Clinical and neuropsychological assessment of Alzheimer's disease. Neurology 1989;39:1159–1165.
31. Welsh KA, Butters N, Mohs RC, et al. The Consortium to establish a registry for Alzheimer's Disease (CERAD). Part V. A normative study of the neuropsychological battery. Neurology 1994;44:609–614.
32. Benton AL, Hamsher Kd. Multilingual Aphasia Examination. Iowa City, IA: University of Iowa, 1976.
33. Mattis S. Dementia Rating Scale. Odessa, FL: Psychological Assessment Resources, 1988.
34. Hambleton RK, Swaminathan H. Item response theory. Principles and applications. Boston, MA: Kluwer-Nijhoff Publishing, 1985.
35. Hambleton RK, Swaminathan H, Rogers HJ. Fundamentals of item response theory. Newbury Park, CA: Sage Publications, 1991.
36. Visser PJ, Scheltens P, Verhey FR, et al. Medial temporal lobe atrophy and memory dysfunction as predictors for dementia in subjects with mild cognitive impairment. J Neurol 1999;246:477–485.
37. Jack CR, Jr., Petersen RC, Xu YC, et al. Prediction of AD with MRI-based hippocampal volume in mild cognitive impairment. Neurology 1999;52:1397–1403.
38. Jellinger KA. The pathology of ischemic vascular dementia: an update. J Neurol Sci 2002;204:153–157.
39. Mungas D, Reed BR, Jagust WJ, et al. Volumetric MRI predicts rate of cognitive decline related to AD and cerebrovascular disease. Neurology 2002;59:867–873.

15

White Matter Hyperintensities and Cognition

David J. Moser, Jason E. Kanz, and Kelly D. Garrett

1. INTRODUCTION

Despite the well-established relationship between cerebrovascular disease (CVD) and cognitive decline, confusion remains regarding the clinical importance of the white matter hyperintensities (WMH), also called leukoaraiosis *(1)*, that frequently appear on neuroimaging. These phenomena, when occurring in patients who have risk factors for vascular disease and stroke, are typically interpreted as evidence of small-vessel ischemic disease *(2)*, although they can also be the result of other processes. However, the clinical significance of these changes is a matter of debate in both the scientific literature and the daily work of clinicians. This point is illustrated by the fact that although one clinician may consider WMH on magnetic resonance imaging (MRI) as validation of the working diagnosis of vascular dementia (VaD), another may interpret a nearly identical scan as "normal for patient's age" and move on to consider other causes of cognitive decline. That this situation exists is hardly surprising, because of the contradictory literature on the topic and the variable importance of WMH in the various sets of diagnostic criteria for vascular-related cognitive conditions. This chapter represents an attempt to summarize the existing literature on this topic, as well as present key issues for continued research and debate.

2. WHY IS THE LITERATURE SO VARIABLE REGARDING THE RELATIONSHIP OF WMH AND COGNITION?

WMH can develop in the periventricular region, throughout the white matter, and in subcortical structures and have a predilection for the frontal subcortical region. It is believed that they affect cognitive function primarily through the disruption of subcortical-cortical connections, similar to other diseases that affect the white matter. During the past two decades, many studies have demonstrated a significant relationship between WMH severity and cognitive function in patients ranging from the healthy elderly to those with VaD *(3–11)*. However, there also exists a surprisingly large number of negative studies in this area *(12–15)*, raising the question about why this literature is seemingly so inconsistent.

The answer to this question almost certainly lies in the variable methodology across studies published on this topic. One major division, particularly among earlier studies, was whether neuroimaging was conducted with MRI or computed tomography (CT). Bowler and coauthors *(16)* pointed out that CT-based measures of WMH are more strongly related to cognitive function than MRI-based measures. However, this may result in part because in the studies employing CT, detected lesions were likely to have been larger than those in using MRI *(4)*. Furthermore, even in studies that do employ the more sensitive MRI-based methodology, measurement of WMH remains variable. As discussed

From: *Current Clinical Neurology*
Vascular Dementia: Cerebrovascular Mechanisms and Clinical Management
Edited by: R. H. Paul, R. Cohen, B. R. Ott, and S. Salloway © Humana Press Inc., Totowa, NJ

in Section 5.2., measurements of WMH volume range from visual rating scales to highly specific quantitative methods, with each of these having its own advantages and drawbacks, as well as differing effects on the resulting correlations found between white matter abnormalities and cognition.

Unfortunately, an equal or perhaps even greater magnitude of methodological variability exists regarding the assessment of cognitive functioning in this literature. Cognitive batteries have varied widely in both sensitivity and the nature of the cognitive abilities being tested. Assessing cognition with the Mini-Mental State Examination (MMSE) or another basic cognitive screening instrument, for example, simply does not allow for detection of subtle and varied forms of cognitive dysfunction as effectively as would the use of a comprehensive neuropsychological battery *(6)*. Alternatively, use of a comprehensive battery carries its own problems. When challenged to analyze a large number of cognitive variables while also controlling for multiple statistical tests, some investigators have chosen to group tests and create summary scores for a given cognitive domain, such as executive function. Although certainly defensible, the method can create a situation in which significant findings on an individual test may be obscured *(16)*. Finally, the literature in this topic has suffered from the types of variability common to most areas of research: inconsistent inclusion/exclusion criteria and dramatic differences in sample size across studies *(4,16)*. Despite the inconsistency in the literature, the preponderance of evidence does support the existence of a relationship between WMH and cognition. The importance of this relationship lies in WMH not only being evident in patients with severe cognitive disorders, such as VaD but also being associated with subtle forms of cognitive dysfunction among relatively intact individuals who are at risk for progressive decline. Understanding the clinical significance of WMH across the range of cognitive decline, from mild dysfunction to frank dementia, is critical to the development of interventions aimed at preventing or at least attenuating vascular-related cognitive disorders. Following is a brief review of some of the key studies in this area.

3. NONDEMENTED SAMPLES

In 2000, Gunning and colleagues *(8)* conducted a meta-analysis of 23 studies published between 1984 and 1998 on the relationship between WMH and cognition in adults without dementia. Their results indicated that severity of WMH was modestly associated with global cognitive functioning and also with more specific aspects of cognition, including processing speed, immediate and delayed memory, and executive function, defined in this study as tests of "planning, mental flexibility, and ability to inhibit prepotent responses." In comparing these relationships, there was some evidence to suggest that WMH were *most* strongly associated with speed and executive functioning. Of note, WMH severity was *not* significantly associated with performance on tests of general intelligence. Furthermore, partialling out the effects of age did not significantly affect the relationships between WMH and cognition. The authors noted that the pattern of cognitive dysfunction observed in elders without dementia is similar to that seen in patients with demyelinating illnesses, such as multiple sclerosis, suggesting that WMH may affect cognition primarily via detrimental effects on interneuronal connectivity. In particular, that WMH was most strongly associated with performance on tests of processing speed would be consistent with this theory.

One of the hallmark studies in this area—and one that was included in the meta-analysis discussed above—was conducted by Breteler and coinvestigators as part of the Rotterdam Study in 1994 *(6)*. Before then, most studies on this topic were limited by several problems, including small sample size, various forms of sampling bias, and that most of them involved patients who had already developed dementia. Although such studies yielded important results, they did not shed light on the much earlier stages of vascular-related cognitive impairment, knowledge about which could have important implications for treatment.

Breteler studied 90 elderly subjects, 65–84 yr of age, drawn from the general population. None of the subjects met criteria for dementia, and none had suffered stroke. To measure WMH burden, subjects underwent brain MRI, and scans were subsequently graded 0, 1, or 2; a score of 0 corresponded to absent or minimal periventricular hyperintensities, fewer than five punctate lesions, and no confluent lesions; 1 indicated moderate periventricular hyperintensities or more than five punctate lesions, but no confluent lesions; 2 indicated severe periventricular hyperintensity and/or the presence of confluent white matter lesions (WMLs). Neuropsychological functioning was assessed with a comprehensive battery, including tests of general mental status, intelligence, memory, executive function, and attention.

Despite being based on a nondemented general population sample, the results of this study were striking. Twenty-three subjects had moderate or severe WMH (grades 1 or 2). Additionally, when compared to subjects with a WMH grade of 0, those with grade 1 or 2 performed worse on all neuropsychological tests, with the exception of one intellectual subtest of abstract thinking ability. After controlling for age and gender, the direction of these results was unchanged, but group differences remained significant only for four tests of executive control, attention, processing speed, and memory (Trails A and B, word fluency, and delayed list recall). These findings laid the groundwork for additional research focusing on the degree to which WMH were associated with the earliest stages of vascular cognitive impairment. Indeed, as discussed in the next paragraph, subsequent research suggested that WMH might be associated with cognitive decline even before the point at which such decline becomes measurable with objective tests.

Studying more than 1000 elderly subjects without dementia drawn from two large cohort studies, de Groot and coauthors sought to determine the relationship between subjective cognitive complaints and WMH severity *(9)*. Subjects underwent brain MRI, which was used to produce semiquantitative measurements of subcortical and periventricular WMLs. They also completed the Cognitive Failure Questionnaire, which includes questions on cognitive problems (e.g., being forgetful of names) and were administered a broad battery of objective neuropsychological tests. Results indicated that severity of WMLs was associated with subjects' reports of cognitive problems, particularly with subjects' reports that these problems had worsened during the previous 5-yr period. Surprisingly, not only were more severe WMLs found in subjects reporting cognitive problems, but also this was particularly true among those subjects with *above-average* cognitive performance. The authors found that the relationship between WMLs and cognition assumed a dose-dependent pattern. Specifically, starting at the milder end of the WMLs severity distribution were subjects with no reported cognitive problems and good objective cognitive performance, followed by subjects who reported cognitive problems but showed no measurable cognitive dysfunction, and then by subjects who reported cognitive problems that progressed during the previous 5 yr *and* showed measurable cognitive dysfunction. The results of this intriguing study served as evidence that reports of progressive cognitive problems may be an early warning sign of impending cognitive decline related to WMLs, even in patients who do not show measurable cognitive dysfunction at the time the cognitive problems are reported.

4. WMH AND COGNITION IN DEMENTIA

The findings that WMHs are associated with cognitive ability in nondemented samples may render obvious the fact that this relationship would also exist in patients with VaD. However, this remains an important issue to consider. Specifically, in a large proportion of cases of VaD, WMH represent only one aspect of the abnormality seen on neuroimaging, because many of these scans will also reveal large-vessel stroke, lacunar infarcts, atrophy, and other markers of neurological insult. Therefore, if one seeks to gain a better understanding of the specific relationship of WMH to cognition across the full range of cognitive impairment, studies that help tease apart the relative contributions of these vascular-related phenomena become essential.

In 2002, Cohen et al. published data on subcortical hyperintensities and neuropsychological functioning in 24 patients with VaD *(10)*. All subjects, 55 yr of age or more, met National Institute of

Neurological Disorders and Stroke-Association Internationale pour la Recherche et l'Enseignement en Neurosciences (NINDS-AIREN) *(17)* criteria for VaD and all had MMSE scores between 9 and 24, inclusive. Subcortical hyperintensity volumes were calculated from MRI using semiautomated thresholding methodology to select pixel values representing abnormal brain tissue in the subcortical white matter, thalamus, and basal ganglia. These computer-generated volumes were verified visually, and then hyperintensity volumes were expressed as a percentage of whole brain volume (excluding ventricles). Neuropsychological assessment consisted of a comprehensive battery of tasks, including tests of general mental status, intelligence, verbal and nonverbal learning and recall, visuospatial/constructive skills, language, executive functioning, and attention.

MRI results indicated that all subjects with VaD had significant WMH, and a minority also had cortical infarcts and/or infarcts in the thalamus or basal ganglia. Analysis of the neuropsychological data revealed that, on average, this group had dementia of moderate severity, with performance across all cognitive domains that was significantly inferior to that of healthy individuals of similar age.

Across all subjects with dementia, amount of subcortical hyperintensity was strongly and significantly associated with performance on tests of executive function, attention, and psychomotor speed. However, to examine the specific relationship of WMH to cognition, it was necessary to analyze these data after excluding those subjects with infarcts in the cortical and/or subcortical grey matter. Again, a strong and significant correlation was found between hyperintensity volume and performance across a group of tests of executive function, attention, and psychomotor speed. Follow-up analyses revealed that digit symbol and grooved pegboard performance accounted for the majority of the variance in this relationship, suggesting a strong association of WMH with speed, focused attention, working memory, rapid information processing, and fine-motor control.

Interestingly, when whole brain volume was analyzed in relation to cognition in this study, an entirely different pattern was found, representing a double dissociation. Specifically, whereas WMH severity was strongly associated with executive function, speed, and attention, whole brain volume was not. In contrast, whole brain volume shared strong associations with performance on tests of general mental status, language, memory, and visuospatial/constructive function. It is important to note that subcortical hyperintensity volume was correlated with whole brain volume but accounted for less than 20% of the variance in this variable. This suggests that diminished whole brain volume and related aspects of cognitive dysfunction should not be attributed to subcortical ischemic disease alone.

Although the studies discussed provide strong evidence for the clinical importance of WMH across the range of cognitive decline, debate continues regarding the amount of WMH that is necessary to cause impairment, how WMH should be measured, and, ultimately, how assessment of WMH should factor into the development of new diagnostic criteria for vascular-related cognitive disorders. These issues are discussed in Section 5.

5. ISSUES FOR CONTINUED RESEARCH AND DEBATE

5.1. WMH Thresholds: How Much WMH is Sufficient to Cause Cognitive Impairment?

Given the studies mentioned in the previous section and others like them, it is now generally accepted that WMH are associated with declining cognitive performance, ranging from subtle dysfunction to frank dementia. However, the field of vascular-related cognitive decline is in the midst of significant controversy, centering on what will constitute the most effective set of diagnostic criteria for such disorders. The criteria currently used in the clinical diagnosis of VaD and other forms of dementia sprang directly from research on Alzheimer's disease (AD) *(18)*. The cornerstone of this Alzheimer's-based diagnosis is early and progressive memory dysfunction, a symptom that often does not appear in vascular-related cognitive decline until other aspects of cognition, particularly executive function, have become significantly impaired. Furthermore, even diagnostic criteria created specifically for VaD (e.g., NINDS-AIREN *[17]* and State of California Alzheimer's Disease

Diagnostic and Treatment Centers [SCADDTCs] *[19]* criteria) have proved unacceptable because patients must be significantly impaired, to the point of dementia, before being diagnosed. In a potentially preventable or at least alterable process such as vascular-related cognitive decline, it is important that patients be identified as early as possible, giving maximum opportunity for treatment *(18)*.

Therefore, the field is currently moving away from formal VaD criteria toward criteria for a group of vascular-related cognitive conditions, collectively called vascular cognitive impairment (VCI) *(20)* that range from mild impairment to dementia. Although many researchers accept this as a positive development, the challenges involved in selecting appropriate diagnostic criteria remain at least as daunting as they have previously been. A major part of this process will be deciding to what degree WMH should be a part of these criteria and how these abnormalities should be measured. In the NINDS-AIREN *(17)* criteria, a condition in which 25% of the white matter is affected by WMH is considered sufficient to cause dementia. Although including such a specific threshold is certainly useful in helping researchers speak a common language, there is simply no empirical support for it *(18)*.

The reason for this lack of empirical support lies partly in the inherent heterogeneity of patients and research subjects. If all individuals possessed of the same premorbid cognitive ability, environment, education, and presence and severity of various medical conditions, perhaps it would then be possible to determine the precise amount of WMH necessary to cause varying degrees of cognitive impairment. However, even in carefully selected samples, individuals have vastly different histories, including variable levels of premorbid functioning, differing patterns of vascular risk factors, and other factors, such as substance abuse, head injury, and psychiatric conditions. Furthermore, the *location* of WMHs may be just as important as volume regarding effects on cognition. The question of how much WMH is necessary to cause cognitive impairment then becomes akin to asking how much luggage a person can carry before he or she becomes walking impaired. The answer, of course, depends on the specific person in question. This example is somewhat oversimplified, of course, because it is possible to gain some degree of statistical control over potential confounding factors, but the task remains extremely difficult. Given the current state of the literature, it is clear that there are not yet sufficient data to include a specific WMH threshold in the diagnostic criteria for VCI. For now, it will be important for clinicians and researchers to appreciate the relationship between subcortical ischemic changes and cognition and that even relatively small infarct volumes are associated with cognitive decline.

5.2. How Should WMH Be Measured?

There are currently two main techniques used to measure WMH. The first and more common of these involves the use of visual rating scales, in which a trained rater views the film (usually one section per subject) and assigns a WMH severity grade based on predefined criteria and an ordinal scale. Numerous scales exist for this type of analysis, and they share the advantage of being time and cost effective in comparison with more technologically complex methods. Drawbacks to the visual rating scale techniques include the ordinal scales on which they are based possibly causing result data to be restricted in range, and the somewhat subjective nature of the process invites issues of interrater and intrarater reliability. Additionally, because these methods are based on ordinal scales, outcome variables typically must be analyzed using nonparametric techniques, which are frequently less powerful than their parametric counterparts *(21)*.

Although many investigators prefer the relative simplicity of using visual rating scales, the large number of existing scales and the differences between them can not only make studies difficult to compare but also question results. In 1997, Mänytlä and coinvestigators subjected scans from 395 poststroke patients to 13 different visual rating scales to determine the consistency with which the various methods would rate WMH severity *(22)*. The results, only part of which are summarized here, indicated that the scales differed considerably. The authors found that, at best, more than 80% of the patients received equivalent WMH grades, but in other cases, this value went as low as 18% for

WMH and below 1% for periventricular hyperintensities. Furthermore, it was clear that some of the scales were limited by ceiling and/or floor effects. Having no gold standard (e.g., histopathology) to which to compare the visual rating scales, there was not a firm conclusion regarding which of the scales may have been superior to the others. However, it was concluded that enough inconsistency existed among them to consider this a contributing factor to the highly mixed findings in research on WMH and cognition.

The second, more recently developed method of measuring WMH severity involves using computer-based techniques to obtain an actual WMH volume. One such method is commonly termed "region of interest" (ROI) methodology, in which the investigator views the scan on a computer (usually multiple images from each subject) and manually traces WMH with the mouse and cursor. Once an ROI is traced, the computer will produce a volume of that region based on the section thickness and the number of pixels residing in the traced area. The resulting values are then summed for all sampled sections, producing a total WMH volume.

A second computer-based technique for measuring WMH volume is termed "thresholding." In such techniques, a computer program is used to measure the intensity of each pixel. The number of pixels exceeding a predefined intensity is counted, and, again, a WMH volume is obtained by summing the values from all selected samples. One drawback to this procedure involves setting the threshold above which a pixel will be considered to be hyperintense. This is most commonly done by visually assessing one initial section and selecting areas that are representative of healthy vs abnormal white matter and then using these intensity values as a guide by which the computer program will identify areas of healthy and abnormal white matter on all other sections for that subject. Unfortunately, this predefined intensity threshold may not apply perfectly to the other sections and can result in error resulting from factors such as artifact and ambiguity between grey and white matter zones. It is common practice to visually verify the hyperintense regions selected with this type of program to try to ensure that they do, in fact, represent WMH and not other phenomena, but even with this verification the process is far from flawless.

Because of the respective advantages and drawbacks to visual rating scales and computer-mediated methods, the question arises whether one should be considered state-of-the-art and incorporated into future diagnostic criteria for VCI. Research comparing the two directly is limited but does include a study recently published by Garrett and coinvestigators *(21)*. The authors studied 36 patients with VaD and subjected their MRI scans to visual ratings of periventricular and deep WMHs that produced a value from 0 to 9, with high numbers indicating greater severity. These scans were also analyzed with computer-mediated thresholding methodology, followed by visual verification of selected areas of WMH. Results indicated that interrater reliability was slightly higher for the thresholding technique, but this difference was relatively small. More importantly, the authors found that the WMH volumes that were obtained via the thresholding technique correlated much more strongly with neuropsychological performance than did the visual ratings. This was particularly true when the thresholding-based WMH volumes were corrected for whole brain volume, something than cannot be readily done with visual ratings. As in the Mänytlä study *(22)* it was not possible without histopathology to truly determine which of these techniques is superior, but the authors concluded that computer-mediated methods are likely to yield more accurate estimates of WMH severity.

Although computer-based methods may be an improvement on visual rating scales in assessing WMH burden, it is not yet clear that the margin by which they are superior outweighs the drawbacks inherent in using them. They are certainly more costly and take much more time than visual rating scales. Even though most researchers may not find it overly burdensome to adapt computer-based methods to obtain relatively specific measures of WMH burden, it is simply not yet practical to expect the same of clinicians who are generally under different time constraints. Furthermore, in many parts of the world, clinicians are forced to practice with entirely inadequate neuroimaging resources, not to mention having access to the additional technology necessary to obtain specific computer-based WMH volumes. It is important that such factors are considered as diagnostic criteria are developed for VCI, because these criteria will be most valuable if they are broadly useful to clinicians and researchers alike. Therefore, until technology allows for more rapid processing and analysis of scans, it is best for these criteria to at least allow for, if not require, visual ratings of phenomena such as WMH.

6. SUMMARY

Despite inconsistencies in the literature, it is currently accepted that WMH share at least a modest relationship with cognitive performance, particularly executive dysfunction, in conditions ranging from very mild cognitive decline to VaD. To date, it has not been possible to determine the specific amount of WMH necessary to cause cognitive impairment, but it has been found that even relatively mild WMH can have deleterious effects on cognition. Issues for continued debate and research include how WMH should be assessed and incorporated into the diagnostic criteria for Vascular Cognitive Impairment.

REFERENCES

1. Hachinski VC, Potter P, Merskey H. Leukoaraiosis: an ancient term for a new problem. Can J Neurologic Sci 1986;13(Suppl 4):383–384.
2. Pantoni L, Garcia JH. Pathogenesis of leukoaraiosis: a review. Stroke 1993;28:652–659.
3. Almkvist O, Wahlund L, Andersson-Lundman G, et al. White-matter hyperintensity and neuropsychological functions in dementia and healthy aging. Arch Neurol 1992;49:626–632.
4. Boone KB, Miller BL, Lesser IM, et al. Neuropsychological correlates of white-matter lesions in healthy elderly subjects. A threshold effect. Arch Neurol 1992;49:549–554.
5. Breteler MMB, van Swieten JC, Bots ML, et al. Cerebral white matter lesions, vascular risk factors, and cognitive function in a population-based study: The Rotterdam Study. Neurology 1994;44:1246–1252.
6. Breteler MB, Amerongen NM, van Swieten JC, et al. Cognitive correlates of ventricular enlargement and cerebral white matter lesions on Magnetic Resonance Imaging: The Rotterdam Study. Stroke 1994;25:1109–1115.
7. Kertesz A, Polk M, Carr T. Cognition and white matter changes on magnetic resonance imaging in dementia. Arch Neurol 1994;47:387–391.
8. Gunning-Dixon FM, Raz N. The cognitive correlates of white matter abnormalities in normal aging: a quantitative review. Neuropsychology 2000;14:224–232.
9. deGroot JC, de Leeuw FE, Oudkerk M, Hofman A, Jolles J, Breteler MMB. Cerebral white matter lesions and subjective cognitive dysfunction: The Rotterdam Scan Study. Neurology 2001;56:1539–1545.
10. Cohen RA, Paul RH, Ott BR, et al. The relationship of subcortical MRI hyperintensities and brain volume to cognitive function in vascular dementia. J Intl Neuropsycholog Soc 2002;8:743–752.
11. Kramer JH, Reed BR, Mungas D, Weiner MW, Chui HC. Executive dysfunction in subcortical ischaemic white matter disease. J Neurol Neurosurg Psychiatry 2002;72:217–220.
12. Hershey LA, Modic MT, Greenough PG, Jaffe DF. Magnetic resonance imaging in vascular dementia. Neurology 1987;37:29–36.
13. Rao SM, Mittenberg W, Bernardin L, et al. Neuropsychological test findings in subjects with leukoaraiosis. Arch Neurol 1989;46:40–44.
14. Mirsen TR, Lee DH, Wong CJ, et al. Clinical correlates of white-matter changes on magnetic resonance imaging scans of the brain. Arch Neurol 1991;48:1015–1021.
15. Erkinjuntti T, Gao F, Lee DH, et al. Lack of difference in brain hyperintensities between patients with early Alzheimer's disease and control subjects. Arch Neurol 1994;51:260–268.
16. Bowler JV, Steenhuis R, Hachinski V. Conceptual background to vascular cognitive impairment. Alzheimer Dis Assoc Disord 1999;13(Suppl 3):S30–S37.
17. Roman GC, Tatemichi TK, Erkinjuntti T, et al. Vascular dementia: diagnostic criteria for research studies. Report of the NINDS/AIREN International Workshop. Neurology 1993;43:250–260.
18. Bowler JV. The concept of vascular cognitive impairment. J Neurologic Sci 2002;203-204:11–15.
19. Chui HC, Victoroff JI, Margolin D, et al. Criteria for the diagnosis of ischemic vascular dementia proposed by the State of California Alzheimer's Disease Diagnostic and Treatment Centers. Neurology 1992;42:473–480.
20. Hachinski VC, Bowler JV. Vascular dementia. Neurology 1993;43:2159–2160.
21. Garrett KD, Cohen RA, Paul RH, Moser DJ, Malloy PF, Shah P. Computer-mediated measurement and subjective ratings of white matter hyperintensities in vascular dementia: relationships to neuropsychological performance. Clinical Neuropsychologist, in press.
22. Mänytlä R, Erkinjuntti T, Salonen O, et al. Variable agreement between visual rating scales for white matter hyperintensities on MRI. Comparison of 13 rating scales in a post-stroke cohort. Stroke 1997;28:1614–1623.

16

Poststroke Dementia

The Role of Strategic Infarcts

Anelyssa D'Abreu and Brian R. Ott

1. INTRODUCTION

Poststroke dementia is a syndrome characterized by the acute onset of deficits in multiple cognitive domains, often including memory, after a clinical stroke, in a patient with nonrecognizable prestroke cognitive impairment. The interaction of various factors is necessary to produce its symptoms, and different clinical-pathologic correlates may lead to this diagnosis. At least two different mechanisms are responsible for poststroke dementia: strategic infarcts and mixed dementia resulting from the association with Alzheimer's pathology.

Strategic infarcts are lesions placed in areas that control or participate in cognition and behavior, such as the thalamus, basal ganglia, angular gyrus, and inferomedial temporal lobes. In a strict sense, this constitutes the most convincing case of vascular dementia (VaD). Another basis for strategic infarction is a stroke in a susceptible brain, leading to the development of dementia. For instance, patients with prior subclinical infarcts may develop dementia, not necessarily resulting from the lesion location *per se* but from the summation effect from all those affected areas.

This chapter focuses on poststroke dementia in relation to strategic infarcts. The authors discuss the clinical determinants for the development of dementia, secondary to acute stroke, followed by descriptions of the most common cognitive and neuropsychiatric manifestations of strategically located strokes.

2. CLINICAL DETERMINANTS OF POSTSTROKE DEMENTIA

Poststroke dementia is a frequent complication of stroke, and, in large series, its incidence oscillates around 30% (13.6–31.8%) *(1–6)*. The wide range of variability probably reflects the differences in the inclusion/exclusion criteria within the studies, such as history of prior clinical stroke, use of standardized or validated battery tests to exclude prestroke dementia, type of imaging study selected (computed tomography [CT] vs magnetic resonance imaging [MRI]), and presence of aphasia. The presence of dementia before clinical stroke is often unrecognized. For example, Hénon et al. evaluated the cognitive function of patients with presumed poststroke dementia and found that at least one-sixth of the patients had unrecognizable dementia before stroke *(7)*.

It is important to mention that poststroke dementia does not necessarily develop in the immediate poststroke period, and subclinical cases of Alzheimer's disease (AD) may be recognizable only after ischemic pathology has occurred. In a population-based study in Rochester, MN, retrospective data indicated the risk of dementia in the first year after a stroke is approximately nine times that of the general population and twice the annual rate thereafter *(8)*.

From: *Current Clinical Neurology*
Vascular Dementia: Cerebrovascular Mechanisms and Clinical Management
Edited by: R. H. Paul, R. Cohen, B. R. Ott, and S. Salloway © Humana Press Inc., Totowa, NJ

Controversy exists over whether dementia after a strategic stroke is necessarily static (unless associated with AD pathology as suggested by some authors) *(9)* or if dementia after stroke may also follow a progressive course. Szirmai et al. followed 21 patients after vascular events in the thalamus from 2 mo to 5 yr *(10)*. They observed that many patients demonstrated cognitive decline during the course of years, which was presumed secondary to Wallerian degeneration of the thalamo-cortical connections. Neither the number of the patients in which progression was observed nor neuropathological data to rule out associated Alzheimer pathology was available.

For up to 4 yr, Tatemichi et al. followed a group of poststroke patients without dementia older than 60 yr and age-matched controls, without a history of stroke, with annual evaluations, including neurological, neuropsychological, and functional assessment *(11)*. The incidence of dementia in the poststroke group was 8.4 per 100 person yr, whereas in the control group, the incidence was 1.3 per 100 person year. All the control group patients who developed dementia carried a diagnosis of AD. The relative risk of developing dementia associated with stroke when compared to the control group after 52 mo follow-up was 5.5% (95% CI, 2.5 to 11.1). Autopsy was performed in one patient in the poststroke group, which did not demonstrate any neuritic plaques or neurofibrillary tangles.

It is generally believed that poststroke dementia is a multifactorial process, resulting from the interaction of various clinical determinants. A summation effect of having more than one correlate has been demonstrated *(2)*. Host factors, cooccurrence of AD, demographics, and stroke characteristics, such as lesion location and volume, render an individual susceptible to the development of poststroke dementia *(12)*.

2.1. Demographic Factors

Age is one of the most consistent clinical determinants of poststroke dementia *(1–6,11)*. In one series, the mean age of patients with dementia was 76.9 yr, whereas the group without dementia was 65.4 yr ($p < 0.0001$) *(2)*. In another series, both univariate and multivariate analysis demonstrated significant association between the development of poststroke dementia and older age *(1)*.

Likewise, *low level of education* is a notable risk factor for poststroke dementia. Forty percent of patients with dementia had less than 8 yr of schooling, in comparison with 32.4% in the group without dementia ($p = 0.02$) *(1)*. Likewise, there is a threefold increased risk when patients with less than or equal to 8 yr of education are compared to patients with 13 yr or more of education *(11)*. In another study, the odds ratio was 4.1 for less than or equal to 8 yr of education and 3.0 for 9–12 yr of education, compared to those with 13 yr or more *(5)*. Other series using a cut off of less than or equal to 6 yr of education have demonstrated similar results *(2–4,13)*.

Nonwhite race (non-Hispanic blacks, Hispanic, and others) plays an important role in poststroke dementia *(1,5)*. Other studies did not consider race as part of the analysis *(3,4)* most likely because of the more homogeneous population, and one study showing a racial effect did not reach statistical significance *(11)*.

Female sex was shown in one study to correlate with poststroke dementia *(14)*. In a second study, women with a major hemispheric stroke syndrome had a disproportionately higher risk of dementia *(5)*. Nonetheless, in most other series, sex is not related to dementia *(1,2,4,11)*.

2.2. Cardiovascular Risk Factors

Recognized vascular risk factors, such as *diabetes mellitus*, *hypertension*, *hypercholesterolemia*, *atrial fibrillation*, *high homocysteine levels*, *smoking*, and *prior myocardial infarct*, have been variably related to poststroke dementia. Diabetes, as well as smoking *(4)*, was significantly associated with poststroke dementia in some studies *(1,5,6,15)* but not in others *(3)*. Hypertension, high homocysteine levels, and hypercholesterolemia correlate with dementia in logistic regression analysis *(3)*. Ischemic heart disease in one series was individually correlated with dementia but not in another *(1,3)*. Atrial fibrillation *(3,6,14)*, as well as nephropathy (3), has been demonstrated in logistic regression analysis to correlate with poststroke dementia.

Unlike these vascular risk factors, a *history of prior cerebrovascular event* has been invariably correlated with poststroke dementia, with an odds ratio as high as 2.7 *(1,4,5)*. Curiously, transient ischemic attacks (TIA) do not directly increase the risk of occurrence of poststroke dementia *(4)*, even though 20% of patients with a clinical diagnosis of TIA have documented diffusion-weighted MRI abnormalities if performed in less than 3 d of the event *(16)*. One may speculate that the majority of TIA cases do not, *per se*, represent damage to the cerebral hemispheres

In one study, the development of intercurrent *global cerebral hypoxic-ischemic disorders*, such as seizures, sepsis, cardiac arrhythmia, and congestive heart failure, was an independent risk factor in the development of dementia after stroke, even after adjustment for other recognized risk factors *(17)*.

2.3. Neurologic Examination

Neurologic examination findings most frequently encountered in patients with dementia when compared to patients without dementia after stroke are frontal release signs, visual neglect, hemiparesis, gait impairment, and urinary incontinence *(1,4)*. Neither aphasia nor hemianopia was related to dementia in any study of neurologic signs in dementia *(1)*. Intact orientation after stroke is a good prognostic factor and usually suggests preserved cognitive function *(18)*.

2.4. Lesion Location and Stroke Features

In a series of 251 patients examined 3 mo after stroke, 66 patients (26.3%) were diagnosed with dementia. Thirty-six percent had a left hemisphere stroke, compared with 25% with right-sided lesions and 13.8% with brainstem/cerebellar infarction. Even after adjustment for aphasia, the odds ratio for left hemispheric infarct was still higher than for right hemispheric infarcts *(1)*. These findings have been corroborated by other studies *(4,5)*. In Singapore, 12 patients had dementia after one clinical stroke, without radiographic evidence of prior strokes. All but one had *left-sided lesions (10)*. In a retrospective population-based study evaluating the incidence of VaD, 12% of the patients had a temporal relationship between stroke and the development of dementia. Thirty-two percent of those patients had *bilateral lesions*, either cortical or subcortical. However, cortical lesions outnumbered subcortical lesions *(19)*. Bilateral lesions were also more frequently encountered in patients with dementia than in patients without it *(20)*.

Major hemispheric stroke syndrome, which reflects *stroke size,* as well as *laterality*, is also associated with dementia *(4,5)*. In a study group of 337 patients, 107 (31.8%) were diagnosed with poststroke dementia. Logistic regression, excluding patients with aphasia, demonstrated major dominant syndrome (OR 4.6; 95% CI 1.5–14.7) and low level of education (OR, 1.1; 95% CI 1.05–1.22) as significant correlates of poststroke dementia *(4)*.

Radiological studies have confirmed these findings and suggest other possible correlates, such as infarct volume, association of white matter disease, and hippocampal atrophy. Pohjasvaara et al. evaluated the MRI correlates of dementia in a series of patients with ischemic stroke *(13)*. Regardless of side of lesion, v*olume of infarcts* in any superior middle cerebral artery (MCA) territory and left thalamocortical connection was different between the population with dementia and the population without dementia. Mean volume of infarct was 37.7 cm^3 in patients with dementia and 22.5 cm^3 in patients without dementia ($p = 0.002$).

Considering *vascular territories*, infarcts in anterior cerebral artery (ACA) and posterior cerebral artery (PCA) territories vs other territories are more frequently associated with dementia *(1,5)*. This comes as no surprise as these vessels are responsible for the blood supply of areas such as the thalamus, basal ganglia, limbic system, and major interhemispheric and intrahemispheric pathways. As discussed in Section 3., injuries in those areas are responsible for multiple neurobehavioral syndromes and cognitive deficits.

The *stroke mechanism* most often associated with dementia is lacunar infarct *(10)*, whereas patients with cardioembolic infarcts may be less likely to develop dementia *(1)*. Nevertheless, these findings are not universal *(6)*. Concomitant white matter abnormalities have been more frequently reported in patients with dementia than in the populations without dementia after stroke *(2,13,15)*.

2.5. *Hippocampal Atrophy*

The presence of moderate or severe *hippocampal atrophy* compared with absence or minimal atrophy is more frequent in patients with dementia than in patients without dementia, after stroke *(2,13)*. Patients who had a stroke and medial temporal lobe atrophy have a higher incidence of poststroke dementia than do patients with no atrophy. This likely reflects the presence of concurrent AD, because numerous studies have shown a relationship between hippocampal atrophy and early AD. Nevertheless, medial temporal lobe atrophy was not an independent risk factor for the development of poststroke dementia in one study *(15)*.

3. STRATEGIC INFARCTION

In 1993, a report of the National Institute of Neurological Disorders and Stroke-Association Internationale pour la Recherche et l'Enseignement en Neurosciences (NINDS-AIREN) international workshop was published, with diagnostic criteria for research studies in VaD *(21)*. The guidelines highlighted the variability of pathological subtypes and clinical course, which could be progressive, static, or remitting; the association of other clinical findings, such as gait disorder and incontinence; the need for a temporal relationship with a stroke syndrome; and the importance of brain imaging.

In this diagnostic scheme, the neuropathologic classification of VaD would be associated with various types of lesions, including strategic single infarct dementia, constituting well-defined clinical syndromes, resulting from small, localized injury to functionally important cortical and subcortical areas.

McPherson and Cummings *(22)* believe four different areas are responsible for the development of strategic infarct dementia: the angular gyrus, the caudate nucleus, globus pallidus, and thalamus. However, other authors also believe that areas such as the occipital lobe, genu of the internal capsule, corpus callosum, and mesial temporal lobes *(10,23,24)* as sites of strategic infarcts.

Understanding how large cortical lesions, especially in the MCA territory, may lead to pronounced neurobehavioral changes is obvious to the clinician. On the other hand, the mechanism of subcortical dementia is not as well understood. Interruption of frontal-subcortical circuits is a widely accepted explanation *(25)*. The general organization of these circuits includes the frontal lobes, striatum, globus pallidus/substantia nigra, and the thalamus. Three different circuits have been associated with behavior control: dorsolateral circuit, lateral orbital cortex, and anterior cingulate cortex. Each includes interconnections between different areas of the frontal lobes, caudate, and distinct thalamic nuclei.

According to Cummings *(25)* some rules apply for these circuits:

- Behavioral disturbances simulate the ones observed with pure frontal lobe lesions.
- Lesions in different areas of the same circuit will produce similar symptoms.
- Simultaneous lesions in different circuit structures produce analogous effects.
- Symptoms may result from dysfunction of circuit structures by changing its effects in distant structures within the circuit.
- Circuit structures may participate in noncircuit behavioral syndromes because of their connection with noncircuit areas.

Thalamocortical disconnection is an important concept. Studies using positron emission tomography (PET) scans in patients with unilateral thalamic lesions demonstrated ipsilateral cortical hypometabolism. Contralateral hypometabolism has also been observed when patients are compared to controls *(26,27)*. The amount of neuropsychologic impairment is proportional to the degree of metabolic change *(27)*. As the genu of the internal capsule carries important pathways from the limbic system, including corticothalamic and thalamocortical fibers, the same model of disconnection between subcortical and cortical structures would apply *(28,29)*.

Right-sided subcortical lesions produce neglect. In a recent study, 16 patients with spatial neglect, no associated visual field deficits, and lesions restricted to either the basal ganglia or thalamus were compared with 16 controls with right basal ganglia or thalamic lesions but no neglect. By superimposing the lesions in between the groups and subtracting the controls from the affected patients, the right hemispheric putamen, pulvinar, and, to a lesser extent, the caudate nucleus were more frequently lesioned in the patients with neglect than in the controls *(30)*. Because these areas have a direct anatomical connection with the superior temporal gyrus (the cortical area that correlates with spatial neglect), the authors concluded that a possible cortical-subcortical network is involved in spatial neglect.

3.1. Caudate Infarcts

Caplan et al. *(31)*, evaluated 18 patients with caudate infarcts, and only 4 of them did not present behavioral or cognitive dysfunction. Motor abnormalities were usually absent or slight and, when present, were characterized by decreased spontaneous movement and reduced associative movements. Eleven patients were dysarthric. The most frequent abnormality was abulia, followed by restlessness and hyperactivity, contralateral neglect (only observed in right-sided lesions), and language deficits, such as word finding difficulties. Two patients with left-sided infarcts had "poor memory," and two others with right-sided lesions had visuospatial and constructional abnormalities.

The cognitive domains mostly affected in caudate infarcts are decreased problem-solving ability, impaired recent and remote memory with preservation of recognition memory, and decreased attention *(32)*. Patients with dorsal lesions characteristically present with decreased spontaneous activity and affective symptoms with psychotic features, whereas ventromedial lesions mostly lead to disinhibition and impulsivity.

Godefroy et al. questioned these findings after evaluating 10 patients with presumed unilateral lenticulostriate infarct on CT. Patients underwent neuropsychological testing and MRI studies. According to the findings, patients with neuropsychological abnormalities had associated cortical lesions on MRI, not previously observed on CT, whereas caudate lesions accounted only for the disturbances observed on a crossed tapping test *(33)*.

A more recent study, which also included MRI examination, did not corroborate their results *(34)*. In a series of 25 patients after ischemic caudate infarcts, isolated left caudate strokes were associated with cognitive and behavioral abnormalities but minimal motor abnormalities. The most common abnormalities included aphasic syndromes (global, transcortical, and nonfluent aphasias with impaired repetition), anomia, visual and verbal amnesia, ideomotor, and buccolingual apraxia. These findings were more prominent in infarcts at the lateral lenticulostriatum rather than anterior lenticulostriate infarcts, which demonstrated only confusion and disorientation.

Right-sided lesions were associated with visual neglect, decreased spontaneity, flat affect, and frontal dysfunction, also more pronounced at the lateral lenticulostriate territory. Motor deficits were more frequently observed in this group, most likely because of the higher rate of extension to anterior limb of internal capsule. Right-sided anterior lenticular infarcts produced confusion and abulia. The three patients with bilateral caudate strokes demonstrated acute confusional state and disorientation.

Two important points are worth mentioning. First, in none of the studies cited were the patients described as having dementia. However, the deficits were persistent in the majority of the cases after prolonged follow-up, and behavioral abnormalities prompted institutionalization in some cases. Tatemichi et al. reported a case of clear dementia after caudate infarct, with extension to the anterior corona radiata, anterior internal capsule, and putamen *(29)*. Second, few of the patients discussed had isolated lesions of the caudate nucleus, and extension toward internal capsule or putamen was frequently observed.

3.2. Lenticular Nucleus

Isolated lenticular strokes are relatively uncommon, and few reports in the literature are available. Bilateral pallidal lesions cause a frontal lobe syndrome *(35)*. Left putaminal-pallidal infarction may induce persistent word-finding difficulty *(36)*. Putaminal lesions are also associated with hemispatial neglect in the absence of visual field deficits *(30)*.

3.3. Capsular Genu

The primary clinical manifestations of genu infarction are acute confusional state, with fluctuating alertness, inattention, memory loss, abulia, and psychomotor retardation, in the acute stage. Chronic impairments include verbal and visuospatial memory deficits, decreased verbal fluency, and constructional impairment *(28,29,37)*. Lesions are mostly left-sided and at the inferior portion of the genu, in the territory supplied by the anterior perforating arteries, arising from the apex of the internal carotid artery or anterior cerebral artery. Patients with acute cognitive deficits, without the development of dementia, have considerable improvement during long-time follow-up *(38)*. On the other hand, association of infarct with white matter lesions (WMLs) or coexistent cortical lesions carry a worse prognosis *(36)*.

3.4. Thalamus

In a series of 12 patients with strategic single infarct dementia, 8 had thalamic infarct *(10)*. Among cases of thalamic infarction, memory dysfunction usually follows the pattern left-verbal and right-nonverbal *(39)* and has been primarily reported with lesions in two of the four main arterial territories of the thalamus: the tuberothalamic artery and the paramedian artery. The tuberothalamic artery comes off the posterior communicating artery and supplies the anterolateral thalamus, including the ventral anterior nucleus and part of the ventral lateral nucleus. The paramedian artery arises from the P1 segment of the posterior cerebral artery, and its territory includes the medial upper midbrain and medial thalamus, including most of the dorsomedial nucleus and the intralaminar nuclear group *(40,41)*. Both the tuberothalamic and the paramedian arteries supply hippocampal- and amygdala-related components of the thalamus that have been suggested to be critical for memory function, including the mamillothalamic tract, the ventroamygdalofugal pathway, and the dorsomedial nucleus *(42–44)*. Involvement of the mamillothalamic tract is particularly associated with amnestic syndrome *(45,46)*.

Features accompanying memory deficits in thalamic infarction vary with lesion site. The main presenting features in tuberothalamic infarctions are cognitive deficits, including aphasia with left-sided lesions and neglect and visuospatial processing impairments with right-sided lesions, along with transient motor and sensory signs, as well as a facial paresis for emotional movements.

Paramedian infarctions typically begin with somnolence and supranuclear vertical gaze paresis. Neuropsychological deficits, including amnesia, appear as the patient improves. Severe neurobehavioral abnormalities, simulating prefrontal lesions, may follow, such as decreased motivation, arousal, initiation, attention, and executive function *(39)*. Hemiparesis, hemiataxia, and delayed abnormal movements may also occur *(39,40)*. Disturbance of naming and perseveration may be observed but not cortical aphasia *(39)*. Bilateral paramedian infarcts resulted in severe dementia, characterized by verbal, visual memory impairment, and retrieval deficits in seven of nine patients in one series *(47)*.

Because of the common blood supply through the posterior circulation, strokes involving the thalamus, with subsequent memory disturbance, may be accompanied by infarction of the medial temporal lobe.

Posterior choroidal artery infarcts affect the lateral geniculate body, pulvinar, posterior thalamus, hippocampus, and parahippocampal gyrus. The main clinical findings in these patients are visual field defects, sensorimotor dysfunction, and, rarely, memory disturbances and transcortical

Table 1
Syndromes of Unilateral Amnesic Stroke

Vascular territory	Memory-related anatomic structures involved	Common associated symptoms	Reported cases	Laterality
Posterior cerebral artery	Hippocampus, parahippocampal gyrus, collateral isthmus	Hemi- or quadrantanopia pure alexia, color anomia	51	47 left, 4 right
Thalamus: Paramedian artery (PmA)	Mamillothalamic tract, ventroamygdalofugal pathway, dorsomedial nucleus	Somnolence, vertical gaze paresis, hemiparesis, hemiataxia (PmA)	42 infarcts	33 left, 9 right
Tuberothalamic artery (TtA)		Visuospatial deficits, emotional facial paresis, aphasia (TtA)	11 hemorrhages	8 left, 3 right
Anterior choroidal artery	Amygdala, anterior hippocampus, genu and posterior internal capsule	Hemiparesis, hemiataxia, hemisensory and hemi-visual deficit	4	4 left

Reprinted with permission from ref. *50*.

aphasia (in left-sided lesions) *(48)*. Thalamogeniculate infarcts rarely result in neurobehavioral syndromes *(40)*.

3.5. Angular Gyrus

The most frequent clinical symptomatology observed with angular gyrus lesions is Gerstman syndrome *(49)* (acalculia, right-left confusion, agraphia, and finger agnosia), with or without fluent aphasia, alexia with agraphia, and constructional disturbance. One reported patient with left angular gyrus stroke also had deficits in attention, language visual, and verbal memory *(10)*. The clinical features of the Gerstman syndrome can also be seen in Alzheimer's disease (AD) *(22)*.

3.6. Temporal, Occipital, and Frontal Lobes

Amnesia can occur with left anterior choroidal artery (AChA) infarction. When the infarct is confined to the mesial temporal lobe, amnesia may arise in relative isolation; when the ischemic lesion includes the posterior limb of the internal capsule and the lateral geniculate body, accompanying hemimotor, hemisensory, and hemivisual deficits may appear *(50)*.

The AChA artery arises from the internal carotid artery shortly after the takeoff of the posterior communicating artery *(51,52)*. Inferolateral branches of the AChA supply the posteromedial half of the amygdala, the anterior hippocampus, and the fascia dentata *(51)*. A rich anastomotic net exists with the PCA in this area, and, in the absence of a PCA hippocampal branch, the AChA may additionally supply the middle portion and tail of the hippocampus *(52)*.

Evidence from a series of consecutive PCA stroke patients suggests that PCA infarctions produce memory disturbance only when lesions extend to posteromedial temporal lobe structures critical for normal memory function *(53)*. Amnesia resulting form unilateral PCA stroke reflects the degree of involvement of the different branches of the PCA territory. Lesions involving the occipitotemporal or calcarine branches, supplying the optic radiations or calcarine cortex, produce hemianopic or quadrantanopsic visual field defects, usually affecting the superior visual field *(54)*.

Although bilateral temporolimbic lesions are most likely to be affected in case of severe, persistent amnesia, cases of amnestic stroke have been reported with single stroke lesions *(50)* (*see* Table 1). Radiographic examples of "amnesic stroke" are illustrated in Figs. 1–3 *(50)*.

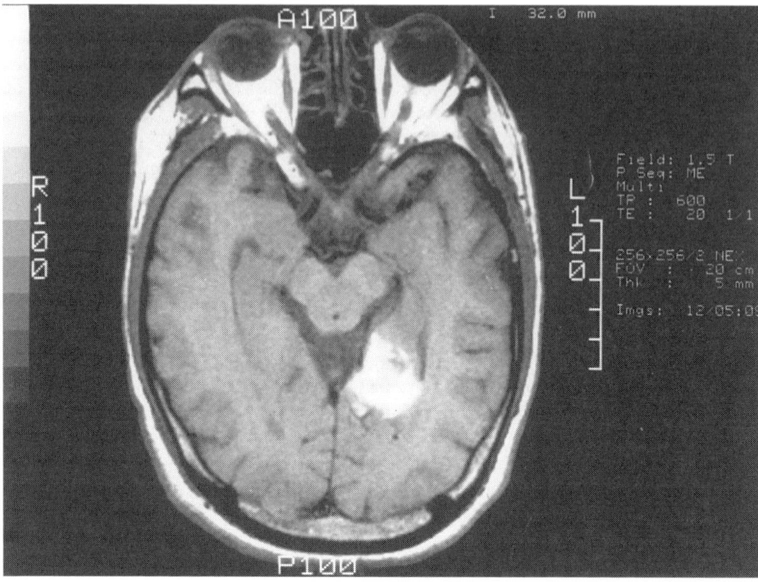

Fig. 1. T1-weighted magnetic resonance imaging (MRI) axial view (TR, 600 ms; TE, 20ms) of patient with persistent amnesia. Region of hemorrhage, ischemia, and edema involves middle and posterior portions of left hippocampus and parahippocampal gyrus.

Alexia without agraphia appears if the paraventricular white matter of the left occipital lobe has been damaged, disconnecting both interhemispheric and intrahemispheric visual pathways to the angular gyrus *(55,56)*. Involvement of the mesial occipitotemporal junction of the left hemisphere may result in color anomia *(55)*. Aphasia is rarely observed in PCA stroke but has been reported and is usually either transcortical sensory (usually with lesions of the dorsomedial and ventrolateral thalamic nuclei) or amnestic *(57)*.

Infarcts of the anterior cerebral artery mainly produce prolonged mutism, acute confusional state (right-sided lesions), abulia, decreased verbal fluency, and sphincter incontinence. Abulia is usually persistent. The areas most often involved in abulia and mutism are the cingulate gyrus and supplementary motor area *(58)*. Transcortical motor aphasia may follow mutism or may be present from onset and normally correlates with lesions in the supplementary motor area *(59)*. Bilateral lesions may result in akinetic mutism (which can be persistent or transitory), incontinence, bilateral grasp reflex, and functional-dependent outcome *(58,59)*.

4. SUMMARY

The most convincing evidence that dementia has been caused by stroke comes from careful clinicopathologic and clinicoradiologic correlation between specific stroke lesions and observations of abnormal cognition and behavior. Knowledge about strategic infarction provides a firm basis on which to determine cause-and-effect relationships with dementia symptoms. The closer the time proximity of the stroke lesion and the suspected behavioral outcome, the more confident one may be about the vascular basis of the dementia.

Strokes in the temporolimbic pathways are important contributors to the development of persistent amnesia. Left hemisphere lesions are more commonly associated with poststroke dementia through involvement of language circuits. Other strategic areas of infarction causing recognizable brain-behavior syndromes include thalamus, caudate and lenticular nuclei, capsular genu, angular gyrus, occipital junction area, and prefrontal lobes.

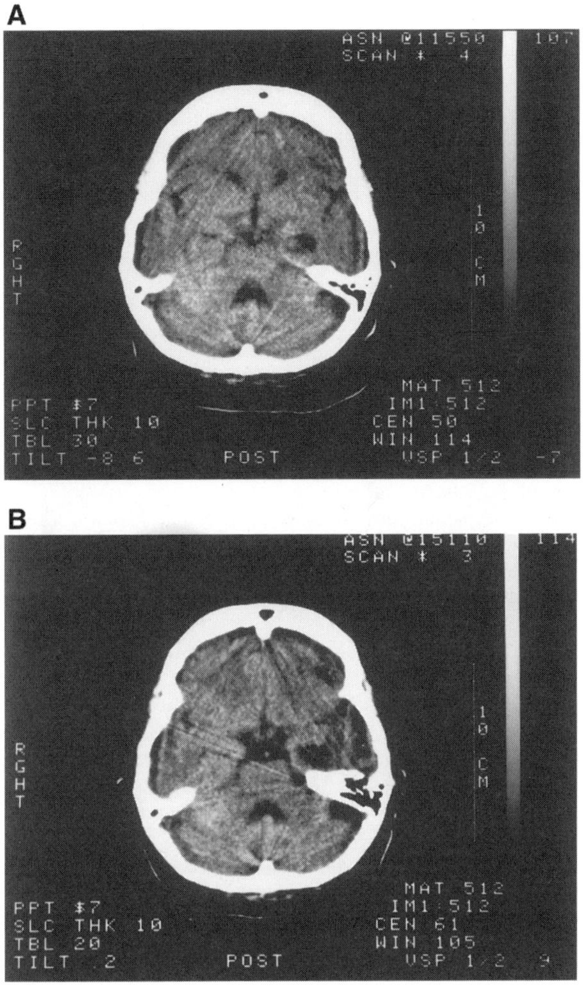

Fig. 2. Nonenhanced computed tomography axial views of patient with persistent amnesia. Region of ischemia involves left anterior hippocampus and amygdala.

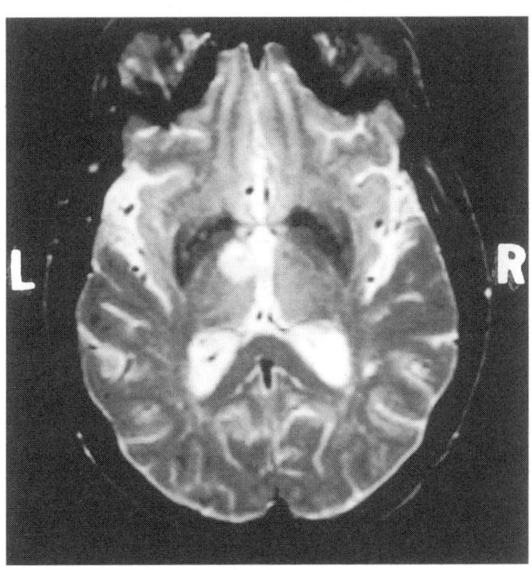

Fig. 3. T2-weighted magnetic resonance imaging (MRI) axial view (TR, 2500 ms; TE, 80 ms) of patient with persistent amnesia. Region of ischemia involves ventral anterior nucleus of left thalamus.

REFERENCES

1. Tatemichi TK, Desmond DW, Paik M, et al. Clinical determinants of dementia related to stroke. Ann Neurol 1993;33: 568–575.
2. Pohjasvaara T, Mäntylä R, Salonen O, et al. MRI correlates of dementia after first clinical ischemic stroke. J Neurol Sci 2000;181:111–117.
3. Barba R, Martínez-Espinosa S, Rodrígues-García E, et al. Poststroke dementia. Clinical features and risk factors. Stroke 2000;31:1494–1501.
4. Pohjasvaara T, Erkinjuntti T, Ylikoski R, et al. Clinical determinants of poststroke dementia. Stroke 1998;29:75–81.
5. Desmond DW, Moroney JT, Paik MC, et al. Frequency and clinical determinants of dementia after ischemic stroke. Neurology 200;54:1124–1131.
6. Censori B, Manara O, Agostini C, et al. Dementia after first stroke. Stroke 1996;27:1205–1210.
7. Hénon H, Pasquier F, Durieu I, et al. Preexisting dementia in stroke patients. Baseline frequency, associated factors and outcome. Stroke 1997;28:1932–1939.
8. Kokmen E, Whisnant JP, O'Fallon WM, et al. Dementia after ischemic stroke: a population-based study in Rochester, Minnesota (1960-1984). Neurology 1996;46:154–159.
9. Pasquier F, Didier L. Why are stroke patients prone to develop dementia. J Neurol 1997;244:135–142.
10. Auchus AP, Chen CPLH, Sodagar SN, et al. Single stroke dementia: insights from 12 cases in Singapore. J Neurol Sci 2002;203-204:85–89.
11. Tatemichi TK, Paik M, Beigelli MS, et al. Risk of dementia after stroke in a hospitalized cohort: results of a longitudinal study. Neurology 1994;44:1885–1891.
12. Tatemichi TK. How acute brain failure becomes chronic: a view of the mechanisms of dementia related to stroke. Neurology 1990;40:1652–1659.
13. Pohjasvaara T, Mäntylä R, Salonen O, et al. How complex interactions of ischemic brain infarcts, white matter lesions, and atrophy relate to poststroke dementia. Arch Neurol 2000;57:1295–1300.
14. Instar D, Di Carlo A, Paracusic G, et al. Incidence and determinants of poststroke dementia as defined by an informant interview method in a hospital-based stroke registry. Stroke 1998;29:2087–2093.
15. Cordoliani-Mackowiak MA, Hénon H, Pruvo JP, et al. Poststroke dementia—influence of hippocampal atrophy. Arch Neurol 2003;60:585–590.
16. Crisostomo RA, Garcia MM, Tong DC. Detection of diffusion-weighted MRI abnormalities in patients with transient ischemic attack: correlation with clinical characteristics. Stroke 2003;34:932–937.
17. Moroney JT, Bagiella E, Desmond DW, et al. Risk factors for incident dementia after stroke. Role of hypoxic and ischemic disorders. Stroke 1996;27:1283–1289.
18. Desmond DW, Tatemichi TK, Figueroa M, et al. Disorientation following stroke: frequency, course and clinical correlates. J Neurol 1994;241:585–591.
19. Knopman DS, Rocca WA, Cha RH, et al. Incidence of vascular dementia in Rochester, Minn, 1985-1989. Arch Neurol. 2002;59:1605–1610.
20. Laduner G, Iliff LD, Lechner H. Clinical factors associated with dementia in ischemic stroke. J Neurol Neurosurg Psychiatry 1982;45:97–101.
21. Román GC, Tatemichi TK, Erkinjuntti T, et al. Vascular dementia: diagnostic criteria for research studies. Report of the NINDS-AIREN International Workshop. Neurology 1993;43:250–260.
22. McPherson SE, Cummings JL. Neuropsychological aspects of vascular dementia. Brain Cogn 1996;31:269–282.
23. Ferro J. Hyperacute cognitive stroke syndromes. J Neurol 2001;248:841–849.
24. Leys D, Erkinjuntti T, Desmond DW, et al. Vascular dementia: the role of cerebral infarcts. Alzheimer Dis Assoc Disord 1999;13(S3):S38–S48.
25. Cummings JL. Frontal-subcortical circuits and human behavior. Arch Neurol 1993;50:873–880.
26. Baron JC, D'Antona R, Pantano P, et al. Effects of thalamic stroke on energy metabolism of the cerebral cortex. A positron tomography study in man. Brain 1986;109:1243–1259.
27. Baron JC, Levasseur M, Mazoyer B, et al. Thalamocortical diaschisis: positron emission tomography in humans. J Neurol Neurosurg Psychiatry 1992;55:935–942.
28. Tatemichi TK, Desmond DW, Prohovnik I, et al. Confusion and memory loss from capsular genu infarction: a thalamocortical disconnection syndrome? Neurology 1992;42:1966–1979.
29. Tatemichi TK, Desmond DW, Prohovnik I. Strategic infarcts in vascular dementia. A clinical and brain imaging experience. Drug Research 1995;45:371–385.
30. Karnath HO, Himmelbach M, Rorden C. The subcortical anatomy of human spatial neglect: putamen, caudate nucleus and pulvinar. Brain 2002;125:350–360.
31. Caplan LR, Schmahmann JD, Kase CS, et al. Caudate infarcts. Arch Neurol 1990;47:133–143.
32. Mendez MF, Adams NL, Lewandowski KS. Neurobehavioral changes associated with caudate lesions. Neurology 1989;39:349–354.

33. Godefroy O, Rousseaux M, Leys D, et al. Frontal lobe dysfunction in unilateral lenticulostriate infarcts. Prominent role of cortical lesions. Arch Neurol 1992;49:1285–1289.
34. Kumral E, Evyapan D, Balkir K. Acute caudate vascular lesions. Stroke 1999;30:100–108.
35. Strub RL. Frontal lobe syndrome in a patient with bilateral globus pallidus lesions. Arch Neurol 1989;46:1024–1027.
36. Pantoni L, Basile AM, Romanelli M, et al. Abulia and cognitive impairment in two patients with capsular genu infarct. Acta Neurol Scand 2001;104:185–190.
37. Russmann H, Vingerhoets F, Ghika J, et al. Acute infarction limited to the lenticular nucleus. Clinical, etiologic and topographic features. Arch Neurol 2003;60:351–355.
38. Madureira S, Guerreiro M, Ferro JM. A follow-up study of cognitive impairment due to inferior capsular genu infarction. J Neurol 1999;246:764–769.
39. Stuss DT, Guberman A, Nelson R, Larochelle S. The neuropsychology of paramedian thalamic infarction. Brain Cogn 1988;8:348–378.
40. Bogousslavsky J, Regli F, Uske A. Thalamic infarcts: clinical syndromes, etiology, and prognosis. Neurology 1988; 38:837–848.
41. Castaigne P, Lhermitte F, Buge A, Escourolle R, Hauw JJ, Lyon-Caen O. Paramedian thalamic and midbrain infarcts: clinical and neuropathological study. Ann Neurol 1981;10:127–148.
42. Graff-Radford NR, Tranel D, Van Hoesen GW, Brandt JP. Diencephalic amnesia. Brain 1990;113:1–25.
43. Bogousslavsky J, Regli F, Assal G. The syndrome of unilateral tuberothalamic artery territory infarction. Stroke 1986; 17:434–441.
44. von Cramon DY, Hebel N, Schuri U. A contribution to the anatomical basis of thalamic amnesia. Brain 1985;108:993–1008.
45. Van Der Werf YD, Witter MP, Uylings HBM, Jolles J. Neuropsychology of infarctions in the thalamus: a review. Neuropsychologia 2000;38:613–627.
46. Van Der Werf YD, Scheltens P, Lindeboom J, et al. Deficits of memory, executive functioning and attention following infarction in the thalamus; a study of 22 cases with localized lesions. Neuropsychologia 2003;41:1330–1344.
47. Szirmai I, Vastagh I, Szombathelyi E, Kamondi A. Strategic infarcts of the thalamus in vascular dementia. J Neurol Sci 2002;203-204:91–97.
48. Neau JP, Bogousslavsky J. The syndrome of posterior choroidal artery territory infarction. Ann Neurol. 1996;39: 779–788
49. Mayer E, Martory MD, Pegna AJ, et al. A pure case of Gerstmann syndrome with a subangular lesion. Brain 1999;122:1107–1120.
50. Ott BR, Saver JL. Unilateral amnesic stroke. Six new cases and review of the literature. Stroke 1993;24:1033–1042.
51. Rhoton AL, Fujii K, Fradd B. Microsurgical anatomy of the anterior choroidal artery. Surg Neurol 1979;12:171–187.
52. Hussein S, Renella RR, Dietz H. Microsurgical anatomy of the anterior choroidal artery. Acta Neurochir 1988;92:19–28.
53. von Cramon DY, Hebel N, Schuri U. Verbal memory and learning in unilateral posterior cerebral infarction. Brain 1988;111:1061–1077.
54. Pessin MS, Lathi ES, Cohen MB, Kwan ES, Hedges TR, Caplan LR. Clinical features and mechanism of occipital infarction. Ann Neurol 1987;21:290–299.
55. Damasio AR, Damasio H. The anatomic basis of pure alexia. Neurology 1983;33:1573–1583.
56. De Renzi E, Zambolin A, Crisi G. The pattern of neuropsychological impairment associated with left posterior cerebral artery infarcts. Brain 1987;110:1099–1116.
57. Servan J, Verstichel P, Catala M, et al. Aphasia and infarction of the posterior cerebral artery territory. J Neurol 1995; 242:87–92.
58. Kumral E, Bayulkem G, Evyapan D, Yunten N. Spectrum of anterior cerebral artery territory infarction: clinical and MRI findings. Eur J Neurol. 2002;9:615–624.
59. Bogousslavsky J, Regli F. Anterior cerebral artery territory infarction in the Lausanne Stroke Registry. Arch Neurol 1990;47:144–150.

V Interactions Between Vascular Dementia and Alzheimer's Disease

17

Understanding Incidence and Prevalence Rates in Mixed Dementia

John Gunstad and Jeffrey Browndyke

1. INTRODUCTION

Countries throughout the world are reporting increased life-spans and lower birth rates. These sociodemographic changes result in the elderly, particularly the oldest old, comprising an increasingly larger segment of the population *(1)*. Consequently, dementia is projected to be one of the major health-care problems of future decades *(2)*.

Alzheimer's disease (AD) and vascular dementia (VaD) have long been considered the most prevalent forms of dementia *(3)*. More recently, increased attention has been given to the co-occurrence of AD and VaD, typically referred to as mixed dementia (MD). Although first described in the 1960s, MD has received relatively little attention until recently *(4)*.

It has been speculated that MD may be the most common form of dementia *(5)*, but its "true" prevalence remains unknown. A growing number of studies report the frequency of MD within their samples of patients with dementia or in the community at large, but these studies were designed to detect AD or VaD, not MD. The goals of this chapter are to present the incidence/prevalence rates of MD reported in past studies, to identify possible methodological concerns of these studies, and to suggest future directions for MD studies. To accomplish these goals, this chapter has been divided into five sections:

2. RATES OF MIXED DEMENTIA

2.1. *Terminology Review*

The prevalence of a disorder may be defined as the "fraction (proportion) of a group possessing a clinical outcome at a given point in time and is measured by a single examination or survey of a group" *(6)*. Incidence rates refer to the "fraction or proportion of a group initially free of the outcome which develops the outcome over a given period of time" *(6)*. To put these definitions into more concrete terms, incidence rates refer to the number of examined persons that develop MD within a particular time period, whereas prevalence rates refer to the number of individuals who develop MD and survive until the time of assessment. Incidence studies are typically longitudinal, requiring researchers to assess the same sample on at least two occasions. Prevalence studies assess participants at a single time point, establishing a "point prevalence" for the condition of interest.

2.2. *Incidence Rates*

Few studies have examined the incidence of MD. Reported incidence rates of MD and combined MD /VaD are presented in Tables 1 and 2.

From: *Current Clinical Neurology*
Vascular Dementia: Cerebrovascular Mechanisms and Clinical Management
Edited by: R. H. Paul, R. Cohen, B. R. Ott, and S. Salloway © Humana Press Inc., Totowa, NJ

Table 1
Standardized Incidence Rates of Dementia in Studies Separating Mixed Dementia From Vascular Dementia

Study	Population	*n*	Age	Follow-up (yr)	Total [a]	AD [b]	VaD [c]	MD [d]
Aronson et al., 1991 *(7)*	New York City, United States	442	75–85	8	2.4	1.0	—	0.7
Fratiglioni et al., 1997 *(8)*	Stockholm, Sweden	987	75+	3	5.0	3.7	0.8	0.2
Liu et al., 1998 *(9)*	Southern Taiwan	2175	65+	2	1.4	0.6	0.4	0.2
Lopez et al., 2003 *(10)*	Multisite, United States	2831	65+	11	2.3	1.6	0.3	0.4

[a] Number of dementia cases per 100 persons.
[b] Number of dementia cases per 100 persons attributed to Alzheimer's disease (AD).
[c] Number of dementia cases per 100 persons attributed to vascular dementia (VaD).
[d] Number of dementia cases per 100 persons attributed to mixed dementia (MD).

Table 2
Standardized Incidence Rates of Dementia in Studies Including Mixed Dementia With Vascular Dementia

Study	Population	*n*	Age	Follow-up (yr)	Total [a]	AD [b]	VaD/MD [c]
Tsolaki et al., 1999 *(11)*	Pylea[d] Greece	380	70+	2–4	5.7	4.0	1.4
Kawas et al., 2000 *(12)*	Baltimore, United States	1236	55–97	2–13	1.7	1.2	0.2

[a] Number of dementia cases per 100 persons.
[b] Number of dementia cases per 100 persons attributed to Alzheimer's disease (AD).
[c] Number of dementia cases per 100 persons attributed to vascular dementia (VaD) or mixed dementia (MD).
[d] Unable to provide standardized rate.

Standardized incidence rates were used to promote comparison across studies. Rates were standardized by dividing the total number of incident cases by the average number of years to follow-up *(13)*. This value was then standardized to incidence per 100 cases. It should be noted that this method assumes a constant incidence rate over time (e.g., 100 incident cases during 10 yr, 10 cases/yr), even though MD rates increase with age *(14,15)*. Despite this potential statistical artifact, standardized incidence rates allow greater comparability across studies than cases per patient years (e.g., cases per 1000 patient yr) because of the differential influence of long-enrolled participants.

Using this method, the incidence rates of any type of dementia range from 1.5 to 5.0 cases per 100 persons, with MD incidence ranging from 0.2 to 0.7 cases per 100 persons/yr. Overall dementia incidence rates for studies combining MD and VaD range from 1.7 to 5.7, with MD /VaD incidence ranging from 0.2 to 1.4 cases per 100 persons/yr. Not appearing in the tables, the Sydney Older Persons Study found incidence rates of 3.3 for mixed AD and 1.4 for mixed VaD during an average of 3-yr follow-up *(16)*. It is unclear how these groups may overlap.

Table 3
Dementia Prevalence Rates

Study	Population	*n*	Age	Total [a]	AD [b]	VaD [c]	MD [d]
Brayne et al., 1989 *(17)*	Cambridgeshire, England	365	70–79	7.9	4.1	2.5	0.3
O'Conner et al., 1989 *(18)*	Cambridge, England	2311	75+	10.5	7.9	2.2	0.3
Rocca et al., 1991 *(19)*	Appignano, Italy	751	60+	6.2	2.6	2.2	0.8
Skoog et al., 1993 *(20)*	Gothenberg, Sweden	494	85+	29.8	13.0	11.5	2.4
White et al., 1996 *(21)*	Honolulu, United States	3734	71–93	6.0	2.1	1.8	0.6
Andersen et al., 1997 *(22)*	Odense, Denmark	3346	65–84	7.1	4.7	1.3	0.1
Shiba et al., 1999 *(23)*	Hanazono-mura, Japan	201	65+	8.5	3.5	3.0	1.8
von Strauss et al., 1999 *(24)*	Stockholm, Sweden	1424	77+	25.1	19.2	4.4	0.0
Wang et al., 2000 *(25)*	Beijing, China	5003	60+	2.7	1.4	1.0	.002
Ikeda et al., 2001 *(26)*	Nakayama, Japan	1162	65+	5.2	1.8	2.4	0.1
Yamada et al., 2001 *(27)*	Amino, Japan	3715	65–99	3.8	2.1	1.0	0.2
Benedetti et al., 2002 *(28)*	Buttapietra, Italy	222	75+	15.8	6.8	3.6	1.4
Herrara et al., 2002 *(29)*	Catanduva, Brazil	1656	65–96	7.1	3.9	0.7	1.0
Yamada et al., 2002 *(30)*	Campo Grande, Brazil	157	70–100	12.1	5.7	0.6	4.5

[a] Number of dementia cases per 100 persons.
[b] Number of dementia cases per 100 persons attributed to Alzheimer's disease.
[c] Number of dementia cases per 100 persons attributed to vascular dementia.
[d] Number of dementia cases per 100 persons attributed to MD.

2.3. *Prevalence Rates of Mixed Dementia*

Relative to other forms of dementia, few studies have examined the prevalence rates of MD. Reported prevalence rates of MD are presented in Table 3. Prevalence rates for all dementia range from 2.7 to 29.8 cases per 100 persons, with MD prevalence ranging from 0.0 to 4.5 cases per 100 persons.

Table 4 presents studies that reported the prevalence rates of MD by age group. Results suggest that MD becomes more prevalent with age, with a possible decline in the oldest old. This decline may reflect an increased mortality risk in persons with vascular pathology.

A similar pattern is found in those studies reporting the combined prevalence of MD and VaD across the age span (*see* Table 5).

Table 4
Dementia Prevalence Rates by Age in Studies Separating Mixed Dementia and Vascular Dementia

Study	Population	Age	*n*	Total [a]	AD [b]	VaD [c]	MD [d]
Manubens et al., 1995 *(14)*	Pamplona, Spain	72–74	146	6.3	0.6	3.0	1.3
		75–79	311	11.8	8.2	1.9	0.3
		80–84	302	17.3	10.6	2.2	2.2
		85–89	279	25.6	17.8	0.9	4.6
		90–91	89	34.7	25.0	6.1	2.3
Vas et al., 2001 *(15)*	Bombay, India	<49	12,099	0.0	0.0	0.0	0.0
		50–54	3,933	0.08	0.0	0.05	0.0
		55–59	2,422	0.04	0.04	0.0	0.0
		60–64	2,112	0.3	0.05	0.1	0.1
		65–69	1,751	0.9	0.5	0.2	0.2
		70–74	1,157	2.4	1.6	0.4	0.2
		75–79	481	5.0	2.9	1.2	0.4
		80–84	336	5.1	3.9	0.6	0.9
		85+	208	3.9	2.9	1.0	0.0

[a] Number of dementia cases per 100 persons.
[b] Number of dementia cases per 100 persons attributed to Alzheimer's disease (AD).
[c] Number of dementia cases per 100 persons attributed to vascular dementia (VaD).
[d] Number of dementia cases per 100 persons attributed to mixed dementia (MD).

Table 5
Dementia Prevalence Rates by Age in Studies Combining Mixed Dementia and Vascular Dementia

Study	Population	Age	Total [a]	AD [b]	VaD/MD [c]
Sulkava et al., 1985 *(31)*	Finland	30–64	0.3	0.03	0.08
		65–74	4.2	1.7	1.9
		75–84	10.7	6.3	4.3
		85+	17.3	14.8	2.5

[a] Number of dementia cases per 100 persons.
[b] Number of dementia cases per 100 persons attributed to Alzheimer's disease (AD).
[c] Number of dementia cases per 100 persons attributed to vascular dementia (VaD) or mixed dementia (MD).

2.4. *Rates of Mixed Dementia in Clinicopathological Studies*

Clinicopathological studies may be categorized as being either prospective or retrospective examinations of a disorder. Prospective studies select individuals and follow them over time to identify the frequency of a given clinical outcome. Retrospective studies identify persons with a given clinical outcome and gather information about the past *(13)*.

MD clinicopathological rates are presented in Table 6 and range from 2.9 to 54.2%. MD rates in prospective studies range from 2.9 to 31.3%, whereas retrospective rates range from 6.0 to 54.2%.

Table 6
Mixed Dementia Prevalence Rates in Clinicopathological Studies

Study	Study type	*n*	AD [a]	VaD [b]	MD [c]
Jellinger et al., 1990 *(32)*	Retrospective	675	60.0	15.7	7.9
Mirra et al., 1991 *(33)*	Retrospective	142	41.5	2.1	28.1
Gilleard et al., 1992 *(34)*	Prospective	64	37.5	32.8	15.6
Mendez, 1992 *(35)*[d]	Retrospective	650	60.0	—	6.0
Giannakopoulos et al., 1994 *(36)*	Retrospective	127	45.7	8.7	45.7
Ince et al., 1995 *(37)*	Prospective	69	60.9	5.8	2.9
Victoroff et al., 1995 *(38)*	Retrospective	196	33.7	1.5	7.7
Snowdon et al., 1997 *(39)*	Prospective	102	36.2	1.0	23.5
Bowler et al., 1998 *(40)*	Prospective	122	38.5	4.1	18.0
Nolan et al., 1998 *(41)*	Retrospective	87	50.5	0.0	36.8
Lim et al., 1999 *(42)*	Prospective	134	25.3	3.0	31.3
Kammoun et al., 2000 *(43)*	Retrospective	120	17.5	28.3	54.2
Barker et al., 2002 *(44)*	Retrospective	382	41.6	3.1	11.3
Jellinger, 2003 *(45)*	Prospective	950	33.0	8.6	3.6

[a] Percentage of dementia cases attributed to Alzheimer's disease (AD).
[b] Percentage of dementia cases attributed to vascular dementia (VaD).
[c] Percentage of dementia cases attributed to mixed dementia (MD).
[d] Rate for pure VaD unavailable.

3. METHODOLOGICAL ISSUES

As shown in Section 2., recent years have seen a growing number of studies report MD incidence and/or prevalence rates. Despite this interest, few studies have been specifically designed to detect the presence of MD. As a result, methodological concerns specific to MD are not accounted for in these studies. Concerns including the absence of established definition for MD, limits of instrumentation, differential mortality rates, possible selection bias, and low incidence rate likely result in an underestimation of the actual incidence and prevalence of MD. Each of these concerns is briefly discussed in the following sections.

3.1. *Lack of Established Criteria for Mixed Dementia*

Although researchers more or less agree that MD is the co-occurrence of AD and VaD, operational definitions vary widely across studies. Past definitions include:

- A clinical dementia syndrome consistent with AD but with history of stroke *(8)*.
- History of acute focal neurologic symptoms/signs without a clear temporal connection with the evolution of the dementia *(20)*.
- Clinical history and Hachinski score of 5 or 6 *(46)*.
- The Neuroepidemiology Branch of the National Institute of Neurological Disorders and Stroke-Association Internationale pour la Recherche et l'Enseignement en Neurosciences (NINDS-AIREN) criteria for AD with cerebrovascular disease (CVD) *(29)*.
- Alzheimer's Disease Diagnostic Treatment Center (ADDTC) criteria *(21)*.

There are also no established criteria for the identification of MD in clinicopathological studies. It absence may be the largest limiting factor in using these studies to identify MD prevalence *(47)* and limits comparison across studies *(40)*. Past definitions include:

- The Consortium to Establish a Registry for Alzheimer's Disease (CERAD) protocol for AD and more than 100 mL combined infarct volume *(37)*.
- Presence of senile plaques and neurofibrillary tangles in excess of 5 mm^2 in the hippocampal formation/ neocortex and the presence of multifocal cerebral infarcts *(36)*.
- The presence of moderate or severe concentrations of neuritic plaques in the neocortex and two or more gross cortical infarcts or two or more gross subcortical infarcts *(35)*.

Conclusions regarding clinicopathological studies are further complicated by the use of different criteria at various sites within the same study *(38)* or changing criteria over time *(41)*. Further complicating these studies, many persons exhibit neuropathological changes at autopsy similar to those found in AD, VaD, or MD but do not meet clinical criteria for dementia *(36,37)*.

3.2. *Measurement Limitations*

The limitations of cognitive screening instruments in detecting dementia are well known *(48)*. Instrument selection is critical, because different measures have different conceptualizations of cognitive impairment *(49)*. Screening instruments also vary in their psychometric properties, often with less than desirable reliability/validity, sensitivity/specificity, and degree of regression to the mean over multiple assessments. Studies also use different cutoffs on similar instruments, further limiting comparison. For example, many dementia studies use a form of the Mini-Mental State Examination (MMSE) to screen participants, although cutoff scores for impairment range from 23 to 17 total correct *(8,25)*.

Concerns regarding instrumentation or measurement issues are not limited to incidence and prevalence studies of MD. Standard practices in autopsy studies may also distort the prevalence rates of different forms of dementia. Korczyn *(5)* describes potential concerns in using pathological studies to detect dementia, including using only half the brain for analysis, failure to include myelin stains, and slicing at 5- to 10-mm intervals (perhaps missing lacunes between slices).

3.3. *Differential Mortality for Mixed Dementia?*

Although unknown, the mortality rate of individuals with MD is likely elevated. All persons with dementia have a higher mortality rate than their counterparts without dementia *(50)*, and individuals suffering from VaD are at greatest risk *(51)*. If MD progression is more similar to VaD than AD *(52)*, it is appropriate to assume an elevated mortality rate for MD. If so, more persons with MD would die before assessment than other types of dementia (i.e., AD) and thus underestimate its prevalence.

Methodological and statistical procedures have been developed to allow researchers to estimate dementia in persons who die between assessment time points *(53)*. However, these methods can distort observed rates, because a single source of information (e.g., death certificate or informant) rarely provides sufficient information to accurately diagnose antemortem dementia *(53)*.

3.4. *Selection Bias*

Obtaining a representative sample is a difficult task, because prevalence rates are influenced by many factors. One factor is the compliance rates of potential participants. Epidemiological studies often overrepresent younger, healthier individuals *(6)*, perhaps reflecting the less positive attitude toward study participation in older persons with cognitive impairment *(54)*. Another factor affecting sample composition is the method by which persons are enrolled. For example, dementia prevalence is higher in institutional settings than community-based samples *(55)*. Rates of different kinds of dementia are also believed to vary by geographic region *(19)*. Although these factors are well known, their effects on observed prevalence rates of MD remain unclear.

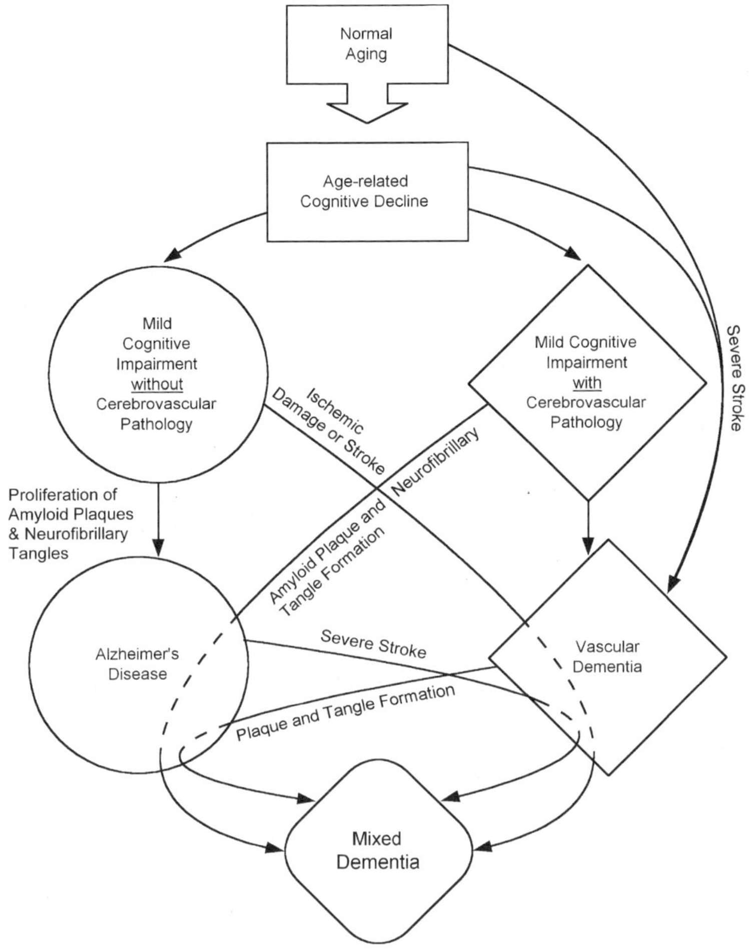

Fig. 1. Possible clinical course of MD.

As in clinical studies of MD, recruiting a representative sample is important in clinicopathological studies. Neuropathological studies are often conducted on samples of persons originally referred to a memory disorders clinic, and higher rates of AD are found in memory clinic samples than in community samples *(56)*. Furthermore, persons with AD may be more likely to participate in necropsy studies *(52)*. It remains unclear how these tendencies influence observed MD rates.

3.5. *Low Incidence Rates*

Accurate determination of the incidence of disorders with low incidence rates is difficult. Although MD is not a rare condition (its incidence similar to stroke in the general population, 0.15 per 100 cases per year *[57]*), its incidence is much lower than AD or geriatric depression (4.6 per 100 persons per year *[58]*). A large sample size is required to compensate for this low incidence rate, typically larger than those employed in past studies.

4. DEVELOPMENT OF MIXED DEMENTIA

Another obstacle in determining the true incidence and prevalence rates of MD is the development of the disorder, because MD may look different to the clinician or pathologist at different points in time (*see* Fig. 1). Persons identified as having MD at autopsy likely move from one diagnostic category to another in the years before death, reflecting the progression of neurodegenerative and vascular pathology over time.

For example, early in the disease course, a person may be diagnosed with mild cognitive impairment (MCI) or vascular cognitive impairment no dementia (VCI-ND) *(59,60)*. With the passing of additional time and exacerbation of vascular problems, persons may be diagnosed with VaD (given the similarities between VaD and MD progression *[52]*). Finally, these vascular problems cause a proliferation of senile plaques and neurofibrillary tangles, resulting in the neuropathological changes consistent with MD. If this hypothesized development is accurate, an individual's death at different stages of the disorder would result in different neuropathological findings, despite the possibility that all represent the same underlying disorder.

Support for this progression may be found in clinical studies of persons with mild cognitive dysfunction who later develop dementia. Persons with VCI-ND progress to MD, AD, or VaD *(60)*. Individuals with vascular problems and cognitive difficulties progress to AD at approximately the same rate as those with MCI *(59)*. Persons with MCI progress to VaD at a higher rate than controls, not just AD *(61)*.

These findings may be interpreted in many ways. One interpretation is that these findings reflect the need for better diagnostic criteria and more sensitive instrumentation. Another, more optimistic, perspective is that these findings are accurate and hint at the "synergistic" interaction between vascular and degenerative processes of the brain *(62)*. Such optimism appears warranted, because both vascular and degenerative lesions influence cognitive performance in persons with dementia and controls and most demented persons exhibit mixed pathology at autopsy *(63)*.

5. FUTURE DIRECTIONS

Dementia researchers have devoted increased resources to cross-cultural and genetic studies in recent years. This attention is well-founded, because a better understanding of cross-cultural dementia rates and the likely genetic contribution to cognitive impairment may offer insight into the etiology of all dementia syndromes, including MD.

5.1. *Cultural Issues in Mixed Dementia*

It is believed that nearly 75% of all persons with dementia in 2020 will reside in a developing nation *(64)*. Despite the methodological difficulties involved in conducting studies in third-world regions *(65)*, determination of the incidence and prevalence of dementia in various countries may yield important etiological clues *(3)*. In addition to studying people in developing nations, further attention is also needed in examining underserved populations within developed nations. For example, relatively little is known about dementia rates in Native American populations *(66)*.

5.2. *Genetics and Mixed Dementia*

The search for possible genetic factors in dementia recently has received considerable attention. The presence of the apolipoprotein E4 (apo E4) allele is frequently associated with increased risk for AD *(67)*. Studies also report a relationship between apo E4 and VaD *(68)*, although this finding is inconsistent *(69)*. Currently, no large studies have examined the relationship between apo E4 and MD. However, apo E4 has been linked to coronary heart disease *(70)* and atherosclerosis *(71)*, suggesting the possibility of a common mechanism *(72)*. Finally, no study has examined the possibility of the genetic factors associated with increased risk for vascular pathology (e.g., angiotensin peptide receptors) being associated with MD, AD, and VaD.

6. CONCLUSION

Although it has been speculated that MD may be the most common form of dementia, its "true" prevalence remains unknown. MD incidence rates range from 0.2 to 0.7 cases per 100 persons per year, with prevalence estimates ranging to 4.5% of the elderly population. MD neuropathological estimates vary widely, ranging from 2.9 to 54.2% of cases. Because of methodological issues and the hypothesized development of the disorder, past studies likely underestimate MD prevalence. Epidemiological studies are needed to better understand this disorder, with special attention given to diverse populations and possible genetic factors.

REFERENCES

1. U.S. Department of Commerce, Economics, and Statistics Administration, Bureau of the Census (1999). International brief. World population at a glance: 1998 and beyond. Available at Website: (http://www.census.gov/ipc/prod/wp98/ib98-4.pdf). Accessed May 27, 2003.
2. U.S. Department of Health and Human Services, National Institutes of Health. (2002). Alzheimer's Disease: Unraveling the Mystery (NIH Publication No. 02-3782).
3. Jorm A. Cross-national comparisons of the occurrence of Alzheimer's and vascular dementias. Eur Arch Psychiatry Clin Neurosci 1991;240:218–222.
4. Zekry D, Hauw J, Gold G. Mixed dementia: epidemiology, diagnosis, and treatment. J Amer Geriatric Soc 2002;50: 1431–1438.
5. Korczyn A. Mixed dementia:the most common form of dementia. Ann NY Acad Sci 2002;977:129–134.
6. Fletcher R, Fletcher S, Wagner E. Clinical Epidemiology: The Essentials. Baltimore, MD:Williams & Wilkins, 1991.
7. Aronson M, Ooj W, Geva D, Masur D, Blau A, Frishman W. Dementia: age-dependent incidence, prevalence, and mortality in the old old. Arch Intern Med 1991;151:989–992.
8. Fratiglioni L, Biitanen M, von Strauss E, Tontodonati V, Herlitz A, Winblad B. Very old women at highest risk of dementia and Alzheimer's disease: incidence data from the Kungsholmen Project, Stockholm. Neurology 1997;48:133–138.
9. Liu C, Lai C, Tai C, Lin R, Yen Y, Howng S. Incidence and subtypes of dementia in southern Taiwan: impact of sociodemographic factors. Neurology, 1998;50:1573–1579.
10. Lopez O, Kuller L, Fitzpatrick A, Ives D, Becker J, Beauchamp N. Evaluation of dementia in the Cardiovascular Health Cognition Study. Neuroepidemiology, 2003;22:1–12.
11. Tsolaki M, Fountoulakis C, Pavlopoulos I, Chatzi E, Kazis A. Prevalence and incidence of Alzheimer's disease and other dementing disorders in Pylea, Greece. Amer J Alzheimer Dis, 1999;14:138–146.
12. Kawas C, Gray S, Brookmeyer R, Fozard J, Zonderman A. Age-specific incidence rates of Alzheimer's disease: The Baltimore Longitudinal Study of Aging. Neurology 1999;54:2072–2077.
13. Elwood J. Critical Appraisal of Epidemiological Studies and Clinical Trials. 2nd Ed. New York, NY: Oxford University Press, 1998.
14. Manubens J, Martinez-Lage J, Lacruz F, et al. Prevalence of Alzheimer's disease and other dementing disorders in Pamplona, Spain. Neuroepidemiology 1995;14:155–164.
15. Vas C, Pinto C, Panikker D, et al. Prevalence of dementia in an urban Indian population. Intl Psychogeriatric 2001;13: 439–450.
16. Waite L, Broe G, Grayson D, Creasey H. The incidence of dementia in an Australian community population: The Sydney Older Persons Study. Intl J Geriatric Psychiatry, 2001;16:680–689.
17. Brayne C, Calloway P. An epidemiological study of dementia in a rural population of elderly women. Br J Psychiatry 1989;155:214–219.
18. O'Connor D, Politt A, Hyde J, et al. The prevalence of dementia as measured by the Cambridge Mental Disorders of the Elderly Examination. Acta Psychiatrica Scandinavia 1989;79:190–198.
19. Rocca W, Hofman A, Brayne C, et al. The prevalence of vascular dementia in Europe: facts and fragments from the 1980-1990 studies. Ann Neurol 1991;30:817–824.
20. Skoog I, Nilsson L, Palmertz B, Andreasson L, Svanborg A. A population-based study of dementia in 85-year-olds. N Engl J Med 1993;328:153–158.
21. White L, Petrovitch H, Ross W, et al. Prevalence of dementia in older Japanese-American men in Hawaii: The Honolulu-Asia Aging Study. JAMA 1996;276:955–960.
22. Anderson K, Lolk A, Nielsen H, Andersen J, Olsen C, Kragh-Sorensen P. Prevalence of very mild to severe dementia in Denmark. Acta Neurologica Scandinavia 1997;96:82–87.
23. Shiba M, Shimogaito J, Kose A, et al. Prevalence of dementia in the rural village of Hanazono-mura, Japan. Neuroepidemiology 1999;18:32–36.
24. von Strauss E, Viitanen M, De Ronchi D, Winblad B, Fratiglioni L. Aging and the occurrence of dementia: findings from a population-based cohort with a large sample of nonagenarians. Arch Neurol 1999;56:587–592.
25. Wang W, Wu S, Cheng X, et al. Prevalence of Alzheimer's disease and other dementing disorders in an urban community of Beijing, China. Neuroepidemiology 2000;19:194–200.
26. Ikeda M, Hokoishi K, Maki M, et al. Increased prevalence of vascular dementia in Japan: a community-based epidemiological study. Neurology 2001;57:839–844.

27. Yamada T, Hattori H, Miura A, Tanaba M, Yamori Y. Prevalence of Alzheimer's disease, vascular dementia and dementia with Lewy bodies in a Japanese population. Psychiatry Clin Neurosci 2001;55:21–25.
28. Benedetti M, Salviati A, Filipponi S, et al. Prevalence of dementia and Apolipoprotein E genotype distribution in the elderly of Buttapietra, Verona Province, Italy. Neuropepidemiology 2002;21:174–180.
29. Herrara E, Caramelli P, Silveira A, Nitrini R. Epidemiologic survey of dementia in a community-dwelling Brazilian population. Alzheimer Dis Assoc Disord 2002;16:103–108.
30. Yamada T, Kadekaru H, Matsumoto S, et al. Prevalence of dementia in the older Japanese-Brazilian population. Psychiatry Clin Neurosci 2002;56:71–75.
31. Sulkava R, Wikstrom J, Aromaa A, et al. Prevalence of severe dementia in Finland. Neurology, 1995;35:1025–1029.
32. Jellinger K, Danielczyk W, Fischer P, Gabriel E. Clinicopathological analysis of dementia disorders in the elderly. J Neurolog Sci 1990;95:239–258.
33. Mirra S, Heman A, McKeel D, et al. The Consortium to Establish a Registry for Alzheimer's Disease (CERAD): Part II. Standardization of the neuropathological assessment f Alzheimer's disease. Neurology 1991;41:479–486.
34. Gilleard C, Kellett J, Coles J, Millard P, Honavar M, Lantos P. The St. George's dementia bed investigation study: a comparison of clinical and pathological diagnosis. Acta Psychiatrica Scand 1992;85:264–269.
35. Mendez M, Mastri A, Sung J, Frey W. Clinically diagnosed Alzheimer's disease: neuropathologic findings in 650 cases. Alzheimer's Dis Assoc Disord 1992;6:35–43.
36. Giannakopoulos P, Hof P, Mottier S, Michel J, Bouras C. Neuropathological changes in the cerebral cortex of 1258 cases from a geriatric hospital: retrospective clinicopathological evaluation of a 10-year autopsy population. Acta Neuropathologica 2994;87:456–468.
37. Ince P, McArthur F, Bjertness E, Torvik A, Candy J, Edwardson J. Neuropathological diagnoses in elderly patients in Oslo: Alzheimer's disease, Lewy body disease, vascular lesions. Dementia 1995;6:162–168.
38. Victoroff J, Mack W, Lyness S, Chui H. Multicenter clinicopathological correlation in dementia. Amer J Psychiatry 1995;152:1476–1484.
39. Snowdon D, Greiner L, Mortimer J, Riley K, Greiner P, Markesbery W. Brain infarction and the clinical expression of Alzheimer disease: the Nun Study. JAMA 1997;277:813–817.
40. Bowler J, Munoz D, Merskey H, Hachinski V. Fallacies in the pathological confirmation of diagnosis of Alzheimer's disease. J Neurol Neurosurg Psychiatry 1998;64:18–24.
41. Nolan K, Lino M, Seligmann A, Blass J. Absence of vascular dementia in an autopsy series from a dementia clinic. J Amer Geriatric Soc 1998;46:597–604.
42. Lim A, Tsuang D, Kukull W, et al. Clinico-neuropathological correlation of Alzheimer's disease in a community-based case series. J Amer Geriatric Soc 1999;47:564–569.
43. Kammoun S, Gold G, Bouras C, et al. Immediate causes of death of demented and non-demented elderly. Acta Neurologica Scand, 2000;176:96–99.
44. Barker W, Luis C, Kashuba A, et al. Relative frequencies of Alzheimer's disease, Lewy body, vascular and frontotemporal dementia, and hippocampal sclerosis in the state of Florida brain bank. Alzheimer Dis Assoc Disord 2002; 16:203–212.
45. Jellinger K. Is Alzheimer's disease a vascular disorder? J Alzheimer Dis 2003;5:247–250.
46. Rocca W, Bonaiuto S, Lippi A, et al. Prevalence of clinically diagnosed Alzheimer's disease and other dementia disorders: a door-to-door survey in Appignano, Macerata Province, Italy. Neurology 1990;40:626–631.
47. Hauw J, Duyckaerts C. Dementia, the fate of brain? Neuropathological point of view. Comptes Rendus Biologies 2002; 325:655–664.
48. Wind A, Schellevis F, Van Staveren G, Scholten R, Jonker C, Van Eijk J. Limitations of the Mini-Mental State Examination in diagnosing dementia in general practice. Intl J Geriatric Psychiatry 1997;12:101–108.
49. Clarke M, Jagger C, Anderson J, Battcock T, Kelly F, Stern M. The prevalence of dementia in a total population: A comparison of two screening instruments. Age Ageing 1991;20:396–403.
50. Noale M, Maggi S, Minicuci N, et al. Dementia and disability: impact on mortality. The Italian longitudinal study on aging. Dementia Geriatric Cogn Disord 2003;16:7–14.
51. Knopman D, Rocca W, Cha R, Edland S, Kokmen E. Survival study of vascular dementia in Rochester, Minnesota. Arch Neurol 2003;60:85–90.
52. Bowler J, Eliasziw M, Steenhuis R, et al. Comparative evolution of Alzheimer disease, vascular dementia, and mixed dementia. Arch Neurol 1997;54:697–703.
53. Stewart M, McDowell I, Hill G, Aylesworth R. Estimating antemortem cognitive status of deceased subjects in a longitudinal study of dementia. Intl Psychogeriatric 2001;13:99–W106.
54. von Strauss E, Fratiglioni L, Jorm A, Viitanen M, Winblad B. Attitudes and participation of the elderly in population surveys: data from a longitudinal study on aging and dementia in Stockholm. J Clin Epidemiol 1998;51:181–187.
55. Matthews F, Dening T, UK Medical Research Council Cognitive Function and Ageing Study. Prevalence of dementia in institutional care. Lancet 2002;360:225–226.
56. Massoud F, Devi G, Stern Y, et al. A clinicopathological comparison of community-based and clinic-based cohorts of patients with dementia. Arch Neurol 1999;56:1368–1373.

57. Brown R, Whisnant J, Sicks J, O'Fallon W, Wiebers D. Stroke incidence, prevalence, and survival: secular trends in Rochester, Minnesota, through 1989. Stroke 1996;27:373–380.
58. Schoevers R, Beekman A, Deeg D, Geerlings M, Jonker C, Van Tilburg W. Risk factors for depression in later life: Results of a prospective community based study (AMSTEL). Journal of Affective Disorders, 2000;59:127–137.
59. Larrieu S, Letenneur L, Orgogozo J, et al. Incidence and outcome of mild cognitive impairment in a population-based prospective cohort. Neurol 2002;59:1594–1599.
60. Wentzel C, Rockwood K, MacKnight C, et al. Progression of impairment in patients with vascular cognitive impairment without dementia. Neurology 2001;4:714–716.
61. Meyer J, Xu G, Thornby J, Chowdhury M, Quach M. Is mild cognitive impairment prodromal for vascular dementia like Alzheimer's disease? Stroke 2002;33:1981–1985.
62. Zekry D, Duyckaerts C, Moulias R, et al. Degenerative and vascular lesions of the brain have synergistic effects in dementia of the elderly. Acta Neuropathologica 2002;103:481–487.
63. Neuropathology group of the medical research council cognitive function and ageing study (MRC CFAS). Pathological correlates of late-onset dementia in a multicentre, community-based population in England and Wales. Lancet 2001; 357:169–175.
64. 10/66 Dementia Research Group. Dementia in developing countries: A consensus statement from the 10/66 Dementia Research Group. Intl J Geriatric Psychiatry 2000;15:14–20.
65. 10/66 Dementia Research Group. Methodological issues for population-based research into dementia in developing countries: a position paper from the 10/66 Dementia Research Group. Intl J Geriatric Psychiatry 2000;15:21–30.
66. Eastwood M, Rifat S, Roberts D. The epidemiology of dementia in North America. European Arch Psychiatry Clin Neurosci 2001;240:207–211.
67. Bennett D, Wilson R, Schneider J, et al. Apolipoprotein E epsilon4 allele, AD pathology, and the clinical expression of Alzheimer's disease. Neurology 2003;60:246–252.
68. Katzman R, Zhang M, Chen P, et al. Effects of apolipoprotein E on dementia and aging in the Shanghai Survey of Dementia. Neurology 1997;49:779–785.
69. Traykov L, Rigaud A, Baudic S, Smagghe A, Boller F, Forette F. Apolipoprotein E epsilon 4 allele frequency in demented and cognitively impaired patients with and without cerebrovascular disease. J Neurolog Sci 2002;203–204:177–181.
70. Wilson P, Myers R, Larson M, Ordovas J, Wolf P, Schaefer E. Apolipoprotein E alleles, dyslipidemia, and coronary heart disease: the Framingham offspring study. JAMA 1994;272:1666–1771.
71. Davignon J, Gregg R, Sing C. Apolipoprotein E polymorphism and atherosclerosis. Arteriosclerosis 1988;8:1–21.
72. Skoog I, Kalaria R, Breteler M. Vascular factors and Alzheimer disease. Alzheimer Dis Assoc Disord 1999;13:S106–S114.

18

Vascular Basement Membrane Abnormalities and Alzheimer's Disease

Edward G. Stopa, Brian D. Zipser, and John E. Donahue

1. INTRODUCTION

There is a growing consensus that microvascular damage is an important contributing factor to the pathogenesis of dementia *(1)*. Increased vascular tortuosity and narrowing is a frequent consequence of normal aging and is significantly worsened by Alzheimer's disease (AD). Furthermore, late-onset sporadic AD, which comprises approximately 90% of AD cases, has been associated with homozygosity for the circulating plasma high-density lipoprotein apo E4. This chapter describes some of the recent work that has been conducted to suggest an association between damage to the microvasculature within the central nervous system (CNS) and AD development.

2. APO E AND SPORADIC ALZHEIMER'S DISEASE

Apo E is a 299-amino acid protein that is a well-known determinant of lipid transport and metabolism *(2)*. In humans, there are three protein isoforms of apo E (E2, E3, and E4) that differ by a single amino acid and are encoded by different gene alleles (ε2, ε3, and ε4). The identification of the apo E genotype as a risk factor for developing the late-onset sporadic form of AD represents a major breakthrough in our understanding of AD *(3)*. Apo E4 is believed to play a role in approximately 50% of AD cases and is second only to aging in importance *(4,5)*. In addition to being a risk factor for sporadic AD, the ε4 allele is also a risk factor for atherosclerosis *(6)*, CVD *(7)*, stroke *(8)*, poor clinical outcome after head injury *(9)*, and spontaneous intracerebral hemorrhage *(10)*. The mechanisms by which apo E4 confers these risks remain unknown, but their elucidation may be critical toward the development of therapeutic targets for these disorders. Interestingly, ethnic differences demonstrating no effect of apo E4 on the risk of AD have been observed in people of African-American and Hispanic origins *(11)*.

3. VASCULAR RISK FACTORS AND ALZHEIMER'S DISEASE

The incidence of AD is increased in patients with underlying vascular risk factors, such as coronary artery disease *(12)*, hypertension *(13)*, diabetes *(14)*, and elevated serum cholesterol *(15)*. Sparks et al. have shown that abundant senile plaques are found in the brains of patients without dementia dying with, or as a result of, critical coronary artery disease, compared to subjects without heart disease *(16)*. They also observed an increase in the densities of senile plaques and neurofibrillary tangles, which are the neuropathologic hallmarks of AD, in individuals with hypertension without critical coronary artery disease. These observations suggest that vascular risk factors and AD may be

From: *Current Clinical Neurology*
Vascular Dementia: Cerebrovascular Mechanisms and Clinical Management
Edited by: R. H. Paul, R. Cohen, B. R. Ott, and S. Salloway © Humana Press Inc., Totowa, NJ

related. In the Nun Study *(17)*, cases of AD with infarcts had fewer tangles than AD cases without infarcts, indicating that infarcts and AD may be parallel processes that have additive effects on the development of clinical dementia. Atherosclerosis, arteriolosclerosis, and amyloid angiopathy often occur simultaneously, making it difficult to assess their respective influence on the degree of cognitive impairment in a given patient.

Hypertensive arteriolosclerosis (small-vessel disease) is one of the most consistently observed magnetic resonance imaging (MRI) and autopsy findings in the brains of elderly patients *(18,19)*. Ironically, such changes are often seen in the absence of a well-documented clinical history of systemic hypertension, suggesting that local organ-specific factors may be more critical for the development of these vascular changes than diastolic or systolic blood pressure elevation *(18)*. Vascular dementia (VaD) is consistently associated with chronic hypertension *(20–23)*. However, the role of hypertension in the development of AD is more complicated to elucidate. In some individuals with hypertension, there is an increase in senile plaques and neurofibrillary tangles. Skoog has theorized that patients suffering from chronic hypertension during their midlife have a greater likelihood of developing AD at an older age *(24)*. Positron emission tomography (PET) scans performed on patients with hypertension have consistently confirmed a reduction in cerebral blood flow (CBF). This reduced CBF is most severe in areas that are predisposed to the development of AD, such as the hippocampus and amygdala *(25–27)*. The resultant decrease in nutrient delivery may be insufficient to meet the metabolic demands of neurons and may also have a deleterious effect on the cerebral microvasculature, further compounding the problem.

4. MICROVASCULAR INJURY IN ALZHEIMER'S DISEASE

Most work on the aging of the cerebral vasculature in humans has focused on the atherosclerotic changes of large caliber vessels, the lipohyalinosis/arteriolosclerosis resulting from chronic hypertension, and the amyloid angiopathy resulting from β amyloid deposition. However, the pathologic alterations of capillaries in the aging brain have not been well studied.

Microvascular disease is a common autopsy finding in the brains of elderly patients, and significant microvascular pathology, including reduced vascular density, atrophic and coiling vessels, glomerular loop formations, and vascular amyloid deposits, have been described in AD *(28)*. Aging animals also exhibit more subtle alterations of arteriolar and capillary morphology. Such alterations are characterized by changes in connective tissue and smooth muscle *(29)*, thickening of the basement membrane *(30)*, thinning and loss of the endothelial cells *(31)*, an increase in endothelial pinocytotic vesicles *(32)*, loss of endothelial mitochondria *(33)*, and an increase in pericytes *(34)*. The laminar and regional distribution of these microvascular alterations typically correlates with the presence of neuropathological lesions (neurofibrillary tangles and amyloid deposits), suggesting a role for microvascular damage in AD pathology *(28,35)*. Both extrinsic (fibronectin) *(36)* and intrinsic (heparan sulfate proteoglycans *[37,38]*, type IV collagen *[39]*, and laminin *[40,41]*) components of the vascular basement membrane have been found within senile plaques. Pericytes share the immunophenotype of microglia and are, therefore, ideally situated within the microvasculature to uptake and process the amyloid precursor protein and deposit β amyloid in a fashion analogous to other systemic and cerebral amyloidoses *(34)*.

Microvascular endothelial cells in patients with AD become activated and have increased expression of intercellular adhesion molecule-1 (ICAM-1), suggesting an inflammatory phenotype in this disease *(42)*. Brain microvessel preparations from patients with AD have been observed to perturb signal transduction cascades *(43–46)*, produce reactive oxygen species (ROS) and nitric oxide *(47)*, express the inflammatory mediator CAP-37 *(48)*, and cause neuronal death in vitro *(49)*.

5. MICROVASCULAR INJURY AND OXIDATIVE STRESS

Considerable clinical and experimental data have shown that cerebral perfusion is progressively decreased during increased aging and that this decrease in brain blood flow is significantly greater in AD *(25–27)*. De la Torre has hypothesized that advanced aging together with a comorbid condition, such as a vascular risk factor, which further decreases cerebral perfusion, promotes a critically attained threshold of cerebral hypoperfusion (CATCH) *(1)*. With time, CATCH induces brain capillary degeneration, causing an increase in basal nitric oxide levels and suboptimal delivery of energy substrates to neuronal tissue *(50)*. Because glucose is the main fuel of brain cells, its impaired delivery, with the deficient delivery of oxygen, compromises neuronal stability when the supply for aerobic glycolysis fails to meet brain tissue demand. The outcome of CATCH is a metabolic cascade that involves, among other things, mitochondrial dysfunction, oxidative stress, decreased adenosine triphosphate (ATP) production, abnormal protein synthesis, cell ionic pump deficiency, signal transduction defects, and neurotransmission failure. These events contribute to the progressive cognitive decline characteristic of patients with AD, as well as regional anatomic pathology, consisting of synaptic loss, senile plaques, neurofibrillary tangles, tissue atrophy, and neurodegeneration. The concept of CATCH explains the heterogeneous clinical pattern that characterizes AD, because it provides compelling evidence that multiple different pathophysiologic vascular risk factors, in the presence of advanced aging, can lead to AD.

6. AGRIN AND THE CEREBRAL MICROVASCULAR BASEMENT MEMBRANE

Heparan-sulfate proteoglycans (HSPGs) are ubiquitously present within the extracellular matrix (ECM) and basement membrane (BM) of most tissues, where they serve both structural and functional roles. The distribution of HSPGs correlates with the characteristic lesions of AD, the senile (amyloid) plaques and neurofibrillary tangles *(37,38)*. HSPGs may be directly involved in the formation and/or persistence of amyloid plaques *(51)*. Moreover, the amyloid precursor protein (APP) binds heparan sulfate, suggesting that the interaction of APP with HSPG in the extracellular matrix may stimulate the effects of APP on neurite outgrowth *(52)*. APP-proteoglycan interactions may disturb normal APP function and contribute to the neuritic outgrowth surrounding the core of senile plaques *(53)*.

Agrin is a multidomain HSPG with a predicted core molecular weight of approximately 200 kDa *(54,55)* (Fig. 1). The amino-terminal half of agrin contains a laminin-binding domain *(56)*, regions homologous to protease-inhibitors and growth factor-binding proteins *(57,58)*, and three sites for heparan-sulfate side chain addition. One or more of these sites is used, because native agrin is approximately 500 kDa *(59,60)*. In addition, these glycosaminoglycan (GAG) chains can mediate binding to the β amyloid peptide *(61)*.

Agrin was first isolated from the basal laminae of the Torpedo electric organ *(62)*. It was identified by its ability to organize the aggregation of myotube acetylcholine receptors and other postsynaptic elements beneath the nerve terminal *(62–64)*. In the peripheral nervous system, agrin is a key determinant of synapse formation at the neuromuscular junction and serves as an integral part of the dystrophin-associated protein complex in skeletal muscle *(65–67)* (Fig. 2E). Agrin's role in the CNS remains unknown. Its presence in neurons of the brain and retina *(68)* argues that it may be required for synapse formation there as well. Agrin phosphorylates and activates the transcription factor cyclic adenosine monophosphate (cAMP) response element-binding protein (CREB), which suggests that agrin in CNS neurons might influence gene expression *(69)*.

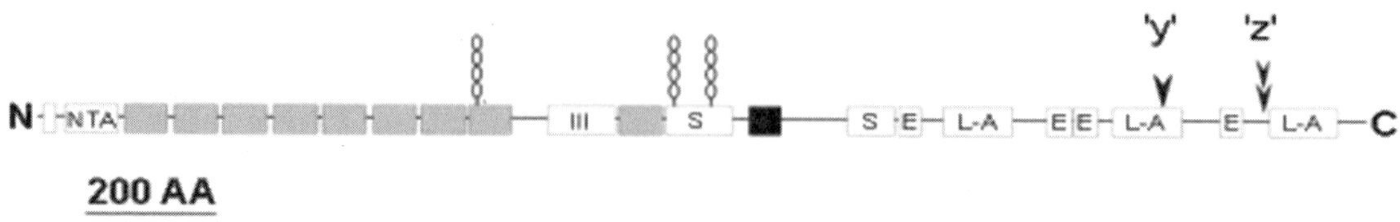

Fig. 1. The structural organization of agrin. The N-terminal portion of the molecule has a laminin-binding (NTA) domain, nine Kazel-type protease inhibitor repeats (shaded), a region homologous to domain III of laminin B chains (III), a serine- and threonine-rich domain (S), and a 38-amino acid hydrophobic region believed to be a signal sequence. The C-terminal portion has four epidermal growth factor (EGF)-like cysteine repeats (E), a serine-threonine-rich domain, and three regions homologous to G-domains of the laminin A chain (L-A or 'G'). Arrowheads indicate two important sites of alternative exon splicing. At the *y* site a 4-amino acid insert can be present, whereas at the *z* site, there can be the 8, the 11, both, or no inserts, resulting in '8', '11', '19', or '0' forms. (The *y* and *z* sites are denoted *A* and *B*, respectively, in chick agrin.) The 8- and 11-amino acid inserts are uniquely expressed in the nervous system.

However, of particular interest to this chapter is the recent observation that agrin is found in the basal lamina of the cerebral microvasculature, where it binds with the extracellular matrix molecule laminin *(70)*. The ubiquitous abundance of agrin within the cerebral microvascular basement membrane suggests an important role in blood–brain barrier formation and function *(71)*. During chick and rat development, agrin accumulates on brain microvessels around the time the vasculature becomes impermeable. Anti-agrin immunoreactivity completely ensheathes all microvessels labeled with anti-von Willebrand factor and codistributes with antilaminin immunoreactivity *(70)*. A similar staining pattern for agrin and laminin is found in microvessels of the testis and thymus, tissues that also contain blood–tissue barriers. In contrast, little or no agrin immunoreactivity is observed on capillaries in muscle and other tissues *(70)*.

More recent studies have demonstrated the existence of several isoforms of the protein with differing specificity and signaling capabilities *(72)*. Differential staining and electroblotting suggest that the agrin isoforms expressed on brain microvessels lack the 8- and 11-amino acid sequences that confer high potency in acetylcholine receptor clustering *(70)*. These results indicate that different agrin isoforms may function as important players in the formation and maintenance of cerebral microvascular impermeability.

Fig. 2. *(opposite page)* **(A)** Aged control brain section labeled with anti-agrin antibody. Agrin immunoreactivity is prominent within the cerebral microvasculature (large arrows) and also is evident in selected neurons (small arrows). Prefrontal cortex, A10 (×200). **(B)** A higher magnification of the control brain section in Fig. 2A. Agrin immunoreactivity is evident within the cytoplasm of the neuronal soma and processes (large arrows). Occasional neurons also demonstrate staining of the nucleus. Note the presence of rare, agrin-immunoreactive puncta (small arrows) in the neuropil, which are often adjacent to blood vessels, A10 (×600). **(C)** Prefrontal cortex (A10) of a patient with Alzheimer's disease (AD) immunostained with anti-agrin antibody. Note the robust staining of neuritic and diffuse plaques (large arrows) and blood vessels. In contrast to aged control cases (e.g., Fig. 2A), blood vessels in AD had attenuated diameters and a more ragged profile (small arrows) (×200). **(D)** A higher magnification of AD brain illustrating two neuritic plaques with surrounding puncta of agrin immunoreactivity (large arrows). Circumferential puncta of immunoreactivity also can be seen in plaques surrounding and adjacent to cerebral capillaries (small arrows), A10 (×600).

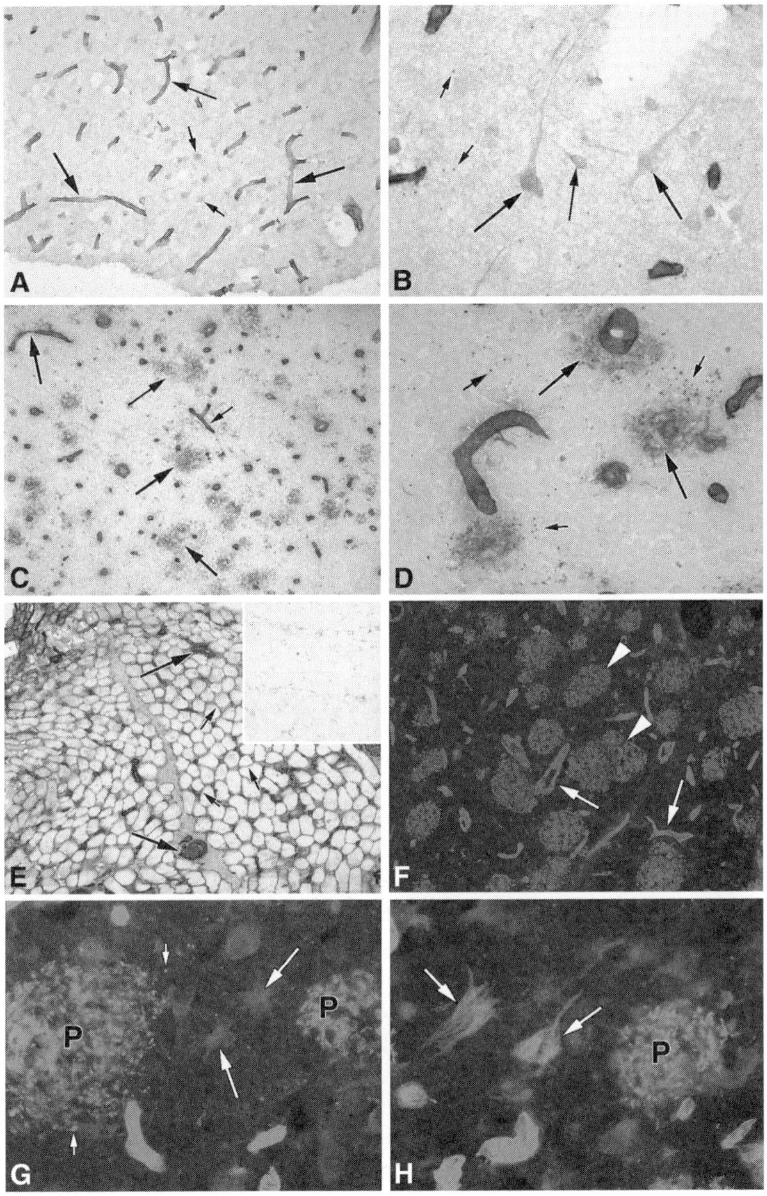

Fig. 2. *(continued)* **(E)** Normal infant skeletal muscle labeled with anti-agrin antibody. Note the uniform agrin immunoreactivity of the basement membranes surrounding individual muscle fibers (small arrows) and capillaries (large arrows). (*Inset*) The same skeletal muscle after the primary antibody was preabsorbed with 10^{-6} M agrin protein. There is essentially complete abolishment of agrin immunoreactivity. Quadriceps muscle, (×200). **(F)** Amygdala of a patient with AD labeled with anti-agrin antibody. Note the robust staining of neuritic and diffuse plaques (arrowheads) and blood vessels. Blood vessels in this AD case have attenuated diameters and ragged profiles (arrows) (×200). **(G)** A higher magnification of the AD amygdala seen in Fig. 2F illustrating two neuritic plaques (P) with surrounding puncta of agrin immunoreactivity (small arrows). Agrin immunoreactivity also may be seen in reactive gemistocytic astrocytes and their stellate processes (large arrows) (×600). **(H)** Another high-magnification photomicrograph of the AD amygdala seen in Fig. 2F showing agrin immunoreactivity within two neurofibrillary tangles (arrows). Note the fine wisps of paired helical filaments conforming to the shape of the neurons they are within. An agrin-stained neuritic plaque (P) is also present (×600).

7. AGRIN IN ALZHEIMER'S DISEASE

In normal human brain, agrin is widely expressed within neurons of multiple brain areas and robustly stains microvascular basement membranes *(71,73)* (Fig. 2A–B). Studies in AD patients reveal that agrin is highly concentrated in both diffuse and neuritic plaques, as well as in neurofibrillary tangles *(71,73)* (Fig. 2C–D,F–H). Unlike controls, patients with AD have microvascular alterations characterized by thinning and fragmentation of the basal lamina *(71,73)* (Fig. 2C,F). Agrin is also distributed in a granular, punctate fashion within each plaque and around microvessels (Fig. 2D,G), suggesting that the agrin in senile plaques originated from fragmentation of the microvascular basal lamina *(71)*. The changes in the distribution of agrin immunoreactivity in AD correspond with an alteration in the solubility properties of agrin; approximately 50% of agrin from AD brains was insoluble in 1% sodium dodecyl sulfate at pH 7.0, whereas all agrin in normal brain was soluble *(73)*. The overall concentration of both soluble and insoluble again is also increased in AD, as compared with non-AD brains *(71)*. Comparative immunohistochemical analyses of the expression of agrin, perlecan, glypican-1, and syndecans 1-3 support a premier role for agrin in AD and suggest that agrin may protect the protein aggregates in senile plaques and neurofibrillary tangles against extracellular proteolytic degradation, leading to the persistence of these deposits *(74)*. Agrin is able to accelerate β amyloid fibril formation and protect β amyloid (1-40) from proteolysis in vitro, suggesting that agrin may be an important factor in the progression of β amyloid peptide aggregation *(61)*.

8. VASCULAR RISK FACTORS, APO E GENOTYPE, AND ALZHEIMER'S DISEASE

Numerous epidemiological and clinical studies in humans and experimental studies in animals and in vitro cell cultures have provided evidence for a relationship among vascular risk factors, apo E genotype, and AD. Recently, concentrations of soluble agrin in AD brains increased with increasing severity of AD, as measured with agrin enzyme-linked immunosorbent assay (ELISA) studies *(71)*. Apo E4/4 homozygotes had smaller capillary basement membrane surface areas of agrin immunoreactivity than Apo E3/3 homozygotes *(75)*. One possible explanation for the increased concentration of soluble agrin, coupled with the reduction in basement membrane surface area in apo E4/4 brains is that the loss of agrin in the basement membrane contributes to the deposition of β amyloid by a yet to be determined mechanism. As β amyloid increases, so does the fraction of insoluble agrin, thereby further limiting the bioavailability of soluble agrin. This may hypothetically lead to a compensatory increase in agrin production by glial cells and/or neurons, ultimately causing an overall increase in both soluble and insoluble agrin. Figure 2G shows reactive astrocytes in AD staining for agrin, supporting the previous idea that glial cells upregulate agrin production in AD. These results provide further support for an association among microvascular changes, the apo E4/4 genotype, and AD. It is extremely important to determine the nature of the multiple potential links between APOE and AD, so that new treatment strategies can be devised and appropriate existing treatment strategies therapeutically employed.

9. CONCLUSION

This chapter provided evidence that microvascular damage is an important component of the pathology in AD and that these microvascular changes are more severe in brains that are homozygous for the apo E4 allele. As mentioned, the mechanisms by which apo E4 confers the risk of severe microvascular damage remain unknown, but their elucidation may be critical toward the development of therapeutic targets for these disorders. The role of agrin in the mammalian brain deserves further elucidation as well. A wealth of literature indicates that agrin is essential for the formation of synapses at the neuromuscular junction. It is unclear if this is also true in the brain, because intact synapses have been observed in the brains of agrin knockout mice *(76)*. However, these mice are nonviable at birth, so it is difficult to know if the synapses present are functionally normal. Loss of agrin within the cerebral capillary basement membrane may lead to a pathologic increase in blood–brain barrier permeability. This will point to the need for developing novel treatment modalities designed to stabilize agrin within the basement membrane and repair damaged endothelial cells.

REFERENCES

1. de la Torre JC. Critically attained threshold of cerebral hypoperfusion: the CATCH hypothesis of Alzheimer's pathogenesis. Neurobiol Aging 2000;21:331–342
2. Mahley RW. Apolipoprotein E: cholesterol transport protein with expanding role in cell biology. Science 1988;240:622–630.
3. Strittmatter WJ, Roses AD. Apolipoprotein E and Alzheimer's disease. Annu Rev Neurosci 1996;19:53–77.
4. Slooter AJ, Tang MX, van Duijn CM, et al. Apolipoprotein E epsilon4 and the risk of dementia with stroke. A population-based investigation. JAMA 1997;277:818–821.
5. Weisgraber KH, Roses AD, Strittmatter WJ. The role of apolipoprotein E in the nervous system. Curr Opin Lipidol 1994;5:110–116.
6. Kobori S, Nakamura N, Uzawa H, Shichiri M. Influence of apolipoprotein E polymorphism on plasma lipid and apolipoprotein levels, and clinical characteristics of type III hyperlipoproteinemia due to apolipoprotein E phenotype E2/2 in Japan. Atherosclerosis 1988;69:81–88.
7. Eto M, Watanabe K, Makino I. Increased frequencies of apolipoprotein epsilon 2 and epsilon 4 alleles in patients with ischemic heart disease. Clin Genet 1989;36:183–188.
8. Kessler C, Spitzer C, Stauske D, et al. The apolipoprotein E and beta-fibrinogen G/A-455 gene polymorphisms are associated with ischemic stroke involving large-vessel disease. Arterioscler Thromb Vasc Biol 1007;17:2880–2884.
9. Friedman G, Froom P, Sazbon L, et al. Apolipoprotein E-epsilon4 genotype predicts a poor outcome in survivors of traumatic brain injury. Neurology 1999;52:244–248.
10. McCarron MO, Hoffmann KL, DeLong DM, et al. Intracerebral hemorrhage outcome: apolipoprotein E genotype, hematoma, and edema volumes. Neurology 1999;53:2176–2179.
11. Tang MX, Stern Y, Marder K, et al. The APOE-epsilon4 allele and the risk of Alzheimer disease among African Americans, whites, and Hispanics. JAMA 1998;279:751-5.
12. Aronson MK, Ooi WL, Morgenstern H, et al. Women, myocardial infarction, and dementia in the very old. Neurology 1990;40:1102–1106.
13. Cacciatore F, Abete P, Ferrara N, et al. The role of blood pressure in cognitive impairment in an elderly population. Osservatorio Geriatrico Campano Group. J Hypertens 1997;15:135–142.
14. Ott A, Stolk RP, van Harskamp F, Pols HA, Hofman A, Breteler MM. Diabetes mellitus and the risk of dementia: The Rotterdam Study. Neurology 1999;53:1937–1942.
15. Graves AB, van Duijn CM, Chandra V, et al. Alcohol and tobacco consumption as risk factors for Alzheimer's disease: a collaborative re-analysis of case-control studies. EURODEM Risk Factors Research Group. Int J Epidemiol 1991;20(Suppl):S48–S57.
16. Sparks DL, Scheff SW, Liu H, Landers TM, Coyne CM, Hunsaker JC, 3rd. Increased incidence of neurofibrillary tangles (NFT) in non-demented individuals with hypertension. J Neurol Sci 1995;131:162–169.
17. Snowdon DA, Greiner LH, Mortimer JA, Riley KP, Greiner PA, Markesbery WR. Brain infarction and the clinical expression of Alzheimer disease. The Nun Study. JAMA 1997;277:813–817.
18. Lammie GA, Brannan F, Slattery J, Warlow C. Nonhypertensive cerebral small-vessel disease. An autopsy study. Stroke 1997;28:2222–2229.
19. Erkinjuntti T, Gao F, Lee DH, Eliasziw M, Merskey H, Hachinski VC. Lack of difference in brain hyperintensities between patients with early Alzheimer's disease and control subjects. Arch Neurol 1994;51:260–268.
20. Forette F, Rigaud AS, Morin M, Gisselbrecht M, Bert P. Assessing vascular dementia. Neth J Med 1995;47:185–194.
21. Fujishima M, Tsuchihashi T. Hypertension and dementia. Clin Exp Hypertens 1999;21:927–935.
22. Hebert R, Brayne C. Epidemiology of vascular dementia. Neuroepidemiology 1995;14:240–257.
23. Lis CG, Gaviria M. Vascular dementia, hypertension, and the brain. Neurol Res 1997;19:471–480.
24. Skoog I. The relationship between blood pressure and dementia: a review. Biomed Pharmacother 1997;51:367–375.
25. Fujii K, Sadoshima S, Okada Y, et al. Cerebral blood flow and metabolism in normotensive and hypertensive patients with transient neurologic deficits. Stroke 1990;21:283–290.
26. Nakane H, Ibayashi S, Fujii K, Irie K, Sadoshima S, Fujishima M. Cerebral blood flow and metabolism in hypertensive patients with cerebral infarction. Angiology 1995;46:801–810.
27. Nobili F, Rodriguez G, Marenco S, et al. Regional cerebral blood flow in chronic hypertension. A correlative study. Stroke 1993;24:1148–1153.
28. Buee L, Hof PR, Delacourte A. Brain microvascular changes in Alzheimer's disease and other dementias. Ann N Y Acad Sci 1997;826:7–24.

29. Perry G, Smith MA, McCann CE, Siedlak SL, Jones PK, Friedland RP. Cerebrovascular muscle atrophy is a feature of Alzheimer's disease. Brain Res 1998;791:63–66.
30. Mancardi GL, Perdelli F, Rivano C, Leonardi A, Bugiani O. Thickening of the basement membrane of cortical capillaries in Alzheimer's disease. Acta Neuropathol (Berl) 1980;49:79–83.
31. Thomas T, Thomas G, McLendon C, Sutton T, Mullan M. beta-Amyloid-mediated vasoactivity and vascular endothelial damage. Nature 1996;380:168–171.
32. Claudio L. Ultrastructural features of the blood-brain barrier in biopsy tissue from Alzheimer's disease patients. Acta Neuropathol (Berl) 1996;91:6–14.
33. Mancardi GL, Tabaton M, Liwnicz BH. Endothelial mitochondrial content of cerebral cortical capillaries in Alzheimer's disease. An ultrastructural quantitative study. Eur Neurol 1985;24:49–52.
34. Perlmutter LS, Myers MA, Barron E. Vascular basement membrane components and the lesions of Alzheimer's disease: light and electron microscopic analyses. Microsc Res Tech 1994;28:204–215.
35. Kalaria RN. Cerebrovascular degeneration is related to amyloid-beta protein deposition in Alzheimer's disease. Ann N Y Acad Sci 1997;826:263–271.
36. Westermark GT, Norling B, Westermark P. Fibronectin and basement membrane components in renal amyloid deposits in patients with primary and secondary amyloidosis. Clin Exp Immunol 1991;86:150–156.
37. Perry G, Siedlak SL, Richey P, et al. Association of heparan sulfate proteoglycan with the neurofibrillary tangles of Alzheimer's disease. J Neurosci 1991;11:3679–3683.
38. Snow AD, Mar H, Nochlin D, et al. The presence of heparan sulfate proteoglycans in the neuritic plaques and congophilic angiopathy in Alzheimer's disease. Am J Pathol 1988;133:456–463.
39. Roll FJ, Madri JA, Albert J, Furthmayr H. Codistribution of collagen types IV and AB2 in basement membranes and mesangium of the kidney. An immunoferritin study of ultrathin frozen sections. J Cell Biol 1980;85:597–616.
40. Murtomaki S, Risteli J, Risteli L, Koivisto UM, Johansson S, Liesi P. Laminin and its neurite outgrowth-promoting domain in the brain in Alzheimer's disease and Down's syndrome patients. J Neurosci Res 1992;32:261–273.
41. McGeer PL, Zhu SG, Dedhar S. Immunostaining of human brain capillaries by antibodies to very late antigens. J Neuroimmunol 1990;26:213–218.
42. Frohman EM, Frohman TC, Gupta S, de Fougerolles A, van den Noort S. Expression of intercellular adhesion molecule 1 (ICAM-1) in Alzheimer's disease. J Neurol Sci 1991;106:105–111.
43. Cashman RE, Grammas P. cAMP-dependent protein kinase in cerebral microvessels in aging and Alzheimer disease. Mol Chem Neuropathol 1995;26:247–258.
44. Grammas P, Roher AE, Ball MJ. Increased accumulation of cAMP in cerebral microvessels in Alzheimer's disease. Neurobiol Aging 1994;15:113–116.
45. Grammas P, Moore P, Botchlet T, et al. Cerebral microvessels in Alzheimer's have reduced protein kinase C activity. Neurobiol Aging 1995;16:563–569.
46. Kalaria RN, Harik SI. Reduced glucose transporter at the blood-brain barrier and in cerebral cortex in Alzheimer disease. J Neurochem 1989;53:1083–1088.
47. Dorheim MA, Tracey WR, Pollock JS, Grammas P. Nitric oxide synthase activity is elevated in brain microvessels in Alzheimer's disease. Biochem Biophys Res Commun 1994;205:659–665.
48. Grammas P. A damaged microcirculation contributes to neuronal cell death in Alzheimer's disease. Neurobiol Aging 2002;21:199–205.
49. Grammas P, Moore P, Weigel PH. Microvessels from Alzheimer's disease brains kill neurons in vitro. Am J Pathol 1999;154:337–342.
50. de la Torre JC, Stefano G.B. Evidence that Alzheimer's disease is a microvascular disorder: the role of constitutive nitric oxide. Brain Res Brain Res Rev 2002;34:119–136.
51. Snow AD, Sekiguchi R, Nochlin D, et al. An important role of heparan sulfate proteoglycan (Perlecan) in a model system for the deposition and persistence of fibrillar A beta-amyloid in rat brain. Neuron 1994;12:219–234.
52. Small DH, Nurcombe V, Reed G, et al. A heparin-binding domain in the amyloid protein precursor of Alzheimer's disease is involved in the regulation of neurite outgrowth. J Neurosci 1994;14:2117–2127.
53. Small DH, Williamson T, Reed G, et al. The role of heparan sulfate proteoglycans in the pathogenesis of Alzheimer's disease. Ann N Y Acad Sci 1996;777:316–321.
54. Rupp F, Ozcelik T, Linial M, Peterson K, Francke U, Scheller R. Structure and chromosomal localization of the mammalian agrin gene. J Neurosci 1992;12:3535–3544.
55. Tsim KW, Ruegg MA, Escher G, Kroger S, McMahan UJ. cDNA that encodes active agrin. Neuron 1992;8:677–689.
56. Denzer AJ, Brandenberger R, Gesemann M, Chiquet M, Ruegg MA. Agrin binds to the nerve-muscle basal lamina via laminin. J Cell Biol 1997;137:671–683.
57. Patthy L, Nikolics K. Functions of agrin and agrin-related proteins. Trends Neurosci 1993;16:76–81.
58. Biroc SL, Payan DG, Fisher JM. Isoforms of agrin are widely expressed in the developing rat and may function as protease inhibitors. Brain Res Dev Brain Res 1993;75:119–129.

59. Denzer AJ, Gesemann M, Schumacher B, Ruegg MA. An amino-terminal extension is required for the secretion of chick agrin and its binding to extracellular matrix. J Cell Biol 1995;131:1547–1560.
60. Tsen G, Halfter W, Kroger S, Cole GJ. Agrin is a heparan sulfate proteoglycan. J Biol Chem 1995;270:3392–3329.
61. Cotman SL, Halfter W, Cole GJ. Agrin binds to beta-amyloid (Abeta), accelerates abeta fibril formation, and is localized to Abeta deposits in Alzheimer's disease brain. Mol Cell Neurosci 2002;15:183–198.
62. Nitkin RM, Smith MA, Magill C, et al. Identification of agrin, a synaptic organizing protein from Torpedo electric organ. J Cell Biol 1987;105:2471–2478.
63. Reist NE, Magill C, McMahan UJ. Agrin-like molecules at synaptic sites in normal, denervated, and damaged skeletal muscles. J Cell Biol 1987;105:2457–2469.
64. Wallace BG. Agrin-induced specializations contain cytoplasmic, membrane, and extracellular matrix-associated components of the postsynaptic apparatus. J Neurosci 1989;9:1294–1302.
65. Campanelli JT, Roberds SL, Campbell KP, Scheller RH. A role for dystrophin-associated glycoproteins and utrophin in agrin-induced AChR clustering. Cell 1994;77:663–674.
66. Fallon JR, Hall ZW. Building synapses: agrin and dystroglycan stick together. Trends Neurosci 1994;17:469–473.
67. Deyst KA, Bowe MA, Leszyk JD, Fallon JR. The alpha-dystroglycan-beta-dystroglycan complex. Membrane organization and relationship to an agrin receptor. J Biol Chem 1995;270:25,956–25,959.
68. Kroger S, Horton SE, Honig LS. The developing avian retina expresses agrin isoforms during synaptogenesis. J Neurobiol 1996;29:165–182.
69. Ru-Rong J, Böse CM, Lesuisse C, et al. Specific agrin isoforms induce cAMP response element binding protein phosphorylation in hippocampal neurons. J Neurosci 1998;18: 9695–9702.
70. Barber AJ, Lieth E. Agrin accumulates in the brain microvascular basal lamina during development of the blood-brain barrier. Dev Dyn 1997;208:62–74.
71. Berzin TM, Zipser BD, Rafii MS, et al. Agrin and microvascular damage in Alzheimer's disease. Neurobiol Aging 2002;21:349–355.
72. Bowen DC, Sugiyama J, Ferns M, Hall ZW. Neural agrin activates a high-affinity receptor in C2 muscle cells that is unresponsive to muscle agrin. J Neurosci 1996;16:3791–3797.
73. Donahue JE, Berzin TM, Rafii MS, et al. Agrin in Alzheimer's disease: altered solubility and abnormal distribution within microvasculature and brain parenchyma. Proc Natl Acad Sci USA 1999;96:6468–6472.
74. Verbeek MM, Otte-Holler I, van den Born J, et al. Agrin is a major heparan sulfate proteoglycan accumulating in Alzheimer's disease brain. Am J Pathol 1999;155:2115–2125. 1999.
75. Salloway S, Gur T, Berzin T, et al. Effect of APOE genotype on microvascular basement membrane in Alzheimer's disease. J Neurol Sci 2002;203-204:183–187.
76. Serpinskaya AS, Feng G, Sanes JR, Craig AM. Synapse formation by hippocampal neurons from agrin-deficient mice. Dev Biol 1999;205:65–78.

19

Amyloid Beta and the Cerebral Vasculature

Paula Grammas

1. INTRODUCTION

The vascular pattern of amyloid beta (Aβ) deposition in the brain is commonly referred to as cerebral amyloid angiopathy (CAA) *(1)*. CAA is an important cause of cerebral hemorrhages and may lead to ischemic infarction and dementia *(2)*. A pure form of CAA, without parenchymal lesions, has been documented in hereditary cerebral hemorrhage, Dutch type, sporadic idiopathic CAA and in cerebrovascular malformations *(3–5)*. Cerebrovascular amyloid deposition is associated with aging, and CAA is an important feature of several disorders associated with mutations in the amyloid precursor protein (APP) gene, as well as in Down's syndrome and Alzheimer's disease (AD) *(6–8)*. Indeed, CAA is a key pathologic finding in 80–90% of AD cases *(9,10)*. A recent study of 201 autopsy cases of elderly Japanese shows that the incidence and severity of CAA are significantly higher in AD cases compared to non-AD cases *(11)*. Also, some genetic risk factors associated with the AD are involved in the pathogenesis of CAA, including apolipoprotein E (apoE) genotype, presenilin 1, and α_1-antichymotrypsin *(12–14)*.

The genetic factors that regulate Aβ deposition in the vasculature have not been defined. A study examining the relationship between apo E genotype and the relative extent of Aβ accumulation in the brain demonstrates that expression of apo Eε4 leads to a higher level of Aβ in the vasculature compared to Aβ levels in the brain parenchyma *(15)*. In addition, the severity of CAA among apo Eε4 carriers is significantly higher than among non-ε4 carriers *(11)*. The Dutch, Flemish, Italian, and Arctic mutations in the APP gene that render Aβ resistant to proteolysis by neprilysin, a peptidase important for the catabolism of Aβ in the brain, are associated with CAA *(16)*. Also, Yamada and colleagues *(17)* demonstrate an association between a polymorphism of the gene encoding for neprilysin and an increased risk of CAA. It is likely that multiple mechanisms contribute to the deposition of Aβ in brain blood vessel walls, including endogenous vascular synthesis, blood-to-brain transport, and impaired clearance of brain Aβ.

2. MECHANISMS OF VASCULAR Aβ DEPOSITION

The events and/or processes that regulate Aβ availability in the cerebral vasculature, systemic circulation, and the brain could contribute to the deposition of vascular Aβ observed in CAA and AD.

2.1. *Endogenous Vascular Synthesis of Aβ*

APP mRNA is expressed throughout cerebral vessel walls. The demonstration of APP-mRNA at all vascular sites where amyloid formation occurs supports an important contribution for locally derived Aβ to cerebrovascular amyloidosis *(18)*. The notion that Aβ deposition in AD results from

From: *Current Clinical Neurology*
Vascular Dementia: Cerebrovascular Mechanisms and Clinical Management
Edited by: R. H. Paul, R. Cohen, B. R. Ott, and S. Salloway © Humana Press Inc., Totowa, NJ

vascular production of Aβ is supported by data showing that proteins elevated in the AD brain, specifically in AD blood vessels, increase secretion and/or expression of APP in endothelial cells. For example, thrombin, a multifunctional coagulant and inflammatory mediator, has been detected in both brain vessel walls and senile plaques in AD *(19,20)*. This protease, via activation of cell surface thrombin receptors, induces APP secretion from endothelial cells *(21)*. The inflammatory cytokine interleukin (IL)-1 also upregulates APP gene expression in endothelial cells *(22)*. A causal role for IL-1 in vascular Aβ deposition in AD is supported by the author's data showing that isolated brain microvessels from patients with AD express high levels of several inflammatory cytokines, including IL-1 *(23)*. The presence in the vessel wall of both APP mRNA and high levels of proteins that regulate APP expression in endothelial cells implicate the vasculature as a source of vascular Aβ in AD.

2.2. Transport of Aβ Across the Blood–Brain Barrier

Increased transport of circulating Aβ across the blood–brain barrier (BBB) is also a potential mechanism for exacerbating cerebral amyloidosis *(24–26)*. The idea that vascular Aβ derives from blood borne Aβ is supported by studies demonstrating specific mechanisms for brain capillary sequestration and BBB transport of ^{125}I-Aβ1–40 synthetic peptide and its complexes with apolipoprotein J and apoE4 *(24,27,28)*. It has been suggested that the receptor for advanced glycation end products (RAGE) on the brain vascular endothelium facilitates influx of Aβ into the brain from the systemic circulation *(25,29)*. The possibility that this RAGE-mediated transport contributes to elevated levels of Aβ in the brain and vasculature in AD is supported by data showing elevated expression of RAGE in cells of Aβ containing vessels *(30)*.

Another potential factor that can influence blood to brain transport of Aβ and is pathogenically relevant in AD is aging. Indeed, aging is the most important risk for the development of AD. In a study using an intravenous injection of labeled Aβ, Zlokovic and colleagues *(31)* show that compared to adult animals, aged squirrel monkeys show increased transendothelial transport of blood-borne Aβ1–40, as well as increased microvascular Aβ accumulation. Similarly, in a more recent study, this group demonstrates enhanced cerebrovascular sequestration of blood-borne Aβ in aged nonhuman primates *(32)*. Brain microvascular sequestration of Aβ is also found in rodents *(33,34)*.

2.3. Impaired Clearance of Brain Aβ

It has been suggested that cerebral amyloidosis in sporadic AD is a "storage" disease caused by inefficient clearance of the peptide that is produced at normal levels *(26)*. Both physical and biochemical abnormalities in brain blood vessels could contribute to vascular Aβ accumulation. For example, Aβ is eliminated from the extracellular spaces of the human brain by a perivascular route, draining along the walls of cortical arteries to leptomeningeal arteries *(35)*. A study using serial sections shows that cortical arteries feeding capillary beds with Aβ angiopathy are occluded by thrombi, suggesting that Aβ normally eliminated from the brain along vascular pathways may become blocked in the AD or aged brain, resulting in CAA *(36)*.

Biochemical mechanisms that govern elimination of Aβ peptide from the brain are poorly understood. Intracerebral microinjections of radioiodinated Aβ1–40 in young mice results in rapid clearance of the peptide, mainly by vascular transport across the BBB *(37)*. This clearance is inhibited by antibodies against low-density lipoprotein receptor-related protein-1 (LRP-1) and α_2-macroglobulin *(26)*. LRP-1 is abundant in the brain microvessels of young mice and is downregulated in vessels from older animals. Also, clearance is significantly reduced in apoE knockout mice *(37)*. The demonstration of a correlation between regional Aβ accumulation in brains of AD and downregulation of vascular LRP-1 supports its importance in AD *(37)*. Also, using single photon emission computed tomography (SPECT) to assess elimination of Aβ peptide from the brains of squirrel monkeys, an age-dependent increase in Aβ deposition has been documented, suggesting that with age, impaired Aβ clearance across the BBB may contribute to the development of CAA *(38)*.

The presence of Aβ in brain blood vessels has important consequences for the pathophysiology of endothelial cells and smooth muscle cells (SMC) and thus for vascular function.

3. FUNCTIONAL EFFECTS OF Aβ ON ENDOTHELIAL AND SMOOTH MUSCLE CELLS

There is extensive literature documenting changes in the biochemical properties and functional behavior of endothelial and SMC in brain blood vessels in AD. It is also well appreciated that the overwhelming majority of AD cases demonstrate significant amyloid angiopathy. The specific parameters of endothelial cell and SMC function that are altered or impaired by Aβ are discussed below.

3.1. Aβ and Vascular Endothelial Cell Functions and Properties

Aβ exerts a range of effects on endothelial cells, including changes in signal transduction pathways, enzyme activity, cellular behaviors, and apoptosis.

Abnormalities in signal transduction cascades have been documented in the cerebral microcirculation in AD *(39–42)*. The author's laboratory has shown a profound decrease in protein kinase C (PKC) activity in microvessels isolated from AD brains compared to brain vessels from age-matched non-AD controls *(41)*. Accumulation of Aβ peptide in the cerebral vasculature may play a significant role in the downregulation of PKC seen in the AD cerebral vasculature because exposure of cultured brain endothelial cells to Aβ1–40 causes changes in enzyme translocation and a decrease in the membrane-bound activity of PKCα, one of the primary PKC isoforms in endothelial cells *(43)*. Also, the serine-threonine signal kinase Akt, which is important for endothelial cell survival as well as endothelial nitric oxide synthase (eNOS) activation, is altered by exposure to Aβ1–42 *(44)*.

Because NO produced in large amounts is neurotoxic, disruption of the NOS system in the cerebral vasculature could contribute to neuronal cell death in AD. The author has shown that brain microvessels isolated from AD microvessels have high levels of inducible NOS (iNOS) and release large amounts of NO *(45)*. Aβ inhibits NOS activity by subtracting nicotinamide adenine dinucleotide phosphate (NADPH) availability *(46)*. The amyloid peptides Aβ1–42 and Aβ25–35 strongly inhibit the activity of constitutive eNOS in cell free systems *(46)*. This could link Aβ to the overexpression of iNOS in AD because of the molecular cross-talk between NOS isoforms, where repression of constitutive NOS results in enhanced expression of iNOS.

Aβ can also affect endothelial cell behaviors. Plaque-derived amyloid inhibits rat brain endothelial cell proliferation in vitro by 40% *(47)*. Amyloid fractions from AD brains, although not directly cytotoxic to brain endothelial cells, inhibit endothelial replication and, therefore, could alter the ability of vessels to repair and regenerate after injury. Aβ can also affect monocyte-endothelial cell interactions and induce migration of monocytes across the endothelium. Exposure of human brain microvascular endothelial cells to Aβ results in increased adherence and transmigration of monocytes *(48,49)*.

Several studies show that Aβ induces apoptosis in endothelial cells *(50–54)*. Exposure of human endothelial cells to Aβ evokes an apoptotic response characterized by morphological changes and fragmentation of DNA *(51)*. Aβ has also been found in cerebral endothelial cells to induce translocation of the apoptosis regulator termed second-mitochondria-derived activator of caspase (Smac) from the intramembranous compartment of the mitochondria to the cytosol, via AP-1/Bim activation. Aβ25–35, a cytotoxic fragment of Aβ, induces mitochondrial dysfunction, caspase activation and cerebral endothelial cell death *(54)*.

3.2. Effects of Aβ on Smooth Muscle Cell Function

Aβ affects both the physical and the biochemical properties of SMC. Structural and functional disruption of vascular SMC has been documented in a transgenic mouse model of amyloid angiopathy. In these mice, before the onset of SMC death, the arrangement of SMC becomes disorganized in pial vessels heavily invested with Aβ *(55)*. Furthermore, these structurally abnormal vessels are also functionally compromised and are unable to respond appropriately to the application of endothelial-dependent and endothelial-independent vasodilators *(55)*. Thus, Aβ can alter SMC structure and affect vessel wall integrity, stability, and reactivity.

In SMC, some of the structural pathology induced by Aβ may result from activation of proteolytic mechanisms. Therefore, pathogenic forms of Aβ stimulate the expression of urokinase-type plasminogen activator in human cerebral SMC *(56)*. Also, Aβ induces the expression and activation of matrix metalloproteinase (MMP)-2 in human cerebral SMC *(57)*. This increase in MMP-2 activation is largely caused by increased expression of membrane-type-1 (MT1)-MMP. The importance of this mechanism for mediating SMC injury is suggested by data showing that treatment with MMP inhibitors increases SMC viability in the presence of pathogenic Aβ *(57)*.

4. Aβ AND CEREBROVASCULAR INFLAMMATION

Numerous inflammatory mediators have been documented in pathologically vulnerable areas of the AD brain *(58)*. Also, anti-inflammatory drugs reduce the risk of AD pathology and enhance cognitive performance in both human and animal studies *(59–64)*. Emerging data suggest that the brain microvasculature may be an important source of inflammatory mediators in AD *(23,45,65–67)*. Results from the author's laboratory demonstrate that vessels from AD brains release significantly higher levels of IL-1β, IL-6, tumor necrosis factor-α (TNF-α), and transforming growth factor-β (TGF-β) compared to microvessels from non-AD brains *(23,67)*. Previous work from the author's laboratory demonstrates that in the AD brain, blood vessels express the inflammatory mediator cationic antimicrobial protein 37 kDa (CAP37) *(66)*. Also, the author has shown a significant overexpression of iNOS in microvessels isolated from AD brains *(45)*. This NOS isoform is not usually present in endothelial cells, but can be induced in endothelial cells by inflammatory stimuli. In addition, the intercellular adhesion molecule-1 (ICAM-1), a surface glycoprotein expressed by endothelial cells during inflammation, has been shown on brain endothelial cells in AD *(65)*.

In most AD cases, the cerebrovasculature is heavily invested with Aβ, suggesting that Aβ may play a causal role in the development of vascular inflammation. In human endothelial cells, Aβ induces an inflammatory cascade that includes secretion of interferon-γ, IL-1β, and CD40 expression *(68)*. Treatment of cerebral endothelial cell cultures with Aβ results in the induction of CAP37 expression *(66)*. Mullan and colleagues have explored the proinflammatory and vasoactive effects of Aβ in the cerebrovasculature and document that freshly solubilized Aβ potentiates endothelin-1 induced vasoconstriction in isolated cerebral arteries *(69)*. The Aβ induced response is antagonized by the anti-inflammatory effects of statins, as well as by drugs that inhibit cyclooxygenase *(69,70)*.

A similar proinflammatory response to Aβ resulting in increased production of PGE_2, and $PGF_{2\alpha}$ has been shown in isolated human brain microvessels *(69)*. However, a causal role for Aβ in mediating vascular or parenchymal inflammation has not been definitively determined. Indeed, in a recent study showing a discordant effect of anti-inflammatory drugs on Aβ and cyclooxygenase concludes that inflammation and cerebral amyloidosis are not connected *(71)*. Further work is required to address this important issue.

5. CONCLUSIONS

Increasing evidence supports the idea that the cerebral microcirculation is pathologically altered in AD and that a dysfunctional microcirculation contributes to the pathogenesis of neuronal cell death in AD. The evolution of vascular dysfunction and the factors that affect this process have yet to be defined. Because of the high incidence of CAA in AD and the numerous effects of Aβ on vascular cell function, Aβ is strongly implicated as an important mediator of vascular pathology in AD.

ACKNOWLEDGMENTS

The author thanks Theresa Rush and Melanie Beery for their administrative assistance. This work was supported in part by NIH AG 15964 and NIH AG 020569 (Grammas) and a grant from the Alzheimer's Association (Grammas). Dr. Grammas is the recipient of the Presbyterian Health Foundation Chair in Neuroscience.

REFERENCES

1. Matsubara E, Shoji M, Abe K, Frangione B, Ghiso J. Vascular amyloidosis in neurodegenerative conditions. Drug News Perspect 2002;15:439–444.
2. Ghiso J, Frangione B. Cerebral amyloidosis, amyloid angiopathy, and their relationship to stroke and dementia. J Alzheimer Dis 2001;3:65–73.
3. Levy E, Carman MD, Fernandez-Madrid IJ, et al. Mutation of the Alzheimer's disease amyloid gene in hereditary cerebral hemorrhage, Dutch type. Science 1990;248:1124–1126.
4. Vinters HV. Cerebral amyloid angiopathy. A critical review. Stroke 1987;18:311–324.
5. Ghiso J, Wisniewski T, Frangione B. Unifying features of systemic and cerebral amyloidosis. Mol Neurobiol 1994;8: 49–64.
6. Donahue JE, Khurana JS, Adelman LS. Intracerebral hemorrhage in two patients with Down's syndrome and cerebral amyloid angiopathy. Acta Neuropathol 1998;95:213–216.
7. Jellinger KA. Alzheimer disease and cerebrovascular pathology: an update. J Neural Transm 2002;109:813–836.
8. Revesz T, Holton JL, Lashley T, et al. Sporadic and familial cerebral amyloid angiopathies. Brain Pathol 2002;12: 343–357.
9. Mandybur TI. The incidence of cerebral amyloid angiopathy in Alzheimer's disease. Neurology 1975;25:120–126.
10. Ellis RJ, Olichney JM, Thal LJ, et al. Cerebral amyloid angiopathy in the brains of patients with Alzheimer's disease: The CERAD experience, part XV. Neurology 1996;46:1592–1596.
11. Yamada M. Risk factors for cerebral amyloid angiopathy in the elderly. Ann N Y Acad Sci 2002;977:37–44.
12. Premkumar DRD, Cohen DL, Hedera P, Friedland RP, Kalaria RN. Apolipoprotein E ε4 in cerebral amyloid angiopathy and cerebrovascular pathology associated with Alzheimer's disease. Am J Pathol 1996;148:2083–2095.
13. Yamada M, Sodeyama N, Itoh Y, et al. Association of presenilin-1 polymorphism with cerebral amyloid angiopathy in elderly. Stroke 1997;28:2219–2221.
14. Yamada M, Sodeyama N, Itoh Y, et al. Association of alpha1-antichymotrypsin polymorphism with cerebral amyloid angiopathy. Ann Neurol 1998;44:129–131.
15. Chalmers K, Wilcock GK, Love S. APOE var epsilon 4 influences the pathological phenotype of Alzheimer's disease by favouring cerebrovascular over parenchymal accumulation of Abeta protein. Neuropathol Appl Neurobiol 2003;29: 231–238.
16. Tsubuki S, Takaki Y, Saido TC. Dutch, Flemish, Italian, and Arctic mutations of APP and resistance of A β to physiologically relevant proteolytic degradation. Lancet 2003;361:1957–1958.
17. Yamada M, Sodeyama N, Itoh Y, et al. Association of neprilysin polymorphism with cerebral amyloid angiopathy. J Neurol Neurosurg Psychiatry 2003;74:749–751.
18. Natte R, de Boer WI, Maat-Schieman ML, et al. Amyloid beta precursor protein-mRNA is expressed throughout cerebral vessel walls. Brain Res 1999;828:179–183.
19. Akiyama H, Ikeda K, Kondo H, McGeer PL. Thrombin accumulation in brains of patients with Alzheimer's disease. Neurosci Lett 1992;146:152–154.
20. McGeer PL, Klegeris A, Walker DG, Yasuhara O, McGeer EG. Pathological proteins in senile plaques. Tohoku J Exp Med 1994;174:269–277.
21. Ciallella JR, Figueiredo H, Smith-Swintosky V, McGillis JP. Thrombin induces surface and intracellular secretion of amyloid precursor protein from human endothelial cells. Thromb Haemost 1999;81:630–637.
22. Forloni G, Demicheli F, Giorgi S, Bendotti C, Angeretti N. Expression of amyloid precursor protein mRNAs in endothelial, neuronal and glial cells: modulation by interleukin-1. Brain Res Mol Brain Res 1992;16:128–134.
23. Grammas P, Ovase R. Inflammatory factors are elevated in brain microvessels in Alzheimer's disease. Neurobiol Aging 2001;22:837–842.
24. Zlokovic BV, Martel CL, Matsubara E, et al. Glycoprotein 330/megalin: probable role in receptor-mediated transport of apolipoprotein J alone and in a complex with Alzheimer disease amyloid beta at the blood-brain and blood-cerebrospinal fluid barriers. Proc Natl Acad Sci 1996;93:4229–4234.
25. Mackic JB, Stins M, McComb JG, et al. Human blood-brain barrier receptors for Alzheimer's amyloid-β. J Clin Invest 1998;102:734–743.
26. Grammas P, Yamada M, Zlokovic B. The cerebromicrovascular: a key player in the pathogenesis of Alzheimer's disease. J Alzheimer Dis 2002;4:217–223.

27. Zlokovic BV, Ghiso J, Mackic JB, McComb JG, Weiss MH, Frangione B. Blood-brain barrier transport of circulating Alzheimer's amyloid beta. Biochem Biophys Res Commun 1993;197:1034–1040.
28. Martel CL, Mackic JB, Matsubara E, et al. Isoform-specific effects of apolipoproteins E2, E3, and E4 on cerebral capillary sequestration and blood-brain barrier transport of circulating Alzheimer's amyloid beta. J Neurochem 1997;69: 1995–2004.
29. Deane R, Du Yan S, Submamaryan RK, et al. RAGE mediates amyloid-beta peptide transport across the blood-brain barrier and accumulation in brain. Nat Med 2003;9:907–913.
30. Yan SD, Stern D, Kane MD, Kuo YM, Lampert HC, Roher AE. RAGE-Ab interactions in the pathophysiology of Alzheimer's disease. Restor Neurol Neurosci 1998;12:167–173.
31. Mackic JB, Weiss MH, Miao W, et al. Cerebrovascular accumulation and increased blood-brain barrier permeability to circulating Alzheimer's amyloid beta peptide in aged squirrel monkey with cerebral amyloid angiopathy. J Neurochem 1998;70:210–215.
32. Mackic JB, Bading J, Ghiso J, et al. Circulating amyloid-beta peptide crosses the blood-brain barrier in aged monkeys and contributes to Alzheimer's disease lesions. Vascul Pharmacol 2002;38:303–313.
33. Maness LM, Banks WA, Podlisny MB, Selkoe DJ, Kastin AJ. Passage of human amyloid beta-protein 1-40 across the murine blood-brain barrier. Life Sci 1994;55:1643–1650.
34. Poduslo JF, Curran GL, Haggard JJ, Biere AL, Selkoe DJ. Permeability and residual plasma volume of human, Dutch variant, and rat amyloid beta-protein 1-40 at the blood-brain barrier. Neurobiol Res 1997;4:27–34.
35. Preston SD, Steart PV, Wilkinson A, Nicoll JA, Weller RO. Capillary and arterial cerebral amyloid angiopathy in Alzheimer's disease: defining the perivascular route for the elimination of amyloid beta from the human brain. Neuropathol Appl Neurobiol 2003;29:106–117.
36. Weller RO, Yow HY, Preston SD, Mazanti I, Nicoll JA. Cerebrovascular disease is a major factor in the failure of elimination of Abeta from the aging human brain: implications for therapy of Alzheimer's disease. Ann NY Acad Sci 2002;977:162–168.
37. Shibata M, Yamada S, Kumar SR, et al. Clearance of Alzheimer's amyloid-ss(1-40) peptide from brain by LDL receptor-related protein-1 at the blood-brain barrier. J Clin Invest 2000;106:1489–1499.
38. Bading JR, Yamada S, Mackic JB, et al. Brain clearance of Alzheimer's amyloid-beta40 in the squirrel monkey: a SPECT study in a primate model of cerebral amyloid angiopathy. J Drug Target 2002;10:359–368.
39. Grammas P, Roher A, Ball MJ. Increased accumulation of cAMP in cerebral microvessels in Alzheimer's disease. Neurobiol Aging 1994;15:113–116.
40. Cashman RE, Grammas P. cAMP-dependent protein kinase in cerebral microvessels in aging and Alzheimer's disease. Mol Chem Neuropathol 1995;26:247–258.
41. Grammas P, Moore P, Botchlet T, et al. Cerebral microvessels in Alzheimer's have reduced protein kinase C activity. Neurobiol Aging 1995;16:563–569.
42. Moore P, White J, Christiansen V, Grammas P. Protein kinase C-ζ activity but not level is decreased in Alzheimer's disease microvessels. Neurosci Lett 1998;254:29–32.
43. Pakaski M, Balaspiri L, Checler F, Kasa P. Human amyloid-beta causes changes in the level of endothelial protein kinase C and to alpha isoform in vitro. Neurochem Int 2003;41:409–414.
44. Suhara T, Magrane J, Rosen K, et al. Abeta42 generation is toxic to endothelial cells and inhibits eNOS function through an Akt/GSK-3beta signaling-dependent mechanism. Neurobiol Aging 2003;24:437–451.
45. Dorheim MA, Tracey WR, Pollock JS, Grammas P. Nitric oxide is elevated in Alzheimer's brain microvessels. Biochem Biophy Res Commun 1994;205:659–665.
46. Venturini G, Colasanti Persichini T, Fioravanti E, Ascenzi P, Palomba L, Cantoni O. Musci G. Beta amyloid inhibits NOS activity by subtracting NADPH availability. FASEB J 2002;16:1970–1972.
47. Grammas P, Botchlet T, Fugate R, Ball MJ, Roher AE. Alzheimer disease amyloid proteins inhibit brain endothelial cell proliferation in vitro. Dementia 1995;6:126–130.
48. Giri R, Shen Y, Stins M, et al. Beta-amyloid-induced migration of monocytes across human brain endothelial cells involves RAGE and PECAM-1. Am J Physiol 2000;279:1772–1781.
49. Giri R, Selvaraj S, Miller CA, et al. Effect of endothelial cell polarity on beta-amyloid-reduced migration of monocytes across normal and AD endothelium. Am J Physiol 2002;283:C895–C904.
50. Blanc EM, Toborek M, Mark RJ, Hennig B, Mattson MP. Amyloid beta-peptide induces cell monolayer albumin permeability, impairs glucose transport, and induces apoptosis in vascular endothelial cells. J Neurochem 1997;68:1870–1881.
51. Hase M, Araki S, Hayashi H. Fragments of amyloid beta induce apoptosis in vascular endothelial cells. Endothelium 1997;5:221–229.
52. Xu J, Chen S, Ka G, et al. Amyloid beta peptide-induced cerebral endothelial cell death involves mitochondrial dysfunction and caspase activation. J Cereb Blood Flow Metab 2001;21:702–710.
53. Munoz FJ, Opazo C, Gil-Gomez G, et al. Vitamin E but not 17beta-estradiol protects against vascular toxicity induced by beta-amyloid wild type and the Dutch amyloid variant. J Neurosci 2002;22:3081–3089.
54. Yin KJ, Lee JM, Chen SD, Xu J, Hsu CY. Amyloid-beta induces Smac release via AP—1/Bim activation in cerebral endothelial cells. J Neurosci 2002;22:9764–9770.

55. Christie R, Yamada M, Moskowitz M, Hyman B. Structural and functional disruption of vascular smooth muscle cells in a transgenic mouse model of amyloid angiopathy. Am J Pathol 2001;158:1065–1071.
56. Davis J, Wagner MR, Zhang W, Xu F, Van Nostrand WE. Amyloid beta-protein stimulates the expression of urokinase-type plasminogen activator (uPA) and its receptor (uPAR) in human cerebrovascular smooth muscle cells. J Biol Chem 2003;278:19,054–19,061.
57. Jung SS, Zhang W, Van Nostrand WE. Pathogenic Abeta induces the expression and activation of matrix metalloproteinase-2 in human cerebrovascular smooth muscle cells. J Neurochem 2003;85:1208–1215.
58. Neuroinflammation Working Group. Inflammation and Alzheimer's disease. Neurobiol Aging 2000;21:383–421.
59. McGeer PL, Schulzer M, McGeer EG. Arthritis and anti-inflammatory agents as possible protective factors for Alzheimer's disease: a review of 17 epidemiologic studies. Neurology 1996;47:425–432.
60. Hull M, Fiebich BL, Schumann G, Lieb K, Bauer J. Anti-inflammatory substances—a new therapeutic option in Alzheimer's disease. Drug Discovery Today 1999;4:275–282.
61. Halliday GM, Shepard CE, McCann H, et al. Effect of anti-inflammatory medications on neuropathological findings in Alzheimer's disease. Arch Neurol 2000;57:831–836.
62. Lim GP, Yang F, Chu T, et al. Ibuprofen suppresses plaque pathology and inflammation in a mouse model for Alzheimer's disease. J Neurosci 2000;20:5709–5714.
63. Gupta A, Pansari K. Inflammation and Alzheimer's disease. Int J Clin Pract 2003;57:36–39.
64. Launer L. Nonsteroidal anti-inflammatory drug use and the risk for Alzheimer's disease: dissecting the epidemiological evidence. Drugs 2003;63:731–739.
65. Frohman EM, Frohman TC, Gupta S, de Fourgerolles A, Van Den Noort S. Expression of intercellular adhesion molecule (ICAM-1) in Alzheimer's disease. J Neurol Sci 1991;106:105–111.
66. Pereira HA, Kumar P, Grammas P. Expression of CAP37, a novel inflammatory mediator in Alzheimer's disease. Neurobiol Aging 1996;17:753–759.
67. Grammas P, Ovase R. Cerebrovascular transforming growth factor-β contributes to inflammation in the Alzheimer's disease brain. Am J Pathol 2002;160:1583–1587.
68. Suo Z, Tan J, Placzek A, Crawford F, Fang C, Mullan M. Alzheimer: β-amyloid peptides induce inflammatory cascade in human vascular cells: the roles of cytokines, and CD40. Brain Res 1998;807:110–117.
69. Townsend KP, Obregon D, Quadros A, et al. Proinflammatory and vasoactive effects of Abeta in the cerebrovasculature. Ann NY Acad Sci 2002;977:65–76.
70. Paris D, Townsend KP, Humphrey J, Obregon DF, Yokota K, Mullan M. Statins inhibit A beta-neurotoxicity in vitro and A beta-induced vasoconstriction and inflammation in rat aorta. Atherosclerosis 2002;161:293–299.
71. Quinn J, Montine T, Morrow J, Woodward WR, Kulhanek D, Eckenstein F. Inflammation and cerebral amyloidosis are disconnected in an animal model of Alzheimer's disease. J Neuroimmunol 2003;173:32–41.

20

Cerebrovascular Disease and the Expression of Alzheimer's Disease

Margaret M. Esiri and Zsuzsanna Nagy

1. INTRODUCTION

This chapter reviews clinicopathological studies that illuminate the manner in which cerebrovascular disease (CVD) and Alzheimer's disease (AD) pathology may interact to produce dementia. It does not consider the role of congophilic angiopathy, which is examined in Chapter 19. Central to the view put forward here is the idea that altered functional performance in cognition with aging depends on brain reserve capacity falling below a certain threshold or pathology exceeding a tolerance threshold (or both): brain reserve capacity is reduced with ageing while the burden of AD and vascular pathology rises; at some point, the reserve capacity is exhausted and combinations of AD pathology and CVD then cause dementia.

The idea that dementia is a condition that develops when brain reserve capacity for cognitive processing is exhausted is one that has been current for more than 30 yr. In seminal studies by Tomlinson et al. *(1)*, volumes of cerebral ischemic necrosis or densities of neurofibrillary tangles exceeded certain thresholds if dementia, caused by CVD or AD, respectively, was present. The same concept applies in another neurodegenerative disease—loss of substantia nigra neurons sufficient to reduce dopaminergic input to the striatum by 75% or more is required for Parkinson's disease to become symptomatic *(2)*.

Remarkably, the components of the human brain can survive and function relatively effectively for up to 100 yr or more. It is hardly surprising that with time it becomes possible to detect potentially deleterious changes in the brain. Although the details of how these changes are produced are still being worked out, a major factor is likely to be free radical damage resulting from sustained energy generation in both neurons and the cellular components of blood vessel walls during the course of a lifetime. The main focus of damage sustained by the brain as it ages are modest loss and shrinkage of neurons at some (although not all) sites (reviewed in ref. *3*), various forms of ischemic damage *(4)*, and pathology of the type that is seen in AD *(4)*. In a recent autopsy study in an unselected community-based population of elderly people in the United Kingdom, 78% had evidence of CVD and 70% had some degree of Alzheimer-type pathology. Parkinson's disease pathology was much less common, being found in 11% *(4)*. Loss of cortical synapses accompanies the shrinkage of neurons *(5)*. Cross-sectional studies of the brains of people dying at different ages suggests that some of these changes develop gradually, probably throughout decades *(6)*. Some of the risk factors for their development, both environmental and genetic, have been identified. Functional imaging studies indicate that as the brain ages it may alter the way in which it employs networks of neuronal connections to achieve a given task. For example, in motor performance, more regions become activated when car-

From: *Current Clinical Neurology*
Vascular Dementia: Cerebrovascular Mechanisms and Clinical Management
Edited by: R. H. Paul, R. Cohen, B. R. Ott, and S. Salloway © Humana Press Inc., Totowa, NJ

rying out a grasping action in older than in younger subjects *(7)*. Similarly, although both young and older subjects activate the left hippocampus when retrieving autobiographical event memories, the older subjects also activate the right hippocampus to a significantly greater extent than young subjects when performing this task *(8)*. Although little is known about the mechanisms controlling such adaptive changes, it is suggested that reserve capacity can be called on with aging to enable function to be effectively maintained in healthy subjects. The premise underlying this chapter is that such adaptive changes gradually become unable to maintain normal cognitive function as disease of one or more types robs the brain of its reserve capacity. The early clinicopathological literature is certainly consistent with this idea, but firm evidence supporting it was lacking because the quantitative data linking cognition and pathology were relatively rudimentary. More recent studies are starting to provide more substantial support and have important implications for preventing or minimizing rates of progression of dementia.

2. HOW AD AND CVD EACH PRODUCE DEMENTIA

Only when we have clear evidence of how AD and CVD each produce dementia can we improve understanding of how their interaction can also promote dementia. Early studies of brain structure and dementia established that both AD pathology and CVD can be associated with dementia, but later studies revealed the quantitative manner of this association. This required the development of rating instruments sensitive for detection of mild, as well as severe, dementia in life and a method of quantifying the relevant pathology. By applying both tools to the same individuals in longitudinal studies, we now have some idea of which elements of the complex AD pathology are particularly related to dementia severity. In CVD, we are at a more preliminary stage of understanding, with less widely applied clinical measures that are sensitive to the types of deficits CVD produces and no well-developed and widely applied scoring system for quantifying the heterogeneous forms of CVD encountered. Although there is general agreement that in AD neuritic pathology, as seen in neurofibrillary tangles (NFT), neuropil threads, and neuritic plaques, is highly correlated with the severity of dementia *(9–11)* , there is less agreement about which forms of CVD are particularly liable to produce dementia. Early studies emphasized that a large volume of cerebral tissue needed to be infarcted if someone with CVD was to be diagnosed with dementia *(1)*. The risk of dementia was believed to be greater after multiple strokes *(12)*. However, more recent studies have emphasized the important contribution of subcortical CVD, affecting small blood vessels, as described in Binswanger's disease and in the form of lacunes, to dementia *(13,14)*.

Some studies indicate that the most commonly observed neuropathologic abnormalities in vascular dementia (VaD) are lacunar infarcts and microinfarcts (in >50% of patients with dementia) *(14)* throughout the central nervous system (CNS) with predominant subcortical lesions in the basal ganglia and white matter or in strategically important brain regions, such as the thalamus and hippocampus *(15,16)*. There is also evidence of remote hippocampal injury *(14)* and hippocampal sclerosis, often accompanied by other cerebrovascular lesions *(15–18)*. Thus, VaD correlates with widespread small ischemic lesions distributed throughout the CNS *(13–16)*. Some studies also indicate that although amyloid angiopathy does not relate to amyloid plaque burden in the brain of patients with AD, it increases the frequency of small-vessel lesions and cerebral hemorrhages and infarcts and correlates with dementia *(4,19–21)*.

3. HOW AD AND CVD INTERACT TO CAUSE DEMENTIA

The frequent co-occurrence of AD and CVD pathologies in the same brain has long been recognized *(22,23)*. The occurrence of multiple pathologies makes clinical diagnosis of these patients exceedingly difficult *(24,25)* and neuropathological examination may be the only possible way to distinguish between AD with and without VaD *(26)*. This latter recognition prompted several studies trying to define the exact pathological substrates of VaD, with or without concomitant AD. The

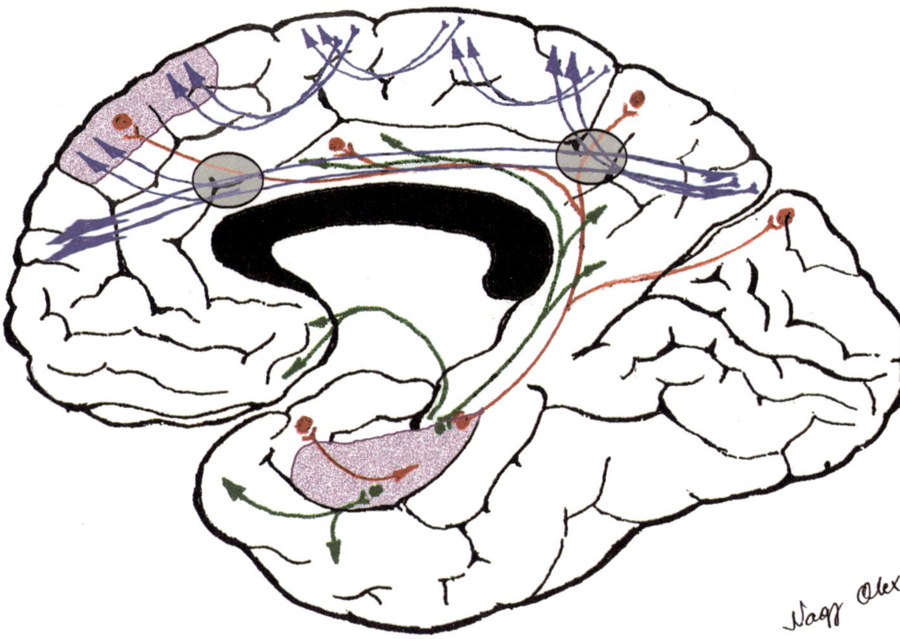

Fig. 1. It is suggested in this chapter that cerebral cortical and hippocampal interconnections are interrupted in the cerebral cortex and hippocampus by Alzheimer's disease (AD) pathology and principally in the white matter by cerebrovascular disease (CVD). In this cartoon of a cerebral hemisphere, the interruptions in connections caused by AD are indicated in purple and the interruptions in connections caused by CVD in gray.

authors undertook such a study on archival cases without significant AD pathology. A group of relatively uncommon cases of dementia in which vascular disease was the only form of pathology present was compared with a group of cases which had CVD mainly clinically in the form of strokes. These latter cases did not have dementia. The authors compared forms of vascular disease between the two groups and found that small-vessel subcortical disease was much more common in those who were demented, whereas major infarcts were more common in those with strokes and no dementia *(27)*. Unfortunately, there are no widely applied criteria characterizing small-vessel disease, thus limiting useful comparisons between studies on the relative importance of this common feature of elderly brains and its significance in promoting dementia. A recent study urges the need for development of consensus pathologic diagnostic criteria for assessment of small-vessel disease *(28)*.

The simplest form of interaction between AD and CVD in causing dementia would be simple summation of their effects. This is an entirely plausible possibility. NFT, neuritic plaques, loss of nerve cells, and loss of synapses in AD interfere with cortico-cortical and hippocampal-cortical connections by reducing communication between nerve cells. Because AD pathology also affects subcortical nuclei, such as the nucleus basalis, raphe nuclei, and locus ceruleus that are required for normal cortical function, deficiencies in these neurotransmitter systems further add to impaired communications. CVD that affects white matter diffusely is likely to compound the problems by interrupting cortico-cortical and subcortico-cortical axons or their myelin sheaths (*see* Fig. 1). CVD that affects gray matter may have numerous effects, depending on the region of the brain involved, e.g., strategically located infarcts may give rise to memory deficits if centered on hippocampi or anterior thalamus, but infarcts affecting basal ganglia or small regions of frontal cortex may be asymptomatic. Hippocampal damage consist-

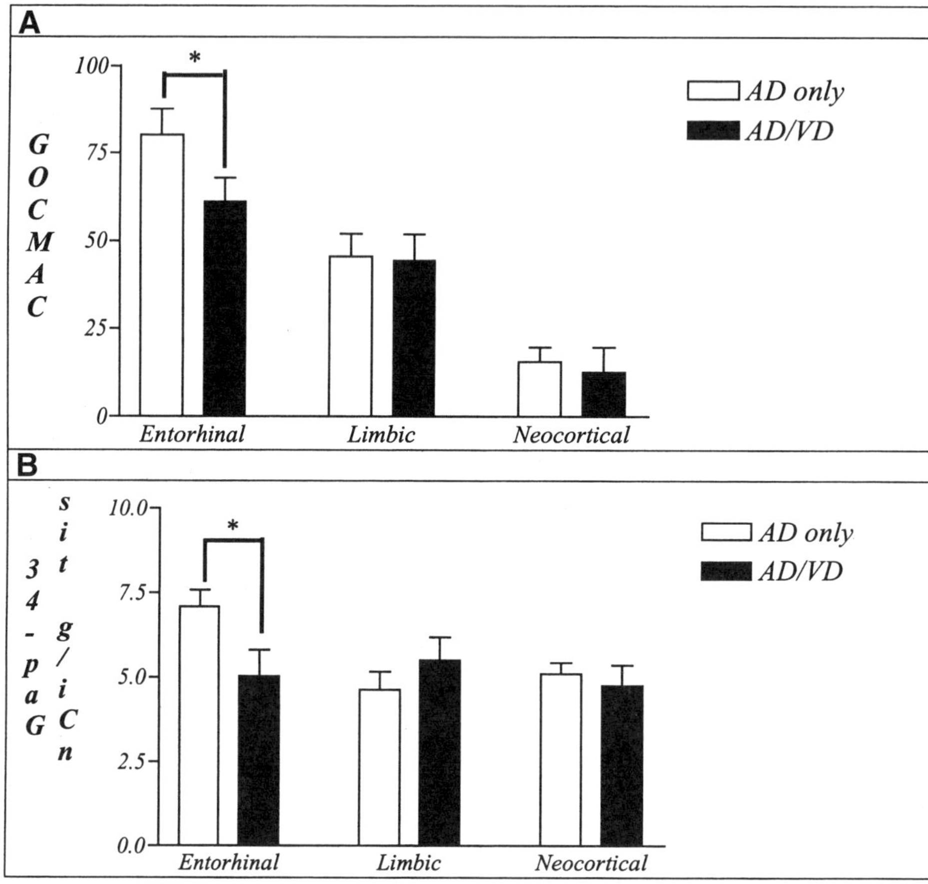

Fig. 2. (A) Comparison of CAMCOG scores, a measure of cognitive functioning (normal score 80–107) in cases with and without CVD at early (entorhinal), intermediate (limbic), and late (neocortical) stages of Alzheimer's disease (AD) *(30)*. Cognitive function is significantly reduced (*) by the presence of additional cerebrovascular disease (CVD) only at the entorhinal stage of AD. **(B)** Comparison of GAP-43 immunoreactivity expressed as nCi/g of radioactivity following reaction with an ^{35}S-labelled secondary antibody in cases with and without CVD at early (entorhinal), intermediate (limbic), and late (neocortical) stages of AD *(30)*. There is a significant reduction (*) in immunoreactivity for GAP-43, a measure of synaptic plasticity, in the entorhinal stage of AD in the presence of CVD.

ing of neuronal loss in the CA1 sector but falling short of frank infarction has also been documented in VaD and can give rise to a dementia syndrome similar to that of AD *(18)*. In mixed dementia, strategic infarcts have a role in the mechanism of cognitive impairment *(29)*.

The pathology of AD is restricted in location, is mild, and is asymptomatic. Thus, in the first two (entorhinal) most locally restricted stages of the Braak classification of AD pathology *(30)*, there is no significant interference to cognitive performance. However, at this stage, cognition is significantly depressed if additional CVD is present *(31)* (*see* Fig. 2A). In the intermediate two (limbic) Braak stages, in which NFT formation affects the hippocampus, as well as entorhinal cortex, symptoms start to appear when this is the only pathology present. Cognitive scores are moderately reduced but not significantly more so if additional CVD is present (*see* Fig. 2A). In the most advanced two

Braak stages in which neocortex, as well as hippocampus and entorhinal cortex, contains numerous NFT, cognitive performance is profoundly impaired and no more so if additional CVD is present (*see* Fig. 2A). These observations are corroborated in other studies *(32,33)*. Thus, additional CVD has the greatest opportunity to influence cognitive performance in conjunction with AD pathology when the latter is mild and, on its own, asymptomatic. The implications of this observation for preventing dementia are considerable: preventing CVD can delay onset of symptoms of AD until the pathology has progressed to involve at least the hippocampus; the course of AD is not likely to be altered in terms of rate of progression but is likely to be symptomatically more long lasting.

Additionally, in late-stage AD, the extent of neurofibrillary pathology for a given severity of cognitive decline is significantly lowered in the presence of vascular disease *(34,35)*. In the authors' studies, they found that the presence of additional vascular disease augmented the accumulation of hyperphosphorylated tau affecting paired helical filaments (PHF) formation in the hippocampus in cases with mild AD changes and reduced the extent of PHF formation with severe AD pathology *(36)*. GAP-43 immunoreactivity, a marker of synaptic plasticity, was significantly reduced in the hippocampus in the early (entorhinal) stages of AD if CVD was also present (Fig. 2B). The authors have also found that the relationship between PHF formation and cognitive decline was lost in patients with additional vascular pathology.

4. CONCLUSION

CVD influences expression of AD differently, depending on the stage of the AD pathology. Its greatest clinical effect is seen at the early stages of the development of AD. Whether it influences the evolution of AD pathology is another question.

REFERENCES

1. Tomlinson BE, Blessed G, Roth M. Observations on the brains of demented old people. J Neurol Sci 1970;11:205–242.
2. Bernheimer H, Birkmayer W, Hornykiewicz O, et al. Brain dopamine and the syndromes of Parkinson and Huntington. Clinical, morphological and neurochemical correlations. J Neurol Sci 1973;20:415–455.
3. Esiri MM. Dementia and normal aging: neuropathology. In: Huppert F, Brayne C, O'Connor DW, ed. Dementia and Normal Aging. Cambridge, UK: Cambridge University Press, 1994, pp. 385–436.
4. Pathological correlates of late-onset dementia in a multicentre, community-based population in England and Wales. Neuropathology Group of the Medical Research Council Cognitive Function and Ageing Study (MRC CFAS). Lancet 2001;357:169–175.
5. Masliah E, Mallory M, Hansen L, et al. Quantitative synaptic alterations in the human neocortex during normal aging. Neurology 1993;43:192–197.
6. Ohm TG, Muller H, Braak H, Bohl J. Close-meshed prevalence rates of different stages as a tool to uncover the rate of Alzheimer's disease-related neurofibrillary changes. Neuroscience 1995;64:209–217.
7. Ward NS, Frackowiak RS. Age-related changes in the neural correlates of motor performance. Brain 2003;126:873–888.
8. Maguire EA, Frith CD. Aging affects the engagement of the hippocampus during autobiographical memory retrieval. Brain 2003;126:1511–1523.
9. Nagy Z, Esiri MM, Jobst KA, et al. Relative roles of plaques and tangles in the dementia of Alzheimer's disease: correlations using three sets of neuropathological criteria. Dementia 1995;6:21–31.
10. Arriagada PV, Growdon JH, Hedley-Whyte ET, Hyman BT. Neurofibrillary tangles but not senile plaques parallel duration and severity of Alzheimer's disease. Neurology 1992;42:631–639.
11. McKee AC, Kosik KS, Kowall NW. Neuritic pathology and dementia in Alzheimer's disease. Ann Neurol 1991;30:156–165.
12. del Ser T, Bermejo F, Portera A, et al. Vascular dementia. A clinicopathological study. J Neurol Sci 1990;96:1–17.
13. Esiri MM, Wilcock GK, Morris JH. Neuropathological assessment of the lesions of significance in vascular dementia. J Neurol Neurosurg Psychiatry 1997;63:749–753.
14. Vinters HV, Ellis WG, Zarow C, et al. Neuropathologic substrates of ischemic vascular dementia. J Neuropathol Exp Neurol 2000;59:931–945.
15. Jellinger KA. The pathology of ischemic-vascular dementia: an update. J Neurol Sci 2002;203–204:153–157.
16. Jellinger KA. Vascular-ischemic dementia: an update. J Neural Transm (Suppl) 2002;62:1–23.
17. Leverenz JB, Agustin CM, Tsuang D, et al. Clinical and neuropathological characteristics of hippocampal sclerosis: a community-based study. Arch Neurol 2002;59:1099–1106.

18. Kril JJ, Patel S, Harding AJ, Halliday GM. Patients with vascular dementia due to microvascular pathology have significant hippocampal neuronal loss. J Neurol Neurosurg Psychiatry 2002;72:747–751.
19. Jellinger KA. Alzheimer disease and cerebrovascular pathology: an update. J Neural Transm 2002;109:813–836.
20. Pfeifer LA, White LR, Ross GW, et al. Cerebral amyloid angiopathy and cognitive function: the HAAS autopsy study. Neurology 2002;58:1629–1634.
21. Suter OC, Sunthorn T, Kraftsik R, et al. Cerebral hypoperfusion generates cortical watershed microinfarcts in Alzheimer disease. Stroke 2002;33:1986–1992.
22. Fratiglioni L, Launer LJ, Andersen K, et al. Incidence of dementia and major subtypes in Europe: a collaborative study of population-based cohorts. Neurologic Diseases in the Elderly Research Group. Neurology 2000;54:S10–S15.
23. Morris JH. Vascular dementia. In: Esiri MM, Morris JH, eds. The Neuropathology of Dementia. Cambridge, UK: Cambridge University Press, 1997, pp. 137–173.
24. O'Brien JT, Erkinjuntti T, Reisberg B, et al. Vascular cognitive impairment. Lancet Neurol 2003;2:89–98.
25. Knopman DS, Parisi JE, Boeve BF, et al. Vascular dementia in a population-based autopsy study. Arch Neurol 2003;60: 569–575.
26. Dickson DW. Neuropathology of Alzheimer's disease and other dementias. Clin Geriatr Med 2001;17:209–228.
27. Esiri MM. Which vascular lesions are of importance in vascular dementia? Ann NY Acad Sci 2000;903:239–243.
28. Halliday G, Ng T, Rodriguez M, et al. Consensus neuropathological diagnosis of common dementia syndromes: testing and standardising the use of multiple diagnostic criteria. Acta Neuropathol (Berl) 2002;104:72–78.
29. Zekry D, Duyckaerts C, Belmin J, et al. The vascular lesions in vascular and mixed dementia: the weight of functional neuroanatomy. Neurobiol Aging 2003;24:213–219.
30. Braak H, Braak E. Neuropathological stageing of Alzheimer-related changes. Acta Neuropathol (Berl) 1991;82:239–259.
31. Esiri MM, Nagy Z, Smith MZ, et al. Cerebrovascular disease and threshold for dementia in the early stages of Alzheimer's disease. Lancet 1999;354:919–920.
32. Goulding JM, Signorini DF, Chatterjee S, et al. Inverse relation between Braak stage and cerebrovascular pathology in Alzheimer predominant dementia. J Neurol Neurosurg Psychiatry 1999;67:654–657.
33. Snowdon DA, Greiner LH, Mortimer JA, et al. Brain infarction and the clinical expression of Alzheimer disease. The Nun Study. JAMA 1997;277:813–817.
34. Zekry D, Duyckaerts C, Belmin J, et al. Alzheimer's disease and brain infarcts in the elderly. Agreement with neuropathology. J Neurol 2002;249:1529–1534.
35. Zekry D, Duyckaerts C, Moulias R, et al. Degenerative and vascular lesions of the brain have synergistic effects in dementia of the elderly. Acta Neuropathol (Berl) 2002;103:481–487.
36. Smith MZ, Nagy Z, Barnetson L, et al. Coexisting pathologies in the brain: influence of vascular disease and Parkinson's disease on Alzheimer's pathology in the hippocampus. Acta Neuropathol (Berl) 2000;100:87–94.

21

The Neuropsychological Differentiation Between Alzheimer's Disease and Subcortical Vascular Dementia

David J. Libon, Stephen Scheinthal, Dana L. Penney, and Rod Swenson

1. INTRODUCTION

Our orientation regarding the dementias has changed during the past 30 yr. For example, in the not too distant past, illnesses such as Alzheimer's disease (AD) and Pick's disease were believed to be rare, if not obscure, illnesses *(1)*. This viewpoint is juxtaposed to contemporaneous ideas put forth by Katzman and colleagues *(2)* who believed that AD was not only prevalent but represented a major public health problem. During the past 10 yr, the diagnosis of dementia has become increasingly complex, requiring the consideration of an array of conditions, including AD, vascular dementia (VaD), dementia with Lewy body (DLB), frontal-temporal dementia (FTD), cortical basilar degeneration (CBD), and subcortical dementias, such as progressive supernuclear palsy (PSP) and Parkinson's disease.

The impetus for the current interest in VaD stems from the availability of magnetic resonance imaging (MRI) technology. Although there is considerable debate and controversy regarding issues such as *does white matter matter* or *does VaD exist*, interest in vascular syndromes, particularly as they relate to dementia, has a long tradition in neurological science. Beginning in the 1840s, French neurologist Max Durand-Fardel (for review, *see* ref. *3)* made original descriptions of three types of vascular lesions—lacunar infarcts, *etat crible*, and *atrophe interstitelle du cerveau*. Durand-Fardel characterized a *lacune* as a small cavity in the brain "without any change in consistency or color from which it was possible to remove a little cellular tissue containing very small vessels with a thin forceps." Durand-Fardel characterized lacunar lesions as healed infarcts, separate from other vascular lesions. He used the term *etat crible* (i.e., a sieve-like state) to describe occasions where the subcortical white matter was "riddled with a number of little holes, with sharp edges, usually surrounded by a quite normal white matter, without any change in color or consistency." Finally, Durand-Fardel described *atrophe interstitelle du cerbeau* (interstitial atrophy of the brain) as: "alterations of the cerebral pulp...different from infarctions...not due to a change in the consistency of the brain but a rarefaction of the pulp." This type of lesion is analogous to Hachinski et al.'s *(4)* description of leukoaraiosis, a term that describes the white matter alterations (WMA) seen on modern imaging studies of older adults *(3)*. Pierre Marie is credited with introducing the term *etat lacunaire (3)*. He separated lacunes from *etat crible*, largely accepting Durand-Fardel's description of this phenomenon. Moreover, Marie provided precise macroscopic, as well as histological, descriptions of lacunes.

From: *Current Clinical Neurology*
Vascular Dementia: Cerebrovascular Mechanisms and Clinical Management
Edited by: R. H. Paul, R. Cohen, B. R. Ott, and S. Salloway © Humana Press Inc., Totowa, NJ

This nosology, constructed without the aid of imaging technology we now take for granted, is still relevant today *(5)*.

Despite Durand-Fardel's insightful work, historical accounts of VaD often begin with the small series of cases described by Binswanger in 1884 *(6,7)*. Binswanger suggested that WMA were caused by vascular insufficiency that could impair mental functioning. He coined the term *encephalitis subcorticalis chronica progressiva* to describe this syndrome *(6,7)*. Microscopic information regarding these patients was never published; nonetheless, in 1902, Alzheimer *(8)* made observations that substantiated Binswanger's findings. Case descriptions provided by Olszewski *(9)* and Caplan and Schoene *(10)* have supported the clinical and neuropathological observations of both Binswanger and Alzheimer.

Throughout most of the 20th century, dementia associated with arteriosclerosis was believed to cause widespread cortical atrophy secondary to an attenuation of brain perfusion. Hachinski and colleagues *(11,12)* proved that this was not true and introduced the term of multiinfarct dementia (MID). However, after Hachinski's seminal work, the term MID was used to denote almost all presentations of VaD. Indeed, until the introduction of the diagnostic criteria from the Alzheimer's Disease Diagnostic and Treatment Centers (ADDTC) *(13)* and National Institute of Neurological Disorders and Stroke-Association Internationale pour la Recherche et l'Enseignement en Neurosciences (NINDS-AIREN) criteria *(14)*, Hachinski's Ischemic Scale *(11,12)* was the convention by which MID or VaD was typically defined.

Until recently, Binswanger's disease or dementia associated with subcortical WMAs was viewed as a rather obscure illness or even marginalized as an epiphenomenon. Newer research is changing this perception, but many questions remain. Our current interest in VaD in general, and subcortical WMA in particular, owes a substantial debt to French neurological science. Many of these original observations have withstood the test of time. Perhaps it is time to recall another bit of French wisdom, *plus ça change, plus c'est le même* (the more things change, the more things stay the same).

2. OVERLAP BETWEEN VASCULAR DEMENTIA AND ALZHEIMER'S DISEASE

A traditional perspective regarding the diagnosis of dementia suggests that specific pathological changes in the brain should result in a specific clinical presentation. However, there is research indicating that among patients suffering from dementia, the relationship between pathology and clinical presentation may not be linear or direct. Indeed, some of the most interesting research to emerge during the last several years addresses mixed diagnoses and suggests that vascular disease may alter the development and distribution of the senile plaques and neurofibrillary tangles (NFT) associated with AD.

For example, Nagy and colleagues *(15)* found that patients who met pathological criteria for AD *and* displayed evidence of cardiovascular disease (CVD) had lower numbers of senile plaques and NFT when compared to patients with AD who presented with minimal or no cerebrovascular pathology. Nagy and colleagues *(15)* described several cerebrovascular alterations, including single infarcts, small macroscopic infarcts, multiple microinfarcts, and cribriform alterations, tissue rarefaction, and white matter myelin pallor. They speculated that neuropathologic evidence of vascular lesions could have a significant impact regarding the clinical expression of these patients' dementia, because these patients had less AD pathology. Similarly, Snowdon and colleagues *(16)* reported that patients with AD with evidence of CVD, primarily involving subcortical infarcts, presented with fewer NFT throughout the cortex.

Other studies have shown that the incidence of so-called pure AD may be much lower than previously reported. For example, Victoroff and colleagues *(17)* indicated that 86% of their patients diagnosed with AD in life also displayed evidence of other possible dementing disorders, including CVD. Bowler and colleagues *(18)* found that on autopsy, only 44% of their cases had pure AD without any other coexisting causes of dementia. More recently, Crystal and colleagues *(19)* reported that of their patients diagnosed in life with AD, only half of these patients actually met neuropathological criteria for AD. However, of the patients who met pathological criteria for AD, many also presented with a variety of cerebrovascular lesions that could have contributed to the dementia. Such research has even led some to speculate that AD might even be a type of vascular disorder *(20)*. Clearly, more research is necessary to resolve this issue.

3. NEUROPSYCHOLOGY OF SUBCORTICAL VASCULAR DEMENTIA

Throughout the past decade, there have been many studies examining the neuropsychological profile associated with subcortical vascular lesions. Overall, there is a relationship between increased subcortical periventricular and deep WMA and subcortical lacunar infarctions and greater impairment on tests of executive control, with some relative sparing on tests of memory and language *(21–24)*. Yet there has been little effort to interpret or integrate these findings within any larger context. Some authors have invoked the construct of working memory *(25)* to describe the mechanism that underlies executive control deficits associated with subcortical pathology. However, we believe deficits in establishing and maintaining a mental set is a more parsimonious construct that helps explain executive control impairment and, perhaps, elements of the declarative memory disorder associated with subcortical VaD *(26,27)*.

We characterize the ability to establish and maintain a mental set as the ability of patients to appreciate and understand the nature of a task and to respond within the context of that task until the task is completed. Described in Sections 3.1.–3.3. are several recent studies from our laboratory that attempt to elucidate the parameters regarding the difficulty patients with subcortical VaD exhibit on tests of executive control, memory, and language.

3.1. *Executive Control*

Lamar and colleagues *(28)* studied deficits in establishing and maintaining mental set by looking at the perseverative behavior produced by patients with AD and subcortical VaD primarily associated with WMA. Two interesting findings emerged from this study. First, and perhaps not surprisingly, the overall number of perseverations was greater in patients with moderate to severe subcortical vascular lesions as compared to patients with AD. Second, and more interesting, the *type* of perseverations made by patients with moderate to severe subcortical WMA was distinctive. For example, patients with subcortical VaD often produced *hyperkinetic/interminable perseverations* (i.e., persisting in the production of responses even when there was no command to do so). The perseverations generated by patients with AD were different. For example, when asked to *write* the sentence "three squares and two circles," these patients might produce an *activity perseveration,* whereby they would *draw* three squares and two circles; or an *element perseveration,* such as drawing a circle when asked to produce a square.

The mechanisms that underlie these difficulties in maintaining mental set were different. Among patients with subcortical VaD, *hyperkinetic/interminable perseverations* were correlated with poor performance on tests of motor functions. This suggests that impaired regulation of motor behavior may be the mechanism responsible for their difficulty. In the AD group *activity/element* perseverations were correlated with poorer performance on the Boston Naming Test and reduced output on the animal word list generation task. This suggests that problems in the response selection of lexical/semantic information may underlie their difficulty.

In another study Giovannetti and colleagues *(29)* examined problems in establishing and maintaining mental set with the Wechsler Adult Intelligence Scale-Revised (WAIS-R) Similarities subtest, a test of verbal concept formation. Zero-point responses were recoded into two broad categories, *in-set* vs *out-of-set* errors. An *in-set error* was coded when a response was vague but retained some superordinate relationship (i.e., dog-lion—*they're alive*). By contrast, an *out-of-set* error was coded when no superordinate relationship was conveyed (i.e., dog-lion—*one barks and the other growls*). Overall, it was found that patients with subcortical VaD made more out-of-set errors, whereas patients with AD made more in-set errors. When these two types of errors were included in a factor analysis with other neuropsychological tests, out-of-set errors loaded with variables consistent with gross deficits in establishing and maintaining mental set, such as perseverations made on the Graphical Sequence Test *(28)* or errors made on clock drawing *(30)*. Similar to Lamar and colleagues *(28)*, in-set errors loaded with variables related to problems in the selection of lexical/semantic information.

More recently, Lamar and colleagues *(31)* investigated the capacity of patients with dementia to establish and maintain a complex mental set using the Boston Revision of the Wechsler Memory Scale Mental Control subtest. This test consists of tasks such as asking patients to identify letters that rhyme with the word *key* and to identify printed letters that contain a curved line. In this study, tasks were divided into three equal sections and all errors and correct responses were summed separately for each of the three sections on each task. However, in the AD group, performance declined from the first to the middle sections of these tasks but remained stable when the middle portion of the test was compared to the latter portion of the test. In the VaD group, errors accumulated and performance declined throughout all three sections of the task. In a second experiment, the number of responses generated over time on tests of letter fluency tasks (FAS) was examined. Each 1-min letter trial was divided into four 15-s intervals, and the number of responses generated for each interval was compared. Interestingly, when performance was controlled for total output, the percentage of correct responses generated by patients with AD within each quadrant was no different from normal control participants. By contrast, patients with VaD tended to generate their maximum output during the first 15-s epoch.

We believe that when viewed as a whole, executive control deficits associated with subcortical VaD tend to be pandemic, capable of compromising virtually all areas of cognitive functioning. By contrast, the executive control deficits associated with AD are more restricted and context specific, that is related to lexical/semantic operations. These findings are consistent with the theoretical constructs put forth by Luria *(32)* and recent research suggesting that subcortical gray matter structures, such as the caudate, help to modulate or gate frontal lobe activity *(26,27)*. In this context, it is intriguing to speculate whether subcortical WMA are capable of acting as a surrogate or in an analogous fashion as subcortical gray matter structures regarding the etiology of executive control deficits associated with VaD. This is another area for future research.

3.2. Memory and Learning

Recent research also shows that patients with subcortical WMA retain some capacity to learn new information, a profile different from AD *(33–37)*. On the nine-word dementia version of the California Verbal Learning Test (CVLT) *(34,38)* patients with AD display poor retention, rapid forgetting, little to no benefit from cued recall or recognition test conditions, and many intrusion errors. However, patients with subcortical VaD produce a different profile. They obtain higher scores on measures of delayed free and cued recall memory and produce improvement on the recognition discriminability index. The profile produced by patients with VaD is similar to the profile produced by patients with Parkinson's disease and Huntington's disease *(39–41)*.

Davis and colleagues *(42)* have investigated the mechanisms that underlie the types of errors produced on the immediate free recall portion of the nine-word CVLT. They define *initial intrusions* as denoting the first time an intrusion error is produced. A *trans-trial perseveration* is coded when intrusions reoccurred in later free recall learning trials. Finally, *within-trial perseverations* are scored when patients repeated a response that was produced earlier in any single free recall learning trial. Similar to our previous work regarding executive control deficits in dementia *(28,29,31)*, Davis and colleagues *(42)* speculated that deficits in the response selection of lexical/semantic information might be the mechanism that underlies the production of initial and trans-trial errors; whereas poor self-monitoring might be responsible for the production of within-trial perseverations. Partial support was found for this prediction is that *initial* intrusion errors were correlated with poor scores on the animal word list generation Association Index (*see* Carew et al. *[43]*), a measure of the lexical-semantic organization.

Davis and colleagues *(42)* also examined the distribution of false positive responses produced by patients with AD and subcortical VaD on the CVLT-9 word delayed recognition task. Within-group analyses indicated that as a percentage of the total number of foils endorsed, patients with subcortical VaD endorse more interference (list B) foils than semantic or unrelated foils. By contrast, patients with AD endorsed more semantic and unrelated foils. Also, there was a significant correlation between the production of interference (list B) foils and the production of perseverations, as measured with the Graphical Sequence Test *(28)*. Similar to the research of Lamar and colleagues *(28,31)* and Giovannetti and colleagues *(29)*, Davis and colleagues *(42)* concluded that on serial list learning tests deficits in executive control and lexical/semantic knowledge underlie many of the errors produced by VaD and AD, respectively.

3.3. *Language/Semantic Knowledge*

Deficits of language and semantic knowledge in patients with subcortical VaD have not been extensively studied. Carew and colleagues *(43)* designed a paradigm to measure the lexical/semantic organization on the animal word list generation task, a popular test that is often part of the neuropsychological work-up for dementia. On this task, patients are given 60 s to generate animal names (animal categories are not supplied). Carew and colleagues *(43)* coded all responses on the following six categories: size (big or small), geographic location (foreign or North America), diet (herbivore, carnivore, or omnivore), zoological class (insect, mammal, bird, etc.), habitat (farm, Africa/jungle, widespread, etc.), and biological order/related groupings (feline, canine, bovine, etc.). An Association Index was calculated by totaling the number of shared attributes between successive responses and then dividing by the number of total responses. The authors believe that the Association Index provides a measure of the lexical/semantic organization between successive responses independent of the number of words produced. Carew and colleagues *(43)* found that the total number of responses made by patients with AD and subcortical VaD did not differ. Regarding the Association Index, normal control participants and patients with subcortical VaD did not differ. However, both groups obtained higher scores on this measure as compared to patients with AD. Carew and colleagues *(43)* interpreted their data as consistent with the idea that lexical/semantic knowledge is relatively intact in subcortical VaD as compared to AD.

In conclusion, the studies reviewed suggest that dementia associated with moderate to severe MRI-WMA can be differentiated from dementia associated with little or mild MRI-WMA. The neuropsychological profile associated with subcortical WMA revolves around poor performance on tests of executive control but relatively better performance on delayed-recognition tasks. Semantic knowledge can be relatively intact among patients with substantial subcortical WMA. Several preliminary conclusions might be drawn from these data. First, from an anatomic perspective, the pattern of performance produced by patients with moderate to severe MRI-WMA could be caused by a disruption of the frontal-basal ganglia-thalamic pathways *(44,45)*. Second, from a clinical perspective, these data suggest that to identify or diagnose subcortical VaD, dissociation between tests of executive control vs tests of memory/ language should be obtained. However, exactly how severe or what volume of MRI-WMA is necessary to produce this profile?

4. THE RESEARCH CRITERIA FOR SUBCORTICAL VASCULAR DEMENTIA

Erkinjuntti and colleagues *(46)* have proposed some modification to the existing diagnostic criteria for VaD. These changes focus on subcortical VaD associated with radiological evidence of periventricular and deep WMAs and/or lacunar stroke. Clinically, to diagnose subcortical VaD as proposed by Erkinjuntti and colleagues *(46)*, two broad criteria must be satisfied—radiological evidence of subcortical CVD, sufficient to be associated with dementia, and a profile on neuropsychological tests showing greater impairment on tests of executive control and less impairment on tests of delayed-recognition memory. However, as stated in Section 3.3., it is unclear exactly how much WMA is necessary to produce this kind of profile on neuropsychological tests. We now present data that will attempt to address this issue.

The authors' goal is to provide some concrete operational guidelines for a putative diagnosis of subcortical VaD, as suggested by Erkinjuntti and colleagues *(46)*. In the data presented in Section 6., MRI-WMA were measured using the 40-point leukoaraiosis scale of Junque *(47,48)*. Measures of executive control, memory, and language were drawn from the studies discussed in Section 3. If dementia seen in conjunction with subcortical WMA is associated with a relative dissociation on tests of executive control vs memory as suggested by Erkinjuntti and colleagues *(46)*, then it is reasonable to expect that patients with minimal to mild MRI-WMA will present with greater impairment on tests of delayed-recognition memory and, perhaps language as compared to tests of executive control. Conversely, patients with severe MRI-WMA should yield the opposite profile (i.e., greater impairment on tests of executive control as compared to tests of delayed recognition memory/language).

In the data presented in Section 6., patients with dementia are divided into mild, moderate, and severe white matter groups on the basis of the severity of their MRI WMAs as measured with the leukoaraiosis scale of Junque *(47,48)*. The prediction to be tested is that there should be a statistically significant interaction between the severity of MRI-WMA and performance on neuropsychological tests of executive control and memory/language.

5. METHODS

5.1. *Patients*

A total of 105 patients were studied. All patients were clinically diagnosed with either AD or VaD and were enrolled from the Crozer-Chester Medical Center Alexander Silberman Geriatric Assessment Program, an outpatient dementia evaluation program. All patients were examined by a neurologist, neuropsychologist, psychiatrist, geriatrician, and social worker. An MRI study of the brain and appropriate diagnostic laboratory studies were obtained to evaluate for reversible causes of dementia. A clinical diagnosis was determined at an interdisciplinary team conference. On the basis of team diagnosis, 55 patients with National Institute of Neurological and Communicative Diseases and Stroke/Alzheimer's Disease and Related Disorders Association (NINCDS/ADRDA) probable AD *(49)*, and 50 patients with probable/possible ischemic VaD) using ADDTC criteria *(13)* were studied. Patients with AD and IVD with cortical cerebrovascular accidents (CVAs) on MRI scans were excluded. Patients were excluded if there was any history of head injury, substance abuse, major psychiatric disorders (including major depression), epilepsy, or B_{12}, folate, or thyroid deficiency. This information was gathered from a knowledgeable family member.

5.2. *MRI Protocol*

All MRI scans were conducted on a Siemens 1.5 Tesla machine. Both T1- (TR - 500 ms, TE - 15 ms) and T2- (TR - 4000 ms, TE - 90 ms) weighted studies were obtained. The severity of WMA was quantified using the 40-point leukoaraiosis scale described by Junque and colleagues *(47,48)*. This scale divides each hemisphere into five areas: the frontal centrum semiovale, the parietal centrum semiovale, the white matter around the frontal horns, the white matter around the body of the lateral ventricles, and the white matter around the atrium and occipital horns. The severity of WMA was then graded from 0 to 4 and summed across all 10 areas. Leukoaraiosis scores were calculated by two board-certified neuroradiologists who were blind to all clinical information (inter-rater reliability, $r = 0.98, p < 0.001$) *(35)*. Patient's leukoaraiosis scores ranged from 1 to 28.

Table 1
Demographic Information and Junque Leukoaraiosis Scores

	Age	Education	MMSE	GDS	Junque LA score
Mild MRI-WMA	76.56 (5.43)	12.15 (2.54)	21.80 (3.62)	5.44 (3.80)	3.76 (2.75)
Moderate WMA	78.83 (5.44)	11.64 (2.68)	21.36 (3.74)	7.00 (4.06)	12.83 (2.30)
Severe MRI-WMA	77.00 (6.73)	11.20 (3.43)	20.20 (4.81)	5.80 (2.51)	22.07 (3.03)

Abbr: MMSE, Mini-Mental State Examination; GDS, geriatric depression scale; LA, Junque leukoaraiosis scale; MRI-WMA, periventricular and deep white matter alterations.

5.3. *Patient Groups*

To test the direct association between white matter severity and neuropsychological functioning, patients who were diagnosed with either AD or VaD were recategorized into three groups based on their leukoaraiosis scale *(47,48)*, i.e., a mild WMA group (Junque scores, 0–8, $n = 54$), a moderate WMA group (Junque scores, 8–17, $n = 36$), and a severe WMA group (Junque scores, 18–28, $n = 15$). There were no between-group differences among these three groups with respect to age, education, level of dementia as assessed with the Mini-Mental State Examination (MMSE) *(50)*, and depression as assessed with the Geriatric Depression Scale (GDS) *(51)* (*see* Table 1).

5.4. *Neuropsychological Assessment*

5.4.1. *Executive Systems Functioning (WMS-Accuracy)*

Executive systems functioning (WMS-Accuracy) was assessed with the Boston Revision of the Wechsler Memory Scale-Mental Control subtest (WMS-MC) *(31)*. In addition to the three tasks that comprise the standard WMS-MC subtest *(52)* (i.e., counting from 20 to 1, reciting the alphabet, and adding serial 3's), the Boston Revision of the WMS-MC *(31)* subtest includes four additional tasks: reciting the months of the year forward and backward, an alphabet rhyming task that requires patients to identify letters that rhyme with the word "key," and an alphabet visualization task that requires patients to visualize and identify all block printed letters that contain curved lines. Patients were allowed to work as long as necessary on these tasks provided they were working meaningfully. The dependent variable derived from this test was an accuracy index (AcI) derived only from the three non-automatized tasks (i.e., months backward, alphabet rhyming, and alphabet visualization). These accuracy indices were based on the following algorithm:

$$\text{AcI} = [1 - (\text{false positives} + \text{misses/no. possible correct})] \times 100.$$

This algorithm yielded a percentage score ranging from 0–100, such that patients obtaining a score of 100% correct identified all targets and made no false positive responses or misses. A composite score was calculated by averaging the WMS-Mental Control AcI's for all three tasks for each patient.

5.4.2. *Visuoconstructional Functioning (Clock Errors)*

Visuoconstructional functioning (clock errors) was assessed by asking patients to draw the face of a clock with the hands set for "ten after eleven" to command and copy *(53)*. Following procedures described by Libon and colleagues *(30)*, errors related to graphomotor impairment, errors in hand/number placement, and errors related to executive control impairment were scored as either 1 (i.e., present) or 0 (i.e., absent). The dependent variable derived from this test was the total number of errors summed across the command and copy test conditions.

5.4.3. *Language/Semantic Functioning (Animal Association Index)*

Language/semantic functioning (animal association index) was assessed with the animal word list generation task *(43,54)*. On this task, patients were given 1 min to generate animal names. The

Table 2
Neuropsychological Data: Test Scores and z-Scores

	MRI-WMA		
	Mild	Moderate	Severe
WMS Accuracy Index			
Test score	69.6 (16.2)	57.7 (21.9)	33.7 (20.8)
z-score	–2.0 (1.5)	–3.1 (2.0)	–5.4 (1.9)
Clock Drawing Errors			
Test score	3.4 (1.6)	5.4 (2.5)	7.1 (2.8)
z-score	1.2 (1.0)	2.5 (1.6)	3.6 (1.8)
WLG-AI			
Test score	2.7 (.87)	3.3 (.70)	3.7 (.73)
z-score	–1.6 (1.7)	–.41 (1.4)	.45 (1.5)
CVLT-discrim			
Test score	67.3 (12.4)	75.7 (14.9)	80.2 (7.8)
z-score	–5.8 (2.5)	–4.1 (3.1)	–3.1 (1.6)

Abbr: MRI-WMA, periventricular and deep white matter alterations; WMS Accuracy Index, WMS Mental Control non-automatized accuracy index (AcI); The clock drawing scale is based on errors. A positive z-score signals impaired performance; WLG-AI, animal word list generation association index (AI); CVLT-discrim, CVLT recognition discriminability index.

dependent variable derived from the animal fluency task was the total association index (animal-AI). The animal-AI is a special scoring technique that measures the semantic organization between successive responses. A high score on this measure is believed to reflect generally intact semantic memory stores. Complete details regarding how the animal-AI index is calculated can be found in Carew and colleagues *(43)*.

5.4.4. Declarative Memory (CVLT-Recognition Discrimination)

Declarative memory was assessed with the nine-word dementia version of the CVLT *(34,38)*. The dependent variable used in the present research was the delayed recognition discriminability index (CVLT-discrim).

5.5. Statistical Analysis

Using z-scores based on the performance of a normal control group (n = 18), two indices were created from the four neuropsychological dependent variables described (*see* Table 2). An executive control index was created by averaging the z-scores from the WMS-Mental Control Accuracy Index and total clock drawing errors. A memory/language index was created by averaging the z-scores from the CVLT-discrim index and the animal Association Index. The authors' prediction regarding the dissociation between tests of executive control vs memory/language among patients with mild, moderate, and severe MRI-WMA was tested with a 3 (white matter groups) × 2 (executive control and memory/ language indices) repeated measures analysis of variance (ANOVA). Simple correlations between the Junque leukoaraiosis scale and all neuropsychological measures were also conducted.

6. RESULTS

6.1. Correlation Analyses

Pearson Product Moment correlations between the Junque leukoaraiosis scale indicated little association between the MMSE and the Junque scale (r = –0.220, ns). By contrast, all four neuro-

Table 3
Between-Group Performance on the Executive Control vs Memory/Language Indices: *z*-Scores (Means and Standard Deviations)

	MRI-WMA				
	Mild	Moderate	Severe	Significance	*p*
Executive Control Index (*z*-scores)	–1.4 (.90)	–2.7 (1.6)	–4.5 (1.5)	Mild < moderate	< 0.006
				Mild < severe	< 0.001
				Moderate < severe	< 0.001
Memory/Language Index (*z*-scores)	–3.9 (1.6)	–1.7 (1.5)	–1.4 (.88)	Mild > moderate	< 0.001
				Mild > severe	< 0.001
				Moderate = severe	ns

Abbr: MRI-WMA, periventricular and deep white matter alterations.

psychological variables were significantly related to the severity of MRI-WMA. Thus, as the leukoaraiosis scale increased, patients obtained low scores on the WMS Mental Control Accuracy Index ($r = -0.554$, $p < 0.001$) and made more errors on their clock drawings ($r = 0.531$, $p < 0.001$). Increasing amounts of MRI-WMA also resulted in relatively better scores on the animal fluency Association Index ($r = 0.455$, $p < 0.001$) and on the CVLT-discrim index ($r = 0.348$, $p < 0.001$).

Our prediction regarding the dissociation between executive control vs memory/language test performance across groups of patients with mild, moderate, and severe MRI-WMA was tested with a 3 × 2 repeated measures ANOVA. This analysis yielded a significant two-way interaction (F[4,116] = 22.73, $p < 0.001$). Neither main effect was significant.

6.2. *Between-Group Comparisons*

Between-group follow-up analyses were first conducted with two separate univariate ANOVAs (*see* Table 3). Both of these analyses were highly significant (executive control - F[2, 62] = 27.13, $p < 0.001$; memory/language - F[2, 62] = 19.24, $p < 0.001$). Between-group pairwise comparisons were conducted with Tukey tests (significance – $p < 0.01$). For the executive control index, the mild MRI-WMA group obtained a better score than either the moderate MRI-WMA ($p < 0.006$) or severe MRI-WMA group ($p < 0.001$). Also, the moderate MRI-WMA group obtained a better score than the severe MRI-WMA group ($p < 0.001$).

On the memory/language index, the mild MRI-WMA displayed greater impairment than both the moderate MRI-WMA group ($p < 0.001$) and the severe MRI-WMA group ($p < 0.001$). There was no difference on this index between the moderate and severe MRI-WMA groups.

6.3. *Within-Group Comparisons*

Within-group comparisons were conducted with paired *t*-tests (significance set for $p < 0.01$). Participants in the mild MRI-WMA group obtained a significantly lower score, i.e., demonstrating worse test performance on the memory/language index compared to the executive control index ($t[30] = 8.29$, $p < 0.001$). The opposite profile was observed in the severe MRI-WMA group such that these participants obtained a lower score on the executive control index as compared to the memory/language index ($t[15] = 6.97$, $p < 0.001$). There was no within-group difference between the executive control and memory/language indices in the moderate MRI-WMA group (*see* Table 4).

7. SUMMARY AND CONCLUSIONS

Several conclusions can be drawn from these data. First, increased levels of subcortical MRI-WMA as measured with the Junque leukoaraiosis scale resulted in significant impairment on tests of executive control, whereas performance on tests of memory and language were relatively spared. An

Table 4
Within-Group Performance on the Executive Control vs Memory/Language Indices: *z*-Scores (Means and Standard Deviations)

	Memory/language index	Executive control index	Significance
Mild MRI-WMA Group	−3.9 (1.6)	−1.4 (.90)	$p < 0.001$
Moderate MRI-WMA Group	−1.7 (1.5)	−2.7 (1.6)	ns
Severe MRI WMA Group	−1.4 (.88)	−4.5 (1.5)	$p < 0.001$

Abbr: MRI-WMA, periventricular and deep white matter alterations.

association between subcortical WMA and poor performance on tests of executive control has been described by other researchers *(24)*. The mechanism that underlies the executive control deficits associated with MRI-WMA revolves around problems in establishing and maintaining mental set as operationalized by an increased number of perseverations *(28)* and an increased number of omission and commission errors. These errors occur as participants with dementia attempt to maintain mental set for the task at hand *(31)*.

The correlations between MRI-WMA and performance on the animal AI and CVLT-discrim measures suggest relatively *better* performance on these tests as MRI-WMA increases. This may appear to be counterintuitive. Deficits in memory/semantic organization are, of course, usually associated with AD. One possible explanation for the positive correlations between MRI-WMA and performance on tests of memory/language is that this reflects either the absence or some altered distribution of senile plaques and NFT *(15,16)*. Such a suggestion is controversial and requires greater research.

Second, can these data be used to provide some operational guidelines regarding Erkinjuntti's criteria for the diagnosis of subcortical VaD? From a statistical viewpoint, some interesting relationships between subcortical white matter alterations as measured with the Junque leukoaraiosis scale and neuropsychological tests emerged from the data described above. Between-group, as well as within-group, comparisons regarding the mild MRI-WMA group revealed that performance on the memory/language index was approximately *twice* as impaired as compared to the executive control index. Similar comparisons regarding the severe MRI-WMA group revealed the opposite profile, i.e., their score on the executive index was approximately twice as impaired as compared to the memory/language index. The profile of neuropsychological test performance observed in the moderate MRI-WMA is revealing for two reasons. First, there was no difference in the severity of impairment on tests of executive versus memory/language. Second, as demonstrated by the between-group analyses, executive control test performance becomes more impaired in relation to increasing MRI-WMA, whereas performance on tests of memory/language improves. These data offer further evidence that vascular pathology might be influencing the presence and/or distribution of senile plaques and NFT.

Does this dissociation regarding performance on tests of executive control and memory/language in relation to MRI-WMA provide the basis of an operational definition of subcortical VaD as suggested by Erkinjuntti and colleagues *(46)*? Using the methodology described above, the authors identified 15 patients from their sample of 105 patients who exhibited striking impairment on tests of executive control as compared to memory and language. However, this represents only approximately 15% of the sample. Also, the mean leukoaraiosis score of this group was high (i.e., a mean of 22.07) and represents slightly more than 50% of the total subcortical white matter as measured by the Junque LA scale *(47,48)*. Although it certainly appears that white matter does *matter* for this group of patients, it may be overly conservative to limit the diagnosis of subcortical VaD to these guidelines.

Alternatively, Roman and colleagues *(14)* have suggested that perhaps only 25% of white matter needs to be involved to be judged clinically significant. In terms of the Junque leukoaraiosis scale this would be defined as a score of 10. This guideline is consistent with a mean and standard deviation of the Junque leukoaraiosis scale of the moderate MRI-WMA group (i.e., M = 12.8; SD = 2.3, respectively). As noted above, this group produced equal impairment on tests of executive control vs memory/language. This profile does not necessarily satisfy some of the requirements to diagnose subcortical VaD as suggested by Erkinjuntti and colleagues *(46)*. Nonetheless, a profile of equal impairment on tests of executive control vs memory/language is not what is expected in AD for which a dense anterograde amnesia is the hallmark neuropsychological feature of the disease. Therefore, the authors maintain that a moderate degree of MRI-WMA (i.e., a Junque leukoaraiosis score between 10 and 15 is likely sufficient to alter the neuropsychological presentation of patients with putative AD vs subcortical VaD). They also maintain that this characterization regarding the relationships between neuropsychological test performance and MRI-WMA may be consistent with the findings reported by Nagy and colleagues *(15)* and Snowdon and colleagues *(16)* who have shown that subcortical CVD influences the expression of senile plaques and NFT.

One solution to the problem of diagnosing subcortical VaD might be to diagnose *probable subcortical VaD* when MRI scans indicate severe white matter loss and a striking dissociation on neuropsychological tests of executive control vs memory/language and to diagnose *possible subcortical VaD* when scans show only moderate white matter loss and relatively equal impairment on executive control and memory/language test. However, the authors believe that to set such boundaries is artificial and likely does not represent clinical reality as it exists in nature. Also, trying to graft NINCDS-ADRDA terminology onto the diagnosis of the VaDs has likely created more problems than it has solved.

Another solution to the problem of diagnosing subcortical VaD is to use some combination of neuroradiological and neuropsychological data as a grouping or independent variable without necessarily assigning any diagnostic labels. In their research, the authors used the leukoaraiosis scale of Junque as the means to operationally define subcortical white matter disease. However, they make no claim that this is best or even the optimal method to measure MRI-WMA. Other scales have been proposed *(55–57)*. Indeed, the newly proposed rating scale of Wahlund and colleagues *(57)* has some distinct advantages over other rating scales, including the Junque scale *(47,48)*.

Dementia continues to be a worldwide public health problem. The data presented above suggests that dementia associated with moderate to severe periventricular and deep WMA is associated with a pattern of performance on neuropsychological tests that is distinctly different than AD. The authors' proposal to use neuroradiological criteria as a grouping variable is made to achieve greater diagnostic specificity. Medications for many of the dementias are now available. The authors believe that research combining neuropsychological and neuroradiological data in the manner suggested above might be a powerful tool to predict outcome regarding pharmacological treatment.

REFERENCES

1. Merit HH. A Textbook of Neurology, 5th Ed. Philadelphia, PA: Lea and Febiger, 1973.
2. Katzman R. The prevalence and malignancy of Alzheimer's disease: a major killer. Arch Neurol 1976;33:217–218.
3. Hauw JJ. The history of lacunes. In: Donnan GA, Norrving, B, Bamford, JM, Bogousslavsky J, eds. Lacunar and Other Subcortical Infarctions. New York, NY: Oxford Medical Publications, 1995, pp. 3–15.
4. Hachinski VC, Potter P, Merskey H. Leuko-araiosis. Arch Neurol 1987;44:21–23.
5. Wallin A, Blennow K. Heterogeneity of vascular dementia: Mechanisms and subgroups. J Geriatric Psychiatry Neurol 1993;6:177–188.
6. Blass JP, Hoyer S, Nitsch RA. Translation of Otto Binswanger's article, The Delineation of the Generalized Progressive Paralyses. Arch Neurol 1991;48:961.
7. Schorer CE, Rodin E. Binswanger's disease: a complete translation. J Geriatric Psychiatric Neurol 1990;3:61–66.
8. Roman GC. A historical review of the concept of vascular dementia: Lessons from the past for the future. Alzheimer Dis Assoc Disord 1999;13(Suppl 3):S4–S8.
9. Olszewski J. Subcortical arteriosclerotic encephalopathy. Word Neurol 1965;3:359–313.
10. Caplan LR, Schoene W. Clinical features of subcortical arteriosclerotic encephalopathy (Binswanger's disease). Neurology 1978;28:1206–1215.

11. Hachinski VC, Lassen NA, Marshall J. Multi-Infarct dementia: a cause of mental deterioration in the elderly. Lancet 1974;27:207.
12. Hachinski VC, Iliff LD, Zilhka E, et al. Cerebral blood flow in dementia. Arch Neurol 1975;32:632–637.
13. Chui H, Victoroff J, Margolin D, Jagust W, Shankle R, Katzman R. Criteria for the diagnosis of ischemic vascular dementia proposed by the State of California Alzheimer's Disease Diagnostic and Treatment Centers. Neurology 1992; 42:473–480.
14. Roman GC, Tatemichi TK, Erkinjuntti T, et al. Vascular dementia: diagnostic criteria for research studies. Report of the NINDS-AIREN international workshop. Neurology 1993;43:250–260.
15. Nagy Z, Esir, MM, Jobst KA, et al. The effects of additional pathology on the cognitive deficits in Alzheimer disease. J Neuropathol Exper Neurol 1997;56:165–170.
16. Snowdon DA, Greiner LH, Mortimer JA, Riley KP, Greiner PA, Markesbery WR. Brain infarction and the clinical expression of Alzheimer disease. The Nun Study. JAMA 1997;277:813–817.
17. Victoroff J, Mack WJ, Lyness SA, Chui HC. Multicenter clinicopathological correlation in dementia. Amer J Psychiatry 1995;152:1476–1484.
18. Bowler JV, Munoz DG, Hachinski VH. Fallacies in the pathological confirmation of the diagnosis of Alzheimer's disease. J Neurol Neurosurg Psychiatry 1998;64:18–24.
19. Crystal HA, Dickson D, Davies P, Masur D, Grober E, Lipton RB. The relative frequency of Dementia of Unknown Aetiology' increases with age and is nearly 50% in nonagenarians. Arch Neurol 2000;57:713–719.
20. de la Torre JC. Alzheimer's disease as a vascular disorder: nosological evidence. Stroke 2002;33:1152–1162.
21. Ishii N, Nishihara Y, Imamura T. Why do frontal lobe symptoms predominate in vascular dementia with lacunes? Neurology 1986;36:340–345.
22. Libon DJ, Bogdanoff B, Bonavita J, et al. Neuropsychological deficits associated with Ischaemic Vascular Dementia caused by periventricular and deep white matter alterations. Arch Clin Neuropsychol 1997;12:239–250.
23. Libon DJ, Bogdanoff B, Swenson R, et al. Neuropsychological profile associated with subcortical white matter alterations and Parkinson's disease: implications for the diagnosis of dementia. Arch Clin Neuropsychol 2001;16:19–32.
24. Looi CL, Sachdev PS. Differentiation of vascular dementia from Alzheimer's disease on neuropsychological tests. Neurology 1999;53:670–678.
25. Owen AM, James M, Leigh PN, et al. Fronto-striatal cognitive deficits at different stages of Parkinson's disease. Brain 1992;115:1727–1751.
26. Beiser DG, Houk JC. Model of cortical-basal ganglionic processing: encoding the serial order of events. J Neurophysiol 1998;79:3168–3188.
27. Frank MJ, Loughry B, O'Reilly RC. Interactions between frontal cortex and basal ganglia in working memory. Cogn Affect Behav Neurosci 2001;1:137–160.
28. Lamar M, Podell K, Carew TG, et al. Perseverative behavior in Alzheimer's disease and subcortical ischaemic vascular dementia. Neuropsychology 1997;11:523–534.
29. Giovannetti T, Lamar M, Cloud BS, et al. Different underlying mechanisms for deficits in concept formation in dementia. Arch Clin Neuropsychol 2001;16:547–560.
30. Libon DJ, Malamut BL, Swenson R, Cloud BS. Further analyses of clock drawings among demented and non-demented subjects. Arch Clin Neuropsychol 1996;11:193–211.
31. Lamar M, Price C, Davis K, Kaplan E, Libon DJ. Capacity to maintain mental set in dementia. Neuropsychologia 2002; 40:435–445.
32. Luria AR. Higher Cortical Functions in Man. 2nd Ed. New York, NY: Basic Books Inc., 1980.
33. Bernard BA, Wilson RS, Gilley DW, Bennett DA, Fox JH. Memory failure in Binswanger's disease and Alzheimer's disease. Clin Neuropsychologist 1992;6:230–240.
34. Libon DJ, Mattson RE, Glosser G, et al. A nine word dementia version of the California Verbal Learning Test. Clin Neuropsychologist 1996;10:237–244.
35. Libon DJ, Bogdanoff B, Cloud BS, et al. Motor learning and quantitative measures of the hippocampus and subcortical white alterations in Alzheimer's disease and Ischaemic Vascular Dementia. J Clin Exp Neuropsychol 1998;20: 30–41.
36. Tierney MC, Black SE, Szalai JP, et al. Recognition memory and verbal fluency differentiate probable Alzheimer's disease from subcortical ischemic vascular dementia. Arch Neurol 2001;58:1654–1659.
37. Lafosse JM, Reed BR, Mungas D, Sterling SB, Wahbeh H, Jagust WJ. Fluency and memory differences between ischemic vascular dementia and Alzheimer's disease. Neuropsychology 1997;11:514–522.
38. Delis DC, Kramer JH, Kaplan E, Ober BA. The California Verbal Learning Test. New York, NY: Psychology Corporation, 1987.
39. Delis DC, Massman PJ, Butters N, Salmon DP, Cermak LS, Kramer JH. Profiles of demented and amnesic patients on the California Verbal Learning Test: implications for the assessment for the assessment of memory disorders. Psychol Assess 1991;3:19–26.
40. Kramer JH, Delis DC, Blusewicz MJ, Brandt J, Ober BA, Strauss M. Verbal memory errors in Alzheimer's and Huntington's dementias. Devel Neuropsychol 1988;4:1–15.

41. Massman PJ, Delis DC, Butters N, Levin B, Salmon DP. Are all subcortical dementias alike? Verbal learning and memory in Parkinson's and Huntington's disease patient's. J Clin Exp Neuropsychol 1990;12:729–744.
42. Davis KL, Price C, Kaplan E, Libon DJ. Error analysis of the nine-word California Verbal Learning Test (CVLT-9) among older adults with and without dementia. Clin Neuropsychologist 2002;16:81–89.
43. Carew TG, Lamar M, Cloud BS, Grossman M, Libon DJ. Impairment in category fluency in ischaemic vascular dementia. Neuropsychology 1997;11:400–412.
44. Alexander GE, DeLong MR, Strick PL. Parallel organization of functionally segregated circuits linking basal ganglia and cortex. Annu Rev Neurosci 1986;9:357–381.
45. Sultzer DL, Mahler ME, Cummings J, Van Gorp WG, Hinkin CH, Brown C. Cortical abnormalities associated with subcortical lesins in vascular dementia. Arch Neurol 1995;52:773–780.
46. Erkinjuntti T, Inzitari D, Pantoni L, et al. Research criteria for subcortical vascular dementia in clinical trials. J Neurotrans 2000;59:23–30.
47. Junque C, Pujol J, Vendrell P, et al. Leukoaraiosis on magnetic resonance imaging and speed of mental processing. Arch Neurol 1990;47:151–156.
48. Pujol J, Junque C, Vendrell P, Capdevila A, Marti-Vilalta JL. Cognitive correlates of ventricular enlargement in vascular patients with leuko-ariosis. Acta Neurologica Scand 1991;84:237–242.
49. McKhann G, Drachman D, Folstein MF, Katzman R, Price DS, Stadlan EM. Clinical diagnosis of Alzheimer's disease: report of the NINCDS-ADRDA work group under the auspices of the Department of Health and Human Services Task Force on Alzheimer's Disease. Neurology 1984;34:939–943.
50. Folstein MF, Folstein SE, McHugh PR. Mini-Mental State: a practical method for grading the cognitive state of patients for the clinician. J Psychiatric Res 1975;12:189–198.
51. Yesavage J. The use of self-rating depression scales in the elderly. In: L.W. Poon, ed. Handbook of Clinical Memory Assessment of Older Adults. Washington, DC: American Psychological Association, 1986, pp. 213–217.
52. Wechsler D. A standardized memory scale for clinical use. J Psychol 1945;19:87–95.
53. Goodglass H, Kaplan E. The Boston Diagnostic Aphasia Examination. Philadelphia, PA: Lea and Febiger, 1984.
54. Monsch AU, Bondi MW, Butters N, et al. A comparison of category and letter in Alzheimer's and Huntington's disease. Neuropsychology 1994;8:25–30.
55. Schelton PH, Barkhof F, Valk J, et al.. White matter lesions on magnetic resonance imaging in clinically diagnosed Alzheimer's disease. Brain 1992;115:735–748.
56. Ylikoski R, Ylikoski A, Erkinjuntti T, Sulkava R, Raininko R, Tilvis R. White matter changes in healthy elderly persons correlate with attention and speed of mental processing. Arch Neurol 1993;50:818–824.
57. Wahlund LO, Barkhof F, Fazekas F, et al. A new rating scale for age-related white matter changes applicable to MRI and CT. Stroke 2001;32:1318–1322.

VI Clinical Management of Vascular Dementia

22

Pharmacological Treatment of Vascular Dementia

Timo Erkinjuntti, Gustavo Román, Serge Gauthier, and Kenneth Rockwood

1. INTRODUCTION

Disease expression in vascular dementia (VaD) is heterogeneous and provides several potential targets for treatment, including (1) symptomatic improvement of the core symptoms (cognition, function, and behavior), (2) slowing of progression, and (3) treatment of secondary manifestation that affect cognition (e.g., depression, anxiety, and agitation) *(1)*.

In patients with dementia—defined as having decline in two or more intellectual domains with clinically significant effect on daily life activities—the treatment targets are those traditionally defined for Alzheimer's disease (AD) both in clinical research and in practice: control existing symptoms, facilitate adjustment to current disability, and slow progression to more severe stages *(1)*. Current VaD trials have closely used the instruments used in AD trials as recommended by the US Food and Drug Administration (FDA) regulatory specifications *(2)*. The instruments adopted as primary outcome measures for the current generation of clinical trials include the cognitive portion of the Alzheimer's Disease Assessment Scale (ADAS-Cog), the Clinician's Interview-Based Impression of change plus caregiver input (CIBIC-plus), or the Clinical Global Impression of Change (CGIC) *(3)*. The European Commission for Medicinal and Pharmaceutical Compounds (CPMC) mostly requires positive effect on activities of daily living (ADLs) and a responder analysis. To the extent that ADAS-cog and CIBIC-plus measures have proved to be sensitive in AD trials after the cholinergic hypothesis and to the extent that the cholinergic hypothesis is being endorsed in VaD, it is not unreasonable to use the same measures in both patient populations. On the other hand, the CIBIC-plus might be particularly difficult to apply in VaD, a condition with unclear rates of decline and greater variability of disease course. Recently, Quinn et al. *(4)* showed that physicians have most difficulty with CIBIC-plus ratings in AD in the face of clinical improvement. The cause is not entirely clear, but physicians lack a good model of successful disease treatment beyond reversal of the untreated natural history of progression. This is likely to be an even greater problem in VaD, as illustrated in a recently reported clinical trial of memantine in VaD. The ADAS-cog, the primary cognitive outcome measure, was strongly positive, whereas the CIBIC did not reach significance *(5)*.

Moreover, the current tests are relatively insensitive to frontal/subcortical dysfunction, which is likely to be a key cognitive domain, particularly in VaD *(6–8)* This has given rise to proposals to incorporate such testing in future clinical trials and to the development of the vascular equivalent of the ADAS-cog, the VaDAS-cog *(3)*. One of the shortcomings of these trials was the absence of formal measurement of executive function; however, ADLs have been considered a proxy evaluation of executive function. Pohjasvaara et al. *(8)* confirmed that executive dysfunction was the main

From: *Current Clinical Neurology*
Vascular Dementia: Cerebrovascular Mechanisms and Clinical Management
Edited by: R. H. Paul, R. Cohen, B. R. Ott, and S. Salloway © Humana Press Inc., Totowa, NJ

determinant of abnormalities in both basic ADLs and independent ADLs (IADLs) in patients with poststroke VaD. Executive function tests, including IADLs, may be sensitive tools for the diagnosis of VaD and could accurately measure the effects of potential therapies.

The role of mood and behavioral symptoms in VaD studies remains to be clarified to define its use as outcome measures in VaD trials *(9)*. Their rates of emergence and patterns of symptomatic involvement across the continuum of VaD are unclear. Their current use requires assumptions of uncertain validity and in consequence is inappropriate as primary outcome measure.

Much the same can be said about functional ability *(10)*. In contrast to AD, where there are predictable hierarchical losses in ADLs in association with cognitive decline, functional losses in VaD may be more discordant. The heterogeneity of subtypes of VaD and functional rates of decline are not well characterized, again making their use as a primary outcome measure premature. The separation of functional decline related directly to sequelae of stroke may have different significance to functional decline evolving out of disordered cognitive function. The current generation of AD scales do not allow this distinction to be made.

2. HISTORY OF PHARMACOTHERAPY IN VaD

Published data on interventions for patients with dementia believed to have a vascular component go back for decades. The American physician Arthur C. Walsh published on an "anticoagulant-psychotherapy" intervention for a broadly constructed "senility" in which he claimed notable success *(11)*. A vascular etiology, or at least pathogenesis, also underlies the use of several compounds purported to be useful in the symptomatic treatment of VaD. These included antithrombotics, ergot alkaloids, nosotropics, TRH-analog, *Ginkgo biloba* extract, plasma viscosity drugs, hyperbaric oxygen, antioxidants, serotonin and histamine receptor antagonists, vasoactive agents, xanthine derivatives, and calcium antagonists *(1,12–15)*. These studies have mostly had negative results, were based on small numbers, had short treatment periods, had variations in diagnostic criteria and tools, often included mixed populations, and have had variations in the application of clinical endpoints. Currently, there is no widely accepted standard symptomatic treatment of VaD *(12)*. Two drugs that were carefully studied are propentofylline *(16)* and nimodipine *(17)*.

Propentofylline, a glial modulator, is no longer under study, despite its observed beneficial effect on learning and memory *(18)*. Unpublished results of several European and Canadian double-blind, placebo-controlled, randomized, parallel group trials on the efficacy and safety of long-term treatment with propentofylline, compared with placebo, in patients with mild to moderate VaD according to National Institute of Neurological Disorders and Stroke-Association Internationale pour la Recherche et l'Enseignement en Neurosciences (NINDS-AIREN)criteria *(19)* have been shown as a poster *(20)*. This 24-wk study showed a significant symptomatic improvement and long-term efficacy in ADAS-Cog and CIBIC-plus up to 48 wk. In addition, sustained treatment effects for at least 12 wk after withdrawal were present suggesting an effect on disease progression.

Nimodipine, a dihydropyridine calcium-antagonist, was used in subcortical VaD. Nimodipine is held to effect vasodilatation, without a steal effect, to reduce the influx of calcium ions into depolarized neurons. Consequently, it is believed to have a neuroprotective effect that is not directly related to changes in cerebral blood flow (CBF). In addition, the drug has a specific effect on small vessels. Encouraging results from an open-label trial *(17)* led to a subgroup analysis of a larger double-blind, placebo-controlled study known as the Scandinavian Multi-Infarct Dementia trial. Patients were divided between multiinfarct dementia (MID) and subcortical VaD groups, according to computed tomography (CT) findings and were blindly assessed. Nimodipine had a beneficial effect on attention and psychomotor performances in the subcortical group, although no clear advantage was seen in the combined sample *(21,22)*. These preliminary results are currently being tested in an international, multi-center, randomized, double-blind trial enrolling patients with subcortical VaD, defined on a clinical-radiological basis *(23)*. Currently, the Cochrane Collaboration review concluded that there is no convincing evidence that nimodipine is a useful treatment for the symptoms of VaD *(24)*.

3. CURRENT TREATMENT OF VaD

Presently, there is evidence-based data that two types of drugs modulating neurotransmission abnormalities are useful in treating VaD; these neurotransmitter abnormalities are acetylcholine deficit (acetylcholinesterase inhibitors [AChEIs]) and glutamate excess (memantine).

Memantine is a moderate-affinity, voltage-dependent, uncompetitive *N*-methyl-D-aspartate (NMDA) receptor antagonist with fast receptor kinetics *(25)*. Initial data from a double-blind, placebo-controlled nursing home trial in severe dementia of mixed etiology (51% of patients had VaD), showed that memantine (10 mg/d) was well tolerated, improved function, and reduced care dependency in treated patients with severe dementia, compared to patients on placebo *(26)*. Based on the hypothesis of glutamate-induced neurotoxicity in cerebral ischemia, two randomized, placebo-controlled 6-mo trials have studied memantine (20 mg/d) in patients with mild to moderate probable NINDS-AIREN VaD *(5,27)*.

The study MMM 300 randomized 147 patients on memantine and 141 on placebo *(5)*. After 28 wk, the mean ADAS-cog scores were significantly improved relative to placebo: the memantine group mean score had gained an average of 0.4 points, whereas the placebo group mean score declined by 1.6, i.e., a difference of 2.0 points ($p = 0.0016$). The response rate for CIBIC-plus, defined as improved or stable, was 60% with memantine, compared with 52% with placebo ($p = 0.227$). The Gottfries-Bråne-Steen (GBS) Scale and the Nurses' Observation Scale for Geriatric Patients (NOSGER) total scores at week 28 did not differ significantly between the two groups. However, the GBS Scale *intellectual function* subscore and the NOSGER *disturbing behavior* dimension also showed a difference in favor of memantine ($p = 0.04$ and $p = 0.07$, respectively).

A total of 277 patients were randomized on memantine and 271 on placebo in the MMM 500 study *(27)*. At 28 wk, the active group had gained 0.53 and placebo declined by 2.28 points in ADAS-cog, a significant difference of 1.75 ADAS-cog points between the groups ($p < 0.05$). The global assessment CGIC, the MMSE, GBS, or NOSGER did not reveal differences between the groups. Memantine was well tolerated in the two studies. In a post-hoc pooled subgroup analysis of these two studies by baseline severity as assessed by MMSE, the more advanced patients obtained a larger cognitive benefit than did the mildly affected patients. The subgroup with an MMSE score less than 15 at baseline showed an ADAS-cog improvement of 3.2 points over placebo *(28)*. Subgroup analyses by radiological findings at baseline showed that the cognitive treatment effect for memantine was more pronounced in the small-vessel type group of patients who had no signs of cortical infarctions in their brain scans (CT or magnetic resonance imaging [MRI]). In addition, the placebo decline in this group was clearly more pronounced than in patients with (cortical) large-vessel type VaD *(29)*.

4. CHOLINERGIC DYSFUNCTION IN VaD

Cholinergic deficit in VaD, independently of any concomitant AD pathology, has been documented. Cholinergic structures are vulnerable to ischemic damage. Indeed, hippocampal CA1 neurons are particularly susceptible to experimental ischemia, and hippocampal atrophy is common in patients with VaD in the absence of AD *(30)*. Selden et al. *(31)* described two highly organized and discrete bundles of cholinergic fibers in human brains that extend from the nucleus basalis to the cerebral cortex and amygdala. Both pathways travel in the white matter and together carry widespread cholinergic input to the neocortex. Localized strokes may interrupt these cholinergic bundles. Mesulam et al. *(32)* demonstrated cholinergic denervation from pathway lesions, in the absence of AD, in a young patient with cerebral autosomal dominant arteriopathy with subcortical infarcts and leukoencephalopathy (CADASIL), a pure genetic form of VaD.

In experimental rodent models, such as the spontaneously hypertensive stroke-prone rat, there is a significant reduction in cholinergic markers including acetylcholine (ACh) in the neocortex, hippocampus, and cerebrospinal fluid (CSF) *(33)*. White matter infarction in rodent models results in substantial decreases in cholinergic markers, presumably through an impact on cholinergic projection fibers *(34)*. In human disease, there is a reported loss of cholinergic neurons in 70% of AD cases and in 40% of patients with VaD examined neuropathologically and reduced ACh activity in the cortex, hippocampus, striatum, and CSF *(35)*.

5. CHOLINESTERASE INHIBITORS IN VaD

Four cholinesterase inhibitors (AChEIs) have been approved for use in AD: tacrine, donepezil, rivastigmine, and galantamine. In controlled trials, secondary outcomes have varied but often included ADL and behavioral scales. Studies have shown a modest improvement of cognition peaking at 3 mo and decline below the baseline or staring point at 9 to 12 mo. There is good evidence for stabilization of ADL decline for at least 6 mo and improvement of some behaviors associated with AD (predominantly apathy and hallucinations). A description of reasonable therapeutic expectations was published by Winblad et al. *(36)*.

5.1. *Donepezil*

The safety and efficacy of *donepezil* has been studied in the largest clinical trial of pure VaD to date *(37)*. A total of 1,219 subjects were recruited for a 24-wk, randomized, placebo-controlled, multicenter, multinational study divided in two identical trials, 307 *(38)* and 308 *(38,39)*. The patients were randomized to one of three groups: placebo, donepezil 5 mg/d, or donepezil 10 mg/d. The group receiving 10 mg/d initially received 5 mg/d for 4 wk; the dosage was then titrated up to 10 mg/d. Patients with a diagnosis of either possible or probable VaD according to the NINDS-AIREN criteria were eligible for inclusion in the study *(19)*. All patients had brain imaging before the study (CT or MRI) with demonstration of relevant cerebrovascular lesions. Patients with pre-existing AD were excluded, as were patients with the so-called mixed dementia, better defined as AD *plus* CVD. Although patients with concomitant AD may not be totally excluded, the NINDS-AIREN criteria are able to classify patients into probable or possible VaD categories.

Probable VaD was present in 73% of the patients in the two studies. Probable VaD was diagnosed by the presence of mild to moderate dementia, clinical and brain imaging evidence of relevant CVD, and a clear temporal relationship between stroke and cognitive decline, with onset of dementia within 3 mo of a clinically eloquent stroke or a stepwise course. Possible VaD was diagnosed in cases with indolent onset of the cognitive decline and accounted for 27% of the cases. Possible VaD included patients with silent stroke, extensive white matter disease, or an atypical clinical course. There were no differences in trial results between these two subgroups.

Compared with placebo, both donepezil treatment groups showed statistically significant improvement in cognitive functioning measured with the ADAS-cog; the mean changes from baseline score were: donepezil 5 mg/d, –1.90 ($p = 0.001$); donepezil 10 mg/d, –2.33 ($p < 0.001$). The MMSE also showed statistically significant improvement vs placebo. The treated group showed equally significant improvement in global function on the CIBIC-plus and on the CDR-SB. The ADLs showed significant benefits in donepezil-treated patients over placebo using the ADFACS, a measurement of both basic and instrumental ADLs.

Of interest, cognitive decline in untreated patients with VaD in this trial was less severe than in placebo-treated patients with AD during 24 wk of study using similar instruments. These differences were also noted for global effects, measured by the CIBIC-plus version, and, in contrast with AD, patients with VaD showed improvements in global function. In contrast with AD trials, these VaD studies enrolled more men than women (58 vs 38%), their mean age was older (74.5 ± 0.2 vs 72 ± 0.2 yr), and their HIS score more elevated (6.6 ± 0.2 vs < 4), with higher percentages of subjects with hypertension, CVD, diabetes, smoking, hypercholesterolemia, previous stroke, and transient ischemic attacks, suggesting that the two populations are clearly different *(37)*.

Donepezil was generally well tolerated, although more adverse effects were reported in the 10-mg group than in the 5-mg or placebo groups. The adverse effects were assessed as mild to moderate and transient and typically included diarrhea, nausea, arthralgia, leg cramps, anorexia, and headache. The incidence of bradycardia and syncope was not significantly different from the placebo group. The discontinuation rates for the groups were 15% for placebo, 18% for the 5-mg group, and 28% for the 10-mg group. There was no significant interaction with the numerous cardiovascular medications and antithrombotic agents used by this population. Donepezil was effective and well tolerated in the treatment of patients with VaD.

5.2. Galantamine

Galantamine is a cholinesterase inhibitor that also modulates central nicotinic receptors to increase cholinergic neurotransmission. In a randomized, controlled trial, patients diagnosed with probable VaD or with AD combined with CVD received galantamine 24 mg/d ($n = 396$) or placebo ($n = 196$) in a multicenter, double-blind, 6-mo trial *(40)*. Eligible patients met the clinical criteria of probable VaD of the NINDS-AIREN *(19)* or possible AD according to the NINCDS-ADRDA *(41)*. They also showed significant radiological evidence of CVD on CT or MR (i.e., they had AD and CVD). Evidence of CVD on a recent (within 12 mo) scan included multiple large-vessel infarcts or a single, strategically placed infarct (angular gyrus, thalamus, basal forebrain, or territory of the posterior or anterior cerebral artery), or at least two basal ganglia and white-matter lacunae or white-matter changes involving at least 25% of the total white matter. They had to score 10–25 on the MMSE and 12 or more in the ADAS-cog/11 and had to be between ages of 40 and 90 yr.

Primary endpoints were cognition, as measured using the ADAS-cog/11 and global functioning as measured using the CIBIC-plus. Secondary endpoints included assessments of ADLs, using the Disability Assessment in Dementia (DAD), and behavioral symptoms, using the Neuropsychiatric Inventory (NPI) *(40)*.

Analyzing both groups as a whole, galantamine demonstrated efficacy on all outcome measures. Galantamine showed greater efficacy than placebo on ADAS-cog (2.7 points, $p \leq 0.001$) and CIBIC-plus (74 vs 59% of patients remained stable or improved, $p \leq 0.001$). ADLs and behavioral symptoms were also significantly improved compared with placebo (both $p < 0.05$). Galantamine was well tolerated *(40)*. In an open-label extension, the original galantamine group of patients with probable VaD or AD plus CVD showed similar sustained benefits in maintenance of or improvement in cognition (ADS-cog), functional ability (DAD), and behavior (NPI) after 12 mo *(42)*.

Although the study was not designed to detect differences between subgroups, the subgroup of patients with AD plus CVD on galantamine ($n = 188$, 48%) showed greater efficacy than placebo ($n = 97$, 50%) at 6 mo on ADAS-cog ($p \leq 0.001$) and CIBIC-plus ($p = 0.019$) *(40)*. In the open-label extension, patients with AD plus CVD continuously treated with galantamine maintained cognitive abilities at baseline for 12 mo *(43)*.

Probable VaD was diagnosed in 81 (41%) of the placebo patients and in 171 (43%) of the patients on galantamine. In the probable VaD group, ADAS-cog scores improved significantly (mean change from baseline, 2.4 points, $p < 0.0001$) in patients treated with galantamine for 6 mo but not in the patients treated with placebo (mean change from baseline, 0.4; treatment difference vs galantamine 1.9, $p = 0.06$) *(40,44)*. More patients treated with galantamine than with placebo maintained or improved global function (CIBIC-plus, 31% vs 23%); however, it was not statistically significant. In these patients, the cognitive benefits of galantamine were maintained at least up to 12 mo, demonstrating a mean change of –2.1 in the ADAS-cog score compared to baseline *(43)* and the active group was still close baseline at 24 mo *(45)*.

5.3. Rivastigmine

Rivastigmine is an acetylcholinesterase and butyrylcholinesterase inhibitor. The effects of rivastigmine in the treatment of cognitive impairment associated with general VaD remain to be established. In a small study of patients with subcortical VaD, rivastigmine improved cognition (clock-drawing test), reduced caregiver stress, and improved behavior *(46,47)*. Patients with AD with vascular risk factors showed relatively larger effect size in cognitive response (ADAS-cog) than those without vascular risk factors *(48,49)*.

6. CONCLUSIONS

Rigorous control of vascular risk factors is important in primary and secondary prevention of VaD and may be important in ameliorating disease expression in those with mild VaD. Numerous controlled clinical trials on VaD using donepezil, galantamine, and memantine are available. However, as of November 2003, none has obtained approved indication by the Food and Drug Administration or the CPMC. More effective therapies are needed, perhaps using combinations of memantine plus Aches, as well as neuroprotective agents.

REFERENCES

1. Rockwood K, Gauthier S, Erkinjuntti T. Prevention and treatment of vascular dementia. In: Erkinjuntti T, Gauthier S, eds. Vascular Cognitive Impairment. London, UK: Martin Duniz Ltd, 2002, pp. 587–595.
2. Sawada T, Whitehouse PJ. Regulatory guidelines for antidementia drugs. In: Erkinjuntti T, Gauthier S, eds. Vascular Cognitive Impairment. London, UK: Martin Duniz Ltd, 2002, pp. 619–627.
3. Ferris S, Gauthier S. Cognitive outcome measures in vascular dementia. In: Erkinjuntii T, Gauthier S, eds. Vascular Cognitive Impairment. London, UK: Martin Duniz Ltd, 2002, pp. 395–400.
4. Quinn J, Moore M, Benson DF, et al. A videotaped CIBIC for dementia patients: validity and reliability in simulated clinical trial. Neurology 2002;58(3):433–437.
5. Orgogozo J-M., Rigaud A-S., Stöffler A, Möbius H-J, Forette F. Efficacy and safety of Memantine in patients with mild to moderate vascular dementia. A randomized, placebo-controlled trial (MMM 300). Stroke 2002;33:1834–1839.
6. Royall D, Roman G. Executive control function: a rational basis for the diagnosis of vascular dementia. Alzheimer Dis Assoc Disord 1999;13(Suppl 3):69–80.
7. Royall DR. Executive cognitive impairment: a novel perspective on dementia. Neuroepidemiology 2000;19:293–299.
8. Pohjasvaara T, Leskelä M, Vataja R, et al. Post-stroke depression, executive dysfunction and functional outcome. Eur J Neurol 2002;9:269–275.
9. Chui E, Yastrubetskaya O, Williams M. Pharmacotherapy of mood and behavior symptoms. In: Erkinjuntti T, Gauthier S, eds. Vascular Cognitive Impairment. London, UK: Martin Duniz Ltd., 2002, pp. 597–605.
10. Gauthier S, Gélinas I. Evaluation of daily activities in vascular cognitive impairment. In: Erkinjuntti T, Gauthier S, eds. Vascular Cognitive Impairment. London, UK: Martin Duniz Ltd., 2002, pp. 411–416.
11. Walsh AC, Walsh BH, Melaney C. Senile-presenile dementia: follow-up data on an effective psychotherapy-anticoagulant regimen. J Am Geriatr Soc 1978;26:467–470.
12. Doody RS, Stevens JC, Beck C, et al. Practice parameter: management of dementia (an evidence-based review). Report of the Quality Standards Subcommittee of the American Academy of Neurology. Neurology 2001;56:1154–1166.
13. Erkinjuntti T, Rockwood K. Vascular cognitive impairment. Psychogeriatrics 2001;1:27–38.
14. Erkinjuntti T. Cerebrovascular dementia. Pathophysiology, diagnosis and treatment. CNS Drugs 1999;12:35–48.
15. Inzitari D, Lamassa M, Pantoni L. Treatment of vascular dementias. In: Bowler JV, Hachinski V, eds. Vascular Cognitive Impairment Preventable Dementia. Oxford, UK: Oxford University Press, Oxford, 2003, pp. 277–292.
16. Rother M, Erkinjuntti T, Roessner M, Kittner B, Marcusson J, Karlsson I. Propentofylline in the treatment of Alzheimer's disease and vascular dementia. Dementia Geriatr Cogn Disord 1998;9(Suppl 1):36–43.
17. Pantoni L, Carosi M, Amigoni S, Mascalchi M, Inzitari D. A preliminary open trial with nimodipine in patients with cognitive impairment and leukoaraiosis. Clin Neuropharmacol 1996;19:497–506.
18. Mielke R, Möller H-J, Erkinjunti T, Rosenkranz B, Rother M, Kittner B. Propentofylline in the treatment of vascular dementia and Alzheimer-type dementia: overview of phase I and phase II clinical trials. Alzheimer Dis Assoc Disord 1998;12(Suppl 2):29–35.
19. Roman GC, Tatemichi TK, Erkinjuntti T, et al. Vascular dementia: diagnostic criteria for research studies. Report of the NINDS-AIREN International Work Group. Neurology 1993;43:250–260.
20. Pischel T. Long-term-efficacy and safety of propentofylline in patients with vascular dementia. Results of a 12-month placebo-controlled trial [abstract]. Neurobiol Aging 1998;19(Suppl):S182.
21. Pantoni L, Rossi R, Inzitari D, et al. Efficacy and safety of nimodipine in subcortical vascular dementia: a subgroup analysis of the Scandinavian multi-infarct dementia trial. J Neurol Sci 2000;175:124–134.
22. Pantoni L, Bianchi C, Beneke M, Inzitari D, Wallin A, Erkinjunti T. The Scandinavian multi-infarct dementia trial: a double-blind, placebo-controlled trial on nimodipine in multi-infarct dementia. J Neurol Sci 2000;175:116–123.
23. Erkinjuntti T, Inzitari D, Pantoni L, et al. Research criteria for subcortical vascular dementia in clinical trials. J Neural Transm 2000;59(Suppl):23–30.

24. Lopez-Arieta BJ. Nimodipine for primary degenerative, mixed and vascular dementia. Cochrane Database Sys Rev 2001;1:CD000147.
25. Görtelmeyer R, Erbler H. Memantine in treatment of mild to moderate dementia syndrome. Drug Res 1992;42:904–912.
26. Winblad B, Poritis N. Clinical improvement in a placebo-controlled trial with memantine in care-dependent patients with severe dementia [abstract]. Neurobiol Aging 1998;19(Suppl):S303.
27. Wilcock G, Möbius HJ, Stöffler A, on behalf of the MMM 500 group. A double-blind, placebo-controlled multicentre study of memantine in mild to moderate vascular dementia (MMM500). Intl Clin Psychopharmacol 2002;17:297–305.
28. Möbius HJ, Stöffler A. Memantine in vascular dementia. Intl Psychogeriatrics 2003;15(Suppl 1):207–213.
29. Möbius HJ, Stöffler A. New approaches to clinical trials in vascular dementia: Memantine in small vessel disease. Cerebrovasc Dis 2002;13(Suppl 2):61–66.
30. Vinters HV, Ellis WG, Zarow C, et al. Neuropathologic substrates of ischemic vascular dementia. J Neuropathol Exp Neurol 2000;60:658–659.
31. Selden NR, Gitelman DR, Salamon-Murayama N, Parrsh TB, Mesulam MM. Trajectories of cholinergic pathways within the cerebral hemispheres of the human brain. Brain 1998;121:2249–2257.
32. Mesulam M, Siddique T, Cohen B. Cholinergic denervation in a pure multi-infarct state: observations on CADASIL. Neurology 2003;60:1183–1185.
33. Togashi H, Matsumoto K, Yoshida M. Neurochemical profiles in cerebrospinal fluid of stroke-prone spontaneously hypertensive rat. Neurosci Lett 1994;166:117–120.
34. Freidle RL. A comparative histochemical mapping of the distribution of butyrylcholinesterase in the brains of four species of animals, including man. Acta Anat (Basel) 1967;66:161–177.
35. Court JA, Perry EK, Kalaria RN. Neurotransmitter control of the cerebral vasculature and abnormalities in vascular dementia. In: Erkinjuntti T, Gauthier S, eds. Vascular Cognitive Impairment. London, UK: Martin Duniz Ltd., 2002, pp. 167–185.
36. Winblad B, Brodaty H, Gauthier S, et al. Pharmacotherapy of Alzheimer's disease: is there a need to redefine treatment success ? Intl J Geriatr Psychiatry 2001;16:388–390.
37. Pratt RD, Perdomo CA, the Donepezil VaD 307 and 308 Study Groups. Donepezil-treated patients with probable vascular dementia demonstrate cognitive benefits. Ann N Y Acad Sci 2002;977:513–522.
38. Black S, Roman GC, Geldmacher DS, et al. Efficacy and tolerability of Donepezil in vascular dementia. Positive results of a 24-week, multicenter, international, randomized, placebo-controlled clinical trial. Stroke 2003;34:2323–2332.
39. Wilkinson D, Doody R, Helme R, et al. Donepezil in vascular dementia. A randomized, placebo-controlled study. Neurology 2003;61:479–486.
40. Erkinjunti T, Kurz A, Gauthier S, Bullock R, Lilienfeld S, Chandrasekharrao VD. Efficacy of galantamine in probable vascular dementia and Alzheimer's disease combined with cerebrovascular disease: a randomised trial. J Am Ger Soc 2002;359:1283–1290.
41. McKhann G, Drachman D, Folstein M, Katzman R, Price D, Stadlan EM. Clinical diagnosis of Alzheimer's disease: report of the NINCDS-ADRDA Work Group under the auspices of Department of Health and Human Services Task Force on Alzheimer's Disease. Neurology 1984;34:939–944.
42. Erkinjuntti T, Kurz A, Small GW, Bullock R, Lilienfeld S, Damaraju CV. An open-label extension trial of galantamine in patients with probable vascular dementia and mixed dementia. Clin Ther 2003;25:1765–1782.
43. Small G, Erkinjuntti T, Kurz A, Lilienfeld S. Galantamine in the treatment of cognitive decline in patients with vascular dementia or Alzheimer's disease with cerebrovascular disease. CNS Drugs 2003;17:905–914.
44. Erkinjuntti T. Cognitive decline and treatment options for patients with vascular dementia. Acta Neurologica Scand 2002;106(Suppl 178):15–18.
45. Kurz AF, Erkinjuntti T, Small GW, Lilienfeld S, Damarju CV. Long-term safety and cognitive effects of galantamine in the treatment of probable vascular dementia or Alzheimer's disease with cerebrovascular disease. Eur J Neurol 2003; 10:663.
46. Moretti R, Torre P, Antonello RM, Cazzato G. Rivastigmine in subcortical vascular dementia: a comparison trial on efficacy and tolerability for 12 months follow-up. Eur J Neurol 2001;8:361–362.
47. Moretti R, Torre P, Antonello RM, Cazzato G, Bava A. Rivastigmine in subcortical vascular dementia: an open 22-month study. J Neurol Sci 2002;203:141–146.
48. Kumar V, Anand R, Messian J. An efficacy and safety analysis of Exelon in Alzheimer's disease with concurrent vascular risk factors. Eur J Neurol 2000;7:159–169.
49. Erkinjuntti T, Skoog I, Lane R, Andrews C. Rivastigmine in patients with Alzheimer's disease and concurrent hypertension. Intl J Clin Pract 2002;56:791–796.

23

Understanding and Managing Caregiver Burden in Cerebrovascular Disease

Geoffrey Tremont, Jennifer Duncan Davis, and Mary Beth Spitznagel

1. INTRODUCTION

Caregiver burden refers to a range of problems that may occur during the process of providing informal care for an individual with an illness. The association between the demands of caregiving on the caregiver's own physical and mental health and the indirect effect on the care recipient has been well-documented during the past two decades. Nevertheless, these findings have not been routinely applied to the clinical management of cerebrovascular disease (CVD), particularly vascular dementia (VaD). Chronic stressors can include disease-specific characteristics (e.g., level of care needed to complete activities of daily living [ADLs], cognitive and physical limitations, and behavioral disturbance), as well as secondary stressors, such as financial burden and disruption of family relationships. Although factors such as patient characteristics and caregiver demographic variables contribute to caregiver burden, there is strong evidence suggesting that caregivers' perceptions, coping skills, and resources play a major role. Given these findings, psychosocial interventions focused on adjusting caregiver appraisal, improving coping skills, and increasing self-efficacy may be targeted in psychosocial interventions to effectively reduce caregiver burden.

The effects of CVD present a unique challenge for the caregiver, given the variability in cognitive, behavioral, physical, and emotional sequelae that result from the disease. In addition, there is considerable unpredictability in the course of CVD that adds to a caregiver's burden. For example, CVD may include large-vessel acute stroke, repeated vascular events, progressive small-vessel disease, or combinations of disease types. In this chapter, the authors identify the consequences of providing care for a family member with acute or chronic CVD, reviewing the research literature examining effects of stroke and dementia caregiving on physical health, psychological and emotional well-being, and family functioning. A focus on the stroke literature is appropriate, because nearly one-third of stroke survivors meet criteria for dementia, and dementia will evolve among many more individuals after recurrent strokes. Furthermore, information obtained from the Alzheimer's disease (AD) literature has direct application to VaD, given the shared focus of dementia between these two conditions. Nevertheless, VaD produces unique challenges to patients and caregivers, which ultimately affect caregiver burden in this population, and these issues are addressed in this chapter. Because caregiver burden is a complex problem, the authors describe factors associated with increased caregiver burden and those associated with protection from caregiver burden. Finally, intervention approaches for prevention or reduction of caregiver burden and associated problems are discussed. Particular emphasis is placed on interventions that are theoretically based and appear cost-effective.

From: *Current Clinical Neurology*
Vascular Dementia: Cerebrovascular Mechanisms and Clinical Management
Edited by: R. H. Paul, R. Cohen, B. R. Ott, and S. Salloway © Humana Press Inc., Totowa, NJ

2. CONSEQUENCES OF CAREGIVING

Most of the literature examining caregiver burden and its associated consequences on the health and well-being of the caregiver has focused on caregivers of patients with AD or dementia in general. Far fewer studies have specifically targeted stroke caregivers, and only two studies have addressed the differential effect of AD compared to VaD on caregiver burden. This chapter will highlight the effects of caregiving on emotional, physical health, and family functioning in CVD and generate hypotheses for this group by reviewing the consequences of burden for dementia caregivers in general.

1.1. Emotional Health

Caregivers of patients with stroke or dementia frequently experience depression and anxiety. Estimates of depression in stroke caregivers range from 11% to as high as 37% using well-validated self-report instruments of depression *(1–5)*. In a study of 241 caregivers of stroke patients, 79% of caregivers of patients who survived for 1 yr reported poor emotional health, and 42% had elevated scores on measures of depression 1 yr after the stroke *(6)*. Similarly, Wade and colleagues *(4)* reported that increased anxiety in the caregiver was the most commonly reported change 6 mo after stroke.

The rates of mood disturbance in caregivers of stroke survivors are similar to the estimates of depression in dementia caregivers when compared to appropriate age- and gender-based normative data *(7–10)*. Dementia caregivers exhibit significantly higher rates of major depressive disorder and generalized anxiety disorder than age-matched controls *(11–13)*. For example, 25–30% of caregivers in study samples meet diagnostic criteria for major depressive disorder, with similar rates for generalized anxiety disorder *(14)*. Rates of psychotropic medication use among dementia caregivers is also higher than age-matched controls *(15–17)*, providing further evidence of increased incidence of psychiatric problems among dementia caregivers. Studies addressing racial differences in depression among dementia caregivers are limited, although preliminary findings show lower rates of depression among African-American caregivers than among Caucasian caregivers *(7,18)*.

Longitudinal analyses provide insight into the relationship between course of illness and emotional functioning in stroke and dementia caregivers. Wright and colleagues *(19)* compared the emotional status of stroke caregivers, dementia caregivers, and noncaregiver controls at three time points (baseline, 6 mo, and 12 mo). Patient caregivers were significantly more depressed than noncaregiver controls at baseline, but caregivers did not differ from each other. These differences remained stable over time, although there was a high attrition rate among stroke caregivers, possibly disguising an effect. Longitudinal analysis of depressive symptoms indicated an increased frequency of moderate to severe depression in dementia caregivers, compared to stroke caregivers who tended to show decreased severity of depression over time. Interestingly, higher levels of depression in stroke caregivers were significantly correlated with poorer patient functional status at baseline and at 6 mo post stroke but not at 1 yr. In contrast, depression in dementia caregivers was unrelated to patients' functional status, suggesting that different factors may underlie depression in dementia caregivers compared to stroke caregivers.

Together, the literature on emotional consequences of caregiving clearly demonstrates that caregivers are at a heightened risk for depression and associated emotional disturbances. Although the prevalence of depression in dementia and stroke caregivers is quite similar, there is evidence that the course of illness and disease characteristics may affect the chronicity and severity of depression symptoms in caregivers. It is possible that stroke caregivers may become more hopeful as the stroke survivor recovers, thereby reducing depression. In contrast, caregivers of patients with chronic CVD or VaD may show increased depression because the care recipient has not recovered fully or exhibits deteriorating course.

2.2. *Physical Health*

Providing care for a family member after a stroke can result in significant physical health consequences. Stress in dementia caregivers has been consistently shown to affect caregiver physical health, but few studies have specifically addressed the physical health consequences of caring for a stroke survivor. Caregivers of stroke patients are certainly vulnerable to the negative health consequences associated with chronic stress and associated reduction in preventive health behaviors of caregivers. Stroke caregivers report declines in physical health after assuming a caregiver role *(5,20)*, although the significance of these findings is unknown because comparison rates with noncaregivers or dementia caregivers have not been determined. Reese and colleagues *(21)* specifically compared self-reported psychological health and immunological functioning in caregivers of patients with AD and stroke survivors and noncaregivers. Psychological distress was highest in AD caregivers, but there were no differences among the three groups in immunological functioning. In addition to chronic stress, stroke survivors are likely to have physical limitations, such as hemiplegia or hemiparesis, which may increase risk of physical injury for caregivers when performing their duties.

Because few studies have directly evaluated the physical health of stroke caregivers and no studies have examined VaD caregivers, data from studies evaluating the health of dementia caregivers can inform our understanding of the possible negative health consequences associated with caring for an individual with chronic limitations secondary to one or multiple cerebrovascular accidents. Dementia caregivers, particularly spousal caregivers, subjectively rate their health as significantly worse than noncaregivers *(15)*. Some studies have also demonstrated that dementia caregivers experience more physical symptoms and illness, although this has not been a consistent finding *(14)*. Dementia caregivers sleep significantly less and are less active than noncaregivers *(15,22)*. Schulz et al. *(10)* found that dementia caregivers use more medication than noncaregivers. Preliminary research suggests that dementia caregiving is associated with specific physical changes, such as increased systolic blood pressure in male caregivers *(23)* and lower T cell counts in caregivers compared to matched controls *(24)*. Furthermore, caregiver strain was associated with a 63% higher mortality risk in older spousal caregivers *(25)*.

Physical health consequences of stroke caregiving have received little attention, although studies with dementia caregivers show reductions in health-related quality of life, perceived health status, and objective physical measures. Furthermore, it is important to emphasize that many caregivers are older adults and possibly more vulnerable to the negative health consequences of chronic stress.

2.3. *Family Functioning*

Disruption to the family system may be pronounced after a stroke. The acute nature of stroke results in the caregiver assuming a caregiver role without sufficient time to plan for this transition in terms of education and mobilization of resources *(26)*. Consequently, the caregiver may experience changes in his or her ability to function physically, socially, occupationally, and emotionally. For example, the caregiver may no longer be able to return to work because of new caregiver demands and may have difficulty meeting new role obligations (e.g., management of finances, household repairs, and housekeeping). Several authors have reported a fundamental disruption of the family structure after a stroke *(27–30)* and associated negative consequences on marital happiness and role satisfaction *(31)*. Furthermore, Evans and colleagues *(32)* reported that changes and instability in family support and the family system had a greater effect on caregiver burden than behavioral disturbance in the stroke survivor.

Few studies have formally evaluated family roles and family functioning in the context of stroke. Using the Family Assessment Device (FAD) *(33)*, a psychometrically sound measure of family functioning based on the McMaster Model of Family Functioning, Evans et al. *(34)* showed that family factors of affective involvement, problem solving, and communication were significantly associated with treatment adherence and stroke recovery. Families who supported treatment communicated and exchanged information directly and clearly, solved problems effectively, and reported a strong, emotional interest in each other. In contrast, nonsupportive families are associated with deterioration after stroke and reduced treatment adherence *(35,36)*. No studies have examined family functioning as a predictor of either stroke outcome or caregiver functioning. In the dementia literature, high levels of criticism and emotional overinvolvement in caregivers are associated with increased likelihood of depression, greater burden, and fewer positive benefits from caregiving *(37)*. Low family cohesiveness, high family conflict, too rigid or too permeable family boundaries, low levels of family organization, lack of clear communication, and poor spousal support have been seen in families with poor adjustment to dementia caregiving *(38)*.

Overall, the family system is negatively affected after a stroke and dementia, particularly in communication style, family problem-solving, and affective involvement. These changes have important implications for treatment compliance and adherence.

2.4. *Financial*

Caring for stroke survivors and patients with dementia at home results in substantial financial burden for informal caregivers, involving both nonreimbursed expenses and unpaid labor. Based on results from a population-based study of 7,743 stroke survivors, the estimated annual cost of stroke-related informal caregiving approximately $6.1 billion in the United States *(39)*. The annual cost of providing informal care to elderly community-dwelling individual with dementia was estimated to be approximately $18,000 per patient *(40)*, and there is some evidence that caring for patients with dementia may involve costs equal to nursing home care *(41)*.

Data suggest that the cost associated with stroke- and dementia-related caregiving is not only profound but also a commonly reported source of caregiver burden *(42)*. There is some suggestion that the financial burden is greater for caregivers of individuals with CVD compared to caregivers of patients with AD. For example, self-reported financial distress was higher in caregivers of patients with VaD compared to patients with AD *(43)*, possibly related to greater functional impairment and focal neurological signs present in vascular compared to Alzheimer's dementia. In addition, stroke survivors are often younger than patients with dementia and may have been working before the stroke. Financial loss may be incurred both resulting from an extended absence or failure to return to work *(44)*.

In summary, the stress associated with providing care to an individual with acute and chronic CVD can significantly affect the emotional and physical functioning of the caregiver, disrupt the family system, and result in significant financial burden and loss. Therefore, in the clinical setting, caregivers must be routinely screened for mental health problems and given attention for any medical needs. Because problems in the caregiver have important implications for the patient with CVD, caregiver assessments should be conducted as part of providing care for the patient. Otherwise, the caregiver may not seek out his or her own mental health or medical care.

3. FACTORS ASSOCIATED WITH NEGATIVE CONSEQUENCES OF CAREGIVING

The potential for negative consequences in caregiving in physical, emotional, family functioning, social, and financial domains is clearly established. Despite these findings, positive aspects of caregiving have been identified, and not all caregivers respond negatively to assuming a caregiver role *(45)*. As such, more recent studies have attempted to identify important predictors of caregiver burden and poor outcome. Many of the predictors identified are modifiable, arguing for possible effective psychosocial interventions to reduce caregiver burden and maximize recovery, function, and quality of life in the care recipient.

Predictors of caregiver burden in stroke and dementia patient populations are well described, but few studies have specifically examined predictors of burden in VaD caregivers. As such, the following section reviews evidence for predictors of caregiver burden in stroke and proposes how these factors may relate to burden in VaD caregivers.

3.1. Caregiver Factors

3.1.1. Demographic Characteristics

Demographic characteristics, such as age, gender, education, income, and duration of time spent caregiving, have been examined in relation to caregiver burden in stroke. Age predicts caregiver burden, with older caregivers feeling less burdened than their younger counterparts, and younger caregivers being at greater risk for burnout *(5,46)*. Although some studies do not show significant relationships for age, there are factors, such as relationship type, that may disguise any effect *(47,48)*. There is also evidence that socioeconomic status predicts burden. Greater income was related to decreased depression in stroke caregivers *(5)*, and lower income predicted caregiver depression *(48)*. These findings are consistent with the dementia caregiving finding that financial concerns may lead to caregiver strain *(49)*. In addition to having the financial means necessary to provide for another individual, income may indirectly affect the probability of burden. For example, greater income predicts confidence in problem-solving abilities, a factor related to burden *(50)*. The influence of caregiver gender on distress is somewhat controversial. Several studies found women had greater strain *(46,51)*, and in one study, female gender was one of the strongest predictors of depression *(52)*. Again, the literature reveals inconsistencies, with some studies showing no significant relationship between gender and caregiver distress *(6,47,48,50)*. It is notable and not surprising that most studies have a significant majority of female caregivers, which makes it difficult to make firm conclusions about gender effects. Ethnicity may also play a role in caregiver burden. Caregiver burden research in dementia provides evidence that different ethnic groups use different coping strategies and problem-solving methods *(53)*. Caregivers of individuals with stroke may also show differences with ethnicity; Hartke and King *(54)* found Caucasian caregivers reported more problems with anxious vigilance and social involvement, whereas their non-Caucasian counterparts reported greater problems with finances and physical health. In contrast, Grant and colleagues *(50)* found no correlation between ethnicity and caregiver depression, health, or life satisfaction. Finally, duration of caregiving, or length of time since stroke, is consistently unrelated to outcome measures of distress and burden *(46,50)*, suggesting that experience with caregiving does not predict who will feel burdened. Similar findings are seen in the dementia caregiving literature, with some studies demonstrating reduction in burden as the duration of caregiving increases *(55)*.

Overall, the relationship between caregiver demographic characteristics and burden is complex, and there are many inconsistencies in the literature. Reasons for disparate findings include variability in outcome measures, overrepresentation and underrepresentation of certain gender and ethnic groups, and confounding variables associated with demographic characteristics. Despite these inconsistencies, age, gender, socioeconomic status, and ethnicity may interact with dispositional and patient characteristics to increase caregiver vulnerability for burden. These factors should be considered when assessing caregiver burden and designing psychosocial interventions.

3.1.2. Dispositional Factors

Dispositional factors of the caregiver, including effectiveness of coping styles and sense of self-efficacy and caregiving preparedness, may also predict burden. Some caregiver coping styles are associated with poorer outcomes. For example, nonconfronting coping (e.g., confiding in another person or keeping busy) is associated with increased levels of stress and depression *(56)*. Other ineffective coping strategies include venting emotions and ignoring day-to-day activities that are not directly related to caregiving duties *(47)*, which are associated with higher levels of caregiver distress and may reflect poor emotional adjustment. In contrast, more active, healthy coping styles may be protective against caregiver burden. The active coping technique of confronting the problem is associated with less strain and improved mental health for the caregiver, and tactical coping responses (e.g., balancing the caregiver's and care recipient's needs with respect and empathy) are associated with lower levels of stress and depression in stroke caregivers *(46)*.

Similarly, the caregiver's perceived self-efficacy and sense of preparedness to face the challenges of caregiving may affect burden. There are strong connections between high self-efficacy, decreased burden, and better overall mental health in stroke and dementia caregivers *(46,47,57)*. Furthermore, caregiver optimism may be a protective factor against depression *(48)*. Caregivers' perceptions of the stroke survivor's illness may also predict likelihood of burden. One study found that anticipation of a longer illness was associated with higher levels of distress *(47)*. Caregivers' self-perception also plays a role in likelihood of burden. Low caregiver self-esteem and high threat appraisal were predictors of emotional distress *(58)*. Other findings suggest that perceived control over emotions when solving problems is a good predictor of caregiver depressive behavior and health and that negative appraisal of illness impact may be a strong predictor of caregiver depression *(50,52)*. Overall, the literature on dispositional factors provides strong evidence that effective coping strategies, high levels of self-efficacy, and good caregiver preparedness are associated with positive stroke and dementia caregiver functioning.

3.1.3. *Social Support*

Poor social support is another factor identified as a potential predictor of burden in stroke and dementia caregivers. Intuitively, the role of social support is especially important in caregiving, because adequate social relationships may help provide support in practical and emotional matters. In a study assessing distress and burden in caregivers 1 yr poststroke, high rates of disruption in social activities (79%) and leisure time (55%) were reported by caregivers *(6)*. Additionally, 35% reported caregiving had an adverse effect on family relationships, suggesting a high risk of disruption of caregivers' quality of life and family integrity. Similarly, Grant and colleagues *(50)* found that adequate social support is a good predictor of stroke caregiver life satisfaction, and decreased satisfaction with amount of social contact is related to increased burden for stroke and dementia caregivers *(5,13)*. Van den Heuval and colleagues *(46)* found that satisfaction with social support among stroke caregivers was associated with less strain and burnout, higher mental well-being, and greater vitality. When asking stroke caregivers to indicate their most pressing problems, lack of social support and social involvement were the most frequent problem types identified *(54,59)*. Poor social support was most problematic for the more depressed, burdened, and lonely caregivers *(54)*.

Overall, social support is the most consistent protective factor against caregiver burden in CVD and dementia. Interestingly, satisfaction with social support may be a more important predictor of burden than amount of social support. This certainly has implications for interventions, which can be geared toward modified perceptions and appraisals of the support network.

3.2. *Care Recipient Factors*

3.2.1. *Cognitive Changes*

By definition, patients with VaD have prominent cognitive deficits in several domains, and cognitive deficits are common in stroke survivors. Van den Heuval and colleagues *(46)* found that greater severity in cognitive disturbance was associated with increased risk for burnout in stroke caregivers. Vetter and colleagues *(43)* compared caregivers of patients with AD and VaD on measures of caregiver burden and found that overall caregiver burden varied as a function of both illness severity and type of dementia. For the severe dementia group, burden was significantly higher in caregivers of patients with AD than caregivers of patients with VaD. In contrast, self-reported burden was higher in caregivers of mildly to moderately demented patients with VaD, compared to caregivers of mild to moderate patients with AD. Perceptions of illness severity may be also be an important predictor of burden in dementia, and there is evidence that burdened dementia caregivers overestimate the severity of the care recipient's dementia *(60,61)*.

One cognitive change that is relatively common in stroke survivors is aphasia and other speech or language difficulties. Wade and colleagues *(62)* report that at 6 mo poststroke, 12% of stroke survivors are aphasic and 57% have residual speech problems, according to their caregivers. Given the increased potential for communication barriers between the caregiver and the stroke survivor with aphasia, it is logical that these caregivers may experience more burden than caregivers of individuals without aphasia. A recent literature review concluded that caregivers of stroke survivors with aphasia experience more problems than when aphasia is not present, and that caregivers of stroke survivors with aphasia experience poorer overall adjustment to the stroke and more deterioration of marital relationship *(63)*. Despite anecdotal reports of caregivers of stroke survivors with aphasia having more emotional problems, studies employing standardized instruments do not find this difference. Overall, Servaes and colleagues suggest the burden of caregiving may be greater in the presence of aphasia than without it, but caregivers challenged with extra burden are not necessarily more emotionally distraught.

3.2.2. Physical Limitations

There is a contribution of the stroke survivor's physical limitations to caregiver burden. Caregiver stress is associated with patients' level of physical handicap and mobility in the home and community, although it should be noted that stroke survivors with severe cognitive impairment and language dysfunction were excluded from the study *(64)*. In contrast, Anderson and colleagues *(6)* examined factors in care recipients that are associated with distress and burden in caregivers 1 yr poststroke and found only a trend for assistance with basic ADLs to be associated with emotional distress in caregivers. In a review of caregiver distress in stroke, Morrison *(65)* concluded there exists only a moderate relationship between the level of the care recipient's physical disability and resulting distress. Still, others find no relationship at all. McClenahan and Weinman *(47)* found that the stroke survivor's ability to complete ADLs did not explain any of the variance in caregiver distress, and Matson *(57)* revealed that stroke survivor dependency (e.g., help in washing and dressing) was not associated with stress or depression in the caregiver. Obviously, physical disability is less common in the early stages of Alzheimer's dementia. In contrast, individuals with VaD may have physical disability in addition to cognitive impairment, which has the potential of increasing caregiver burden. Overall, there is no consistent relationship between physical disability of the stroke survivor and caregiver burden. This may to some degree reflect the timing of the assessment in relationship to stroke recovery, such that more chronic physical disability may lead to increased caregiver distress.

3.2.3. Mood and Behavior

Personality changes after a stroke are common, affecting two-thirds of stroke patients *(66)*. Changes include depression, irritability, difficulty with self-control, impatience, poor frustration tolerance, increased emotional lability, self-centeredness, and decreased initiative. These changes may be secondary to lesion location, life changes, or a combination of both. Prevalence of poststroke depression is as high as 30% of stroke patients *(67,68)*. Noncompliance of the stroke survivor is frequently reported as the most difficult behavior for caregivers to manage *(54)*. Kinney et al. *(69)* showed that behavioral hassles were related to multiple aspects of stroke caregiver well-being, including depression. Comparing stroke and dementia, mood, and behavioral disturbance in the care recipient correlates with caregiver burden but to a greater degree in dementia *(16)*. Behavior problems can also precipitate institutionalization in patients with dementia *(70)*. Although the impact of mood and behavior problems on stroke caregiver burden has not been well studied, these problems likely contribute to caregiver distress. Because VaD is often associated with depression, apathy, and other neuropsychiatric symptoms, caregivers of these patients may be at heightened risk for burden and distress, and these care recipients may be more likely to be prematurely institutionalized.

Overall, findings from the stroke caregiver literature suggest that social support, active coping styles, sense of self-efficacy, and preparedness for caregiving, may buffer caregivers from distress and burden. In addition, physical limitations, disease severity, and mood and behavioral disturbances may lead to increased levels of distress, particularly in caregivers of patients with dementia.

Table 1
Potential Risk Factors for Caregiver Burden in VaD

	Caregiver	Care recipient
Nonmodifiable	• Older age • Low socioeconomic status • Female gender	• Severe illness • Presence of aphasia
Potentially modifiable	• Passive/avoidant coping strategies • Low self-efficacy • Low self-esteem • Not prepared for the caregiving role • Poor social support	• Mood and behavioral disturbance • Physical limitations • Progression of illness

Therefore, the aim of psychosocial interventions would be to increase factors that protect caregivers from burden and minimize those which contribute to burden (*see* Table 1 for a summary of these variables). Clarifying the specific predictors of caregiver burden in VaD can help to tailor interventions for these caregivers.

4. INTERVENTIONS FOR CAREGIVERS OF PATIENTS WITH CVD

Although there is considerable literature examining the efficacy of psychosocial and other interventions for caregivers of individuals with Alzheimer's dementia, few studies have systematically studied treatment approaches for caregivers of stroke survivors. Furthermore, there are no specific outcome studies examining treatment approaches for VaD caregivers. In this section, caregiver intervention outcome studies are reviewed, emphasizing controlled studies. The authors then discuss how these findings, combined with the dementia caregiver literature, have implications for interventions in chronic CVD and VaD. Finally, the authors present potential future treatment approaches for caregivers of individuals with CVD that have the greatest efficacy, feasibility, and cost-effectiveness.

4.1. *Effects of Caregiver Interventions in CVD and Stroke*

Interventions for caregivers of stroke survivors or individuals with CVD must begin as early as possible after the stroke event or clinical identification. Overly stressed caregivers may negatively affect the rehabilitation process, as well as increase the likelihood for long-term institutional placement *(71)*. Recently published poststroke rehabilitation guidelines recommended that families and involved others should be given information as soon as possible about stroke and the rehabilitation process as well as thorough training in techniques and problem-solving approaches required to provide effective support *(72)*. Once stroke survivors are in the community, the panel recommended that clinicians need to be sensitive to the potential adverse effects of caregiving on family functioning and the health of the caregiver. Working with the patient to avoid negative effects, promote problem solving and to facilitate reintegration of the patient into valued family and social roles was also recommended. Therefore, it is important to identify intervention strategies that can effectively meet these goals for patients with CVD and their caregivers.

4.1.1. *Education and Information Provision*

Clearly, stroke survivors and their caregivers need education and information. There is evidence that poorly informed stroke patients and their families may be less satisfied with their overall care, may be more noncompliant with treatment or medical advice, and may have poorer psychosocial outcomes after stroke *(20,73)*. Although educational programs are an integral part of stroke units and rehabilitation centers, there are consistent reports that stroke survivors and their caregivers are dissatisfied with information they receive about all aspects of stroke, and many have unanswered questions for up to 2 yr after the stroke *(73–76)*. Informational needs of patients and caregivers change over time. For example, Hanger et al. *(75)* found that the most requested information immediately after a stroke included the following: the causes of stroke, the nature of stroke, the association of stress and stroke, and stroke recovery. At 6 mo poststroke, caregivers and patients were most interested in risk for additional stroke and medication. At 2 yr poststroke, the emphasis was on poor memory and concentration, risk for additional stroke, and balance problems.

A few well-controlled studies have investigated whether providing information had an effect on stroke patients and their caregivers. These studies involved information provision alone (i.e., providing brochures, manuals, and booklets) or information provision plus educational sessions (i.e., lectures and question-and-answer sessions). Compared to noneducational controls, patients and caregivers who received educational sessions or other more active learning approaches show significantly increased knowledge about stroke that is sustained for up to 6 mo poststroke *(77,78)*. Patients and caregivers who are simply provided with brochures show no consistent improvement in knowledge *(79)*. In addition to increasing knowledge, it is possible that educational interventions may affect psychosocial outcome for stroke patients and caregivers. There is limited evidence that educational sessions improve depression and hopelessness but do not affect coping skills *(80)*. In contrast, the provision of information alone has no effect on emotional outcome. Information alone or information plus educational sessions do not affect perceived health status, satisfaction with care, disability status, service use, or modification of health-related behaviors *(80)*. Evans et al. *(20)* demonstrated that a group receiving an educational intervention showed less deterioration in family functioning (particularly in problem solving, communication, and global functioning) than a group that did not receive the intervention. These differences were maintained at a 1-yr follow-up. There are no studies investigating whether information provision or educational sessions can improve caregiver or patient functioning in vascular dementia. The AD caregiving literature shows that briefer interventions and those with more generic educational components have a small impact on caregiver distress and burden, although they tend to increase caregivers' knowledge about dementia *(58,81)*.

Overall, the research literature on educational interventions suggests that active learning sessions increase caregivers' and survivors' knowledge about CVD, although it is unlikely that education alone will help survivors and caregivers emotionally cope with the changes after stroke. To increase satisfaction with stroke education, tailoring information provision to the needs of stroke survivors and caregivers appears warranted, including consideration of the timing and content of the information provided. Education may also be an important starting point for involving caregivers in the stroke recovery process and for developing collaborative relationships between medical staff and caregivers. The effects of education on VaD caregivers is unknown but again may serve as an effective initial intervention for this group of caregivers.

4.1.2. Case Management

A practical approach to helping stroke survivors and their caregivers is to make a professional available who can identify and meet their needs. Numerous studies (mostly from the United Kingdom) have investigated the effects of nurse or social worker support for individuals after stroke. Although these studies used randomized designs and had large sample sizes, the amount of intervention (i.e., the number of contacts and services) received by caregivers and stroke survivors was variable, complicating interpretation of the results. Forster and Young *(82)* found minimal improvements in mildly disabled stroke survivors who received intervention from a specialist nurse support program compared to those who had standard care. There were no differences between the groups for any of the caregiver variables. Dennis et al. *(83)* found that compared to standard care, case management services improved stroke patient outcome for social adjustment and trends for depression and helplessness. Both patients and caregivers who received treatment reported higher levels of satisfaction with posthospital care than the control participants. Patients in the treatment group reported greater satisfaction with their posthospital care. Caregivers in the treatment group also showed better outcomes than those in the control, with statistically significant differences for mood symptoms and trends for anxiety and hassles scales. Mant et al. *(84)* investigated the effect of a family support organizer (FSO) for patients and caregivers with stroke. The intervention involved hospital visits, home visits, and telephone calls. On measures of caregiver functioning, the intervention group exhibited more activities and better health-related quality of life than the control group. Caregivers receiving the intervention also showed greater satisfaction with their understanding of stroke, its causes, and how to prevent another stroke. No significant differences were found in patients, except for a secondary analysis showing a somewhat lower frequency of depression among patients in the intervention group compared to the control group. Lincoln et al. *(85)* studied a similar approach to Mant et al. *(84)* and found that patients who received the intervention were significantly more knowledgeable about stroke and measures they could take to reduce future stroke. Caregiver outcome data show no significant differences between the groups in mood, strain, or independent ADLs. Again, caregivers in the FSO group showed greater knowledge of community resources and knowledge about stroke. Goldberg et al. *(86)* examined the efficacy of a yearlong intervention (i.e., weekly telephone contact and monthly home visits by a case manager, home-based treatment as needed from therapeutic recreation, social work, psychology consultants, and access to educational resources) to assist stroke patients and their caregivers after discharge from rehabilitation. The intervention group showed improved activity levels compared to the control group, although psychosocial functioning, quality of life, and stroke recurrence were not different between the groups. One interesting finding of the exit interview with intervention participants is that 35% felt that telephone contacts were more helpful than in-home visits.

Overall, the research on case management for stroke patients and caregivers is methodologically flawed, mostly because of extreme variability in the amount of intervention received by treatment groups. With this limitation in mind, there is evidence of effectiveness of case management for stroke caregivers. Limiting factors of these approaches are the high cost and requirements for a relatively large number of personnel. Case management seems applicable to stroke, but may be too expensive to implement on a large scale or for use with more chronic caregivers. Furthermore, there is evidence from the dementia caregiving literature that these caregivers are hesitant to use social services *(56)*. For VaD caregivers, there is clearly a role for respite services to allow caregivers to tend to their own needs and to have an opportunity for time away from caregiving duties. These services are effective with dementia caregivers, although they may be most effective in conjunction with a psychosocial intervention.

4.1.3. Problem-Solving Interventions

Lazarus and Folkman *(87)* elaborated a model of stress and coping that emphasized the appraisal process. Their model is particularly applicable to the stroke caregiving situation, in which the experience of burden may depend on the caregivers' appraisal of whether they have the coping resources to meet the demands of caregiving. Several studies have examined the efficacy of interventions for stroke caregivers theoretically based on this model. Van den Heuvel et al. *(88)* compared two similar stress-coping interventions (i.e., home visit vs group) to a control group in caregivers of stroke survivors. Compared to many of the other intervention studies, this group of caregivers had been providing care for a longer period (3.5 yr on average). The interventions consisted of discussion of caregivers' reactions to taking on the caregiving role and the consequences to them and the survivor. Active problem solving and active coping were used as strategies. The interventions involved 8 weekly 2-h sessions for 2 mo. Caregivers were also encouraged to develop a telephone network with the other caregivers in the group. Approximately 3 mo after the intervention, the treatment groups did not differ, but both groups showed greater confidence in knowledge about patient care, seeking social support, and self-efficacy compared to the control group. Participants in the treatment groups sought more social support than in the control group. No differences were found for caregiver mental well-being, vitality, or caregiver strain. At 6-mo follow-up *(89)*, findings suggested that caregivers in both intervention groups showed increased caregiver knowledge, increased use of active coping strategies, and increased social support compared to control caregivers. Younger female caregivers benefited most from the intervention. In the long term, control caregivers used less social support whereas those in the intervention groups maintained their level of social support. In a large study of a telephone-based social problem-solving intervention, Grant et al. *(90)* showed that caregivers receiving the intervention had significant improvements in vitality, mental health, and role limitations related to emotional problems compared to sham or usual-care control groups. The intervention group also showed significantly better social problem solving, greater caregiver preparedness, and less depression than the other groups. Although there are no specific studies addressing the efficacy of problem-solving interventions for VaD caregivers, a recent review of the literature concluded that the most effective dementia caregiver interventions included a social problem-solving component *(91)*. Together, findings from problem-solving interventions for stroke caregivers suggest that a focused and brief intervention may have significant beneficial effects on caregivers of stroke, even for caregivers of chronic stroke survivors. In addition, the telephone is an effective method for delivering this type of intervention.

4.1.4. Family-Based Interventions

After a cerebrovascular event, family functioning deteriorates and family functioning is associated with treatment compliance *(34)*. Therefore, caregiver interventions with a primary focus on the family may be particularly helpful. In addition to investigating the effects of educational sessions on family functioning after a stroke, Evans et al. *(77)* included a group of stroke patients and caregivers who received education plus seven sessions of a problem-solving intervention with the caregiver. Compared to standard care, education and education plus counseling groups exhibited improved caregiver knowledge and better family functioning. Caregivers who received counseling showed better personal adjustment and role skills at 1 yr follow-up than the other two groups. No groups showed differences in their use of social resources. Limitations of the study include few outcome measures and inclusion of a predominantly male veteran population. Miller et al. *(92)* pilot tested a family-based intervention delivered by telephone in a group of 63 survivors and caregivers who were identified at hospital admission for acute stroke. Survivors and caregivers were randomly assigned to receive either the intervention or standard medical care. The intervention was based on the McMaster Model of Family Functioning and involved a standardized number of telephone contacts to patients and caregivers during 6 mo, following a standardized treatment manual. The intervention included psychoeducation about stroke and caregiving and encouraged the stroke survivor and caregiver to monitor and identify issues in five areas (i.e., health, mood, cognition, functioning, and family life). Problem-solving and emotional support were used to assist them in dealing with these issues, as needed. Caregivers who received the intervention showed a trend toward less severe depression than the control group. In addition, caregivers who received the intervention perceived significantly better family problem solving, role functioning, and affective responsiveness than control caregivers. Many other aspects of family functioning showed trends in the expected direction. Patients and caregivers who received the intervention reported significantly less perceived criticism in the family than those patients and caregivers who received standard care. A striking finding of this study was that patients and caregivers receiving the intervention had 70% fewer hospital days than did individuals in the control condition and less use of doctor visits and therapy hours. Although these results are quite promising, the sample size was relatively small. A much larger study of the efficacy and cost-effectiveness of this intervention is currently underway.

There are no studies specifically examining family-based treatment of VaD caregivers. However, it is important to note that one of the most effective comprehensive interventions for dementia caregivers included family counseling as a major component *(93,94)*. Furthermore, medical compliance and health behavior change is of great importance in VaD because of the increased need to manage vascular risk factors associated with future deterioration and morbidity. Given the relationship between family functioning and treatment compliance, family-based interventions may be particularly appropriate to increase the likelihood of following medical advice, to positively affect the course of the illness, and to enlist family support in making healthy lifestyle changes.

Aphasia may be particularly disruptive to family functioning, family roles, and interpersonal relationships. Only two studies have examined the effect of intensive interventions involving family caregivers and patients with chronic aphasia. One program *(95)* involved a 5-d residential course, including extensive education about etiology, treatment, and prognosis of aphasia; psychological counseling/family therapy to address personal and interpersonal problems; and intensive speech therapy. Results showed evidence for positive changes in psychological and interpersonal functioning in caregivers after 1 yr but not in neurologic or linguistic functions in the individual with aphasia. Hinckley et al. *(96)* designed a 3-d course for patients with aphasia and their caregivers to provide education about aphasia, to review available resources, and to provide support group discussions. Six-month and 1-yr follow-up information showed that the majority of participants sought new resources, reported increased knowledge about aphasia, and reported modest changes in social independence and participation in social activities. Unfortunately, both studies lacked a control group to compare results. In addition, although these results appear promising, the costs of these types of interventions are prohibitive.

Overall, studies assessing the effect of family-based interventions in CVD demonstrate that family approaches can improve knowledge, personal adjustment and emotional functioning, caregiver skills, and family functioning. These types of interventions may be useful for enhancing medical compliance, improving communication among family members (especially with aphasia), and facilitating family agreement and support about lifestyle changes.

4.1.5. Support and Peer Groups

Although support groups such as stroke clubs are commonly recommended to patients and caregivers after a stroke, little information is available about their efficacy. Peer support may be an effective means of social support for stroke caregivers and serve as protective factor against caregiver burden. Printz-Fedderson *(97)* found no differences on measures of caregiver burden or depression between stroke caregivers who participated in a stroke club vs those who did not, although the sample was small. In contrast, Weltermann et al. *(98)* surveyed 133 members of stroke support groups in Germany and found that the majority of participants met stringent criteria for knowledge of stroke symptoms, risk factors, and when to take action. Although there are no studies investigating support groups for VaD caregivers, a small positive effect has been seen on measures of burden and depression among dementia caregivers who attend support groups *(99)*. Overall, the limited literature on support groups suggest that they may improve knowledge about CVD, but their effectiveness in reducing burden and stress among stroke and dementia caregivers is not fully understood.

4.1.6. Interventions for VaD Caregivers

Although there are no specific studies examining interventions for VaD caregivers, we can speculate on how these interventions might differ from those implemented with stroke survivors and their caregivers. Acute care hospitals and rehabilitation centers are natural starting points for stroke caregivers' interventions. Given the insidious onset of AD (and in many cases of VaD), caregivers may not be seen until later in the caregiving process. Often, dementia caregivers will not seek assistance until they are very stressed *(100)*. Therefore, initial intervention strategies for VaD caregivers may need to focus on addressing and stabilizing emotional functioning of the caregiver before other types of intervention strategies are used. Many of the stroke caregiver interventions involve the stroke survivor as part of the intervention process, whereas dementia patient are not typically included in psychosocial or educational interventions because of significant cognitive impairment and memory dysfunction. In stroke intervention, stroke survivors are typically recovering or improving functioning, whereas dementia typically involves deterioration. Therefore, duration of interventions may need to be longer for patients with VaD to assist caregivers in adjusting to deterioration and other changes in cognition and behavior. Similar to stroke caregivers, part of the interventions for VaD caregivers may include education and support concerning important health behavior change to minimize patients' vascular risk factors and progression of their CVD. Results from studies examining burden and psychological distress in caregivers of stroke survivors suggest that caregivers experience high levels of burden and emotional distress even before the patient is discharged home *(50)*. This is in direct contrast to caregivers of patients with chronic or slowly progressive functional and cognitive changes in which burden, emotional distress, and family disruption may occur much later in the disease course *(43)*.

Findings from the Alzheimer's dementia caregiving literature also provide insight into possible effective intervention approaches for caregivers of individuals with VaD. Although many of the same issues may arise when providing care for an individual with VaD, differences in disease onset, course, behavior change, and management of further decline/risk factors may differ. Knight et al. *(99)* used a meta-analysis to summarize findings of 18 controlled dementia caregiver intervention studies between 1980 and 1990. Results revealed that studies examining individual psychosocial interventions yielded higher average effect sizes than studies investigating group psychosocial interventions for both emotional distress and caregiver burden outcomes. Respite interventions (similar to case management described above) had smaller average effect sizes than psychosocial interventions but greater variability, resulting, at least in part, from the differences in respite interventions (i.e., nursing consults, social services, and support groups). In general, the most effective intervention strategies with Alzheimer's caregivers were comprehensive ones. For example, Mittelman et al. *(93,94)* randomly assigned dementia caregivers to receive either a multifaceted intervention consisting of family and individual counseling sessions, caregiver support groups, and continual access to a counselor. Caregivers assigned to the control condition were provided with usual care involving information about resources without active efforts to arrange services or to provide counseling. Results showed that caregivers who received the intervention had lower levels of depression compared to caregivers receiving standard medical care. The antidepressant effect of the intervention strengthened from 4-mo to 12-mo follow-up, even after accounting for other factors related to depression in caregivers. Several studies in the dementia caregiving literature have also demonstrated that caregiver interventions may increase the time to institutional placement, as well as reduce behavior problems and depression in the care recipients *(94,101,102)*. Overall, caregiver intervention studies in VaD are desperately needed so that clinical practice can be informed. In the meantime, VaD caregivers will need comprehensive counseling, family, and social support services, similar to those currently available to Alzheimer's caregivers, with additional emphasis on enlisting the caregiver in managing vascular risk factors (*see* Table 2 for a listing of intervention components).

5. FUTURE DIRECTIONS OF CEREBROVASCULAR CAREGIVER INTERVENTIONS

It is obvious from the review of interventions for stroke and dementia caregivers that little is known about the most effective way to reduce burden and stress in caregivers of patients with CVD. Based on the limited findings, a few important points for future interventions are worthy of discussion. The most important components of interventions for caregivers include educational sessions, family intervention, problem-solving skills training, self-efficacy, and enhancing social support. The timing and duration of interventions are also important factors to consider, because certain components may be more appropriate for use in various phases of the disease process, and patients with progressive disease may require treatment duration for a longer period. Appropriate interventions will be based on a solid theoretical framework yet be flexible enough to address

Table 2
Important Components (With Examples) for a Comprehensive Intervention for VaD Caregivers

Education	• Assess and reassess educational needs to tailor information provision • Use active learning strategies (e.g., lectures and question-and-answer sessions)
Enhancing social support	• Encourage development of peer network • Encourage use of community resources (e.g., support groups or stroke clubs)
Family counseling	• Help family to agree on needs for care recipient • Identify caregiving roles for family members • Enlist family support to implement healthy lifestyle change (e.g., increase physical activities or cardiac diet)
Problem-solving training	• Apply problem-solving steps to multiple situations to enhance generalization • Point out previous successful problem solving to increase self-efficacy
Coping skills training	• Teach active coping strategies (e.g., problem confrontation and balancing caregiver and care recipient needs) • Prepare caregivers for the challenges of caregiving
Respite	• Provide opportunities for caregivers to tend to their own needs • Provide access to case management resources (e.g., help line)

the spectrum of physical, cognitive, emotional, and behavioral changes that can occur in CVD. An example is a structured intervention approach that uses individually tailored interventions based on assessment and reassessment of caregiver needs and changes in the patient. Cost effectiveness and ease of implementation on a large scale are additional characteristics of successful interventions. Telephone-based interventions are particularly cost effective and can be delivered on a large scale to caregivers who may not otherwise be able to access community resources. Computer-based intervention approaches may also be advantageous, although they lack the interpersonal contact available through other interventions. Ultimately, research on caregivers of patients with CVD should be able to answer the following questions: (1) what are the most effective interventions; (2) what type of caregiver benefits most from the intervention; (3) when is the best time to intervene; and (4) what is the most appropriate duration of the intervention.

REFERENCES

1. Carnwath TCM, Johnson DAW. Psychiatric morbidity among spouses of patients with stroke. Br Med J 1987;294:409–411.
2. Grant JS, Bartolucci AA, Elliot TR, Giger JN. Sociodemographic, physical, and psychosocial characteristics of depressed and non-depressed family caregivers of stroke. Brain Injury 2000;14:1089–1100.
3. Kotila M, Numminen H, Waltimo O, Kaste M. Depression after stroke: results for the FINNSTROKE Study. Stroke 1998;29:368–372.
4. Wade DT, Leigh-Smith J, Hewer RL. Effects of living with and looking after survivors of a stroke. Br Med J 1986;293: 418–420.
5. Schulz R, Tompkins CA, Rau MT. A longitudinal study of the psychosocial impact of stroke on primary support persons. Psychol Aging 1988;3:131–141.
6. Anderson CS, Linto J, Stewart-Wynne EG. A population-based assessment of the impact of burden and caregiving for long-term stroke survivors. Stroke 1995;26:843–849.
7. Haley WE, West C, Wadley VG, et al. Psychological, social, and health impact of caregiving: a comparison of black and white dementia family caregivers and noncaregivers. Psychol Aging 1995;10:540–552.
8. Irwin M, Hauger R, Patterson T, Semple S, Ziegler M, Grant I. Alzheimer caregiver stress: basal natural killer cell activity, pituitary-adrenal cortical function, and sympathetic tone. Ann Behav Med 1997;19:83–90.
9. Rose-Rego SK, Strauss M, Smyth KA. Differences in the perceived well-being of wives and husbands caring for persons with Alzheimer's disease. Gerontology 1998;38:224–230.
10. Schulz R, Newsom J, Mittlemark M, Burton L, Hirsch C, Jackson S. Health effects of caregiving: the caregiver health effects study: an ancillary study of The Cardiovascular Health Study. Ann Behav Med 1997;19:110–116.

11. Dura JR, Stukenberg KW, Kiecolt-Glaser JK. Anxiety and depressive disorders in adult children caring for demented parents. Psychol Aging 1991;6:467–473.
12. Russo J, Vitaliano PP, Brewer DD, Katon W, Becker J. Psychiatric disorders in spouse caregivers of care-recipients with Alzheimer's disease and matched controls: a diathesis-stress model of psychopathology. J Abnormal Psychol 1995;104:197–204.
13. Vitaliano PP, Russo F, Young HM, Teri L, Maiuro RD. Predictors of burden in spouse caregivers of individuals with Alzheimer's disease. Psychol Aging 1991;6:392–402.
14. Schulz R, O'Brien AT, Bookwala J, Fleissner K. Psychiatric and physical morbidity effects of dementia caregiving: prevalence, correlates, and causes. Gerontologist 1995;35:771–791.
15. Baumgarten M, Battista RN, Infante-Rivard C, Hanley JA, Becker R, Gauthier S. The psychological and physical health of family members caring for an elderly person with dementia. J Clin Epidem 1992;45:61–70.
16. Draper BM, Poulos CJ, Cole AM, Poulos RG, Ehrlich F. A comparison of caregivers for elderly stroke and dementia victims. J Amer Geriatric Soc 1992;40:896–901.
17. Kiecolt-Glaser JK, Dura JR, Speicher CE, Trask J, Glaser R. Spousal caregivers of dementia victims: longitudinal changes in immunity and health. Psychosom Med 1991;53:345–362.
18. Miller B, Campbell RT, Farran CJ, Kaufman JE, Davis L. Race, control, mastery, and caregiver distress. J Gerontol B Psychol Sci Soc Sci 1995;50:S374–S382.
19. Wright LK, Hickey JV, Buckwalter, KC, Hendrix, SA, Kelechi T. Emotional and physical health of spouse caregivers of persons with Alzheimer's disease and stroke. J Adv Nurs 1999;30:552–563.
20. Evans RL, Bishop DS, Haselkorn JK. Factors predicting satisfactory home care after stroke. Arch Phys Med Rehab 1991;72:144–147.
21. Reese DR, Gross AM, Smalley DL, Messer SC. Caregivers of Alzheimer's disease and stroke patients: immunological and psychological considerations. Gerontology 1994;34:534–540.
22. Burton LC, Newsom JT, Schulz R, Hirsch CH, German PS. Preventive health behaviors among spousal caregivers. Prevent Med 1997;26:162–169.
23. Moritz DJ, Kasl SV, Ostfeld AM. The health impact of living with a cognitively impaired elderly spouse. J Aging Health 1992;4:244–267.
24. Glaser R, Kiecolt-Glaser JK. Chronic stress modulates the virus-specific immune response to latent herpes simplex type 1. Ann Behav Med 1997;19:78–82.
25. Schulz R, Beach SR. Caregiving as a risk factor for mortality: The Caregiver Health Effects Study. JAMA 1999;282: 2259–2260.
26. Galarneau L. An interdisciplinary approach to mobility and safety education for caregivers and stroke patients. Rehab Nurs 1993;18:395–399.
27. Anderson CS. The quality of life of stroke patients and their caregivers. In: Anderson R, Bury M, eds. Living with Chronic Illness. London, UK: Unwin Hyman, 1988, pp. 14–42.
28. Bishop DS, Epstein NB, Keitner GI, Miller IW, Srinivasan SV. Stroke: morale, family functioning, health status, and functional capacity. Arch Phys Med Rehab 1986;67:84–87.
29. Jongbloed L, Stanton S, Fousek B. Family adaptation to altered roles following a stroke. Can J Occup Ther 1993;60:70–77.
30. Robinson-Smith G, Mahoney C. Coping and marital equilibrium after stroke. J Neurosci Nurs 1995;27:83–89.
31. Enterlante TM, Kern JM. Wives' reported role changes following a husband's stroke: a pilot study. Rehab Nurs 1995;20: 155–160.
32. Evans RL, Northwood LK. Social support needs in adjustment to stroke. Arch Phys Med Rehabil 1983;64:61–64.
33. Epstein NB, Baldwin LM, Bishop DS. The McMaster Family Assessment Device. J Marital Fam Ther 1983;9:171–180.
34. Evans RL, Bishop DS, Matlock AL, Stranahan S, Smith GG, Halar EM. Family interaction and treatment adherence after stroke. Arch Phys Med Rehab 1987;68:513–517.
35. Kane JM. Compliance issues in outpatient treatment. J Clin Psychopharmacol 1985;5:22S–27S.
36. Strickland R, Alston J, Davidson J. Negative influence of families on compliance. Hosp Community Psychiatry 1981;32: 349–350.
37. Wagner AW, Logsdon RG, Pearson JL, Teri L. Caregiver expressed emotion and depression in Alzheimer's disease. Aging Ment Health 1997;1:132–139.
38. Fisher L, Nakell LC, Terry HE, Ransom DC. The California Family Health Project: III. Couple emotional management and adult health. Family Process 1992;231:269–287.
39. Hickenbottom SL, Fendrick AM, Kutcher JS, Kabeto MU, Katz SJ, Langa KM. A national study of the quantity and cost of informal caregiving for the elderly with stroke. Neurology 2002;25:1754–1759.
40. Moore MJ, Zhu CW, Clipp EC. Informal costs of dementia care: estimates for the National Longitudinal Caregiver Study. J Gerontol B Psychol Sci Soc Sci 2001;56:219–228.
41. Rice DP, Fox PJ, Max W, et al. The economic burden of Alzheimer's disease care. Health Aff 1993;12:164–176.
42. Kerr SM, Smith LN. Stroke: an exploration of the experience of informal caregiving. Clin Rehab 2001;15:428–436.
43. Vetter PH, Krauss S, Steiner O, et al. Vascular dementia versus dementia of Alzheimer's type: do they have differential effects on caregivers' burden? J Geront Soc Sci 1999;54B:S93–S98.

44. MacKay A, Nias BC. Strokes in the young and middle-aged: consequences to the family and to society. J Royal Coll Phys London 1979;13:106–112.
45. Beach SR, Schulz R, Yee, JL, Jackson S. Negative and positive health effects of caring for a disabled spouse: longitudinal findings from the caregiver health effects study. Psychol Aging 2000;15:259–271.
46. van den Heuval ETP, de Witte LP, Schure LM, Sanderman R, Meyboom-de Jong B. Risk factors for burn-out in caregivers of stroke patients, and possibilities for intervention. Clin Rehab 2001;15:669–W677.
47. McClenahan R, Weinman J. Determinants of carer distress in non-acute stroke. Int J Lang Commun Disord 1998;33 (Suppl):138–143.
48. Tomkins CA, Schulz R, Rau MT. Post-stroke depression in primary support persons: predicting those at risk. J Consult Clin Psychology 1988;56:502–508.
49. Cantor MH. Strain among caregivers: a study of experience in the United States. Gerontologist 1983;23:597–604.
50. Grant JS, Elliot TR, Giger JN, Bartolucci AA. Social problem-solving abilities, social support, and adjustment among family caregivers of individuals with a stroke. Rehab Psychol 2001;46:44–57.
51. Thommessen B, Aarsland D, Braekhus A, Oksengaard AR, Engedal K, Lakke K. The psychosocial burden on spouses of the elderly with stroke, dementia and Parkinson's disease. Int J Geriatr Psychiatry 2002;17:78–84.
52. King RB, Carlson CE, Shade-Zeldow Y, Bares KK, Roth EJ, Heinemann AW. Transition to home care after stroke: depression, physical health, and adaptive processes in support persons. Res Nurs Health 2001;24:307–323.
53. Wykle M, Segal M. A comparison of Black and White family caregivers experience with dementia. J Natl Black Nurses Assoc 1991;5:29–41.
54. Hartke RJ, King RB. Analysis of problem types and difficulty among older stroke caregivers. Top Stroke Rehab 2002;9: 16–33.
55. Dunkin JJ, Anderson-Hanley C. Dementia caregiver burden: a review of the literature and guidelines for assessment and intervention. Neurology 1998;51:S53–S60.
56. Matson N. Coping, caring, and stress: a study of stroke carers and carers of older confused people. Br J Clin Psychol 1994;33:333–344.
57. Coen RF, Swanwick GR, O'Boyle CA, Coakley D. Behaviour disturbance and other predictors of carer burden in Alzheimer's disease. Int J Geriatr Psychiat 1997;12:331–336.
58. Bakas T, Burgener SC. Predictors of emotional distress, general health, and caregiving outcomes in family caregivers of stroke survivors. Top Stroke Rehab 2002;9:34–45.
59. Denman A. Determining the needs of spouses caring for aphasic partners. Disability Rehab 1998;20:411–423.
60. Hadjistavropoulos T, Taylor S, Tuokko H, Beattie BL. Neuropsychological deficits, caregivers' perception of deficits and caregiver burden. J Am Geriatr Soc 1994;42:308–314.
61. Mangone CA, Sanguinetti RM, Baumann PD, et al. Influence of feelings of burden on the caregiver's perception of the patient's functional status. Dementia 1993;4:287–293.
62. Wade DT, Langton RL, David RM, Enderby PM. Aphasia after stroke: natural history and associated deficits. J Neurol Neurosurg, Psychiatry 1986;49:11–16.
63. Servaes P, Draper B, Conroy P, Bowring G. Informal carers of aphasic stroke patients: Stresses and interventions. Aphasiology 1999;13:889–900.
64. Segal ME, Schall RR. Life satisfaction and caregiving stress for individuals with stroke and their primary caregivers. Rehab Psychol 1996;41:303–320.
65. Morrison V. Predictors of carer distress following stroke. Rev Clin Gerontol 1999;9:265–271.
66. Coughlin AK, Humphrey M. Presenile stroke: long-term outcome for patients and their families. Rheumatol Rehab 1982;21:115–122.
67. Hosking SG, Marsh NV, Friedman PJ. Poststroke depression: prevalence, course, and associated factors. Neuropsychol Rev 1996;6:107–133.
68. Stern RA. Assessment of mood states in aphasia. Sem Speech Lang 1999;20:33–50.
69. Kinney JM, Stephens MAP, Franks MM, Norris VK. Stresses and satisfactions of family caregivers to older stroke patients. J Appl Gerontol 1995;14:3–21.
70. Pruchno R, Michaels JE, Potashnik SL. Predictors of institutionalization among Alzheimer disease victims with caregiving spouses. J Geriatr 1990;45:5259–5266.
71. Han B, Haley WE. Family caregiving for patients with stroke: review and analysis. Stroke 1999;30:1478–1485.
72. Boult C, Brummel-Smith KB. Clinical Practice Committee of the American Geriatrics Society. Post-Stroke Rehabilitation Guidelines. J Am Geriatr Soc 1997;45:881–883.
73. O'Mahoney PG, Rodgers H, Thomson RG, Dobson R, James OFW. Satisfaction with information and advice received by stroke patients. Clin Rehabil 1997;11:68–72.
74. Drummond A, Lincoln N, Juby L. Effects of a stroke unit on knowledge of stroke and experiences in hospital. Health Trends 1996;28:26–30.
75. Hanger HC, Walker G, Paterson LA, McBride S, Sainsbury R. What do patients and their carers want to know about stroke? A two-year follow up study. Clin Rehab 1998;12:45–52.

76. Wellwood I, Dennis MS, Warlow CP. Perceptions and knowledge of stroke amongst surviving patients with stroke and their carers. Age Ageing 1994;24:293–298.
77. Evans RL, Matlock AL, Bishop DS, Stanahan S, Pederson C. Family intervention after stroke: does counseling or education help? Stroke 1988;19:1243–1249.
78. Mant J, Carter J, Wade DT, Winner S. The impact of and information pack on patients with stroke and their carers: a randomized controlled trial. Clin Rehabil 1998;12:465–467.
79. Rodgers H, Bond S, Curless R. Inadequacies in the provision of information to stroke patients and their families. Age Ageing 2001;30:129–133.
80. Forster A, Smith J, Young J, Knapp P, House A, Wright J. Information provision for stroke patients and their caregivers. Cochrane Database Syst Rev 2003;3.
81. Burgener SD, Bakas T, Murray C, Dunahee J, Tossey S. Effective caregiving approaches for patients with Alzheimer's disease. Geriatr Nurs 1998;19:121–126.
82. Forster A, Young J. Specialist nurse support for patients with stroke in the community: a randomized controlled trial. Br Med J 1996;312:1642–1646.
83. Dennis M, O'Rourke S, Slattery J, Staniforth T, Warlow C. Evaluation of a stroke family care worker: results of a randomized controlled trial. Br Med J 1997;314:1071–1076.
84. Mant J, Carter J, Wade DT, Winner S. Family support for stroke: a randomized controlled trial. Lancet N Am 2000;356: 808–813.
85. Lincoln NB, Francis VM, Lilley SA, Sharma JC, Summerfield M. Evaluation of a stroke family support organizer: a randomized controlled trial. Stroke 2003;34:116–121.
86. Goldberg G, Segal ME, Berk SN, Schall RR, Gershkoff AM. Stroke transition after inpatient rehabilitation. Topic Stroke Rehab 1997;4:64–79.
87. Lazarus RS, Folkman S. Stress, Appraisal, and Coping. New York, NY: Springer, 1984.
88. Van den Heuvel ETP, de Witte LP, Nooyen-Haazen I, Sanderman R, Meyboom-de Jong B. Short-term effects of a group support program and an individual support program for caregivers of stroke patients. Patient Educ Couns 2000;40:109–120.
89. Van den Heuvel ETP, Witte LP, Stewart RE, Schure LM, Sanderman R, Meyboom-de Jong B. Long-term effects of a group support program and an individual support program for informal caregivers of stroke patients: Which caregivers benefit the most? Patient Educ Couns 2002;47:291–299.
90. Grant JS, Elliott TR, Weaver M, Bartolucci AA, Newman Giger J. Telephone intervention with family caregivers of stroke survivors after rehabilitation. Stroke 2002;33:2060–2065.
91. Cooke DD, McNally L, Mulligan KT, Harrison MJG, Newman SP. Psychosocial interventions for caregivers of people with dementia: a systematic review. Aging Ment Health 2001;5;120–135.
92. Miller IW, Weiner D, Bishop DS, Johnson B, Albro J. Telephone administered family intervention following stroke. Rehab Psychol 1998;43:323–324.
93. Mittelman MS, Ferris SH, Shulman E, et al. A comprehensive support program: effect on depression in spouse-caregivers of AD patients. Gerontologist 1995;35:792–802.
94. Mittelman MS, Ferris SH, Shulman E, Steinberg G, Levin B. A family intervention to delay nursing home placement of patients with Alzheimer's disease: a randomized controlled trial. JAMA 1996;276:1725–1731.
95. Borenstein P, Linelli S, Wahrborg P. An innovative therapeutic program for aphasia patients and their relatives. Scand J Rehabil Med 1987;19:51–56.
96. Hinckley JJ, Packard MEW, Bardach LG. Alternative family education programming for adults with chronic aphasia. Topic Stroke Rehab 1995;2:53–63.
97. Printz-Fedderssen V. Group process effect on caregiver burden. J Neurosci Nurs 1990;22:164–168.
98. Weltermann BM, Homann J, Rogalewski A, Brach S, Voss S, Ringelstein EB. Stroke knowledge among stroke support group members. Stroke 2000;31:1230–1233.
99. Knight BG, Lutzky SM, Macofsky-Urban F. A meta-analytic review of interventions for caregiver distress: recommendations for future research. Gerontologist 1993;33:240–248.
100. Bass DM, Noelker LS. The influence of family caregiver son elders' use of in-home services: an expanded conceptual framework. J Health Soc Behav 1987;28:184–196.
101. Robinson K, Yates K. Effects of two caregiver-training programs on burden and attitude toward help. Arch Psychiatr Nurs 1994;8:312–319.
102. Teri L, Logsdon RG, Uomoto J, McCurry S. Behavioral treatment of depression in dementia patients: A controlled clinical trial. J Gerontol B Psychol Sci Soc Sci B 1997;52:159–166.

24

Quality of Life in Patients With Vascular Dementia

Rebecca E. Ready and Brian R. Ott

1. INTRODUCTION

Little is known about quality of life (QOL) in vascular dementia (VaD). The past decade has witnessed considerable attention to QOL issues in dementia, but the majority of this work has been conducted with Alzheimer's disease (AD) or mixed dementia samples, with surprisingly scant attention devoted exclusively to VaD populations. Thus, this chapter primarily focuses on future directions for work regarding QOL in VaD, a largely uncharted territory. Current conceptualizations and measurement issues regarding QOL in dementia are reviewed. Hypotheses about QOL in VaD are generated from the literature bases regarding QOL in AD and in stroke patients without dementia, which are two patient populations that share overlapping features with VaD.

2. CONCEPTUALIZATIONS OF QOL IN DEMENTIA

Several definitions and conceptualizations of QOL in dementia have been introduced during the past decade. Lawton's work regarding QOL in dementia has provided much of the theoretical foundation for research in this area. Lawton argued that QOL assessment should include consideration of subjective and objective factors *(1)*. He identified four overarching dimensions that contribute to QOL in dementia: (1) psychologic well-being (e.g., positive and negative affect), (2) behavioral competence (e.g., cognitive and functional abilities), (3) objective environment (e.g., caretakers and living situation), and (4) perceived QOL *(2)*.

Lawton's work was particularly influential in the development of dementia QOL measures. As can been inferred from his model, QOL is highly subjective and multifaceted. Definitions of QOL that are specific to dementia typically include multiple domains, and nearly all of them recognize the centrality of mood, affect, and activity. However, beyond these factors, there is little consensus about additional domains of QOL, and definitions differ primarily in their breadth. Some investigators take a narrow conceptualization of QOL in dementia and focus primarily on affect and activity *(3)*. A broad and encompassing definition was offered by the International Working Group on Harmonization of Dementia Drug Guidelines and includes cognitive function and the ability to perform of activities of daily living (ADLs) in their definition of QOL, in addition to mood and affect *(4)*. Ideal conceptualizations are somewhere between these two extremes and do not confound diagnostic criteria with defining features of QOL.

Optimal measures of QOL recognize that the preserved abilities to experience positive emotions, feelings of belonging, and enjoyment of activities for patients with dementia are important QOL components *(5,6)*. Relative absence of negative emotional experiences, such as depressed mood and anxiety, also are important for QOL. Ideally, measures of QOL should include subscale constructs to assess for differential changes during time or in response to intervention.

From: *Current Clinical Neurology*
Vascular Dementia: Cerebrovascular Mechanisms and Clinical Management
Edited by: R. H. Paul, R. Cohen, B. R. Ott, and S. Salloway © Humana Press Inc., Totowa, NJ

3. MEASURING QOL IN DEMENTIA

Measuring QOL in dementia is difficult because of the subjective nature of the construct and because patients with dementia, by definition, experience cognitive impairments that might interfere with their ability to communicate and accurately report on internal states. Lack of insight refers to the decreased capacity of patients with cognitive impairment to accurately perceive their deficits. Lack of insight is common in dementia *(7–10)* and is another complicating factor in the assessment of QOL, because it may affect the self-reports of patients with dementia. For example, lack of insight is associated with greater disagreement between patient and observer reports of depression *(11)*. As compared to caregiver perceptions, patients with dementia also overestimate their abilities and report less impairment *(7,12)*. Thus, the self-reports of patients with dementia do not always accurately reflect their abilities and recent experiences.

Despite the limitations of data provided by patients with dementia, many investigators argue that QOL assessment should incorporate the patients' perspectives, at least in part *(5,6,13,14)*. Patients with Mini-Mental State Examination (MMSE) scores of less than or equal to 10 can usually participate in an interview about their QOL to some degree. For example, patients with MMSE scores in this range can provide QOL data that are as reliable as caregiver reports *(5,13,15)*. Because patients with mild to moderate dementia are able to provide reliable data about their QOL, efforts should be made to incorporate their opinions and perspectives into QOL assessments, especially because of the highly individual and subjective nature of the construct.

Other investigators rely on reports from proxies, such as family members or caregivers, to measure QOL in dementia *(3,16–18)*. These measures should be used with patients with severe dementia or who are unable to participate in the assessment process. Measuring QOL in patients in the later stages of disease severity and in patients who cannot provide data on their QOL because of language impairment is important, and observer-based instruments have been developed for these purposes *(3)*. For example, on one scale, caregivers, healthcare providers, or residential staff can rate observable behaviors. The behaviors were selected to reflect patients' moods, discomforts, and enjoyments *(18)*.

4. QOL IN VaD

Few dementia QOL studies included patients diagnosed with VaD in their samples, and none conducted subgroup analyses on these patients. For example, in a longitudinal study of caregiver factors and QOL in dementia, patients with VaD were included in the sample, along with AD and mixed dementia cases. Results indicated that several caregiver factors (i.e., personal distress, domestic upset, negative feelings, and the quality of the carer-patient relationship) were predictive of caregiver-rated QOL ratings that were collected 6 mo later, even when decline in cognitive abilities was controlled. In this longitudinal study, psychological well-being was stable and depression decreased in patients diagnosed with dementia, despite significant declines in cognitive status and functional ability. However, analyses did not investigate predictors of QOL separately for VaD, AD, and mixed cases *(16)*.

Another study of QOL in long-term care residents also included patients with VaD, who represented 22% of the sample. Results indicated that disorientation, physical dependency, depression, and anxiolytic treatment were negatively predictive of QOL, but analyses were not conducted separately for diagnostic subgroups of the sample *(17)*.

Thus, current literature on QOL in dementia tells us little about VaD populations. As noted, the majority of work on QOL in dementia has focused on patients with AD, the most common cause of dementia in the elderly. Thus, many of the definitions and conceptualizations for QOL that were reviewed are specific to AD. Although there are many overlapping features between AD and VaD, there also are important differences that may have important implications for QOL. The literature regarding QOL in AD is reviewed, and findings are used to generate hypotheses about QOL in VaD.

In addition to AD, patients with VaD have overlapping features with stroke patients who do not develop dementia *(19)*. There is much greater literature on QOL in stroke patients without relative to patients with VaD. Thus, the literature on QOL in nondemented stroke also is reviewed and used to generate hypotheses about QOL in VaD.

4.1. QOL in AD

Several factors contributing to poor quality of life in elderly patients with mild to severe AD have been investigated, including severity of cognitive impairment, decline in performance of ADLs, and neuropsychiatric symptoms *(3,20–22)*. Depression is one of the most consistent correlates of QOL in AD and is associated with lower ratings of QOL when it is assessed from the perspectives of both patients and caregivers *(5,6,13)*, as well as professional nursing staff *(17,18)*.

In addition to depressive symptoms, severity of cognitive impairment is associated with decreased QOL in AD in some studies. Several cross-sectional studies report lower QOL with greater disease severity *(6,20–22)*, but not all studies find this association *(13,18)*. Furthermore, some aspects of QOL change more than others *(23)*. For example, negative moods increase with dementia severity, but many positive emotional experiences do not decline with greater dementia severity *(3)*.

Performance of ADLs is correlated with QOL ratings of patients with AD in many studies *(3)*. In one report, scores on a measure of basic ADLs were correlated with self- and caregiver-reported QOL for 155 patients with mild to moderate AD. Decreased physical function was also associated with patient and caregiver QOL in AD in this study *(13)*. However, the strength of the association between ADL impairment and QOL is unclear. Evidence indicates that performance of ADLs may be somewhat less strongly associated with QOL than other features of AD *(18,21)*.

Caregiver characteristics have also been associated with QOL in AD. Caregiver burden is correlated with AD patient and caregiver reports of QOL, and caregiver depression correlates with caregiver-reported patient QOL *(13,22)*. Thus, caregiver burden and depression may affect patient QOL. However, it also is possible that these caregiver factors may result in biased reporting from some caregivers. For example, caregivers who are depressed may report lower QOL in patients because of a negative bias in reporting.

4.2. QOL in Stroke

QOL is often measured in victims of stroke, but few studies document cognitive impairment and dementia in their samples *(24)*. In one study that measured cognitive status of patients with stroke, global functional health was the strongest predictor of QOL after ischemic stroke *(24)*. QOL was greater in patients with better cognitive abilities, but cognition was not a significant predictor of QOL.

In a review of 39 studies regarding QOL in stroke published through 2001, Bays found that stroke survivors experienced greater impairment in ADLs, more depressive symptoms, and less social activity as compared to age-matched controls *(25)*. QOL reached a low at 3 mo after stroke and then improved during the next 9 mo, after which time there was stability for the following 2 yr. This may result from functional recovery that occurs within the first year after stroke. However, there was a great deal of heterogeneity in the reports in QOL over time, with many patients reporting little improvement. Depression, functional impairment, and social activities explained between 22 and 73% of the variance in stroke survivors' QOL. Similar to observations in AD, depression was the strongest single predictor of QOL, accounting for 28–40% of the variance. Gender and socioeconomic status were not significantly associated with patients' QOL. Inconsistent findings were reported between QOL and age, comorbid conditions, and stroke location, and no consistent patterns emerged regarding these variables.

In research published since this review, which involved a 3-mo longitudinal study of 215 Chinese victims of stroke, results indicated that functional ability was the strongest QOL predictor. Satisfaction with social support measured 2 wk after the stroke also was a significant QOL predictor at 3 mo *(26)*. Cognitive impairment was not assessed in this study.

4.3. Hypotheses About QOL in VaD

4.3.1. Depression

Depression is a strong QOL predictor in AD and stroke and, thus, is likely to be an important factor that predicts QOL in VaD. It is often noted that mood and personality changes occur earlier and are more severe in VaD than AD *(19,27)*. In a review of the literature in 1996, Ballard et al. concluded that the majority of evidence indicated greater prevalence of depression in VaD relative to AD *(28)*. Since then, results have been mixed, with some studies finding greater depression in VaD *(29,30)* and others reporting no significant differences *(31)*. Thus, depression is at least as common in VaD as AD and may be a strong QOL predictor.

4.3.2. Functional Impairment

Functional impairment in daily living is correlated with QOL in AD and is a significant predictor of QOL in stroke. Thus, impaired functional abilities also are hypothesized to affect QOL in VaD. It is possible that functional impairment will be more predictive of QOL in VaD than AD, because neurologic function is more impaired as a result of cerebrovascular disease (CVD) in VaD *(32)*. Furthermore, executive functions are more impaired in early to moderate VaD relative to AD, whereas memory and language are more impaired in AD *(19,27)*. Because executive dysfunction is a significant predictor of performance of ADLs *(33)*, it is reasonable to hypothesize that ADLs may be more impaired in VaD relative to AD, which, in turn, may lead in poorer QOL.

Functional abilities also may be more impaired in VaD because of greater medical comorbidity than AD. In a large sample of patients with dementia from a managed care organization, patients with VaD had higher prevalence rates than patients with AD for 9 out of 10 cardiovascular conditions and 9 other medical conditions. Patients with VaD also had more inpatient hospital days than patients with AD *(34)*. Other studies also found that general medical health is better in AD and that medical comorbidity is lesser in patients with AD vs VaD *(32,35)*. Associated features of increased medical comorbidity are increased medication use, increased use of healthcare services, more disability and dependence, and greater financial strain. It is conceivable that all of these factors might have a detrimental effect on QOL.

The effect of poor physical health on QOL in dementia has not been investigated, perhaps because the majority of work to date has included patients with AD and, as noted, their health is generally better than patients with VaD. Determining the effect of comorbid medical illness on QOL in dementia is an important task for future research.

4.3.3. Cognitive Impairment

Cognitive impairment is predictive of QOL in AD and is likely to be associated with QOL in VaD. There is inconsistent evidence on the relative rates of decline of cognitive abilities in VaD as compared to AD. Some studies find greater impairment and decline in AD *(32,35)*, and some studies find comparable rates of decline in AD and VaD *(36,37)*. Inconsistent findings likely result from different subgroups of VaD showing different progression patterns *(19)*. In any case, the rate of cognitive decline in VaD is either equal to or less than AD. If the rate of decline of patients with VaD is slower than AD, this might allow for more time to adjust and adapt to current level of impairment, which may contribute to better QOL. This is an issue for future research to address.

4.3.4. Caregiver Factors

Caregiver burden and depression are correlated with the assessment of QOL in AD *(13,22)* and, thus, may be associated with QOL in VaD. However, AD and VaD have differential effects on caregiver burden, depending on the stage of dementia severity. In a study of home care patients with dementia, patients with VaD were more burdensome to caregivers than AD in the early and middle stages of dementia. Patients with VaD were less able to perform basic ADLs and had more severely disturbed day-night rhythms. Patients with VaD also placed a greater financial burden on caregivers than AD. However, for severely impaired patients, AD was more burdensome than VaD *(38)*. Greater caregiver burden in the early to middle stages of VaD may contribute to perceptions of lower patient QOL during these times, relative to patients with AD.

4.3.5. Insight

The association between lack of insight in dementia and QOL is unknown. Insight in VaD appears to be comparable or greater than insight in AD. In a comparison of patients with AD and VaD matched for age, education, and gender, lack of insight did not differ significantly between the two groups *(39)*. Insightfulness in another study was indicated by anxiety and concern or loss of confidence when presented with tasks that patients can no longer accomplish. No differences were found between AD and VaD *(40)*.

However, in a study comparing AD and multiinfarct dementia (MID) cases, insight was measured as a discrepancy between caregiver- and patient-reported impairment in independent living skills (ILS). Patient groups were equated for overall level of impairment in ILS, as measured by a performance-based measure, as well as for age and education. Results indicated that patients with AD had greater loss of insight for ILS than patients with MID. Results were confirmed even when caregiver burden was controlled for in statistical analyses *(41)*. It is possible that greater preserved insight could negatively affect patient perceptions of QOL in VaD, but future research is needed to elucidate the association between insight and QOL.

5. FUTURE DIRECTIONS

VaD is the second leading cause of dementia *(19)*, but little is known about QOL in VaD. Research is this area is a priority, because results will determine how resources should be used to care for patients with VaD to maintain and maximize QOL. QOL will be difficult to study in VaD because it is a heterogeneous disorder, especially compared to AD *(19,27)*. Thus, future investigators should carefully diagnose and characterize VaD samples to determine the subtypes of VaD that are under investigation.

Because of unique characteristics of VaD samples, existing QOL measures developed for AD populations may not be suitable to study QOL in VaD. For example, there is greater incidence of physical illness, functional disability, and caregiver burden in some stages VaD relative to AD. There also may be greater annual costs of care per patient for VaD, as compared to AD *(34)*. Thus, new measures for QOL in VaD need to be developed. Guidance and models should be sought from existing theory and measures of QOL in dementia *(2,42)* and stroke *(25,43)*, as well as through consultation with patients, caregivers, and healthcare professionals who specialize in VaD. Because different QOL dimensions in AD change differentially over time, it is important to develop measures of QOL in VaD that include subscales.

Once QOL measures are developed, investigators can turn their attention to treatment, intervention, and decision-making issues related to QOL in VaD. For example, investigators can determine how QOL affects decisions to care for patients at home vs institutions. They also can determine how to maintain and enhance QOL in VaD. Recent evidence suggests that a multimodal, psychotherapeutic intervention with mild VaD improves patients' clinical condition. In an innovative and flexible intervention that included psychotherapy, occupational therapy, relaxation training, recreational therapy, and physical therapy, patients with mild VaD improved on multiple clinical measures relative to controls. Patients exhibited better cognitive performance, fewer behavioral disturbances and psychiatric symptoms, and participated in more ADLs *(44)*. Interventions such as these have promise to improve QOL for patients with VaD and their caregivers.

In summary, several hypotheses about QOL in VaD can be generated from the literature on QOL in AD and stroke survivors without dementia. Based on this work, hypotheses regarding predictors of QOL in VaD have been proposed. However, the first task of future research is to develop reliable and valid QOL measures in VaD. This will allow investigators to identify means to maintain and enhance patients' life quality.

REFERENCES

1. Lawton MP. Assessing quality of life in Alzheimer disease research. Alzheimer Dis Assoc Disord 1997;11(Suppl 6):91–99.
2. Lawton MP. Quality of life in Alzheimer disease. Alzheimer Dis Assoc Disord 1994;8(Suppl 6):138–150.
3. Albert SM, Castillo-Castaneda CD, Sano M, et al. Quality of life in patients with Alzheimer's disease as reported by patient proxies. J Am Geriatr Soc 1996;44:1342–1347.
4. Whitehouse PJ, Orgogozo JM, Becker RE, et al. Quality-of-life assessment in dementia drug development: position paper from the International Working Group on Harmonization of Dementia Drug Guidelines. Alzheimer Dis Assoc Disord 1997;11:56–60.
5. Brod M, Stewart AL, Sands L, Walton P. Conceptualization and measurement of quality of life in dementia: the dementia quality of life instrument (DQoL). Gerontologist 1999;39:25–35.
6. Ready RE, Ott BR, Grace J, Fernandez I. The Cornell-Brown Scale for Quality of Life in Dementia. Alzheimer Dis Assoc Disord 2002;16:109–115.
7. Ott BR, Lafleche G, Whelihan WM, Buongiorno GW, Albert MS, Fogel BS. Impaired awareness of deficits in Alzheimer's disease. Alzheimer Dis Assoc Disord 1996;10:68–76.
8. Zanetti O, Vallotti B, Frisoni GB, et al. Insight in dementia: when does it occur? Evidence for a nonlinear relationship between insight and cognitive status. J Gerontol 1999;54B:P100–P106.
9. Starkstein SE, Petracca G, Chemerinski E, Kremer J. Syndromic validity of apathy in Alzheimer's disease. Am J Psychiatry 2001;158:872–877.
10. Lopez OL, Becker JT, Somsak D, Dew MA, DeKosky ST. Awareness of cognitive deficits and anosognosia in probable Alzheimer's disease. Eur Neurol 1994;34:277–282.
11. Ott BR, Fogel BS. Measurement of depression in dementia: self vs clinician rating. Int J Geriatr Psychiatry 1992;7:899–904.
12. Vasterling JJ, Seltzer B, Watrous WE. Longitudinal assessment of deficit unawareness in Alzheimer's disease. Neuropsychiatry Neuropsychol Behav Neurol 1997;10:197–202.
13. Logsdon RG, Gibbons LE, McCurry SM, Teri L. Assessing quality of life in older adults with cognitive impairment. Psychosom Med 2002;64:510–519.
14. Selai CE, Trimble MR, Rossor M, Harvey RJ. Assessing quality of life in dementia: preliminary psychometric testing of the Quality of Life Assessment Schedule (QOLAS). Neuropsychological Rehabilitation 2001;11:219–243.
15. Logsdon RG, Gibbons LE, McCurry SM, Teri L. Quality of life in Alzheimer's disease: patient and caregiver reports. J Ment Health Aging1999;5:21–32.
16. Burgener S, Twigg P. Relationships among caregiver factors and quality of life in care recipients with irreversible dementia. Alzheimer Dis Assoc Disord 2002;16:88–102.
17. Gonzales-Salvador T, Lyketsos CG, Baker A, et al. Quality of life in dementia patients in long-term care. Intl J Geriatr Psychiatr 2000;15:181–189.
18. Weiner MF, Martin-Cook K, Svetlik DA, Saine K, Foster B, Fontaine CS. The Quality of Life in Late-Stage Dementia (QUALID) Scale. J Am Med Dir Assoc 2000;1:114–116.
19. Nyenhuis DL, Gorelick PB. Vascular dementia: a contemporary review of epidemiology, diagnosis, prevention, and treatment. J Am Geriatr Soc 1998;46:1437–1448.
20. Kerner DN, Patterson TL, Grant I, Kaplan RM. Validity of the Quality of Well-being Scale for patients with Alzheimer's disease. J Aging Health 1998;10:44–61.
21. Selai CE, Trimble MR, Rossor MN, Harvey RJ, The Quality of Life Assessment Schedule (QOLAS)—A new method for assessing quality of life in dementia. In: Albert SM, Logsdon RG, eds. Assessing Quality of Life in Alzheimer's Disease. New York, NY: Springer Publishing Company, 2000, pp. 31–48.
22. Karlawish JHT, Casarett D, Klocinski J, Clark CM. The relationship between caregivers' global ratings of Alzheimer's disease patients' quality of life, disease severity, and the caregiving experience. J Am Geriatr Soc 2001;49:1066–1070.
23. Albert SM, Michaels K, Padilla M, et al. Functional significance of mild cognitive impairment in elderly patients without a dementia diagnosis. Am J Geriatr Psychiatry 1999;7:213–220.
24. Kwa VIH, Limburg M, de Haan RJ. The role of cognitive impairment in the quality of life after ischaemic stroke. J Neurol 1996;243:599–604.
25. Bays CL. Quality of life of stroke survivors: a research synthesis. J Neurosci Nurs 2001;33:310–316.
26. MacKenzie AE, Change AM. Predictors of quality of life following stroke. Disabil Rehab 2002;24:259–265.
27. Kalaria R. Similarities between Alzheimer's disease and vascular dementia. J Neurol Sci 2002;203-204:29–34.
28. Ballard C, Bannister C, Solis M, Oyebode F, Wilcock G. The prevalence, associations and symptoms of depression amongst dementia sufferers. J Affect Disord 1996;36:135–144.
29. Li YS, Meyer JS, Thornby J. Depressive symptoms among cognitively normal versus cognitively impaired elderly subjects. Int J Geriatr Psychiatry 2001;16:455–461.
30. Aharon-Peretz J, Kloit D, Tomer R. Behavioral differences between white matter lacunar dementia and Alzheimer's disease: a comparison on the Neuropsychiatric Inventory. Dement Geriatr Cogn Disord 2000;11:294–298.
31. Draper B, MacCuspie-Moore C, Brodaty H. Suicidal ideation and the 'wish to die' in dementia patients: the role of depression. Age Ageing 1998;27:503–507.

32. Groves WC, Brandt J, Steinberg M, et al. Vascular dementia and Alzheimer's disease: Is there a difference? A comparison of symptoms by disease duration. J Neuropsychiatry Clin Neurosci 2000;12:305–315.
33. Boyle PA, Malloy PF, Salloway S, Cahn-Weiner DA, Cohen R, Cummings JL. Executive dysfunction and apathy predict functional impairment in Alzheimer disease. Am J Geriatr Psychiatry 2003;11:214–221.
34. Fillit H, Hill J. The costs of vascular dementia: a comparison with Alzheimer's disease. J Neurol Sci 2002;203–204: 35–39.
35. Kittner B, De Deyn PP, Erkinjuntit T. Investigating the natural course and treatment of vascular dementia and Alzheimer's disease. Ann NY Acad Sci 2000;903:535–541.
36. Ballard C, O'Brien J, Morris CM, et al. The progression of cognitive impairment in dementia with Lewy bodies, vascular dementia and Alzheimer's disease. Intl J Geriatr Psychiatry 2001;16:499–503.
37. Ballard C, Patel A, Oyebode F, Wilcock G. Cognitive decline in patients with Alzheimer's disease, vascular dementia and senile dementia of Lewy Body type. Age Ageing 1996;25:209–213.
38. Vetter PH, Krauss S, Steiner O, et al. Vascular dementia versus dementia of Alzheimer's type: do they have differential effects on caregivers' burden? J Gerontol 1999;54B:S93–S98.
39. Verhey FRJ, Ponds RWHM, Rozendaal N, Jolles J. Depression, insight, and personality changes in Alzheimer's disease and vascular dementia. J Geriatr Psychiatry Neurol 1995;8:23–27.
40. Bathgate D, Snowden JS, Varma A, Blackshaw A, Neary D. Behaviour in frontotemporal dementia, Alzheimer's disease and vascular dementia. Acta Neurol Scand 2001;103:367–378.
41. DeBettignies BH, Mahurin RK, Pirozzolo FJ. Insight for impairment in independent living skills in Alzheimer's disease and multi-infarct dementia. J Clin Exp Neuropsychol 1990;12:355–363.
42. Ready RE, Ott BR. Quality of life measures for dementia. Health Qual Life Outcomes 2003;1:11.
43. Williams LS, Weinberger M, Harris LE, Clark DO, Biller J. Development of a stroke-specific quality of life scale. Stroke 1999;30:1362–1369.
44. Kruglov LS. The early stage of vascular dementia: significance of a complete therapeutic program. Int J Geriatr Psychiatry 2003;18:402–406.

25

Approaches to Neuroprotection and Recovery Enhancement After Acute Stroke

Marc Fisher and Magdy Selim

1. INTRODUCTION

The potential relevance of neuroprotective and recovery enhancing therapies after acute ischemic stroke to vascular dementia (VaD) must be considered from several perspectives. The goal of acute neuroprotective therapy for ischemic stroke is to impede one or more aspects of the ischemic cascade of cell injury induced by focal brain ischemia *(1)*. It is presumed that inhibiting the ischemic cascade will reduce the extent of infarction and improve ultimate functional outcome. Recovery-enhancing therapies are designed to enhance brain recovery after stroke and to improve functional outcome but not necessarily to affect infarct size *(2)*. It can be assumed that both neuroprotection and recovery enhancement might lessen the incidence of VaD development after stroke by several mechanisms. This chapter overviews current concepts of ischemic injury related to acute focal brain ischemia and the current status of efforts to develop effective neuroprotective and recovery-enhancing therapies for acute ischemic stroke.

To begin rational development of neuroprotective therapy for acute ischemic stroke, it is important to focus on the likely important mechanisms of cell death related to focal brain ischemia *(3)*. Vascular occlusion induced by local arterial thrombosis or, more commonly, embolization from a distal source in the heart or a more proximal vessel initiates ischemic injury. This vascular occlusion should be considered as the initiating event of a complex number of cellular responses that may be deleterious or self-preservatory in an attempt to salvage injured cells. The balance between mechanisms of cellular survival and death ultimately determines the extent of final infarction. The pathophysiology of ischemic brain injury has been studied for many years, and the complexity of known cellular responses to focal ischemia has increased dramatically over time *(4)*. In regions of low residual cerebral blood flow (CBF), the ischemic core, failure of high-energy metabolism occurs rapidly, followed by commitment to cell death pathways. A primary consequence of high-energy metabolism failure is the loss of ion homeostasis. This loss of ion homeostasis leads to an increase of intracellular calcium, along with other ions and water *(5)*. Calcium accumulates because of the activation of receptor-mediated and voltage-mediated calcium-conducting channels. The activation of glutamate activated channels such as the *N*-methyl-D-aspartate (NMDA) and the α-amino-3-hydroxy-5-methyl-4-isoxazole (AMPA) channels are believed to directly mediate intracellular calcium increases and also activate voltage-mediated calcium-conducting channels *(6)*. The intracellular accumulation of calcium initiates a cytotoxic cascade with the activation of protein kinases, proteases, phospholipases, endonucleases, and proteolytic enzymes, such as calpains and caspases *(7)*. Free radicals are also generated, as well as the formation of excessive amounts of nitric oxide.

From: *Current Clinical Neurology*
Vascular Dementia: Cerebrovascular Mechanisms and Clinical Management
Edited by: R. H. Paul, R. Cohen, B. R. Ott, and S. Salloway © Humana Press Inc., Totowa, NJ

Table 1
Relating Cell Death to Protein Synthesis-Dependent and Nonprotein Synthesis-Related Mechanisms

Nonprotein synthesis-related mechanisms of cell death
1. Depletion of adenosine triphosphate (ATP), disruption of glutamate homeostasis, and activation of glutamate receptors
2. Intracellular calcium overload
3. Free radical generation
4. Activation of phospholipases, leading to oxidation of fatty acids and other lipids
5. Activation of proteases such as calpains
6. Activation of posttranslational prodeath factors.
Protein synthesis-dependent pathways of cell death
1. Expression of proinflammatory mediators of cell death
2. Expression of proapoptotic molecules
3. Expression of other cellular proteins that mediate cell death
4. Expression of metalloproteinases
5. Expression of proapoptotic transcription factors

Oxygen free radicals can interact with nitric oxide to form peroxynitrite, an especially toxic type of free radical. These various cellular consequences of severe brain ischemia rapidly induce cellular necrosis and irreversible injury. Posttranslational activation of intrinsic, cellular prodeath factors may also occur *(8)*. Necrosis is characterized histologically by karyolysis of the cell nucleus and eosinophilic staining and swelling of cytoplasmic structures *(7)*.

Other mechanisms of cell death after focal brain ischemia are programmed cell death and cell death mediated by inflammatory events. Programmed cell death can be triggered by ischemic brain injury, and evidence has implicated release of mitochondrial cytochrome c and activation of caspases as important contributors *(9,10)*. Programmed cell death is distinguished histologically by the appearance of nuclear condensation and fragmentation, along with the development of cytoplasmic appendages *(7)*. One potential way to distinguish between the contributions of necrosis and programmed cell death to tissue injury after focal brain ischemia is to relate these mechanisms to the level of CBF decline and effects on protein synthesis as outlined in Table 1 *(4)*. In brain regions with moderate to severe declines of CBF (i.e., below approximately 25 mL/100 g/min), protein synthesis declines or ceases and the mechanisms of cell death commonly associated with necrosis will likely predominate. In the modestly ischemic zone of CBF decline, protein synthesis mechanisms of cell death that are linked to programmed cell death can occur and may predominate. Thus, in ischemic stroke, it is likely that both types of injury occur and their relative contributions will vary among individual patients in relationship to the range of CBF declines that occur in the ischemic region and also with time *(11)*. For example, in a patient with a large region of severe ischemia, protein synthesis-independent mechanisms of cell death will likely predominate and irreversible injury will likely occur quickly. In another patient with good collateral blood flow and a large region of modest CBF decline, both types of cell death mechanisms may contribute and the evolution of ischemic injury may be much more protracted. The distinction between necrosis and programmed cell death pathways of cellular injury related to CBF levels may be somewhat artificial, because apoptosis-inducing factor can be released from mitochondria without *de novo* protein synthesis and induce a programmed cell death-like mechanism of cell injury *(12)*.

The contribution of inflammatory-mediated mechanisms of cell death to ischemic brain injury after stroke is likely most important after successful reperfusion and is not likely a major factor without reperfusion *(7)*. Cell-mediated inflammatory mechanisms of ischemic injury occur with the recruitment of polymorphonuclear leukocytes and, to a lesser degree, the accumulation of mononuclear white blood cells. The production and release of inflammatory mediators, such as cytokines, prostaglandins, and leukotrienes, may contribute to the inflammatory process *(13)*. These molecules may, in part, be produced by the activation of proinflammatory genes. With reperfusion, the activation of additional pathways of programmed cell death may also occur. The occurrence of so-called "reperfusion injury" has now been documented in both animal stroke models and stroke patients *(14,15)*. It is obvious that the different therapeutic targets must be considered after reperfusion than before reperfusion.

Another approach to consider regarding the tissue and cellular consequences of focal ischemic brain injury is the possibility of exploiting endogenous protective mechanisms that are activated in response to ischemia. Knowledge about self-preservatory mechanisms has been delineated from two major sources, ischemic preconditioning and the study of hibernating animals *(11)*. With ischemic preconditioning, animals are exposed to brief periods of ischemia and then subsequently to more extended and severe periods of ischemia. Ischemic tolerance can be achieved by ischemic preconditioning, and this is related to gene expression initiated by the preconditioning episode *(16,17)*. Precisely which genes and associated proteins are most important for the production of tolerance remains to be determined. It is possible that an array of gene expression is required for optimizing preconditioning, and this might be achieved by the activation of promotor genes. The study of ischemic preconditioning, prosurvival gene expression, and promotors is just beginning and will require many additional experiments before potentially viable therapeutic strategies can be implemented in clinical development. Hibernating animals may also yield important information about how ischemia-tolerant species adapt to conditions of hypoxia and ischemia *(18)*. These species apparently adapt to hypoxic conditions by downregulating energy turnover and by increasing efficiency of adenosine triphosphate (ATP)-producing pathways. Currently, it is unclear how enhancing these adaptive mechanisms can be used as a therapeutic approach for stroke patients, but the lessons learned may lead to the development of new treatment strategies in the future.

2. NEUROPROTECTIVE THERAPIES

A substantial number of compounds with various and disparate inhibitory mechanisms of actions on the ischemic cascade have been developed as "neuroprotective agents" to treat stroke patients. Although several of these agents were neuroprotective in the laboratory, few clinical studies have suggested benefit with them *(19–21)*. Not a single compound to date has achieved unequivocal success when tested in randomized, clinical trials (*see* Table 2). Most neuroprotective strategies employed previously focused on inhibiting one part of the ischemic cascade. A comprehensive review of all neuroprotective agents that have been tested in stroke patients cannot be undertaken in this chapter. The following representative studies highlight the history of clinical research strategies in neuroprotection and different classes of drugs with neuroprotective capabilities.

Gangliosides, which antagonize the damaging effects of excitatory amino acids in experimental ischemia, were heavily investigated in several clinical trials in patients with acute ischemic stroke *(22,23)* without demonstrable benefit. The Sygen in Acute Stroke Study (SASS) *(22)* assessed the safety and efficacy of the ganglioside GM1 vs placebo in 287 patients with acute anterior circulation ischemic stroke. Primary and secondary outcome measures showed no significant difference between treatment arms, and adverse experiences were similar in the two groups. Trials using calcium channel blockers, such as nimodipine, given either orally or intravenously within 12 h of stroke onset also failed to show benefit *(24–26)*. Indeed, intravenous nimodipine was harmful because of associated systemic hypotensive and cardiovascular complications. Activation of γ-aminobutyric acid (GABA)-ergic activity, using the $GABA_A$ receptor agonist clomethiazole, was evaluated in two randomized, placebo-controlled, trials (Clomethiazole Acute Stroke Study [CLASS] and CLASS-Thrombolysis [CLASS-T]) *(27,28)* involving approximately 2500 patients

Table 2
Strategies/Targets of Clinical Neuroprotective Trials to Date

Neuroprotective mechanism(s)	Tested drug
Antagonism of $GABA_A$ receptors	Clomethiazole
Competitive antagonism of NMDA receptors	Selfotel, CPPene
Non-competitive antagonism of NMDA receptors	MK-801, Magnesium,[a] aptiganel
Antagonism of AMPA receptors	NBQX
Antagonism of the polyamine regulatory site of the EAA receptor complex	Eliprodil
Antagonism of the glycine regulatory site	Gavestinel
Antagonism of the opiate receptors	Nalmefene
Blockade of voltage-sensitive calcium channels	Nimodipine, flunarizine, magnesium [a]
Blockade of sodium channels	Sipatrigine, fosphenytoin
Activation of potassium channels	BMS-204352
Activation of the serotonin $5HT_{1A}$ receptors	BAY-3702,[a] SUN-N-4057 [b]
Modulation of glutamate release/uptake	Lamotrigine; ONO-2506
Scavenging of free radicals	tirilazad, NYX 059 [a]
Stabilization of neuronal membranes	Piracetam [a]
Inhibition of nitric oxide synthase	Lubeluzole
Providing trophic factors	Trafermin
Providing antibodies to ICAM-1	Enlimomab
Promoting the synthesis of acetyl choline	Citicoline

[a] Ongoing.
[b] Planned.
Abbr: GABA, γ-aminobutyric acid; NMDA, *N*-methyl-D-aspartate; AMPA, α-amino-3-hydroxy-5-methyl-4-isoxazole; EAA, excitatory amino acid; ICAM-1, intercellular adhesion molecule-1.

worldwide. Although clomethiazole appeared to be safe, no efficacy benefit was found in treated patients. Numerous compounds, which act to modulate excitatory amino acid (EAA) receptors, such as NMDA and AMPA receptor antagonists, have been extensively tested in several randomized clinical trials *(29–32)*. All of these trials failed to show benefit or were terminated prematurely because of lack of efficacy or safety concerns. Other modulators of the EAA release and receptor-gated ion channel complexes, such as the sodium, potassium, or glycine channels, were tested in several randomized clinical trials. The efficacy of sodium channel blockade in limiting acute poststroke brain damage, as measured by magnetic resonance imaging (MRI) was tested in the Sipatrigine In Stroke trial. This trial was halted and its results are yet to be published. The safety and efficacy of maxi-K channel agonist, BMS-204352, was tested in 1978 patients with acute stroke *(33)*. BMS-204352 failed to show superior efficacy compared to placebo. A glycine antagonist, gavestinel, was tested in multiple clinical trials *(34–36)*. There were no significant differences in serious side effects between the drug- and placebo-treated patients, and no statistically significant improvement on the 3-mo outcome measures was demonstrated for gavestinel. Treatment with kappa opiate receptor antagonist, nalmefene, within 6 h of acute ischemic stroke did not result in a significant difference in 3-mo outcome, compared with placebo *(37)*. The ion channel and nitric oxide synthase (NOS) antagonist, lubeluzole, was tested in three randomized clinical trials *(20,38,39)*. The last of which, Combination Therapy with Lubeluzole and t-PA in the Treatment of Acute Ischemic Stroke (LUB-USA-6) *(39)*, was halted prematurely after lack of efficacy was demonstrated for lubeluzole alone.

Several strategies aiming to counterbalance the potentially damaging effects of presumed reperfusion on ischemic tissue have been evaluated in clinical trials as well. Treating acute ischemic stroke patients with methyl tirilazad, iron-dependent peroxidation, and a free radical scavenger within

6 h from ischemic stroke onset has been tested in two multicenter trials in North America *(40,41)*. In the Randomized Trial of Tirilazad mesylate in patients with Acute Stroke (RANTTAS) *(40)*, treatment with 6 mg/kg/d for 3 d beginning at a median of 4.3 h after stroke did not improve functional outcome after 3 mo. A higher dose (12.5–15 mg/kg on the first day, then 10–12 mg/kg/d for 2 d) was tested in RANTTAS II *(41)*. The higher dose regimen was associated with a 14% absolute reduction in mortality and an increase in the proportion of patients who were independent (Barthel Index score >60) at 3 mo. However, these differences were not statistically significant, because only 111 patients were included in RANTTAS II. The study was terminated prematurely because of safety concerns regarding a parallel study in Europe *(42)*. The use of a monoclonal antibody directed against intercellular adhesion molecule-1 (ICAM-1) was tested in the Enlimomab Acute Stroke Trial (EAST) *(43)*. Enlimomab had negative effects and caused more adverse events than placebo, including primarily infections and fever.

Several other "neuroprotective" drugs with novel mechanism(s) of action were tested in stroke patients. The Piracetam in Acute Stroke Study (PASS) *(44)* examined the potential benefit of piracetam vs placebo in the treatment of acute ischemic stroke when given within 12 h after symptom onset. Piracetam is present in the polar heads of phospholipid membrane, and its neuroprotective properties are mediated through its stabilizing effects on the cell membrane by restoring membrane fluidity and maintenance or improvement of membrane-bound cell functions, including ATP production, neurotransmission, and secondary messenger activity. Outcome was similar with both treatments in initial analyses. Post hoc analyses in an early treatment group, presenting within 7 h of stroke onset, showed differences favoring piracetam relative to placebo. The PASS II is currently underway to determine whether the administration of piracetam in aphasic acute stroke patients within 7 h after symptom onset will enhance recovery from aphasia at 4 and 12 wk poststroke *(45)*. The safety and efficacy of basic fibroblast growth factor, trafermin, in reducing infarct volume and promoting functional recovery in acute ischemic stroke patients were tested in two phase III trials *(46)*; both were terminated prematurely by the Data Safety Monitoring Committee after an interim analysis and clinical development in stroke was halted.

The failure of the treatment strategies or compounds discussed does not necessarily translate into the conclusion that neuroprotection cannot be effective. Numerous reasons may account for the lack of positive clinical trials after neuroprotective effects were seen in animal models. It has been suggested that some experimental animal models may be inadequate and that some of the agents evaluated in clinical trials were not adequately tested in preclinical studies. Study design and patients' selection flaws were also responsible for this negative experience with previous neuroprotection trials. For example, various NMDA antagonists produced significant adverse effects at patient plasma levels lower than those affording neuroprotection in animal studies. In most of these trials, patients were treated too late after stroke onset. Again, animal studies indicate that the NMDA antagonists, as a class, have a short window of therapeutic opportunity (60–90 min), yet they were invariably examined in stroke patients between 6 and 12 h after symptom onset. Therefore, it is not surprising that all the drugs in this class of compounds have failed clinically. Most of the neuroprotective drugs tested to date act on mechanisms occurring early in the ischemic cascade and, therefore, are expected to have a short time window for therapeutic efficacy. Other factors accounting for the failure of past neuroprotective trials include underpowered studies or insensitive outcome measures to detect modest treatment benefit and inclusion of a large number of patients with mild or severe deficits in whom treatment effects are hard to assess. The Stroke Therapy Academic Industry Roundtable (STAIR) group has developed guidelines for future neuroprotective drug development and testing in clinical trials to address these concerns *(47,48)*.

Numerous new neuroprotection clinical trials are underway or are expected to begin shortly. Still under investigation are early GABA-ergic activation using diazepam within 0–12 h after stroke onset *(49)*; the safety and feasibility of using transdermal nitric oxide, glyceryl trinitrate *(50)*; the neuroprotective efficacy of intravenous ONO-2506, which acts to modulate the uptake capacity of glutamate transporters and expression of GABA receptors and various astrocytic factors, in patients with acute ischemic stroke; piracetam *(45)*; the $5HT_{1A}$ serotonin agonist, repinotan *(51)*; the nitron spin-trap free radical scavenger, NXY-059; and magnesium.

Magnesium sulfate blocks voltage-gated calcium influx and NMDA receptor-operated calcium channels. It was safe and well tolerated by stroke patients when given as a continuous infusion for 24 h at a dose of 73 mmol *(52)*. A pilot study to determine the safety and feasibility of paramedic-initiated hyperacute magnesium sulfate administration to stroke patients identified in the field was recently completed *(53)*. Clinicians noted patient improvement in 20% of the cases, deterioration in 7%, and no change in 73%. At 3 mo, 67% of patients had good functional outcomes. Investigators concluded that field-based magnesium intervention is safe and feasible, and a large-scale, randomized, controlled trial to test its efficacy will be launched shortly *(54)*. Enrollment was recently completed in a trial to test the neuroprotective efficacy of Ebselen, a glutathione peroxidase-like antioxidant, in patients with cortical ischemic stroke *(55)*. The results are yet to be announced.

Lessons from the past and the rapid pace of accumulating knowledge regarding the pathophysiological, molecular, and biochemical changes in ischemic tissues encourage optimism that effective neuroprotective therapy will become available in the future. Charting progress in the field of neuroprotection, one anticipates that new alternative approaches and strategies for neuroprotection will be pursued, including combining reperfusion strategies with neuroprotective agents to improve tissue recovery and drug delivery, using agents that are tailored to ameliorate the events associated with reperfusion injury, and using multidrug therapy or multipotent drugs to target different aspects of the postischemic cascade simultaneously. Combining pharmacological therapy with nonpharmacological neuroprotective strategies is another plausible approach. Reduction of brain temperature is neuroprotective in experimental stroke models *(56)*. Two small-scale clinical trials *(57,58)* have assessed the safety and feasibility of inducing hypothermia in stroke patients. Moderate hypothermia in acute ischemic stroke is both feasible and safe, and the infarct growth was slightly lower in the hypothermia group than in the control group. However, this difference was not statistically significant. Planning is underway for a large-scale, efficacy trial. Hypothermia can potentially be employed to extend the therapeutic time window for administering neuroprotective therapy or reperfusion strategies. Last, but not least, the concept of neuroprotection is likely to expand to include pharmacological strategies to aid and facilitate recovery and rehabilitation after stroke. Functional imaging studies show that relearning of neurologic function in healthy parts of the brain is essential for reorganization of neuronal function after stroke. Piracetam improves learning and memory *(44)* and, as an adjunct to speech therapy, aphasia. Similarly, amphetamine can promote recovery in animals via its dopaminergic, serotonergic, and noradrenergic actions. Clinical trials assessing the efficacy of piracetam in aphasic stroke patients and D-amphetamine in facilitating poststroke motor recovery are underway.

3. RECOVERY-ENHANCING THERAPY

Another approach to the treatment of stroke patients is to try and enhance functional recovery without affecting the size of the ischemic lesion *(59)*. The natural history of ischemic stroke is for improvement of deficits over time in those patients who survive. This tendency for improvement of initial deficits may relate to the ability of undamaged brain regions to assume functions originally controlled by regions injured by the stroke or for new learning to occur. Brain activation studies, primarily with function of MRI, have demonstrated that brain regions not traditionally assumed to be responsible for a particular activity could become activated after ischemic injury *(59)*. New synapse formation, neurogenesis, and axonal sprouting may contribute to this functional reorganization. Pharmacological enhancement of these processes is possible, and preliminary data suggest that recovery enhancement is an exciting and novel approach to potentially maximizing improvement after stroke *(60)*.

Growth factors have been the most extensively evaluated pharmacological approach for enhancing recovery after stroke. The growth factor basic fibroblast growth factor (bFGF) has a dual treatment effect. When given intravenously early after stroke onset in animal stroke models, it reduces infarct size *(61)*. However, delayed iv initiation of administration of bFGF 24 h after stroke onset does not reduce infarct size but improves functional outcome at 4 wk when assessed by a battery of performance tasks *(62)*. This growth factor was evaluated in two clinical trials, and the overall results were negative *(63,64)*. However, in one of the trials, patients starting treatment intravenously for 24 h who had a later onset of therapy did demonstrate a trend toward improved outcome. Another growth factor, osteogenic protein-1 (OP-1), a bone morphogenic protein, improved delayed functional outcome when given into the cisterna magna, if therapy was initiated at 1 or 4 d after stroke in animals *(65)*. Infarct size was not reduced by this late initiation of OP-1.

A novel approach to enhancing recovery after stroke would be to induce neurogenesis, because it now apparent that neuronal cell proliferation does occur in the adult brain. Several pharmacological interventions have demonstrated the capability to induce neurogenesis and to improve functional outcome in animal stroke models. Nitric oxide is a molecule with documented ability to serve as a chemical messenger and neurotransmitter in the brain. It has been suggested that nitric oxide may play an important role in the proliferation, differentiation, and migration of progenitor cells. This possibility was explored by administering the nitric oxide donor, (Z)-1-(*N*-2-aminoethyl)-*N*-(2-ammonioethyl) amino-1-ium-1,2-diolate (DETA/NONOate) to rats subjected to an embolic stroke model, beginning treatment 24 h after stroke onset *(66)*. Treatment was associated with enhanced cellular proliferation and migration and improved functional outcome 42 d after stroke without an effect on infarct volume. This nitric oxide donor increased brain cyclic guanosine 5'-monophosphate (GMP) levels, so the same group evaluated the effect of sildenafil (Viagra), a phosphodiesterase 5 inhibitor that also increases cGMP levels. Using the same embolic stroke model, it was observed that oral administration of sildenafil for 7 d beginning 2 or 24 h after stroke onset enhanced neurogenesis and improved functional outcome at 28 d *(67)*. Infarct size was not reduced, and cortical cGMP levels were increased. The possibility that a 3-hydroxy-3-methyl-glutaryl-coenzyme A reductase inhibitor (statin) might improve functional outcome after stroke was also evaluated. Statins have many effects that might potentiate brain recovery, including acting as nitric oxide donors, enhancing angiogenesis and improving CBF. Three doses of atorvastatin were administered orally to rats subjected to 2 h of temporary ischemia with the suture occlusion method, beginning 24 h after stroke onset and continuing treatment for 7 d *(68)*. At day 14, the low- and middle-dose groups had improved functional outcome, but the high-dose group did not. Infarct size was not reduced in any of the treated groups. Angiogenesis was enhanced in the two lower dose groups, but not in the high-dose group. Similarly, neuronal cellular proliferation was enhanced, and cGMP levels were increased. The results of these preliminary experiments suggest that currently available, widely prescribed medications, such as sildenafil and atorvastatin, potentially may improve outcome after stroke and deserve further investigation both preclinically and potentially in clinical trials.

The possibility that amphetamines might enhance stroke recovery has been considered for a long time. Amphetamines induce the release of monoamine transmitters, and this may lead to improved recovery. In a rat stroke model, D-amphetamine initiated 3 d after stroke onset improved outcome at day 30 *(69)*. Synaptophysin and GAP-43 levels increased with the D-amphetamine treatment. Two small trials with D-amphetamine suggested a treatment effect on motor function, but this was not confirmed in a third trial. A larger trial of amphetamines to improve stroke outcome is now being conducted and hopefully will determine if this therapeutic approach has merit or not.

Citicoline (CDP-choline) is an interesting molecule that demonstrates neuroprotective effects in animals when initiated shortly after stroke onset *(70)*. Citicoline also likely enhances stroke recovery, probably related to its ability to enhance cell membrane repair. Several large phase III trials were conducted with the initiation of oral citicoline up to 24 h after stroke onset *(19)*. The outcome of these trials was equivocal with no significant effect on the primary outcome measure chosen, but suggestion of benefit on secondary outcome measures. A recent meta-analysis of these citicoline trials evaluated the effect of treatment in patients with moderately severe stroke, NIH score greater than or equal to 8, using as a favorable outcome measure a combined analysis of favorable outcome on the Barthel Index, modified Rankin Scale and the NIH Stroke Scale *(71)*. Using this analysis approach for 3-mo poststroke outcome, 25.2% of citicoline treated patients had a favorable outcome, whereas and only 20.2% of placebo-treated patients had a favorable outcome, $p = 0.0043$. The results of this meta-analysis suggest that citicoline might improve stroke outcome and the late time-to-treatment initiation suggests that this effect is likely to be primarily mediated through recovery enhancement. This favorable treatment effect needs to be prospectively demonstrated in another trial that designates the combined outcome measure as the prespecified primary outcome measure of the trial. Such a trial is currently being planned.

Another potentially exciting and novel approach to enhancement of recovery after stroke is cell-based therapy. Animal studies of cell-based therapies related to transplantation of neural stem cells, postmitotic neuronal cells, and xenogenic stem cells have all demonstrated dramatic effects on enhancing stroke recovery. These cells were delivered locally into the brain by intracisternal administration or most remarkably by intravenous administration and migration to the affected brain region was observed *(72,73)*. Another approach to cell-based therapy is activation of endogenous neural stem cells to enhance stroke recovery *(74)*. Preliminary reports have explored the safety and feasibility of cell-based therapies in stroke patients. Much additional investigative is needed to determine how best to maximize the potential for this approach to enhancing stroke recovery.

It is obvious that the treatment of acute stroke by neuroprotection and the enhancement of stroke recovery are both therapeutic areas that are in their infancy. Much has been learned about how to rationally approach these areas of therapeutic endeavor to maximize the chances for demonstrating treatment responses, and much more will be learned during the next few years. As effective therapies are developed, we can anticipate that they will begin to affect the burden of VaD observed after stroke. Some of the lessons learned may also be applicable to the development of more focused therapies for VaD prevention in other settings.

REFERENCES

1. Fisher M, Schaebitz W. An overview of acute stroke therapy. Arch Int Med 2000;160:3196–4006.
2. Fisher M, Finklestein SP. Pharmacological approaches to stroke recovery. Cerebrovasc Dis 1999;9:29–32.
3. Fisher M. Characterizing the targets of acute stroke treatment. Stroke 1997;28:866–872.
4. Hossmann K-A. Viability thresholds and the penumbra of focal ischemia. Ann Neurol 1994;36:557–565.
5. Kristian T, Siesjo BK. Calcium in ischemic cell death. Stroke 1998;29:705–718.
6. Nietera P, Lipton SA. Excitotoxins in neuronal apoptosis and necrosis. J Cereb Blood Flow Metab 1999;19:583–591.
7. Ye ZR, Liu KF, Garcia JH. Mechanisms of neuronal cell death after ischemic brain injury. In: Fisher M, Bogousslausky J, eds. Current Review of Cerebrovascular Disease. 4th Ed. Philadelphia, PA: Current Medicine, 2001, pp. 15–24.
8. Degracia DJ, Kumar R, Owen CR, et al. Molecular pathways of protein synthesis inhibition during reperfusion: implications for neuronal survival or death. J Cereb Blood Flow Metab 2002;22:127–141.
9. Bresden DE. Neural apoptosis. Ann Neurol 1995;38:839–851.
10. Graham SG, Chen J. Programmed cell death in cerebral ischemia. J Cereb Blood Flow Metab 2001;21:99–109.
11. Fisher M, Ratan R. New perspectives on developing acute stroke therapies. Ann Neurol 2003;53:10–20.
12. Susis SA, Daugar E, Ravagnan, et al. Two distinct pathways leading to nuclear apoptosis. J Exp Med 2000;192:571–580.
13. Rothwell NJ, Hopkins SJ. Cytokines and the nervous system; actions and mechanisms of action. Trends Neurosci 1995; 18:130–136.
14. Li F, Liu KF, Silva, et al. Secondary decline in apparent diffusion coefficient and neurological outcome after a short period of focal brain ischemia in rats. Ann Neurol 2000;48:236–244.
15. Kidwell CS, Saver JL, Mattiello J, et al. Thrombolytic reversal of acute human cerebral ischemic injury shown by diffusion/perfusion magnetic resonance imaging. Ann Neurol 2000;47:462–469.
16. Dawson VL, Dawson TM. Neuronal ischemic preconditioning. Trends Pharmacol Sci 2000;21:423–424.
17. Chen J, Simon R. Ischemic tolerance in the brain. Neurology 1997;48:306–311.

18. Zhou F, Zhu X, Castellani RJ, et al. Hibernation, a model of neuroprotection. Am J Pathol 2001;158:2145–2151.
19. Clark WM, Warach SJ, Pettigrew LC, Gammans RE, Sabounjian LA. A randomized dose-response trial of citicoline in acute ischemic stroke patients. Citicoline Stroke Study Group. Neurology 1997;49:671–678.
20. Grotta J. Lubeluzole treatment of acute ischemic stroke. The US and Canadian Lubeluzole Ischemic Stroke Study Group. Stroke 1997;28:2338–2346.
21. Edaravone Acute Infarction Study Group. Effect of a novel free radical scavenger, edaravone (MCI-186), on acute brain infarction. Cereb Dis 2003;15:222–229.
22. The SASS Trial. Ganglioside GM1 in acute ischemic stroke. Stroke 1994;25:1141–1148.
23. Lenzi GL, Grigoletto F, Gent M, et al. Early treatment of stroke with monosialoganglioside GM-1. Efficacy and safety results of the Early Stroke Trial. Stroke 1994;25:1552–1558.
24. Wahlgren NG, MacMahon D, De Keyser J. The Intravenous Nimodipine West European Trial (INWEST) of nimodipine in the treatment of acute ischemic stroke. Cereb Dis 1994;4:204–210.
25. Ahmed N, Nasman P, Wahlgren NG. Effect of intravenous nimodipine on blood pressure and outcome after acute stroke. Stroke 2000;31:1250–1255.
26. Horn J, de Haan RJ, Vermeulen M, Limburg M. Very Early Nimodipine Use in Stroke (VENUS): a randomized, double-blind, placebo-controlled trial. Stroke 2001;32:461–465.
27. Wahlgren NG, Ranasinha KW, Rosolacci T, et al. Clomethiazole Acute Stroke Study (CLASS): results of a randomized, controlled trial of clomethiazole versus placebo in 1360 acute stroke patients. Stroke 1999;30:21–28.
28. Lyden P, Jacoby M, Schim J, et al. The Clomethiazole Acute Stroke Study in tissue-type plasminogen activator-treated stroke (CLASS-T): final results. Neurology 2001;57:1199–1205.
29. ARTIST +: AMPA Receptor Antagonist Treatment in Ischemic Stroke Trial, YM872 + Alteplase. Ongoing Clinical Trials Session, 27th International Stroke Conference, 2002.
30. ARTIST MRI: AMPA Receptor Antagonist Treatment in Ischemic Stroke Trial-MRI. Ongoing Clinical Trials Session, 27th International Stroke Conference, 2002.
31. Grotta J, Clark W, Coull B, et al. Safety and tolerability of the glutamate antagonist CGS 19755 (Selfotel) in patients with acute ischemic stroke. Results of a phase IIa randomized trial. Stroke 1995;26:602–605.
32. Muir KW, Lees KR. Clinical experiences with excitatory amino acid antagonists. Stroke 1995;26:503–513.
33. Bozik ME, Smith JM, Douglass A, et a. POST: double-blind, placebo controlled, safety and efficacy trials of intravenous BMS-204352 in patients with acute stroke. Ongoing Clinical Trials Session, 25th International Stroke Conference, 2000.
34. The North American Glycine Antagonist in Neuroprotection (GAIN) Investigators. Phase II studies of the glycine antagonist GV150526 in acute stroke: the North American experience. Stroke. 2000;31:358–365.
35. Lees KR, Lavelle JF, Cunha L, et al. GAIN Phase II European Study Group. Glycine antagonist (GV150526) in acute stroke: a multicentre, double-blind placebo-controlled phase II trial. Cereb Dis 2001;11:20–29.
36. Lees KR, Asplund K, Carolei A, et al. Glycine antagonist (gavestinel) in neuroprotection (GAIN International) in patients with acute stroke: a randomised controlled trial. GAIN International Investigators. Lancet 2000;355:1949–1954.
37. Clark WM, Raps EC, Tong DC, Kelly RE. Cervene (Nalmefene) in acute ischemic stroke: final results of a phase III efficacy study. The Cervene Stroke Study Investigators. Stroke 2000;31:1234–1239.
38. Diener HC, Cortens M, Ford G, et al. Lubeluzole in acute ischemic stroke treatment: a double-blind study with an 8-hour inclusion window comparing a 10-mg daily dose of lubeluzole with placebo. Stroke 2000;31:2543–2551.
39. Grotta J. Combination Therapy Stroke Trial: rt-PA +/– Lubeluzole. Stroke 2000;31:278.
40. RANTTAS Investigators. A randomized trial of tirilazad mesylate in patients with acute stroke (RANTTAS). Stroke 1996;27:1453–1458.
41. Haley E. High-dose tirilazad for acute stroke (RANTTAS II). Stroke 1998;29:1256–1257.
42. Peters G, Hwang L, Musch B, Brosse D, Orgogozo J. Safety and efficacy of 6 mg/kg/day tirilazad mesylate with acute ischemic stroke (TESS study). Stroke 1996;27:195.
43. Enlimomab Acute Stroke Trial Investigators. Use of anti-ICAM-1 therapy in ischemic stroke: results of the Enlimomab Acute Stroke Trial. Neurology 2001;57:1428–1434.
44. De Deyn PP, Reuck JD, Deberdt W, Vlietinck R, Orgogozo JM. Treatment of acute ischemic stroke with piracetam. Members of the Piracetam in Acute Stroke Study (PASS) Group. Stroke 1997;28:2347–2352.
45. Major ongoing stroke trials. Stroke 2000;31:2536–2542.
46. Bogousslavsky J, Victor SJ, Salinas EO, et al. European-Australian Fiblast (Trafermin) in Acute Stroke Group. Fiblast (trafermin) in acute stroke: results of the European-Australian phase II/III safety and efficacy trial. Cereb Dis 2002;14: 239–251.
47. Fisher M. Recommendations for advancing development of acute stroke therapies: stroke therapy academic industry roundtable 3. Stroke 2003;34:1539–1546.
48. Stroke Therapy Academic Industry Roundtable II (STAIR-II). Recommendations for clinical trial evaluation of acute stroke therapies. Stroke 200;32:1598–1606.
49. Van Raak L, Hilton A, Kessels F, Lodder J. Implementing the EGASIS trial, an international multicenter acute intervention trial in stroke. Control Clin Trials 2002;23:74–79.

50. Major ongoing stroke trials. Stroke 2002;33:646–655.
51. Repinotan (BAY x3072) in Acute Ischemic Stroke—A Randomized Exposure Controlled Trial. Ongoing Clinical Trials Session, 26th International Stroke Conference.
52. Muir KW, Lees KR. A randomized, double-blind, placebo-controlled pilot trial of intravenous magnesium sulfate in acute stroke. Stroke 1995;26:1183–1188.
53. The Field Administration of Stroke Therapy—Magnesium (FAST-MAG) Phase 3 Trial. Ongoing Clinical Trials Session, 27th International Stroke Conference, 2002.
54. The Field Administration of Stroke Therapy—Magnesium (FAST-MAG) Phase 3 Trial. Ongoing Clinical Trials Session, 28th International Stroke Conference, 2003.
55. Phase III trial of Ebselen. Ongoing Clinical Trials Session, 28th International Stroke Conference, 2003.
56. Kollmar R, Schabitz WR, Heiland S, et al. Neuroprotective effect of delayed moderate hypothermia after focal cerebral ischemia: an MRI study. Stroke 2002;33:1899–1904.
57. The 28th International Stroke Conference. Stroke 2003;34:248.
58. Krieger DW, De Georgia MA, Abou-Chebl A, et al. Cooling for acute ischemic brain damage (cool aid): an open pilot study of induced hypothermia in acute ischemic stroke. Stroke 2001;32:1847–1854.
59. Cramer SC, Nelles G, Benson RR, et al. A functional MRI study of subjects recovered from hemispheric stroke. Stroke 1997;28:2518–2527.
60. Fisher M, Finklestein SP. Pharmacological approaches to stroke recovery. Cereb Dis 1999;9:29–32.
61. Tatlisumak T, Takano K, Carano RAD, Fisher M. Effects of basic fibroblast growth factor on experimental focal ischemia studied by diffusion-weighted and perfusion imaging. Stroke 1996;27:2292–2298.
62. Kawamata T, Alexis NE, Dietrich WD, Finklestein SP. Intracisternal basic fibroblast growth factor enhances behavioral recovery following focal cerebral infarction in the rat. J Cereb Blood Flow Metab 1996;16:542–547.
63. Clark WM, Schim JD, Kasner SE, Victor S. Trafemin in acute ischemic stroke. Neurology 2000;54:A88.
64. Bogousslavsky J, Donnan GA, Fieschi C, et al. Fiblast (Trafenin) in acute stroke: results of the European-Australian phase 2/3 safety and efficacy trial. Cereb Dis 2000;10:16.
65. Kawamata T, Ren J, Chan TCK, Charette M, Finklestein SP. Intracisternal osteogenic protein-1 enhances functional recovery following stroke. Neuroreport 1998;9:1441–1445.
66. Zhang R, Zhang L, Zhang Z, et al. A nitric oxide donor induces neurogenesis and reduces functional deficits after stroke in rats. Ann Neurol 2001;50:602–611.
67. Zhang R, Wang Y, Zhang L, et al. Sildenafil (Viagra) induces neurogenesis and promotes functional recovery after stroke in rats. Stroke 2002;32:2675–2680.
68. Chen J, Zhang Z, Li Y, et al. Statins induce angiogenesis, neurogenesis and synaptogenesis after stroke. Ann Neurol 2003;53:743–751.
69. Stroemer BP, Kent TA, Hulsebosch CE. Enhanced neocortical neural sprouting, synaptogenesis, and behavioral recovery with D-amphetamine therapy after neocortical infarction in rats. Stroke 1998;29:2381–2395.
70. Schabitz WR, Weber J, Takano K, et al. Effects of citicoline on infarct volume, mortality and behavioral outcome. J Neurol Sci 1996;138:21–25.
71. Davalos A, Castillo J, Alvarez-Sabin J, et al. Oral citicoline in acute stroke: an individual patient data pooling analysis of clinical trials. Stroke 2002;33:2850–2857.
72. Modo M, Stroemer P, Tang E, Patel S, Hodges H. Effects of implantation site of stem cell grafts on behavioral recovery from stroke damage. Stroke 2002;33:2270–2278.
73. Chen J, Li Y, Wang L, et al. Therapeutic benefits of intravenous administration of bone marrow stromal cells after cerebral ischemia in rats. Stroke 2001;32:1005–1011.
74. Liu J, Solway K, Messing RO, Sharp FR. Increased neurogenesis in the dentate gyrus after transient global ischemia in gerbils. J Neurosci 1998;18:7768–7778.

Index

B

E

F

G

N

O

P

Q

R

S

T

About the Editors

Robert H. Paul, PhD

Robert Paul is Assistant Director of Outpatient Neuropsychology at The Miriam Hospital and Assistant Professor of Research in the Department of Psychiatry at Brown Medical School. His research program is aimed at the neurobehavioral sequelae of subcortical ischemic vascular disease in the elderly and the interaction between cerebrovascular disease and the development of neurodegenerative dementia. He has authored/co-authored more than 70 peer-reviewed papers and is the principal investigator of studies funded by both federal and private agencies. Dr. Paul also serves as an ad-hoc reviewer for journals in the scientific field and a primary clinical/research supervisor in the Brown Psychology Training Consortium, neuropsychology track.

Ronald Cohen, PhD

Ronald Cohen is Director of Neuropsychology and Co-Director of the Memory Disorders Clinic at The Miriam Hospital in Providence, Rhode Island, and Associate Professor in the Department of Psychiatry and Human Behavior and the Brain Sciences Program at Brown University. He is also an executive committee member of the Magnetic Resonance Foundation for Brown University, and has played an important role in developing functional neuroimaging at this university

Dr. Cohen is author of a book, *The Neuropsychology of Attention*, which is one of the few comprehensive texts on this topic. He has also written a number of chapters for edited books on attention and also on the topic of vascular dementia and the effects of vascular disease on cognitive functions. He is currently the Principal Investigator of a grant from the National Institute of Aging, to study of the effects of cardiovascular disease on the development of neurocognitive dysfunction and vascular dementia in the elderly. He also serves as a co-investigator for Alzheimer's Disease Cooperative Study, a National Institute on Aging (NIA) sponsored multi-center program. He is has published over 90 empirical neuropsychological studies, including a number of brain neuroimaging studies of vascular dementia and related neuropsychological disorders.

Brian R. Ott, MD

Brian Ott is the Director of the Alzheimer's Disease and Memory Disorders Center as well as Associate Chief of Neurology at Memorial Hospital of Rhode Island. His initial research interest in amnesic stoke has expanded over the years into the broader field of dementia, particularly in the area of pathophysiology and management of behavior disorders in dementia. He is the recipient of a grant from the National Institute on Aging to study driving and dementia longitudinally. His research team is also actively involved in clinical trials using experimental medications in the treatment of Alzheimer's disease and mild cognitive impairment. In the area of outcome measures for the treatment of dementia he recently developed the innovative Cornell-Brown Scale for Quality of Life in Dementia.

Stephen Salloway, MD

Stephen Salloway is Director of Neurology and The Memory Disorders Program at Butler Hospital in Providence, Rhode Island, and Associate Professor of Clinical Neurosciences and Psychiatry at Brown Medical School, Rhode Island. Dr Salloway has edited 3 books and more than 75 scientific articles and book chapters. He is a former president of the American Neuropsychiatric Association and serves on national and international committees to help develop criteria for stroke and vascular dementia. He is a scientific reviewer for the National Institutes of Health and for more than 25 journals, universities, and research foundations. Dr Salloway has received numerous grants for his research which focuses on three main areas: (1) clinical trials for prevention and treatment of vascular dementia, Alzheimer's disease, and mild cognitive impairment; (2) studies of cerebral microvascular disease, including CASASIL; and (3) assessment of frontal behavior and executive function. He is the Director of the Brown Combined Residency in Neurology and Psychiatry and co-principal investigator of the Brown Dementia Research Fellowship Program, both in Rhode Island. He lectures widely on dementia and neuropsychiatric disorders.